Rheumatology

Evidence-Based Practice for Physiotherapists and Occupational Therapists

Edited by

Krysia Dziedzic PhD, MCSP
arc Senior Lecturer in Physiotherapy
Arthritis Research Campaign National Primary Care Centre,
Keele University, Keele, UK

and

Alison Hammond PhD, MSc, BSc(Hons), DipCOT, FCOT
Reader in Rheumatology Rehabilitation,
Centre for Health, Sport & Rehabilitation Research,
Faculty of Health & Social Care, University of Salford, Salford
and Consultant Research Therapist – Rheumatology,
Royal Derby Hospital, Derby Hospitals NHS Foundation Trust, Derby, UK

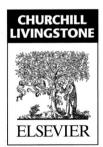

CHURCHILL
LIVINGSTONE

ELSEVIER

EDINBURGH   LONDON   NEW YORK   OXFORD   PHILADELPHIA   ST LOUIS   SYDNEY   TORONTO   2010

CHURCHILL
LIVINGSTONE
ELSEVIER

2010, © Elsevier Ltd. All rights reserved.

No part of this publication may be reproduced or transmitted in any form or by any means, electronic or mechanical, including photocopying, recording, or any information storage and retrieval system, without permission in writing from the publisher. Details on how to seek permission, further information about the Publisher's permissions policies and our arrangements with organizations such as the Copyright Clearance Center and the Copyright Licensing Agency, can be found at our website: HYPERLINK "http://www.elsevier.com/permissions" www.elsevier.com/permissions.

This book and the individual contributions contained in it are protected under copyright by the Publisher (other than as may be noted herein).

ISBN 978-0-443-06934-5

British Library Cataloguing in Publication Data
A catalogue record for this book is available from the British Library

Library of Congress Cataloguing in Publication Data
A catalogue record for this book is available from the Library of Congress

Notice
Knowledge and best practice in this field are constantly changing. As new research and experience broaden our understanding, changes in research methods, professional practices, or medical treatment may become necessary.

Practitioners and researchers must always rely on their own experience and knowledge in evaluating and using any information, methods, compounds, or experiments described herein. In using such information or methods they should be mindful of their own safety and the safety of others, including parties for whom they have a professional responsibility.

With respect to any drug or pharmaceutical products identified, readers are advised to check the most current information provided (i) on procedures featured or (ii) by the manufacturer of each product to be administered, to verify the recommended dose or formula, the method and duration of administration, and contraindications. It is the responsibility of practitioners, relying on their own experience and knowledge of their patients, to make diagnoses, to determine dosages and the best treatment for each individual patient, and to take all appropriate safety precautions.

To the fullest extent of the law, neither the Publisher nor the authors, contributors, or editors, assume any liability for any injury and/or damage to persons or property as a matter of products liability, negligence or otherwise, or from any use or operation of any methods, products, instructions, or ideas contained in the material herein.

 your source for books, journals and multimedia in the health sciences
www.elsevierhealth.com

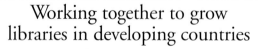

Working together to grow libraries in developing countries

www.elsevier.com | www.bookaid.org | www.sabre.org

ELSEVIER   BOOK AID International   Sabre Foundation

The Publisher's policy is to use paper manufactured from sustainable forests

Printed in China

Rheumatology

This book is dedicated to our next generation of rheumatology practitioners and our patients from whom they seek evidence based rheumatology care.

Commissioning Editor: Rita Demetriou-Swanwick
Development Editor: Veronika Watkins
Project Manager: Sruthi Viswam
Designer/Design Direction: Stewart Larking
Illustration Manager: Merlyn Harvey
Illustrator: Robert Britton and Cactus

Contents

Contributors

Jo Adams PhD MSc DipCOT
Professional Lead and Senior Lecturer in
Occupational Therapy, School of Health
Professions and Rehabilitation Sciences,
University of Southampton, Southampton, UK

Catherine Backman PhD OT(C) FCAOT
Associate Professor, Department of Occupational
Science & Occupational Therapy, The University of
British Columbia, Vancouver, BC, Canada

Lindsay M. Bearne PhD MSc MCSP
Lecturer in Physiotherapy, Academic Department
of Physiotherapy, School of Biomedical and Health
Sciences, Kings College London, Guy's Campus,
London, UK

Ailsa Bosworth
Chief Executive, The National Rheumatoid
Arthritis Society, Westacott Business Center,
Littlewick Green, UK

Jane S. Brandenstein PT
Physical Therapist, Retired, Pennsylvania, USA

Alison Carr PhD
Arc Special Lecturer in Musculoskeletal
Epidemiology, Academic Rheumatology,
University of Nottingham, Nottingham City
Hospital, Nottingham, UK

Mark L. Clemence MPhil Grad Dip Phys MCSP
Clinical Specialist Physiotherapist, Physiotherapy
Department, Torbay Hospital, Torquay, UK

Philip G. Conaghan MBBS PhD FRACP FRCP
Professor of Musculoskeletal Medicine, Section
of Musculoskeletal Disease, Leeds Institute of
Molecular Medicine, University of Leeds &
Honorary Consultant Rheumatologist, Leeds
Teaching Hospitals NHS Trust, Leeds, UK

Janet Cushnaghan MSc MCSP
Research Physiotherapist, MRC Epidemiology
Resource Centre, Southampton General Hospital,
Southampton, UK

Peter Dawes MBChB FRCP
Consultant Rheumatologist, Haywood
Hospital, Stoke on Trent NHS Primary Care
Trust, High Lane, Stoke-on-Trent, UK

Caitlyn Dowson MBChB FRCP
Consultant Rheumatologist, Haywood
Hospital, Stoke on Trent NHS Primary Care
Trust, High Lane, Staffordshire, UK

Krysia Dziedzic PhD MCSP
arc Senior Lecturer in Physiotherapy, Arthritis
Research Campaign National Primary Care
Centre, Primary Care Sciences, Keele University,
Keele, UK

Lynne Goodacre PhD Dip COT
Senior Lecturer Management of Long Term
Conditions, School of Public Health and Clinical
Sciences, University of Central Lancashire,
Preston, UK

Janine Hackett MSc Occupational Therapy BA(Hons) Dip.COT
Senior Lecturer, Department of Occupational
Therapy, University of Derby, Derby, UK

Elizabeth D. Hale BA(Hons) Applied Social Science, MSc Health Psychology, C.Psychol. (Chartered Health Psychologist)
Chartered Health Psychologist, Dudley Group of Hospitals NHS Foundation, UK Trust
Russells Hall Hospital, Dudley; Honorary Research Associate, University of Birmingham, School of Sport and Exercise Sciences, Birmingham, UK

Alison Hammond PhD, MSc, BSc(Hons), DipCOT, FCOT
Reader in Rheumatology Rehabilitation, Centre for Health, Sport & Rehabilitation Research , Faculty of Health & Social Care, University of Salford, Salford and Consultant Research Therapist – Rheumatology, Royal Derby Hospital, Derby Hospitals NHS Foundation Trust, Derby, UK

Janet E. Harkess BSc OT
Head Occupational Therapist, Fife Rheumatic Diseases Unit, Whytemans Brae Hospital, Kirkcaldy, UK

Andrew Hassell MD FRCP MMedEd
Consultant Rheumatologist and Senior Lecturer, Department of Rheumatology, Haywood Hospital, Staffordshire, UK; Director of Undergraduate Programmes, School of Medicine, Keele University, Keele, UK

Kirstie L. Haywood DPhil (Health Sciences and Clinical Evaluation), BSc (Hons) (Physiotherapy) MCSP SRP
Senior Research Fellow (Patient Reported Outcomes), Royal College of Nursing Research Institute, School of Health and Social Studies, University of Warwick, Coventry, UK, Consultant Rheumatologist and Senior Lecturer, Department of Rheumatology, Haywood Hospital, Staffordshire, UK

Michael V. Hurley PhD MCSP
Professor of Physiotherapy, King's College London, Rehabilitation Research Unit (King's College London), Dulwich Community Hospital, Dulwich, London, UK

Bernadette Johnson MCSP
Specialist Paediatric Physiotherapist, Children's Physiotherapy Service, South Staffordshire PCT, Samuel Johnson Hospital, Lichfield, Staffordshire, UK

Rachel Lewis MCSP SRP HT
Clinical Specialist Physiotherapist in Rheumatology, Physiotherapy Dept, Southmead Hospital, Bristol, UK

Christian David Mallen BMedSci BMBS DRCOG DFFP MMedSci MPhil MPCGP PhD
Senior Lecturer in General Practice, Arthritis Research Campaign National Primary Care Centre, Primary Care Sciences, Keele University, Keele, UK

Joseph G. McVeigh PhD DipOrthMed BSc(Hons) Physiotherapy
Lecturer in Physiotherapy, School of Health Sciences, University of Ulster, Jordanstown Northern Ireland, UK

Susan L. Murphy ScD OTR/L
Assistant Professor, Department of Physical Medicine and Rehabilitation, University of Michigan & Research Health Science Specialist, Geriatric Research, Education, and Clinical Center (GRECC), Veterans Affairs Ann Arbor Health Care System, Institute of Gerontology, Ann Arbor, USA

Helen Myers PhD MSc BSc
Research Occupational Therapist, Arthritis Research Campaign National Primary Care Centre, Primary Care Sciences, Keele University, Keele, UK

Karin Niedermann MPH BScPT
Physiotherapist, Head of MSc Programme/Senior Research Fellow Institute of Physiotherapy, University of Applied Sciences, Winterthur, Switzerland; Department of Rheumatology, University Hospital Zurich, Switzerland.

Anne O'Brien MPhil Grad Dip Phys MCSP
Lecturer in Physiotherapy, School of Health and Rehabilitation, MacKay Building, University of Keele, Keele, UK

Rachel O'Brien PhD, MSc DipCOT
Senior Lecturer Faculty of Health & Well Being, Sheffield Hallam University, Broomhall Road, Sheffield, UK

Susan M. Oliver RN, MSc FRCN
Nurse Consultant Rheumatology, Barnstaple, Devon, UK

Dorothy J. Pattison PhD
Research Dietitian, Bone & Joint Research Team, Knowledge Spa, Royal Cornwall Hospitals (NHS) Trust, Treliske, UK

Janet L. Poole PhD OTR/L FAOTA
Professor, Occupational Therapy Graduate Program, University of New Mexico, Occupational Therapy Graduate Program, Albuquerque, NM, USA

Edward Roddy DM MRCP(UK)
Clinical Lecturer & Honorary Consultant
Rheumatologist, Arthritis Research Campaign
National Primary Care Centre, Primary Care
Sciences, Keele University, Keele, UK

Sarah Ryan RGN PhD MSc BSc FRCN
Consultant Nurse Specialist Rheumatology,
Staffordshire Rheumatology Centre, Haywood
Hospital, Stoke on Trent NHS Primary Care Trust,
Stoke on Trent, UK

Benazir Saleem MBChB MRCP
Specialist Registrar in Rheumatology, Leeds
Teaching Hospitals NHS Trust, Section of
Musculoskeletal Disease, Leeds, UK

David G. I. Scott MD FRCP
Consultant Rheumatologist and Honorary
Professor, Clinical Director Comprehensive Local
Research Network for Norfolk and Suffolk; Patient
Involvement Officer Royal College of Physicians;
Chief Medical Advisor to the National Rheumatoid
Arthritis Society; Department of Rheumatology,
Norfolk and Norwich University Hospital,
Norwich, UK

Kay Stevenson MPhil Grad Dip Phys
Consultant Physiotherapist, University Hospital of
North Staffordshire, Stoke on Trent, Staffordshire, UK

Gareth J. Treharne BSc (Hons) PhD
Lecturer, Department of Psychology, University
of Otago, Dunedin, Aotearoa/New Zealand and
Department of Rheumatology, Dudley Group of
Hospitals NHS Foundation Trust, Russells Hall
Hospital Dudley, UK

Deborah E. Turner PhD PGCert Medical ultrasound
BSc(Hons), FCPodMed
arc Senior Lecturer in Podiatry, School of Health,
Glasgow Caledonian University, Glasgow, UK

Adrian White MA MD BM Bch
Clinical Research Fellow, General Practice and
Primary Care, Peninsula Medical School,
Plymouth, UK

Jim Woodburn PhD MPhil BSc FCPodMed
Professor of Rehabilitation, School of Health &
Social Care, Glasgow Caledonian University,
Glasgow, UK

Foreword

The effective management of long term chronic disabling musculoskeletal disorders requires inputs and expertise from several professional groups. One of the heartening trends worldwide over the past decade in rheumatology has been the breaking down of professional barriers between physicians and key health care professionals such as nurses, physiotherapists, occupational therapists and podiatrists amongst others. There is the realisation that only with multidisciplinary working with each group maximising their contribution, can we all achieve optimal patient benefit. Such working requires all groups to share knowledge and it is in this light that this current volume fills a much needed gap. The material in this book will provide students and others in these disciplines with much of the key background information needed to underpin and enhance their role in the joint management of our patients. It deserves to be widely read and its messages used to inform what we do.

Alan J Silman FMed Sci, DSc (Hons) MD,
FRCP, FFPHM
Medical Director UK Arthritis Research Campaign

Preface

The idea for this book arose from a need to produce a rheumatology textbook for physiotherapy and occupational therapy students that was up-to-date and that captured the current trends in rheumatology and evidence-based practice. We were fortunate to have a wide circle of local, national and international collaborators who have provided contributions and in particular, with a patient as co-author, a patient-centred approach (Ch. 2). The hallmark of rheumatology practice is multidisciplinary working so it seemed the obvious approach to combine a textbook for both physiotherapists and occupational therapists, and to enlist contributions from the many members of the rheumatology team. We felt it helpful to construct the book in two parts with one section dealing with the fundamental principles and the other on specific clinical conditions commonly seen by therapists. If we have omitted to cover every one of the 200 musculoskeletal conditions we hope that the book has provided the necessary tools to develop a management plan for those we have neglected.

Whilst we have targeted the undergraduate therapy student, this text will also be a very useful addition for other health care students, therapists specialising in rheumatology, other members of the rheumatology team, and community and hospital-based therapists who treat common rheumatological conditions, such as osteoarthritis.

Krysia Dziedzic
Alison Hammond

Acknowledgements

We would like to thank all the authors for their hard work in producing such interesting and informative contributions. We would like to thank Ailsa Bosworth for her contribution as our patient author and giving the book a patient's perspective in writing chapter two with Susan Oliver. We would like to take the opportunity to thank all supporters of rheumatology and allied health professionals over the many years (patients, rheumatologists, other health care professionals, researchers) who inspired this textbook.

We would like to thank Veronika, Siobhan, Rita and Sruthi from Elsevier who supported us magnificently throughout the editing process with much enthusiasm. We would also like to thank Hilary Jones and Zoe Mayson at Keele for their secretarial and technical support.

In particular we need to thank our family, friends and work colleagues for their support and for picking up the work we had to drop to see this through to its conclusion.

Finally, we can take this opportunity to thank the following who have provided us with funded posts/ research funding at key stages in our own rheumatology careers, which have enabled us to take on this book:

- The Arthritis Research Campaign (KD, AH) And

- The Staffordshire Rheumatology Centre, the Haywood Hospital, Burslem, Stoke on Trent and The Arthritis Research Campaign National Primary Care Centre, Keele University (KD)

- The Rheumatology department, Derby Hospitals NHS Foundation Trust. In particular, Dr R Williams, Dr M Regan, Dr C Deighton, Dr G Summers, and all the members of the Rheumatology MDT (AH).

Chapter 1

Overview of the aims and management of rheumatological conditions: the multidisciplinary approach

CHAPTER CONTENTS

KEY POINTS

- Underpin practice with research
- Be aware of national policy that influences your practice
- Be aware of your local community processes
- Engage patients in design of services
- Explore opportunities to extend roles.

1.1 Rheumatology and the rheumatologist

Krysia Dziedzic PhD MCSP Arthritis Research Campaign National Primary Care Centre, Primary Care Sciences, Keele University, Keele, UK

Peter Dawes MBChB FRCP Haywood Hospital, Stoke on Trent NHS Primary Care Trust, Staffordshire, UK

INTRODUCTION

There are over 200 musculoskeletal conditions affecting millions of adults and children, and it is estimated that up to 30% of all general practice consultations are about musculoskeletal complaints (Department of Health 2006). The ageing population will further

© 2010 Elsevier Ltd
DOI: 10.1016/B978-0-443-06934-5.00001-2

increase the demand for treatment of age-related disorders such as osteoarthritis and osteoporosis (Department of Health 2006). Rheumatology is an exciting and expanding field (BHPR 2004). Its profile has risen dramatically with improved understanding of inflammatory and non-inflammatory conditions, and the availability of powerful and expensive treatments, e.g. anti-TNF therapies.

People with musculoskeletal conditions need a wide range of high-quality support and treatment from simple advice to highly specialised treatments. The Musculoskeletal Services Framework (MSF) (Department of Health 2006) describes best practice, built around evidence and experience. It promotes 'redesign of services, and full exploitation of skills and new roles of all healthcare professionals'; and 'better outcomes for people with musculoskeletal conditions through a more actively managed patient pathway, with explicit sharing of information and responsibility, agreed between all stakeholders in all sectors – patients; the NHS and local authorities; and voluntary/community organisations'. Multidisciplinary services are central to the framework, offering triage, assessment, diagnosis, treatment or rapid referral to other specialists.

THE ROLE OF THE MULTIDISCIPLINARY TEAM

The multidisciplinary team has been shown to be effective in optimising management of patients with arthritis (Vliet Vlieland et al 1997). All patients should have opportunities to access a range of health care professionals (SIGN 2000), including rheumatologist, general practitioner, nurse specialist, physiotherapist, occupational therapist, dietician, podiatrist, health psychologist, social worker and pharmacist. The next section will summarise the individual roles of many of these health care professionals. Following this, the most important member of the rheumatology team, the patient as an expert in living with the condition, will describe their journey (see Ch. 2). Throughout the book members of the multidisciplinary team have contributed chapters on their specific area of specialty, e.g. Chapter 14 on diet and complementary therapies.

THE RHEUMATOLOGIST

Rheumatologists have general medical knowledge, and have additional training and experience in the diagnosis and treatment of arthritis and other diseases of the musculoskeletal system. As well as an empathic approach to patients and the ability to work well within a multidisciplinary team the rheumatologist will often be the team leader. They develop good communication skills and above all the ability to work closely with other health professionals. The team approach to providing care is highly valued by rheumatologists because rheumatology manages longstanding and often incurable conditions.

The majority of musculoskeletal diseases are managed in primary care and rheumatology is mainly an outpatient speciality. Some rheumatology departments hold out-reach clinics in general practice, and some are now sited in primary care trusts. However, there are real advantages for patients with inflammatory arthritis or connective tissue disease in seeing a rheumatologist (BHPR 2004), as some of these are very serious diseases that can be difficult to diagnose and treat. Timing of pharmacological interventions and their safe monitoring is a pre-requisite for managing inflammatory arthritis. Rheumatologists undertake many practical procedures. All would do joint aspiration and injection whilst some develop an interest in ultrasound, nerve conduction studies, arthroscopies, muscle biopsies etc. (BHPR 2004). Others develop expertise in management, research or education.

Some rheumatic diseases are complex requiring monitoring to determine a diagnosis and follow-up to assess change over time. Rheumatologists work closely with patients and the rheumatology team to identify problems, design individualised treatment programmes and help patients and their families cope with the impact of the disease.

Rheumatologists also work closely with orthopaedic surgeons, radiologists, anaesthetists (pain service), and neurosurgeons, and keep the patient's own general practitioner fully informed of progress.

1.2   Nursing

Sarah Ryan RGN PhD MSc BSc FRCN Haywood Hospital, Stoke on Trent NHS Primary Care Trust, Staffordshire, UK

THE RHEUMATOLOGY NURSE

THE ROLE OF THE RHEUMATOLOGY NURSE

The role of the rheumatology nurse has developed from the collection of clinical measurements during drug trials in the 1970's (Bird 1983), to encompass a much broader spectrum of activities. These activities include patient education and counselling, the monitoring of drug therapy, running specialist clinics, patient assessment and management and recommending treatment changes to the rheumatologist and general practitioner (Carr 2001).

Patients are often referred to a rheumatology nurse following diagnosis of an inflammatory rheumatological condition, most commonly rheumatoid arthritis (RA) to commence disease modifying drugs, begin the process of patient education, to obtain symptom control and receive emotional support. At the time of diagnosis the patient can experience a plethora of emotions including anger, shock, grief and denial.

Shaul (1995) demonstrated that in the early stages, women with rheumatoid arthritis needed to have their symptoms explained and managed before they could begin the process of learning coping strategies. The nurse consultation enables partnership, intimacy and reciprocity to evolve, and provides the forum to identify the patient's priorities, providing care that has meaning and relevance to the patient. The key functions of nursing, as described by Wilson Barnett (1985) (Box 1.2.1) will be incorporated into the consultation to promote adaptation to the condition. Education and support will also be offered to family members, if the family does not appreciate the value of the management being advocated, for example exercise to assist with pain, stiffness and fatigue, then the individual may find it difficult to engage in this activity, without the endorsement of their family.

CHARACTERISTICS OF NURSE-LED CLINICS

Hill (1992) describes the characteristics of a nurse led clinic as

- The provision of information and education
- Adopting an holistic approach not task orientated
- The involvement of the multi-disciplinary team

BOX 1.2.1   The key functions of nursing (Wilson Barnett 1985)

- Understanding illness and treatment from the patient's viewpoint
- Providing continuous psychological care during illness and critical events
- Helping patients cope with illness or potential health problems
- Providing comfort
- Co-ordinating treatment and other events affecting the patient.

- Providing symptom management (pain, stiffness and fatigue)
- Fostering patient participation.

A survey of practice in nurse led clinics for patients with RA (Ryan & Hill 2004) demonstrated that nurses are engaged in

- Monitoring of disease status (musculoskeletal examination, initiating and interpreting investigations, referral to other specialists)
- Providing emotional support
- Patient education
- Management of stable disease
- Management of patients on biologic therapies.

The model for clinics for patients with RA has been replicated to other conditions including connective tissue disorders, osteoporosis and chronic pain.

COMMUNITY NURSE LED CLINICS

Nurse led clinics have been replicated in the community and GP practices to provide similar functions including:

- Joint assessment
- Monitoring of the safety and efficacy of drug treatment
- Initiation and interpretation of clinical laboratory data
- Liaison between the patient and the GP (Mooney 1996).

Arthur and Clifford (2004) compared the satisfaction of patients attending drug monitoring within primary and secondary care locations. They found patients reported a higher level of satisfaction with secondary care based drug monitoring. Empathy, specialist knowledge, information provision, technical aspects, time and continuity of care were identified as important attributes contributing to the satisfaction experienced by patients attending secondary care drug monitoring.

THE EFFECTIVENESS OF NURSING INTERVENTIONS

Hill et al (1994) demonstrated the value of a clinic run on true nursing principles. This study was an evaluation of the effectiveness, safety and acceptability of a nurse practitioner in a rheumatology outpatient clinic. Seventy patients with RA were randomly allocated to either the nurse practitioner clinic or a consultant rheumatologist clinic and seen on six occasions over 12 months. On study entry the groups were well matched. At week 48 there was no significant difference between the two groups with both groups showing significant improvement in disease activity. However, the patients in the nurse practitioner cohort showed additional improvements not mirrored in the consultant group. The improvement was in levels of pain, morning stiffness, psychological status and satisfaction with care. One of the most noticeable aspects of the research was the marked difference in the referral patterns of the two practitioners, with the nurse practitioner making greater use of other members of the multi-disciplinary team, such as the physiotherapist. Hill's work demonstrated that the nurse can add something extra to the management of patients with RA, and that extra is something that is valued by the patient.

A randomised controlled trial by Ryan et al (2006) examined the hypothesis that consultation with a consultant nurse specialist in a drug monitor clinic would have a measurable impact on the wellbeing of 71 patients with rheumatoid arthritis. Patients were randomised into two groups over a 3-year period. The intervention group was monitored by the consultant nurse specialist and an outpatient staff nurse reviewed the control group. Patients reviewed by the consultant nurse specialist reported a greater perception of being able to control their arthritis than those managed by the staff nurse. The role of the consultant nurse specialist in helping patients cope with their symptoms through goal setting, pacing, addressing low mood state and advocating exercise may be the nursing tools and expertise through which the 'added value' in influencing control perceptions was achieved. Ten patients from this study were interviewed by an independent researcher to explore ways of coping. The importance of nurse support in relation to enhancing positive control perceptions emerged as a clear theme in the intervention group (Hooper et al 2004).

PROVIDING TELEPHONE ADVICE

Telephone advice lines have become an integral part of rheumatology care and are traditionally run by rheumatology nurses or other health professionals in extended roles (Thwaites 2004). The telephone advice line provides patients with the means of contacting the rheumatology nurse directly involved in their care and is accessed to provide advice of drug therapy and symptom management.

CONCLUSION

The rheumatology nurse utilises specialist knowledge and skills to help the patient address the impact of their condition on a physical, psychological and social level. This is usually achieved through nurse led clinics where the process of education, symptom management and emotional support can commence.

1.3   General practice

Christian David Mallen BMedSci BMBS DRCOG DFFP MMedSci MPhil MPCGP PhD Arthritis Research Campaign National Primary Care Centre, Primary Care Sciences, Keele University, Keele, UK

GENERAL PRACTICE

GENERAL PRACTICE AND THE ROLE OF TRIAGE

Almost all people in the UK are registered with a GP who typically provides treatment for both acute and chronic illnesses as well as providing preventive care and health education. Traditionally, GPs have also acted as gatekeepers to more specialist services, such as those provided in secondary care or by allied health professionals. Over the past few years, however, this model has started to change with the introduction of innovative services such as community matrons and primary care nurse practitioners. Despite significant reorganisation in the health service resulting in the provision of alternative providers of primary care such as NHS Direct and NHS walk-in centres, over 90% of primary care patient contacts still occur in general practice.

Rheumatological conditions are extremely common in general practice, where they account for an estimated one in five consultations (McCormick et al 1995). Consultation rates for musculoskeletal disorders rise with increasing age, with women of all ages consulting more frequently than men. Low back pain is the most frequent reason for consulting a GP in younger age groups and remains a leading cause of work absence, whereas osteoarthritis (particularly of the hip and knee) is the dominant condition managed in older adults (Jordan et al 2007, McCormick et al 1995) accounting for more than two million consultations per year. Referral to secondary care is relatively unusual occurring in approximately 5% of all consultations.

GPs are by name, and training, generalists making it impossible to have in-depth knowledge in all areas, yet given the large workload generated by rheumatological conditions in primary care, it is perhaps surprising that formal clinical training in rheumatology, rehabilitation or orthopaedics does not commonly feature as part of general practice training schemes (Hosie 2000). These unmet educational needs are currently being addressed with the introduction of the first formal curriculum for general practice in 2007. Core competencies for rheumatological disorders have been identified that should be met by all GPs in training (full details are available at www.rcgp.org.uk).

Two recent developments in primary care that have the potential to significantly impact on the delivery of musculoskeletal services in the community are the introduction of GPs with a special interest in rheumatology and practice-based commissioning. These will be discussed in more detail below.

GENERAL PRACTITIONERS WITH A SPECIAL INTEREST

One of the key components of the NHS Plan (2000) was the formal introduction of General Practitioners with a Special Interest (GPwSI). A GPwSI is defined as a general practitioner who supplements their core professional role and undertakes advanced procedures not normally undertaken by their peers (Hay et al 2007). In order to work as a GPwSI, GPs have to first demonstrate that they have the appropriate skills and competencies to deliver an enhanced rheumatological service within a defined quality framework. This enables them to accept direct referrals from other GPs, which has the potential to reduce demand for more specialised secondary care services. Services are provided at a local level, and may include areas such as more specialised joint injection and the management of patients with inflammatory arthropathies.

PRACTICE BASED COMMISSIONING

Another recent development in primary care has been the implementation of practice based commissioning. Practice based commissioning, which is currently only implemented in England, refers to the devolution of commissioning for health related services to GPs (or more usually groups of GPs within

a defined geographical area such as a Primary Care Trust (PCT)). GPs, with the support of their local PCTs, have the potential to hold specific budgets and to be responsible for commissioning key services (a scheme not dissimilar to 'fund holding' which formed the cornerstone of NHS reform in the 1990s). It is envisaged that this will encourage a greater variety of services, from an increased number of providers, in settings that are both closer to home and more convenient for patients and their families. If successful, this scheme has the potential to reduce referrals to secondary care, improve co-ordination of patient services and improve collaboration between local GP practices (Greener et al 2006), however, uptake of practice based commissioning is currently low in many areas and its impact on the provision of services has yet to be evaluated.

TRIAGE

Over the past decade, there has been a dramatic increase in the use of triage (particularly by telephone) in general practice. The term triage refers to the process where calls are received, assessed and managed by giving advice or by referral to a more appropriate service (Lattimer et al 1996). In general practice this is a role typically (although not exclusively) performed by practice nurses.

This system allows practices to prioritise their workload and to fully utilise the clinical skills and experience of the wider primary health care team where appropriate. It is estimated that up to 50% of calls from patients can be handled by telephone advice alone (range 25.5–72.2%) and that triage has the potential to reduce immediate GP surgery consultations and home visits (Bunn 2004). Many practices have introduced a system of telephone triage where patients with a 'new' problem (such as acute low back pain, respiratory tract infection) speak to the practice nurse who gives advice, offers treatment or referral to an appropriate health professional (e.g. GP, physiotherapist, occupational therapist, nurse practitioner) within a predetermined protocol. Although these systems have increased in popularity further research is needed to fully evaluate aspects of safety, cost and patient satisfaction (Bunn et al 2005).

An alterative triage system for patients with rheumatological complaints has been developed by organisations such as Physio Direct (http://www.csp.org.uk/). This system allows patients direct access by telephone to a senior physiotherapist who uses a combination of computerised protocols and their clinical experience to make a diagnosis, discuss management and make an appropriate treatment plan. It also provides patients with the convenience and flexibility of self-referral, and utilises health care professionals with experience and expertise in managing rheumatological disorders. Given the prolonged waits often encountered by patients waiting for physiotherapy, and the benefits associated with prompt treatment, this system has several clear advantages, which also including the potential to reduce GP appointments, reduce non-attendance to physiotherapy clinics and enhanced patient satisfaction, however, its use is currently not universal and it has yet to be fully evaluated.

Over 90% of primary care patient contacts still occur in general practice, and rheumatological conditions are extremely common in primary care. In recent years there has been a dramatic rise in the use of triage and other approaches of direct and self-referral. Future years will see further evaluation of the cost effectiveness of these new initiatives compared with traditional approaches in primary care.

1.4   Physiotherapy

Kay Stevenson M.Phil Grad Dip Phys University Hospital of North Staffordshire, Stoke on Trent, Staffordshire, UK

BACKGROUND

Today many physiotherapists are working at the forefront of services for patients. Extended roles, new ways of working and changing professional boundaries have given physiotherapists greater opportunities than ever before to practice autonomously. This section will discuss some of the opportunities and challenges that physiotherapists may face currently and in the future.

CURRENT CLIMATE

Services for patients are subject to government reforms, which demand improved quality of care and access. The NHS plan for reform (Department of Health 2000) highlighted that services should be

delivered locally, have excellent outcomes, and should be delivered by the most appropriate professional.

Approximately 30% of patients consulting their general practitioner (GP) present with a musculoskeletal condition (DOH 2006a). Physiotherapists have excellent diagnostic and treatment skills for this group of patients, which could be utilised to a greater extent to provide timely management and to assist in the delivery of the '18 week pathway'. This Pathway recommends that patients will be seen and treated within 18 weeks from point of referral to definitive care (Department of Health 2006b). Practice Based Commissioning allows clusters of GP practices to purchase services from their locality. The monies saved from purchasing services locally will then be reinvested to improve services further. Physiotherapists working in primary care will have opportunities to engage with local clusters to influence how and where physiotherapy is delivered.

The Musculoskeletal Strategy – doing it differently (Department of Health 2006a) aims to guide where care should be provided. One of the founding principles is that of the 'Multidisciplinary interface clinic'. This type of clinic acts as a gatekeeper for onward referral to secondary care. Patients are assessed, investigated, diagnosed and referred for treatment, mostly within primary care. Physiotherapists are already working in 'interface' style clinics assessing a range of conditions (Stevenson & Hay 2004). They give opportunities for extended clinical reasoning and the development of additional techniques such as injection therapy (Fig. 1.4.1), prescribing and the use of investigations.

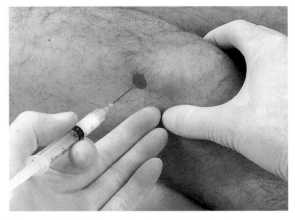

Figure 1.4.1 Injection of the knee joint. Lateral approach with permission From: Hochberg MC et al (eds.) Rheumatology, 4th edn, Elsevier Copyright © 2008.

OPPORTUNITIES

There are many opportunities for physiotherapists to improve care for their patients and extend professional boundaries (CSP 2008). Ten High Impact Changes (Department of Health 2004a) encouraged the extension of roles and working differently. Directives such as Modernising Medical Careers (Department of Health 2003a, Department of Health 2003b) and European Working Time Directive (Department of Health 2004b) will result in further reduction in doctors' hours and provide additional opportunities for physiotherapists.

Physiotherapists have been continually extending their skills and scope and in 2001, Consultant Physiotherapy posts were introduced in recognition of this. These posts combined expert clinical practice, leadership, research and education (Department of Health 2001). The posts are one example of combining aspects of different roles to gain the best care for patients. They have been concerned with delivering expert care, service re-design and integrating research into practice (Department of Health 2001). Post holders work across professional boundaries and utilise the best from each to move services forward. Transformational leadership and facilitating change are key aspects of such posts (Manley 2000).

Physiotherapy now has an increasing body of evidence to support practice (e.g. NICE 2008). Evidence for physiotherapy intervention in rheumatoid arthritis suggests hand exercises and joint protection can improve arm function and hand grip (O' Brien et al 2006). Physiotherapists treating patients with knee osteoarthritis can now be reassured that supervised exercises can improve pain and function when compared to usual care (Hay et al 2006). Where good quality evidence does not exist innovative approaches have been used to engage clinicians in asking appropriate clinical questions, searching the evidence and feeding results back into clinical practice (Stevenson et al 2007). Gaps in the evidence are then highlighted to researchers for consideration for future grant applications.

CHALLENGES

To gain the very best for our patients and be able to develop the services we need to have a great understanding of the political framework within which we sit. More autonomy is being devolved to a local level and it is crucial we understand how to influence local key decision makers around the benefits of physiotherapy and provide them with information that will assist them in their decision making processes. It is clear we need to have good outcome data and robust research evidence to highlight the benefits of our intervention.

In summary, these are both exciting and challenging times for all heath care professionals providing care for patients. Greater political awareness, robust research and patient involvement are key to future success.

1.5 Occupational therapy

Alison Hammond PhD MSc BSc(Hons) DipCOT
FCOT Centre for Rehabilitation and Human Performance Research, University of Salford, Greater Manchester and Derby City General Hospital, Derby Hospitals NHS, Foundation Trust, Derby, UK

OCCUPATIONAL THERAPY

The aims of occupational therapy are to:

- improve a person's ability to perform daily occupations, i.e. activities and valued life roles at work, in the home and with family, at leisure and socially;
- facilitate successful adaptation to disruptions in lifestyle;
- prevent losses of function;
- improve or maintain psychological status (Hammond 2004).

Occupational therapists (OTs) work collaboratively with clients to achieve 'occupational balance' (i.e. a balanced lifestyle) within the context of the person's illness, disability or other limitations. Rheumatology provides the opportunity to apply the full range of OT physical, functional, environmental, psychological and social interventions.

A major focus is self-management education. Many people with arthritis emphasise the frustration arising from pain, fatigue and difficulty performing daily activities and roles. A community survey of older people with osteoarthritis showed 43% had difficulty with household activities and 33% with hobbies and leisure activities (Jordan et al 2000). Within two years of diagnosis 60% of people with rheumatoid arthritis (RA) have difficulties with household, leisure and social activities (Young et al 2000). Over 50% of people with RA will have difficulty with work (reduced hours, difficulty with work roles, long-term sick leave or giving up) by 10 years, with potentially serious personal and financial consequences (Verstappen et al 2004). Hand function in women with RA is only 40% of normal function within 6 months of diagnosis (Hammond et al 2000). Adjusting to living with arthritis or chronic pain conditions, such as fibromyalgia, and adapting roles and lifestyle can lead to differing emotional reactions (e.g. stress, depression, anger) and impact on relationships.

Interventions focus on: maintaining and improving upper limb function through joint protection, hand exercises, assistive devices and splinting; fatigue management; activity and environmental modifications; activities of daily living training; transport and mobility assessment and advice, benefits and community resources advice; and pain and mood management, e.g. through stress management and relaxation training (NICE 2009). Because work problems occur early, OTs should ensure these are systematically identified by the team and timely OT referrals made for ergonomic assessment and vocational rehabilitation to reduce long-term personal, health and social costs. Clients' time use and balance of meaningful activities should be explored and avocational counselling also provided (i.e. advice and practical assistance with leisure, voluntary work and adult education opportunities). Loss of valued activities is associated with poorer psychological status, functional and disease outcomes (Katz & Yelin 1994). People with RA performing fewer valued activities (at work, leisure or in the home) are significantly more likely to be depressed, a predictor for poor outcome (and thus higher health costs) (Katz & Neugebauer 2001).

OTs should provide interventions within the context of individual clients' readiness to make changes in their lives. This can require psychological interventions such as counselling, stress management (e.g. addressing negative thinking), using cognitive-behavioural and motivational strategies, enabling people to explore feelings and beliefs about their condition, its lifestyle impact, their abilities and clarifying goals, to enable concordance with physical and functional interventions. Such approaches are proven effective (NICE 2009). Using a cognitive-behavioural approach is more effective in enabling people to self-manage (Hammond 2004, Hammond & Freeman 2007, Hammond et al 2008, Luqmani et al 2009).

Recent clinical guidelines emphasise skilled rheumatology OT should be available to people with rheumatic conditions (Luqmani et al 2006, 2009, NICE 2009, Scott et al 1998, SIGN 2000, Zhang et al 2007). Rheumatology OT is in short supply nationally. Increasing pressure to reduce time with clients for waiting list management means OTs must ensure evidence-based, effective, efficient practice, such as group cognitive-behavioural patient education programmes, provided collaboratively with physiotherapists and nurses (Hammond et al 2008).

The changing nature of Rheumatology services provides both opportunities and threats. Increasing numbers of clinical specialist posts provide opportunities to: collaborate with academic rheumatology OT researchers furthering the evidence base for rheumatology OT; in developing guidelines; and disseminating specialist practice in 'hub-and-spoke' networks working closely with primary care-based OTs. The growth of OT extended role practice can further enhance team care, identifying and addressing clients' occupational needs rapidly. The increasing shift to primary care-based services poses a risk of losing specialist skills, so all OTs must actively lobby for the continuing need for specialist rheumatology OT, wherever it is located, to enable people with arthritis to lead more meaningful lives.

1.6 Podiatry

Jim Woodburn PhD MPhil BSc FcPod Med School of Health & Social Care, Glasgow Caledonian University, Glasgow, UK

Deborah E. Turner PhD PGCert Medical Ultrasound BSc (Hons) FCPodMed School of Health & Social Care, Glasgow Caledonian University, Glasgow, UK

PODIATRY

The burden of foot disease in rheumatological conditions such as rheumatoid arthritis can be substantial and impact negatively on health related quality of life (ARMA 2007). Impairments such as pain and deformity may be associated directly with primary disease mechanisms such as synovitis and enthesopathy, but complications such as vasculitis also lead to disabling foot problems including ulceration and infection (ARMA 2007). The podiatrist is regarded as a valuable member of the multidisciplinary team however their services are often scarce and poorly accessed (ARMA 2007). Furthermore, foot problems are often neglected during routine clinical assessments further compounding the problem. Requests for podiatry and comfortable footwear are high on priority lists for unmet care for many of these patients (ARMA 2007).

Podiatrists are well-placed to assess, advise and treat patients with foot problems. The overall aims and management can be illustrated by summarising eight patient cases presenting to a typical clinical session in a busy rheumatology outpatient clinic. The first patient is Mrs White, a middle-aged lady with rheumatoid arthritis who presents with well established foot impairments including forefoot pain and deformity and moderately severe flat-footedness, all acquired since the onset of her arthritis. Mrs White attends for routine follow up and has the painful callus overlying her metatarsal heads debrided (removal of tissue to improve the healing potential of the remaining healthy tissue) and her new therapeutic footwear fitted. Mrs White reports immediate improvement in her symptoms as she leaves the clinic.

The next patient is Mr Smith a gentleman with seronegative spondylarthopathy presenting with bilateral plantar heel pain related to enthesopathy. He has responded well to an ultrasound-guided corticosteroid injection and night splint and today is being fitted for a custom made shoe insert. Mr Edwards follows. He is an elderly gentleman with persistent and disabling foot pain associated with hallux rigidus resulting from osteoarthritis at the 1st metatarsophalangeal joint (MTP). On reviewing the case the podiatrist feels he is non responsive to conservative care including orthotics and therapeutic shoes, and non-steroidal antiinflammatory drugs. The podiatrist discusses alternative approaches including surgery and a referral is made to the foot and ankle orthopaedic surgeon.

Before the next patient is seen, one of the rheumatologists brings in Mrs Jones, for an unscheduled consultation. The patient has severe and active RA and is about to start biologic therapy. However, Mrs Jones has a troublesome hammer toe which has a thick callus over the interphalangeal joint. Exquisitely painful the patient has never had this treated. The podiatrist carefully debrides the callused lesion to reveal a small underlying pressure ulcer and, recognising the risks posed by skin infection in patients treated with biologic therapy, recommends delay to systemic therapy until the ulcer is healed. A care plan is developed and the patient booked for follow up foot care.

Mrs Black brings in her 14-year-old daughter, Allison who has polyarticular juvenile idiopathic arthritis. Allison has a troublesome right ankle and is clearly limping as she walks. Following assessment, the podiatrist in consultation with the physiotherapist and paediatric rheumatologist initiates a care plan involving an intra-articular corticosteroid injection to the ankle joint along with joint mobilisation and muscle strengthening, and orthotics to stabilise and control the ankle joint during walking.

The next patient, Mrs Wilson, has been newly diagnosed with RA. Mrs Wilson has just started her methotrexate treatment so has many active joints including those of the feet. The podiatrist carefully provides some personalised advice on joint protection strategies for the feet and dispenses temporary orthoses. The patient's partner is taught how to assist with daily hygiene including nail and skin care. Mrs Wilson is requested to attend for review after her disease is optimally controlled by medication for follow up care if indicated. To reinforce the advice given in clinic, patient information leaflets on foot problems and care are provided. Our podiatrist finishes her list by carrying out a minor surgical procedure for an RA patient with a chronic painful in growing toenail.

During the clinical session our podiatrist, who works as specialist in rheumatology practice, assists the consultant rheumatologist to undertake an ultrasound guided corticosteroid injection to the subtalar joint. They discuss the merits of entering the joint via the sinus tarsi over a medial approach, as well as indications and contra-indications of the technique. This takes place as part of a clinical mentoring scheme as the podiatrist is undertaking training on ultrasound and intra-articular joint injections as part of extended scope practice whilst working towards a consultant grade post.

Underpinning all of these cases are the primary aims of podiatry care to relieve pain, maintain or improve function and to maintain optimal tissue viability and provide wound management. In our examples above our podiatrist is working effectively as part of the multidisciplinary team and is advancing their own knowledge and skills to provide better and more effective patient care. Podiatrists are experts in assessing and evaluating mechanical foot problems and gait as well as understanding underlying systemic and local disease factors that manifest in the feet as part of the rheumatic diseases. They provide physical treatment strategies including orthotics and footwear, nail-care, callus debridement and wound management, injection therapy and minor surgical techniques. Patient education is an integral part of foot care for patients with rheumatic diseases and podiatrists are able to provide advice as well as assistance and training to adapt, self-manage and cope with disabling foot pain. Podiatry, Biomechanics and the rheumatology foot is further detailed in Chapter 13.

1.7   Health psychology

Elizabeth D. Hale BA(Hons), MSc, CPsychol
Dudley Group of Hospitals NHS Trust, Russells Hall
Hospital, Dudley and University of Birmingham, School
of Sport and Exercise Sciences, Birmingham, UK

Gareth J. Treharne BSc (Hons), PhD University
of Otago, Aotearoa/New Zealand and Dudley Group of
Hospitals NHS Trust Russells Hall Hospital Dudley, UK

HEALTH PSYCHOLOGY

WHAT IS PSYCHOLOGY? AND WHAT IS HEALTH PSYCHOLOGY SPECIFICALLY?

The purview of psychology has been defined in many ways over the years. A dictionary of psychology states that 'psychology simply cannot be defined' (Reber 1985). Those who have attempted to define this elusive subject use phrasings akin to 'the science of mind and behaviour' (Gross 1992). The role of psychologists is still commonly misunderstood by health professionals and the general public alike, often provoking mistrust.

This experience of working or studying within a misunderstood discipline might be something that you identify with given that physiotherapy, occupational therapy and advanced specialist nursing are commonly misconstrued professions (see Study activity). One thing that is certain is that the question "And what do you do?" is one which we try to avoid answering at social gatherings. Answering "I'm a psychologist" is usually followed by "Oh, I'd better be careful then!" or "So can you tell what I'm thinking?" To lay these contentions to rest, we are not 'analysing' your behaviour and we are not 'mind readers'. The serious point that this issue raises is that it is very relevant to understand the confusion and possible discomfort that your patients may feel when you

suggest they could benefit from a referral to a psychologist, or if you mention that you will be applying a psychologically-based intervention yourself.

The formal discipline of psychology is over 130 years old. The first psychology laboratory was founded in 1875 at Harvard University in the USA by William James (Kim 2006). Four years later a further psychology laboratory was founded in Leipzig (Germany) by Wilhelm Wundt, who is usually credited as the founding father of modern psychology (Kim 2006). Interestingly, although both Wundt and James were trained in medicine, the application of psychological theory and methods to health and illness is relatively new, particularly in the UK (Division of Health Psychology 2009). In the US the two fields called behavioural medicine and health psychology were formed as recently as the 1970s. Behavioural medicine considers the role of psychology in medicine and includes a wide range of disciplines in its membership and research (Sarafino 1990). Health psychology is a subfield of psychology concerned with physical health. In the UK, health psychology only became officially recognised as a full Division of The British Psychological Society in 1998 when the British Psychological Society's Special Interest Group in Health Psychology was redesignated the Division of Health Psychology and became responsible for the accreditation of courses and training for health psychologists, that is, those psychologists wanting to specialise in aspects of physical health and health promotion (Division of Health Psychology 2009), as detailed in Box 1.7.1.

BOX 1.7.1   Frequently asked question: what is a health psychologist?

In the UK a health psychologist is someone who specialises in the psychology of physical health, having completed accredited undergraduate, masters and doctoral degree programmes (or equivalent). Additionally, evidence of competency in several specified areas (e.g. research, intervention, consultancy) will lead to the title Chartered Health Psychologist and the titular suffix CPsychol, denoting someone who can practice health psychology without further directive supervision. (The need for professional support supervision is, of course, on-going). More information about the role of Health Psychologists is presented by the Division of Health Psychology (2009) and Hale et al (2007).

- Try to write down a definition of your profession in about 20 words or less. Look up the definition as it is described in a dictionary or core textbook and consider the differences between your own thoughts and the points made by the 'formal' definition.
- Next, think about a multidisciplinary team you have encountered. Did they have access to a psychologist or psychological services? If not, how did the team manage their patients' psychological issues when they arose? What suggestions would you make to improve this aspect of care?

The interests and scope of health psychology in the UK remains similar to those originally formulated in the US nearly 30 years earlier; health psychologists apply psychological research and methods to:

- the promotion and maintenance of health
- the prevention and management of illness
- the identification of psychological factors contributing to physical illness
- the improvement of the healthcare system
- the formulation of healthcare policy.

(Division of Health Psychology 2009)

APPLYING HEALTH PSYCHOLOGY RESEARCH

There are currently over 650 active chartered psychologists in the UK who list health as one of their subspecialties (if not their only one; see British Psychological Society 2009). To our knowledge only a few health psychologists have a special interest in rheumatology and even fewer who work in an integrated role combining formal research and clinical practice. The generation and application of health psychology research and practice should be an interdisciplinary and collaborative enterprise, utilising a variety of research methodologies. For example, we have had input on a project by a rheumatology nurse specialist colleague of ours who investigated the experiences of women with rheumatoid arthritis (RA) and how this impacts upon their role as a young mother (Mitton et al 2007). Other such collaborations

are in action, for example between a team including psychologists, a physiotherapist, a biostatistician and a medical doctor who have used their joint expertise to examine the illness perceptions associated with health and behavioural outcomes in people with musculoskeletal hand problems (Hill et al 2007).

As indicated in our brief background to psychology, psychologists have been concerned from the very start that the discipline should be taken seriously and on a par with the natural sciences, hence the early establishment of psychological 'laboratories'. The emphasis was, and continues to be, largely focused upon objective measurement and quantification (Hale et al 2008). The difficulties for psychologists have always been in how to measure something that you cannot objectively see, like motivation, anxiety or depression. Applying the same rigour and methodology as seen in the natural sciences, psychologists continue to find novel, reliable and validated ways of measuring these concepts. Psychology is not 'mind reading'; there are no tricks or special skills that allow us to know how patients are thinking or are likely to behave, unless there is good research evidence to support it. Although it is true to say that psychological research has been dominated by this quantitative approach, there has recently been a growth of interest in the qualitative methodologies, particularly within health psychology and health based research (Hale et al 2008). Adopting the same rigorous approach to research whilst using, for example, structured or semi-structured interviews can provide in-depth perspectives of an experience which might provide knowledge that helps to illuminate a problem or re-shape healthcare policy or practice (Hale et al 2008). In essence practitioners need to critically read and evaluate the existing research literature (the evidence) on the problem they are addressing or the intervention they are intending to implement. New local practice might arise from this evaluation and synthesis. For example, a recent meta-analytic review by Dixon et al (2007) suggested that psychosocial interventions can boost the active coping efforts that people with arthritis engage in. They used the technique called meta-analysis, where the statistical effects seen across several different studies are combined, and found that these interventions are most effective for improving anxiety and joint swelling (recorded as joint counts). Furthermore, they found that depression, functional ability and pain self-efficacy can be improved by psychological intervention but not as consistently across the studies they reviewed. Information on measuring patient reported outcomes such as these can be seen in Chapter 4. We will go on to explain some of these concepts, like anxiety and coping in more detail (see Chs 4–6).

This section has introduced psychology and more specifically health psychology and its role in rheumatology. Concepts and interventions used are explained in more detail in Chapter 11.

1.8   A brief introduction to evidence-based medicine

Adrian White MA MD BM Bch General Practice and Primary Care, Peninsula Medical School, Plymouth, UK

A BRIEF INTRODUCTION TO EVIDENCE-BASED MEDICINE

Patients should receive the best possible treatment that is available for their condition. Evidence based medicine (EBM) is a particular way of deciding what is best. It was first described in the early 1990s and has come to dominate medical practice. While the EBM approach is clearly 'correct', it does have its limitations, and it should not be applied on its own without considering the context, particularly the needs of the individual patient. We shall briefly discuss what EBM involves, and make some suggestions on how it is best applied.

The essential process in choosing a treatment for a patient is: look for the highest quality of evidence on which of the available treatments offer the greatest benefits compared with its harms. The different types of study can be arranged in a hierarchy of their 'quality' (Box 1.8.1), which is based on the scientific rigour of the study. A study that is 'rigorous' is done in a way that the results are not influenced by what the researchers believed beforehand. The most rigorous design is the randomised controlled trial (RCT) and this is regarded as the 'gold standard'.

There are various ways of grading the evidence according to the amount of evidence and its quality, for making decisions. For example, in one system evidence from systematic reviews is graded as level 1a, evidence from one randomized controlled trial as level 1b, down to evidence from expert committee reports which is level IV (Bombadier et al

> **BOX 1.8.1   Hierarchy of evidence (Bomdardier et al 2003)**
>
> - One system for evaluating or grading the strength of evidence was developed for a Cochrane Review
> - Strong evidence: multiple relevant, high quality randomized controlled trials
> - Moderate evidence: one relevant, high quality randomized controlled trial and one or more relevant, low quality randomized controlled trials
> - Limited evidence: one relevant, high quality randomized controlled trial or multiple relevant, low quality randomized controlled trials
> - No evidence: only one relevant, low quality randomized controlled trial, no relevant randomized controlled trials or contradictory outcomes. Contradictory results means less than a third of the studies showed either positive or negative results.

2003). However, health care is not a soulless process that depends purely on reading systematic reviews. When it comes to putting EBM into practice, other factors must be taken into account, particularly the wishes of the patient and the practitioner's clinical judgement in this particular case.

Some of the limitations of EBM are obvious. It will take a huge amount of work to produce randomized controlled trials, let alone systematic reviews, for every possible treatment for every condition. Very often, high quality evidence simply is not available, and a clinical decision has to be made on less rigorous evidence. The fact that randomized controlled trials and systematic reviews have not been done on a particular treatment does not mean it does not work! This is usually summarised in the phrase: Absence of evidence of an effect is not the same as evidence of absence of an effect. When EBM is applied thoughtlessly, useful interventions are likely to be rejected, and many patients will be denied benefit. So, while waiting for the rigorous studies, the principle of EBM is to look for the highest quality evidence available – even if it is only a report from another patient who has benefitted from a particular treatment. The final decision on treatment also has to take other factors into account, such as whether its mechanism is plausible, what it costs, and its safety record.

There are other limitations to EBM. Randomized controlled trials are often done in very restricted circumstances, for example in patients within a certain age range who do not have any other medical condition. The conclusions from these randomized controlled trials may not be applicable to a different group of patients. Additionally, although systematic reviews are supposed to be consistent and reliable, sometimes different reviews reach different conclusions.

Not all decisions require the same level of evidence. For example, taxpayers will want health policies that are based on good evidence of effectiveness, safety and cost. More subtly, a clinician might judge that there is enough evidence to support or condone a patient's choice for a particular treatment, but not enough to recommend the treatment to someone else who has not considered it. It is often said of complementary treatments that the patient's preference might be crucial to success, but this is probably just as true of many conventional treatments that we use every day.

In summary, although EBM may be the best way in theory to choose between different treatments, in practice it will often be necessary to make a case that the 'right' treatment for this particular patient is not the one that is supported by the highest level of evidence. The following chapters have considered the best available evidence whenever possible.

USEFUL WEBSITES

ARMA website accessed 10/11/08
http://www.arma.uk.net.
Chartered Society of Physiotherapy accessed 10/11/08
http://www.csp.org.uk
Department of Health accessed 10/11/08
http://www.dh.gov.uk/en/index.htm.
Arthritis Research Campaign National Primary Care Web site, Critically Appraised Topics accessed 10/11/08
http://www.keele.ac.uk/research/pchs/pcmrc/dissemination/cat/index/htm.
http://www.rcgp-curriculum.org.uk. Accessed March 2009.

References and further reading

ARMA, 2007. Standards of care for people with musculoskeletal foot problems. http://www.arma.uk.net/ (accessed 10.11.08.).

Arthur, V., Clifford, C., 2004. Rheumatology: the expectations and preferences of patients for their follow up monitoring care: a qualitative study to determine the dimensions of patient satisfaction. J. Clin. Nurs. 13, 234–242.

BHPR, 2004. The role of the rheumatologist. Roles in rheumatology British Health Professionals in Rheumatology on line resource http://www.rheumatology.org.uk/bhpr/rolesinrheum/ (accessed March 2009.).

Bird, H.A., 1983. Divided rheumatology care: the advent of the rheumatology practitioner? Ann. Rheum. Dis. 42, 354–355.

Bombardier, C., Bouter, L.M., de Bie, R. A., et al., 2003. Back Group. In: The Cochrane Library issue 3. Update Software, Oxford.

British Psychological Society, 2009. Register of Chartered Psychologists. Online. Available: http://www.bps.org.uk/e-services/find-a-psychologist/register.cfm/ (accessed September 2009)

Bunn, F., Byrne, G., Kendall, S., 2004. Telephone consultation and triage: effects on health care use and patient satisfaction. Cochrane Database Systematic Reviews CD004180.

Bunn, F., Byrne, G., Kendall, S., 2005. The effects of telephone consultation and triage on healthcare use and patient satisfaction: a systematic review. Brit. J. Gen. Pract. 55, 956–961.

Carr, A., 2001. Defining the extended clinical role for allied health professionals in rheumatology. Chesterfield. Arthritis Research Campaign conference proceedings no 12.

CSP, 2008. Charting the future of physiotherapy. Chartered Society of Physiotherapy 14 Bedford Row London WC1R 4ED http://

www.csp.org.uk/director/members/libraryandpublications/csppublications.cfm?item_id=56853683ED91C7CC76535A867964FCE6/ (accessed March 2009.).

Department of Health, 2000. NHS Plan: A plan for investment a plan for reform. Department of Health London http://www.dh.gov.uk/en/Publicationsandstatistics/Publications/PublicationsPolicyAndGuidance/DH_4002960/ (accessed March 2009.).

Department of Health, 2001. Advanced Letter PAM (PTA) Allied healthcare professionals consultant posts. Department of Health London http://www.dh.gov.uk/en/Publicationsandstatistics/Lettersandcirculars/Dearcolleagueletters/DH_4005723/ (accessed March 2009.).

Department of Health, 2003a. Modernising Medical Careers. Department of Health London http://www.dh.gov.uk/en/Publicationsandstatistics/Publications/PublicationsPolicy

AndGuidance/DH_4010460/ (accessed March 2009.).

Department of Health, 2003b. The Foundation Committee of the Academy of Medical Royal Colleges in Co-operation with Modernising Medical Careers in the Department of Heath. Department of Health London http://www.dh.gov. uk/en/Publicationsandstatistics/ Lettersandcirculars/ Dearcolleagueletters/DH_4003085/ (accessed March 2009.).

Department of Health, 2004a. 10 High Impact Changes. Department of Health London http://www.dh.gov. uk/en/Publicationsandstatistics/ Bulletins/theweek/ Chiefexecutivebulletin/DH_ 4088866/ (accessed March 2009.).

Department of Health, 2004b. A Compendium of solutions to implement the working time directive for Doctors in training. Department of Health London http://www.dh.gov. uk/en/Publicationsandstatistics/ Publications/PublicationsPolicy AndGuidance/DH_4082634/ (accessed March 2009.).

Department of Health, 2006. The Musculoskeletal Services Framework A Joint responsibility: doing it differently. Department of Health London http://www.dh.gov.uk/ en/Publicationsandstatistics/ Publications/PublicationsPolicy AndGuidance/DH_4138413/ (accessed March 2009.).

Department of Health, 2006b. Tackling hospital waiting the 18-week patient pathway. An implementation Framework. Department of Health London http://www.dh.gov. uk/en/Publicationsandstatistics/ Publications/PublicationsPolicy AndGuidance/DH_4134668/ (accessed March 2009.).

Division of Health Psychology, 2009. What is Health Psychology? Online.

Available: http://www.health-psychology.org.uk/dhp_home.cfm (accessed September 2009).

Dixon, K.E., Keefe, F.J., Scipio, C. D., et al., 2007. Psychological interventions for arthritis pain management in adults: a meta-analysis. Health Psychol. 26 (3), 241–250.

Greener, I., Mannion, R., 2006. Does practice based commissioning avoid the problems of fundholding?. Brit. Med. J. 333, 1168–1170.

Gross, R., 1992. Psychology: The Science of Mind and Behaviour, third ed. Hodder & Stoughton, London.

Hammond, A., Kidao, R., Young, A., 2000. Hand Impairment and Function in early Rheumatoid Arthritis. Arthritis and Rheumatism 43 (Suppl. 9), S285.

Hammond, A., Freeman, K., 2001. One year outcomes of a randomised controlled trial of an educational-behavioural joint protection programme for people with rheumatoid arthritis.. Rheumatology 40, 1044–1051.

Hammond, A., 2004. What is the role of the occupational therapist? Best Pract. Res. Cl. Rh. 18, 491–505.

Hammond, A., Bryan, J., Hardy, A., et al., 2008. Effects of a modular behavioural arthritis education programme: a pragmatic parallel-group randomized controlled trial. Rheumatology 47 (11), 1712–1718.

Hale, E.D., Treharne, G.J., Peacock, S., et al., 2007. Defining the role of health psychologists in rheumatology. Rheumatology 46 (Suppl. 1), i148. Abstract

Hale, E.D., Treharne, G.J., Kitas, G.D., 2008. Qualitative methodologies I: asking research questions with reflexive insight. Musculoskeletal Care 6, 86–96.

Hay, E., Campbell, A., Linney, S., et al., 2007. Musculoskeletal GPwSI Working Group. Development of a

competency framework for general practitioners with a special interest in musculoskeletal/rheumatology practice. Rheumatology 46, 360–362.

Hay, E.M., Foster, N.E., Thomas, E., et al., 2006. Effectiveness of community physiotherapy and enhanced pharmacy review for knee pain in people aged over 55 presenting to primary care: pragmatic randomised trial. Brit. Med. J. 333 (7576), 995.

Hill, J., 1992. A nurse practitioner rheumatology clinic. Nurs. Stand. 7, 35–37.

Hill, J., Bird, H., Lawton, C., et al., 1994. An evaluation of the effectiveness, safety, and acceptability of a nurse practitioner in a rheumatology outpatient clinic. Brit. J. Rh. 33, 283–288.

Hill, S., Dziedzic, K., Thomas, E., et al., 2007. The illness perceptions associated with health and behavioural outcomes in people with musculoskeletal hand problems: findings from the North Staffordshire Osteoarthritis Project (NorStOP) Rheumatology 46 (6), 944–951.

Hooper, H., Ryan, S., Hassell, A., 2004. The role of social comparison in coping with rheumatoid arthritis: an interview study.. Musculoskeletal Care 2, 195–206.

Hosie, G., 2000. Teaching rheumatology in primary care. Ann. Rheum. Dis. 59, 500–503.

Jordan, J.M., Bernard, S.L., Callahan, L.F., et al., 2000. Self-reported arthritis-related disruptions in sleep and daily life and the use of medical, complementary and self-care strategies for Arthritis: The National Survey of Self-Care and Ageing. Arch. Fam. Med. 9, 143–149.

Jordan, K., Clarke, A., Symmons, D., et al., 2007. Measuring disease prevalence: a comparison of musculoskeletal disease using four general practice consultation databases. Brit. J. Gen. Pract. 57, 7–14.

Katz, P.P., Neugebauer, A., 2001. Does satisfaction with abilities mediate the relationship between the impact of rheumatoid arthritis on valued activities and depression? Arthrit. Care Res. 45, 263–269.

Katz, P., Yelin, E.H., 1994. Life activities of persons with rheumatoid arthritis with and without depressive symptoms. Arthrit. Care Res. 7, 69–77.

Kim A., 2006 Wilhelm Maximilian Wundt. Stanford Encyclopedia of Philosophy. Online. Available: http://www.plato.stanford.edu/entries/wilhelm-wundt/29Jun2007

Lattimer, V., Smith, H., Hungin, P., et al., 1996. Future provision of out of hours primary medical care: a survey with two general practitioner research networks. Brit. Med. J. 312, 352–356.

Luqmani, R., Hennel, S., Estrach, C., et al., 2006. British Society for Rheumatology and British Health Professionals in Rheumatology Guidelines for the management of rheumatoid arthritis (the first 2 years). Rheumatology 45 (9), 1167–1169.

Luqmani, R., Hennel, S., Estrach, C., et al. 2009. British Society for Rheumatology and British Health Professionals in Rheumatology Guidelines for the management of rheumatoid arthritis (after the first 2 years). Rheumatology doi:10.1093/rheumatology/ken450b

McCormick, A., Fleming, D., Charlton, J., 1995. Morbidity statistics from general practice. 4th national study 1991-1992. London, HMSO.

Manley, K., 2000. Organisational culture and consultant nurse outcomes: part 1 organisational culture. Nurs. Stand. 14, 34–38.

Mitton, D.L., Treharne, G.J., Hale, E.D., et al., 2007. The health and life experiences of mothers with rheumatoid arthritis: a phenomenological study. Musculoskeletal Care 5, 191–205.

Mooney, J., 1996. Audit of rheumatology nurse outreach clinics. Rheumatology in Practice. Winter 18-20.

NICE, 2008. National Institute for Health and Clinical Excellence. Osteoarthritis: national clinical guideline for care and management in adults. http://www.nice.org.uk/CG059www.nice.org.uk/CG059/ (accessed March 2009.).

NICE (National Institute of Clinical Excellence), 2009. Rheumatoid arthritis: national clinical guideline for management and treatment in adults. Ch. 6.3 Occupational Therapy. p87-94 http://www.nice.org.uk/nicemedia/pdf/CG59NICEguideline.pdf/. (accessed March 2009.).

O'Brien, A.V., Jones, P., Mullis, R., et al., 2006. Conservative hand therapy treatments in rheumatoid arthritis–a randomized controlled trial. Rheumatology 45, 577–583.

Reber, A.S., 1985. Dictionary of Psychology, third ed.. Penguin, London.

Ryan, S., Hassell, A.B., Lewis, M., et al., 2006. A study into the impact of the expert nurse on the patients attending a drug monitor clinic. J. Adv. Nurs. 53, 277–286.

Ryan, S., Hill, J., 2004. A survey of practice in nurse led rheumatoid arthritis clinics. Rheumatology 43 (Suppl. 2), 411.

Sarafino, E.P., 1990. Health Psychology: Biopsychosocial Interactions, third ed.. John Wiley, New York.

Scott, D.L., Shipley, M., Dawson, A., et al., 1998. The Clinical Management of Rheumatoid Arthritis and Osteoarthritis: Strategies for Improving Clinical Effectiveness. Brit. J. Rheumat. 37, 546–554.

Shaul, M., 1995. From early twinges to mastery: the process of adjustment in living with rheumatoid arthritis. Arthrit. Care Res. 47, 525–531.

SIGN, 2000. Management of Early Rheumatoid Arthritis. SIGN Publication No. 48 ISBN 1899893 37 7 http://www.sign.ac.uk/guidelines/fulltext/48/index.html/. (accessed March 2009.).

Stevenson, K., Bird, L., Sarigiovannis, P., et al., 2007. A new multidisciplinary approach to integrating best evidence into musculoskeletal practice. J. Eval. Clin. Pract. 13, 703–708.

Thwaites, C., 2004. Rheumatology telephone advice lines.. Musculoskeletal Care 2, 120–126.

Verstappen, S.M.M., Jacobs, J.W.G., Verkleij, H., et al., 2004. Overview of work disability in patients with rheumatoid arthritis as observed in transversal and longitudinal studies. Ann. Rheum. Dis. 51 (3), 488–497.

Vliet Vlieland, T.P., Breedveld, F.C., Hazes, J.M., 1997. The two-year follow-up of a randomized comparison of in-patient multidisciplinary team care and routine out-patient care for active rheumatoid arthritis. Brit.J. Rheumat. 36 (1), 82–85.

Wilson Barnett, J., 1985. Key functions in nursing.. Lampada 2, 35–39.

Young, A., Dixey, J., Cox, N., et al., 2000. How does functional disability in early rheumatoid arthritis (RA) affect patients and their lives? Results of 5 years of follow-up in 732 patients from the Early RA Study (ERAS). Rheumatology 39, 603–611.

Zhang, W., Doherty, M., Leeb, B.F., et al., 2007. EULAR Evidence based recommendations for the management of hand osteoarthritis: report of a task force of the EULAR Standing Committee for International Clinical Studies including Therapeutics (ESCISIT). Ann. Rheum. Dis. 66, 377–388.

Chapter 2

The user patient journey

Susan M. Oliver RN MSc FRCN Devon, UK

Ailsa Bosworth The National Rheumatoid Arthritis Society, Westacott Business Center, Littlewick Green Berkshire, UK

KEY POINTS

- The user patient journey is variable and complex
- The costs to the individual are high and are borne silently by the individual
- Individuals who are the recipients of care should be informed of standards and guidelines available and the relevance to their care
- HCPs play an important role in encouraging and supporting patient empowerment
- Process mapping is a useful tool to explore patient experiences of healthcare services and potential strengths and weakness of care provided.

INTRODUCTION

Society as a whole has little understanding of Musculoskeletal Conditions (MSC) and the consequences to the individual. This can have a significant 'knock on' effect to the individual with joint disease particularly, as MSC may cause individuals to stop working, contributing to high levels of claims for Incapacity Benefit, depression and poor self esteem (Department of Health 2006). People with MSC are the second highest group claiming Incapacity Benefit (which, for new claimants since October 2008, is now termed Employment and Support Allowance).

For individuals with MSC (e.g. osteoarthritis, rheumatoid arthritis and back pain) the consequences of their disease, both to the individual and society, are immense (Department of Health 2006). Many individuals fail to seek medical advice despite having significant pain and disability, believing there is "nothing that can be done". This presents challenges when encouraging people to seek medical care as they may be dissuaded by public opinion and have little encouragement from family and friends to do so (Department of Health, 2006, Oliver 2007). Recent patient surveys have identified poor knowledge and support for those with MSC in the workplace and limited educational or financial incentives for support in these areas (The National Rheumatoid Arthritis Society 2004, 2006, 2007).

This chapter will briefly outline an example of patient journeys from a mapping project exploring patient experiences in rheumatoid arthritis (RA), discuss some of the issues related to these and the challenges individuals face in negotiating their healthcare needs.

THE USER–PATIENT JOURNEY – MAPPING PROJECT

A mapping project explored the journeys of patients with early sero-positive RA. Participants were grouped into three disease duration categories (< 1 year; 1–2 years; and >2–3.5 years from diagnosis). The mapping project used qualitative and process mapping principles used in industry but increasingly

© 2010 Elsevier Ltd
DOI: 10.1016/B978-0-443-06934-5.00002-4

applied to healthcare settings. Twenty-two individual patient pathways were mapped retrospectively to explore the user-patient journey and attribute direct and indirect costs to variances in care (Fig. 2.1). An example of one participant map is shown in Figure 2.2. Wide variances in many aspects of care were identified, including access to specialist services, adherence to National Institute of Clinical Excellence (NICE) guidance, support to stay in work and importantly, regular, patient-focussed support to enable active self management (such as telephone advice line services).

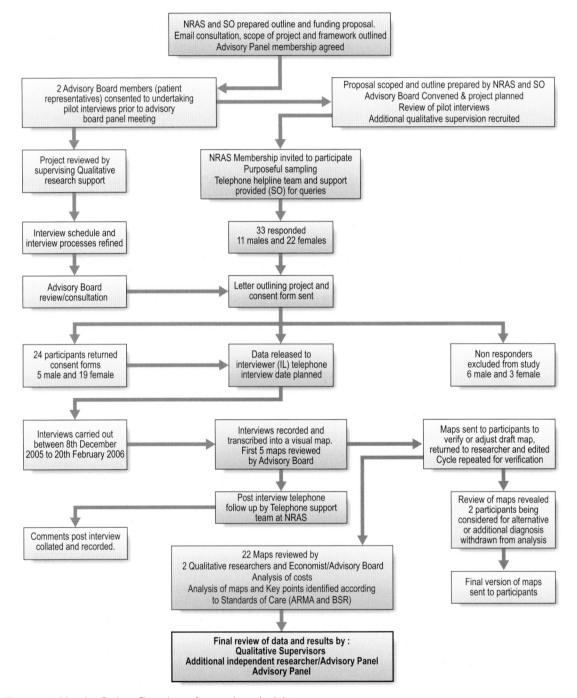

Figure 2.1 Mapping Project: Flow chart of research methodology.

The mapping project demonstrated that indirect costs to the individual were high and borne silently (e.g. job losses). Seven of the 22 participants took early retirement or lost jobs directly due to the RA within the study period (Oliver & Bosworth 2006). These findings are borne out in other observational and quantitative research (Bone and Joint Decade 2005, Hulsemann et al 2005, Woolf et al 2003, 2004).

An additional burden is the time spent waiting to be seen by a consultant. For conditions, such as RA, early referral is essential to improve long-term outcomes. Yet, in the mapping project seven of the

Patient background
1999 patient experienced problems with neck and headaches (GP discussed possible dysphasia): sleepiness (narcolepsy also considered) and depression.

14th February 2002
Patient woke up but unable to move. GP made home visit but not regular GP (locum). Unable to make immediate diagnosis. Suggested issue was due to depression.

New locum GP thought symptoms might indicate Rheumatoid Arthritis. Prescribed anti-inflammatory drug and pain-killers. Referred to Consultant Rheumatologist. Told there would be an 18 month wait. Patient decided to pay for private consultation as she was getting married in May 2002.

April 2002
Patient saw Consultant Rheumatologist who was also unable to confirm RA. Referred back to GP.

May 2002
Went back to GP feeling depressed and concerned that this was 'all in the mind'. GP suggested it might still be a form of arthritis and prescribed steroids. Symptoms improved for a short while.

May 2002
Patient got married and went on honeymoon. However, on her return 'things began to fall apart' and she felt terribly unwell again.

June 2002
Returned to GP who referred patient to National Reumatology Hospital

August 2002
Patient visited on Thursday and admitted the following Tuesday for 3 weeks to undergo tests.
She was taken off all medication, subjected to intensive physiotherapy and eventually diagnosed with RA. Patient describes this as a great relief to at least know what was wrong and referred to the years of uncertainty and depression that included the prescription of drugs such as prozac and seroxat. She recalls one occasion when she fell and was in plaster for 12 weeks because of concerns over possible torn ligaments and wonders whether an earlier investigation might have prevented this.

September 2002
Patient is prescribed sulphasalazine and a programme that required 2-monthly visits supported by monthly tests by her GP. Also prescribed amitriptyline.

December 2002
Patient taken off sulphasalazine as no improvement made and prescribed methotrexate which was to be increased every 2 months till the effective dose was established. Patient recalls spending Christmas 2002 being sick and nauseous.

Patient followed this regime but became progressively worse, eventually becoming bed bound.

May 2003
Patient emergency admission to local hospital with a blood clot. Given steroid injection, tests taken, placed on steroid drip. Found to be intolerant to methotrexate.

May 2003
Transferred from first National hospital to Rheumatologist in her region. Referred to physiotherapist and OT via RA Unit.

Tried a short period of methotrexate injections

July 2003
Patient taken off methotrexate and prescribed leflunomide, 100 mg initial dose then 20 mg regular dosage. Patient reports that this did help for a few months. Fortnightly blood tests at GP.

December 2003
Patient feeling poorly again. Given steroid injection and advised by hospital that she would need to continue with this drug regime until permission approved to try Humira (adalimumab).

Frequent steroid injections given to ease condition

July 2004
Patient prescribed Humira: 40 mg injections fortnightly. Within days patient feeling much better and able to go on holiday

July–December 2004
Patient continues with Humira and steroid injections as needed. Continues to have occasional flare-ups and blood test readings not satisfactory: high ESR– low CPR.

December 2004
Leflunomide 20 mg prescription added to the Humira injections. Patient is still taking daily prescription of amitriptyline. She also takes diazepam as needed when spasms in neck really bad.

December 2005
Patient's current drug regime:
1. Humira (adalimumab) 20 mg/fortnight
2. Leflunomide 20 mg/day
3. Paracetamol up to 8/day as needed for pain
4. Tramadol up to 8/day for arthritic pain (taken with paracetamol)
5. Ibrufen (ibuprofen) up to 4/day (unable to take stronger anti-inflammatory due to stomach cramps caused by length of time on these drugs)
6. Amitriptyline 50 mg/day taken each night
7. Kapake up to 8/day (for migraine)
8. Zimovane 1/night (sleeping tablet)
9. Cod liver oil tablets (suggested by doctor)
10. Stemitel 3 x 5 mg/day (for vertigo as required)

Patient comments
1. Patient forced to give up employment as an In-house Social Worker, a job she had held for 6 years, and an income of between £1000–£2000 per month. She now claims Incapacity Benefit, Disability Allowance, Mobility and Care Allowance.
2. During the period the patient's marriage ended and she was forced to sell the family home as her income could not fund mortgage. It is worth noting that she had moved with her husband in December 2003 from their two-storey home into a bungalow with adaptations to support her condition. This was sold in October 2005 and she now lives with her mother and step-father who help care for her. (See costs below)
3. Occupational Therapist has provided help with special aids such as raised toilet seat, wheelchair, furniture with raising seat, handles, shower chair, soft and hard wrist splints, cutlery, long-handled sponge, etc.
4. Prior to the patient's marriage ending her husband took substantial amounts of time off work resulting in lost earnings. Costs were also incurred through frequent trips/stays. (See below)

Figure 2.2 Patient map. *(Continued)*

Patient costs

1. April 2002 private consultation £80.00
2. March 2003 patient bought electric motor scooter to aid mobility: £1000.00 and needed to change her car to accommodate her electric scooter and change to automatic control: cost £3000.00 allowing for part exchange of previous car.
3. Substantial costs involved in sale of house, agents, solicitor, redemption costs total more than £1000.00.
4. Other aids:
   - shower cubicle £900.00, taps (bathroom and kitchen) £150.00
   - raised oven unit £500.00, kitchen sundries (kettle, knife, etc. £50.00)
   - orthopaedic bed £1000.00
   - gas fire with remote control £350.00
   various personal aids, e.g. electric toothbrush, heat pad, various supports, etc. £?

5. Extra cost for life insurance/mortgage protection, travel insurance, house insurance.
6. Prescription costs: since the patient sold her home she is now required to pay prescription charges because of capital. Currently costing at least £34.00 per month. Intending to buy annual prescription.
7. Food, such as ready meals the patient can prepare herself when left alone: £1000.00 p.a.
8. B & B costs were incurred for patient's husband when staying in area near national hospital at £35.00 per night for approximately 7 nights, totalling £245.00.
9. Travel: journeys to National hospital were 300 miles (return) which at IR rates of 40p/mile amount to £120.00 per trip x 6 visits = £720.00. Visits to Haverfordwest calculated on the same basis amount to £11.20 per trip.

Figure 2.2 Continued.

11 participants seen rapidly, i.e. within 12 weeks of symptom onset, were seen as a result of private referral. The evidence collated from the mapping project is supported by other patient stories, such as those on seen on www.healthtalkonline.org, which is a registered charity describing a range of MSCs and individuals' experiences. There are many patient stories outlined according to disease duration.

One UK study identified average annual direct costs of RA to be £3980 (Cooper et al 2002). Higher costs were associated with those who were either younger, had longer disease duration or more severe disease. A younger group is more likely to be in full-time employment and thus, additional costs relate to loss of work, extended sick leave or reduction in work hours (Merkesdal et al 2005). For example, over a three year period, delays in referral or receiving a definitive diagnosis or treatment for this group identified significant costs. Personal costs for three individuals in this project averaged £1990.27. Some of the variances in treatment costs are outlined in Table 2.1.

Receiving a diagnosis of a long-term condition, such as RA, is a significant life event. The social and psychological impact to the individual varies (Fitzpatrick et al 1988, Oliver & Ryan 2004). Initially, this may be because those receiving the diagnosis are unaware or unable to accept the diagnosis or that they have their own specific health beliefs or coping strategies that have an impact on their perceptions of the diagnosis and the underlying symptoms they are experiencing. Importantly however, evidence suggests that the spectrum of patient need, routes to treatment, advice and support vary dramatically (Bone and Joint Decade 2005). Indeed

Table 2.1 Variances in treatment and personal costs

BIOLOGIC PARTICIPANTS	TOTAL COST TO HEALTH PROVIDER	TOTAL COST TO PATIENT
Patient number (disease duration).		
002 (2–3.6 yrs)	£30,836.21	£3675.47
005 (1–2 yrs)	£1941.03	£2150.70
007 (<1 yr)	£2071.78	£3135.42
010 (2–3.6 yrs)	£21,738.55	£11,097.00
016 (2–3.6yrs)	£24,084.21	£8382.33
023 (2–3.6yrs)	£10,975.30	£413.00
Grand Total	£91,647.08	£28,853.92

DMARD PARTICIPANTS*	TOTAL COST TO HEALTH PROVIDER	TOTAL COST TO PATIENT
Patient number (disease duration).		
004 (<1 yr)	£304.10	£514.00
007 (<1 yr)	£2071.78	£31135.42
009 (2–3.6 yrs)	£3346.32	£444.94
011 (<1 yr)	£1218.56	£11.00
018 (2–3.6 yrs)	£727.60	£348.50
019 (1–2 yrs)	£10,034.56	£2937.60
Grand Total	£17,702.92	£7391.46

(time from diagnosis)
* DMARD = Disease Modifying Anti-Rheumatic Drug

the various patient journeys can, as a result, be confusing and complex to map (Fig. 2.3).

One participant (005) stated "At first the GP very helpful but I was not diagnosed at this time. The second GP good but not particularly clued up on RA and saw this as an old age disease and had no

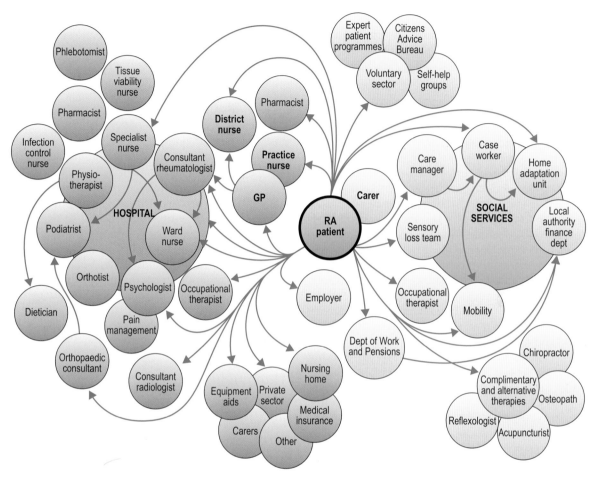

Figure 2.3 The spectrum of contact and needs through a patient journey.

knowledge of medications being prescribed. My current GP has a specialist interest in RA which is wonderful". For the individual, their knowledge and understanding of their condition develops over time. In some circumstances knowledge is gained from interactions with healthcare professionals (Oliver 2004). For others, the general illness experiences learnt through times of exacerbations or temporary remission, form their views and abilities on personal self management strategies (Corben & Rosen, 2005, Department of Health 2001, 2005). The reality is that people with long-term conditions manage much of their care themselves at home with their families and interact with their healthcare team for a few hours per year (Department of Health 2005) (Fig. 2.4).

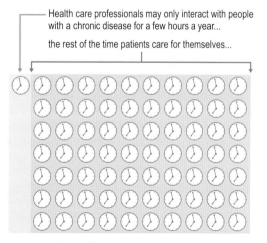

Figure 2.4 Patient self-management.

Some individuals resolved their problems and needs themselves particularly if they were adequately informed of the benefits of the multi-professional team. One participant (009) had to "push hard" for access to a physiotherapist when she wanted advice on walking aids. The same participant asked for splints but ultimately had to purchase them herself. When the issue was raised with the consultant they were advised that the purchased splints "seemed to be doing the trick".

Negotiating healthcare services and accessing the support, information and treatment required can be a challenge. These challenges may be as a result of their point of contact when they receive a diagnosis in a busy clinic environment that is alien to them. This experience is filled with many complex, and sometimes intimidating processes, that are a mystery to those lacking knowledge of healthcare systems. Over time, for most, these experiences should become less intimidating and the threats and challenges of the condition more readily understood and managed.

Participant (024) stated that he "had nothing but praise for the way he has been looked after by all the health professionals and the health service". One participant (021) has subsequently moved from her first hospital but had a less satisfactory experience. The first time she was aware of her diagnosis was when the consultant took her to the RA nurse. As he handed the file to the nurse he told the nurse that the patient had RA. This was the first time it was mentioned.

There are numerous factors that affect the individual's ability to comprehend, retain or accept the information that is provided at the time of diagnosis (Hill 2006). In addition, there are complex issues that affect the initial consultation and information giving process. Some of these include knowledge of the disease prior to seeking a diagnosis, the level of stress and pain experienced at the time of diagnosis, prior health issues, manner of communication at the time of diagnosis, personal health beliefs and the individual's coping styles.

One participant (017) outlined how they were bombarded with information about the condition, drugs, physiotherapy etc as part of a drug trial….. "but very little of this contained advice on what she would experience or how to manage the pain on a day to day basis other than with the use of painkillers".

Education and information giving are not a one stop package but an ongoing part of care. Newly diagnosed individuals may not fully recognise this need in the early phases of the disease (Luqmani et al 2006). The variations in individual needs continue throughout their illness pathway and healthcare professionals (HCPs) need to be continually mindful of opportunities to provide information giving, education and support as and when the individual appears responsive, or requests additional information. HCPs should focus not only on the medical aspects of care but also the social and psychological consequences of disease (Arthritis & Musculoskeletal Alliance 2004, Luqmani et al 2006).

HCPs aim to encourage and support the individual from the first point of contact throughout their healthcare journey, and encourage them to know they are entitled to be an active participant in their treatment choices. At the same time, HCPs need to be mindful of those who are unable or do not wish to make informed decisions about their care. In the changing healthcare system these individuals will need to be considered and appropriate 'safety nets' be in place to ensure they still receive the optimum in care.

FROM NEWLY DIAGNOSED TO ACHIEVING MASTERY IN EMPOWERMENT

It can be seen from the mapping projects that individuals retrospectively understood more about their care and what they should have received. However, the consequences of not having the appropriate management at the right time were significant to the individual. Patient empowerment is high on the healthcare agenda and this should enable individuals to be more informed about their care.

The question is, 'what is empowerment and how do individuals achieve mastery?' Empowerment is defined as: 'To give ability to; enable or permit'. This definition outlines the need to enable or permit patients to take control and this means HCPs must play a key role in providing the help to develop strategies and the right level of support at the right time to facilitate 'empowerment'. If the individual develops effective self-management strategies, their abilities and self-efficacy can be negatively affected if principles fail to be endorsed in the healthcare setting.

The natural course of the disease is variable and an individual's disease path varies dependent upon the actual disease and severity, as well as contributing factors such as:

- Type of onset (e.g. rapid or insidious)
- Time of onset (e.g. stressful life events at the time, loss of job, new baby)

- Age and circumstances at time of presentation
- Social and cultural issues (e.g. level of social support, beliefs about pain and treatment for symptoms)
- Psychological factors (e.g. individual coping styles, health beliefs)
- Other pre-existing or newly presented co-morbidities.

Each of the above aspects can present at different times in the individual's journey. HCPs need to be aware of and ready to provide the appropriate support and guidance that can enable the individual to work their way through these challenges or changes that present. For the individual, recognising their ability to overcome some of these challenges can build their self-esteem and perceptions of self-efficacy.

The relationship between patients and HCPs builds over time and illness experiences, yet the first and specific challenge in the early days of this therapeutic relationship is at the time of diagnosis (Oliver & Ryan 2004). HCPs are aware of the importance of information giving and have to consider issues related to informed consent to treatment. Some individuals will wish to have all the information they can to aid their ability to understand and cope with their newly acquired diagnosis, whilst others need time to adjust and come to terms with the diagnosis or may simply fail to accept the initial diagnosis.

The HCP's expertise is in rapidly assessing the individual and their specific needs at first point of contact and defining how best to support them. However, it still has to be accepted that treatment will need to be started early in the disease process if optimal patient outcomes are to be achieved and this can be particularly difficult for patients who have always had a strong antipathy to taking drugs.

Individuals with RA are likely to have a wide spectrum of needs and meet a wide range of practitioners throughout the life of their disease. They will receive different aspects of care across a wide range of healthcare settings (Fig. 2.3). Yet it is clear that currently, knowledge is poor about how best to provide support and appropriate care for those with RA outside the specialist field of practice (Frank & Chamberlain 2001, Memel & Kirwan 1999, Woolf et al 2003). Individuals who have become adept at negotiating their healthcare needs in specialist services can experience barriers and frustrations when they are perhaps more informed about the management of their disease than for example, their own GP.

Individuals first presenting with joint symptoms in primary care receive widely disparate levels of advice and support. Some receive optimum care and are rapidly referred to specialist services for a diagnosis. Others experience a delay of several months before gaining the same level of management (Oliver & Bosworth 2006, Sanders et al 2004). The mapping project demonstrated that 16 out of the 22 participants received treatment with a disease modifying drug (e.g. methotrexate) within 6 months of first presentation. For those eligible for a biologic therapy (e.g. anti-TNFα inhibitors – adalimumab, etanercept or infliximab), half experienced delays before accessing treatment (ranging from 2–10 months).

Over time, many individuals manage on a day to day basis in their community with the support of their families and local services. Individuals learn to manage their pain and cope with the disability. Individuals who use emotion-focussed coping strategies may end up in a spiral of repeated visits to their doctor and 'learned helplessness' (Ryan et al 2003). The aim of management should be to encourage positive coping styles and self management principles and, hopefully, prevent individuals developing negative health beliefs or coping styles.

GUIDELINES AND STANDARDS

HCPs and patients need a clear framework for practice that will inform and guide them on acceptable standards of care for those with musculoskeletal conditions. Some guidelines have been written with a very strong patient focus under the auspices of patient and professional organisations (Arthritis and Musculoskeletal Alliance 2004, Luqmani et al 2006) and health organisations (National Institute of Clinical Excellence, 2009). Guidelines and standards should encourage individuals with a MSC to develop strategies that can enhance self management and enable them to cascade their own knowledge and expertise of their disease to others. However, such standards and guidelines alone do not ensure equity of access. If we are to encourage individuals to be active participants in their healthcare we need to ensure that information and advice is available at all points of access to health care (Department of Health 2006, Hammond & Badcock 2002). The Arthritis and Musculoskeletal Alliance (ARMA) standards of care provide a reference point for all those providing care, in all healthcare settings and also enable the individual to know what they should expect as they negotiate their complex journey through healthcare.

Patient organisations and volunteer networks can also be a powerful and effective resource in supporting traditional healthcare support. Examples of effective projects include those run by the National Rheumatoid Arthritis Society Volunteer Network and the Arthritis Care self management courses.

CONTINUITY OF CARE

Community care is often the first port of call for most individuals when they are ill. Individuals with a chronic disease may experience various 'health crises'. The problem for them is that many of these crises are not perceived as life threatening and in the current pace of healthcare, individuals with a chronic disease can feel very isolated. Community practitioners at all points in the patient's journey must take responsibility to ensure that they are informed about how to access care for the individual whatever their condition. The ARMA standards of care provide a clear framework for practice not only for the practitioners but also, most importantly, provide information and a rationale for individuals about the care they should be able to expect to receive. At times, there are also unique problems in gaining access to care, as identified by this patient with RA: "My nurse specialist is fantastic and I know I can rely on her to help me but her ever increasing workload means that it is becoming more difficult to get an appointment" (a quote from a patient who participated in a survey exploring implementation of ARMA Standards of Care).

Most individuals will have some experience of being cared for by a nurse or practitioner. These memories may relate to a time as an inpatient receiving day to day care by ward nurses or in outpatient clinics discussing issues such as how to manage pain or receiving information about new medications with a specialist nurse. Experience may equally come from assessment of physical ability by a physiotherapist or discussing the need for splints with an occupational therapist to the on-going care provided by the community teams visiting individuals' own homes. Perceptions and memories of prior aspects of care can alter over time and subsequent illness experiences along the healthcare journey. Such memories are important factors when individuals' are trying to evaluate current experiences or make sense of what to expect in their care and access to services.

Evidence has demonstrated the importance of providing guidance and support to enable individuals with a chronic disease to be informed about their disease, treatments and ultimately how to have an active role in their disease management (Hill & Bird 2003, Homer 2005). People presenting with joint pain are frequently unaware of the standards they should expect, leaving them vulnerable to sub-optimal care.

CONCLUSION – THE USER PATIENT JOURNEY

In this chapter it has only been possible to outline a few key issues in relation to the NRAS mapping project and the importance of the support that individuals need from their HCPs. Understanding the individual's experience of negotiating their pathways through healthcare has recently become an area of intense interest. This is partly due to national and international initiatives to improve service delivery based upon understanding and improving patient flows through the system, using manufacturing principles (often referred to as lean thinking). This has two objectives, firstly to put the patient at the centre of thinking and planning, and secondly, to explore hierarchical and traditional boundaries that prevent high quality care being delivered, which in many cases increase costs and potential bottlenecks (The National Health Service Modernisation Agency 2005).

The process of mapping pathways can also help to identify new ways of delivering services, in particular service redesign. The variances in costs in patient journeys through healthcare are increasingly being scrutinised. Some costs were identified in the mapping project, providing a 'snapshot' of not only health care costs but also, importantly, to the individual. Such individual and societal costs are higher than the costs to healthcare.

IMPROVING THE PATIENT JOURNEY

Musculoskeletal care should no longer be considered a second class specialism in healthcare provision. The consequences to the individual and to society are too high. The ARMA standards of care provide a tool for those with arthritis and health care providers to work with others and ensure they have the expertise to treat, guide and support patients appropriately, recognising the central role the patient has a right to play in their own care. In recent years the role of the nurse and allied healthcare professionals has been recognised as pivotal to providing comprehensive healthcare support to individuals.

In this age of patient choice, risk management and informed decision-making, there are opportunities and threats to the therapeutic relationship that individuals with musculoskeletal conditions should have with their HCPs. Although these principles may be admirable and desirable concepts, the mapping project demonstrates that it can be difficult for individuals to make informed choices through their healthcare journey, particularly for those newly diagnosed who have inadequate knowledge to make choices and limited opportunity to negotiate their healthcare needs.

HCPs and individuals with musculoskeletal conditions need to work together to ensure that patient needs are recognised and high standards of care implemented nationally so that individuals receive the care they deserve.

ACKNOWLEDGEMENT

The authors would also like to thank the Parkinson's Society in Cornwall and Sue Thomas, Nurse Advisor at the Royal College of Nurses. Their work and shared experiences from a mapping project informed the NRAS project. The authors also wish to recognise and thank the full NRAS mapping project advisory board for their advice and support in overseeing the project.

STUDY ACTIVITY

- Consider the potential personal cost implication of having RA (these are often called indirect costs). Include personal costs such as work, adaptations/aids, and mobility issues as well as other factors. Compare your calculations against a research paper discussing indirect costs.
- Consider social and psychological aspects of adjusting to a chronic disease (such as rheumatoid arthritis). List ten possible factors that might affect audits or surveys evaluating patient experiences and satisfaction with care. Evidence has demonstrated the importance of providing guidance and support to enable individuals with a chronic disease to be informed about their disease, treatments and ultimately how to have an active role in their disease management (Hill & Bird 2003, Homer 2005). People presenting with joint pain are frequently unaware of the standards they should expect, leaving them vulnerable to sub-optimal care.

USEFUL WEBSITES

The National Rheumatoid Arthritis Society:
Patient organisation and site for full evidence on mapping project
http://www.rheumatoid.org.uk
The British Health Professionals in Rheumatology
HCP organisation resources, guidelines, bursaries
http://www.rheumatology.org.uk
The Arthritis Research Campaign
Patient information leaflets & HCP resources
http://www.arc.org.uk
Catalzye process mapping:
Process mapping principles
http://www.catalyze.co.uk
The NHS Institute for Innovation & Improvement
Process mapping principles
http://www.institute.nhs.uk
The Health Talk Online Website
Personal experiences of diseases
http://www.healthtalkonline.org

References and further reading

Arthritis and Musculoskeletal Alliance, 2004. Standards of Care for Inflammatory Arthritis, Back Pain and Osteaoarthritis. Arthritis and Musculoskeletal Alliance, London.

Bone and Joint Decade, 2005. European Bone and Joint Health Strategies Project. European Action Towards Better Musculoskeletal Health: A Public Health Strategy to Reduce the Burden of Musculoskeletal Conditions. Bone and Joint Decade, Sweden.

Cooper, N.J., Mugford, M., Symmons, D.P.M., et al., 2002. Total costs and predictors of costs in individuals with early inflammatory polyarthritis; A community-based prospective study. Rheumatology 41, 767–774.

Corben, S., Rosen, R., 2005. Self Management for Long-Term Conditions; Patients' Perspective on the Way Ahead. Kings Fund, London.

Department of Health, 2001. The Expert Patient: A New Approach to Chronic Disease Management for the 21st Century. Department of Health, London.

Department of Health, 2005. Supporting People With Long-Term Conditions: Liberating the Talents of Nurses Who Care for People With Long-Term Conditions. Department of Health, London.

Department of Health, 2006. The Musculoskeletal Services Framework. A Joint Responsibility; Doing it Differently. Department of Health, London.

Fitzpatrick, R., Newman, S., Lamb, R., Shipley, M., 1988. Social relationships and psychological well being in RA. Soc. Sci. Med. 27, 399–403.

Frank, A.O., Chamberlain, M.A., 2001. Keeping our patients at work; implications for the management of those with rheumatoid arthritis and musculoskeletal conditions.. Rheumatology 40, 1201–1205.

Hammond, A., Badcock, L., 2002. Improving education about arthritis; Identifying the educational needs of people with chronic inflammatory arthritis. Rheumatology 41 (Suppl. 87), 216.

Hill, J., 2006. Rheumatology Nursing; a Creative Approach, second ed. John Wiley & Sons, Chichester pp. 151–172.

Hill, J., Bird, H., 2003. Outcomes for patients with RA: a rheumatology nurse practitioner clinic compared to standard outpatient care. Musculoskeletal Care 1 (1), 5–20.

Homer, D., 2005. Addressing psychological and social issues of rheumatoid arthritis within the consultation: a case report. Musculoskeletal Care 3 (1), 54–59.

Hulsemann, J.L., Mittendorf, T., Merkesdal, S., et al., 2005. Direct costs related to rheumatoid arthritis; the patient perspective. Ann. Rheum. Dis. 64, 1456–1461.

Luqmani, R., Hennell, S., Estrach, C., et al., 2006. British Society for Rheumatology and British Health professionals in Rheumatology Guidelines for the management of Rheumatoid Arthritis (the first two years). Rheumatology 45, 1167–1169.

Merkesdal, S., Ruof, J., Huelsemann, J.L., et al., 2005. Indirect cost assessment in patients with rheumatoid arthritis; comparison of data from the health economic patient questionnaire HEQ RA and Insurance claims data. Arthritis Rheum. 53 (2), 234–240.

National Institute of Clinical Excellence (2009) CG79: RHEUMATOID ARTHRITIS National clinical guideline for management and treatment in adults. http://guidance.nice.org.uk/CG79/Guidance/pdf/English

Memel, D., Kirwan, J.R., 1999. General practitioners' knowledge of functional and social factors in patients with rheumatoid arthritis. Health Soc. Care Comm. 7 (6), 387–393.

Oliver, S., Ryan, S., 2004. Effective pain management for patients with arthritis. Nurs. Stand. 18 (50), 43–52.

Oliver, S., 2004. Social and psychological issues in rheumatoid arthritis. Primary Health Care 14 (4), 25–28.

Oliver, S., Bosworth, A., 2006. On behalf of the national rheumatoid arthritis mapping project group. Mapping the patient's journey in rheumatoid arthritis the health and social costs. Ann. Rheum. Dis. 65 (Suppl. II), 597.

Oliver, S., 2007. Best practice in the treatment of patients with rheumatoid arthritis. Nurs. Stand. 21 (42), 47–56.

Ryan, S., Hassell, A., Dawes, P., Kendall, S., 2003. Perceptions of control in patients with rheumatoid arthritis. Nurs. Times 99 (13), 36–38.

Sanders, C., Donovan, J.L., Dieppe, P.A., 2004. Unmet need for joint replacement; a qualitative investigation of barriers to treatment among individuals with severe pain and disability of the hip and knee. Rheumatology 43 (3), 353–357.

The National Health Service Modernisation Agency, 2005. Improvement Leaders Guide; Matching Capacity and Demand; Process and System Thinking. Department of Health, London.

The National Rheumatoid Arthritis Society, 2004. Beyond the Pain: The Social and Psychological Impact of RA. National Rheumatoid Arthritis Society, Berkshire.

The National Rheumatoid Arthritis Society, 2006. Meeting the Standards of Care for Inflammatory Arthritis. A National Pilot Survey of Nras Members on the Arma Standards of Care for Inflammatory Arthritis. The National Rheumatoid Arthritis Society, Berkshire.

The National Rheumatoid Arthritis Society, 2007. I Want to Work....' The National Rheumatoid Arthritis Patient Survey. National Rheumatoid Arthritis Society, Berkshire.

Woolf, A.D., Zeidler, H., Haglund, U.and on behalf of the Arthritis Action Group, , et al., 2004. Musculoskeletal pain in Europe: its impact and a comparison of population and medical perceptions of treatment in eight European countries. Ann. Rheum. Dis. 63, 342–347.

Chapter 3

Initial clinical assessment of patients with possible rheumatic disease

Andrew Hassell MD FRCP MMedEd School of Medicine, Keele University, Keele, UK

Janet Cushnaghan MSc MCSP Epidemiology Resource Centre, Southampton General Hospital, Southampton, UK

CHAPTER CONTENTS

KEY POINTS

- Rheumatic diseases are frequently multi-system and multi-joint conditions and this should be considered in the therapy assessment
- Screening for rheumatic disease in therapy assessments can be undertaken using careful history taking and simple physical tests
- Simple screening questions and physical examinations can guide the clinical assessment.

INTRODUCTION

This chapter describes the key components of screening for rheumatic disease in clinical assessment. It can be used alongside the disease specific chapters following and can be embedded in routine musculoskeletal examinations and assessments of activities of daily living. The chapter draws on the *arc*-funded Handbook on the Clinical Assessment of the Musculoskeletal System (which comes accompanied by a DVD on regional examination) (http://www.arc.org.uk/arthinfo/documents/6321.pdf accessed March 2009).

PRINCIPLES OF RHEUMATOLOGICAL PHYSICAL ASSESSMENT

OVERVIEW

Successful identification and management of rheumatological problems in patients is predicated upon accurate history taking and examination. In this chapter we consider key aspects of history taking,

DOI: 10.1016/B978-0-443-06934-5.00003-6

physical examination and investigations in patients in whom rheumatological disease is suspected. For purposes of this chapter, we interpret rheumatological as pertaining to disorders of the musculoskeletal system (Doherty & Woolf 1999).

JOINT PAIN

By far the commonest symptom with which patients with a rheumatological problem present is pain. For such patients, clinical assessment should first be undertaken to establish answers to the following five questions:

1. Does the problem seem musculoskeletal in nature?
2. Is the problem acute or chronic?
3. Is the problem inflammatory or non-inflammatory?
4. What is the pattern of joint involvement?
5. What is the impact of the symptoms on the patient?

Accurate addressing of the above questions should allow the therapist to go a long way in identifying the problem and appreciating the patient's perspective. Over the next paragraphs, we will briefly expand upon each of these key questions.

1. Does the problem seem musculoskeletal in nature? Patients sometimes present with symptoms they perceive to be arising from their bones or joints when in fact this is not the case. Classic examples are patients with a biliary problem presenting with shoulder pain, patients with angina presenting with left arm pain and/or pins and needles, and patients with intra-abdominal or retro-peritoneal problems presenting with back pain. Careful history taking can often clarify and prevent such confusion.

2. Is the problem acute or chronic? Mode of onset and course is often very helpful in elucidating the nature of a patient's rheumatological problem. The first issue is whether symptoms were related to any physical trauma which could be relevant in their causation – a fall, a possible sports injury, accident, etc. The second issue is the onset and duration. In the absence of injury, acute onset peripheral joint pains often are inflammatory in causation. Peripheral joint symptoms which fluctuate quite markedly are again, often inflammatory. By contrast, pain arising in association with osteoarthritis is often insidious in onset and gradually progressive.

3. Is the problem inflammatory or non-inflammatory? A key aspect of the assessment of a patient presenting with peripheral or spinal joint pain is deciding whether the problem is arising from underlying inflammation as this often has major implications for the diagnosis and management. Prominent joint stiffness, particularly prolonged morning stiffness of the joints (typically in excess of 30 minutes), is suggestive of an inflammatory problem. By contrast, patients with a non-inflammatory problem often report little stiffness. Knee stiffness which comes on after sitting and lasts a minute or two after standing is quite typical of osteoarthritis. Another pointer towards an inflammatory problem which may be reported by patients is joint swelling, particularly swelling which fluctuates. It must be recognised, however, that patients are sometimes not very accurate in reporting joint swelling. Other features suggesting an inflammatory problem include pains, which improve somewhat with activity (particularly in the case of inflammatory back pain) and the presence of systemic upset, e.g. anorexia, weight loss or fever.

4. What is the pattern of joint involvement? This is another highly relevant question. Is the problem monoarticular (one joint), oligoarticular (fewer than five joints) or polyarticular (more than four joints)? Is the joint involvement essentially symmetrical? Are small and large joints involved? If the hands are involved, are the distal interphalanageal (DIP) joints? Taking the information established from points 1-4, one may be able to summarise patients' presentations thus: a 40-year-old woman with a chronic (4 month) fluctuating symmetrical inflammatory arthropathy involving the hands (sparing the DIPs), wrists and feet, with a sub-acute onset. This would be characteristic of a primary inflammatory arthropathy such as rheumatoid arthritis. Alternatively, a 60-year-old man with a one day history of an acute inflammatory arthropathy involving the right knee only would raise the likelihood of acute septic arthritis or crystal arthritis.

5. What is the impact of the symptoms on the patient? No assessment of a patient presenting with musculoskeletal symptoms is complete without an assessment of the impact of the symptoms on the patient's activities and quality of life. Are there specific things the patient can't

do? Some therapists talk of a 'disability ladder', starting with inability of the patient to perform certain activities such as sport or hobbies, then prevention of activities more essential to the patient such as work or looking after the household, through to inability to perform essential activities such as self hygiene or sleeping. Part of this evaluation includes some assessment of the patient's mood. Is the patient depressed? It should be remembered that, as well as joint symptoms resulting in patient depression, there are instances in which joint symptoms can be a physical representation of a patient's depression or mental state, sometimes called somatisation.

Evaluating regional joint pains

In addition to the above approach for a patient presenting with musculoskeletal pain, there are other specific aspects that require assessment in patients presenting with regional joint pains. Are there aspects of the patient's activities, occupational or recreational, which may be causally relevant to their symptoms? More obvious examples include the development of heel pain in someone who does unaccustomed exercise or wears inappropriate footwear (possible plantar fasciitis), or lateral elbow pain in someone who has recently resumed racket sports (lateral epicondylitis). Other important questions for patients with a regional pain problem include exacerbating and relieving factors.

Symptoms in certain joints generally require specific questioning. One example is non-inflammatory mono-articular knee pain. In patients presenting with this, it is important to ask about 'locking' (an acute inability to extend the knee fully, which subsides spontaneously or with some manipulation by the patient – suggests a loose body within the joint) and 'giving way' (the knee acutely letting the patient down). The latter can arise from severe pain but can also be a result of ligamentous instability. In cases of patients presenting with non-inflammatory back pain, it is important to assess for radicular (nerve root compression) or myelopathic (spinal cord compression) problems, by asking about peripheral pins and needles, numbness and weakness, as well as disturbance of control of micturition or bowel evacuation.

MUSCULOSKELETAL RED FLAGS

Red flags are symptoms or signs which raise the possibility of serious underlying disease (Leerar et al 2007, Sizer et al 2007), generally neoplastic (malignant) or infectious. In patients with rheumatological problems, red flags may also reflect inflammatory disease.

Red flags include systemic features such as weight loss and fever, local features of unremitting, boring pain with prominent nocturnal pain, and a past history of cancer. In the case of back pain, the age of presentation can also be a red flag. First onset back pain aged >50 would itself be deemed a red flag (Leerar et al 2007, Sizer et al 2007). The presence of red flags in a patient presenting with musculoskeletal symptoms generally highlights the necessity for further investigation and evaluation.

FURTHER EVALUATION OF THE PATIENT PRESENTING WITH INFLAMMATORY JOINT PAINS

If a patient is thought to be suffering from an inflammatory joint problem it is important to assess other body systems because of the known association of multi-system involvement in the various inflammatory joint conditions. Table 3.1 provides some examples of these associations.

In practice, screening questions might include:

1. Any skin problems or rashes?
2. Any grittiness of the eyes, red eye or visual problems?
3. Do fingers change colour (in the cold)? The classic triad of Raynaud's colour changes consists of the fingers initially going white (as blood fails to gain access to the fingers), then blue (cyanosis of what blood is present), then red (re-entry of blood, e.g. on re-warming).
4. Any hair loss?
5. Any mouth ulcers, dryness of the mouth or swallowing difficulties?
6. Any bowel problems?
7. Any cough or breathlessness?
8. Any miscarriages?
9. Ever any thromboses, clots or DVTs
10. Any migraines?
11. Any genital ulcers?

ASSESSING OSTEOPOROSIS RISK

In certain patients encountered within rheumatological practice, the assessment of risk of osteoporosis and fractures is of great importance, particularly as osteoporosis is itself asymptomatic until a fracture

Table 3.1 Non–articular associations of inflammatory rheumatic diseases

DISEASE	KNOWN NON–ARTICULAR ASSOCIATIONS	TYPICAL SYMPTOMS
Rheumatoid arthritis	Secondary Sjögren's syndrome	Gritty eyes, dry mouth
	Raynaud's phenomenon	Finger/toe colour changes
	Pulmonary fibrosis	Breathlessness
	Anaemia	Fatigue, breathlessness
	Aphthous ulcers	Painful mouth ulcers
Ankylosing spondylitis	Anterior uveitis	Painful red eye with blurring of vision
	Costovertebral involvement	Chest pain and infections
	Apical lung fibrosis	Breathlessness
	Aortic regurgitation	Breathlessness
	Inflammatory bowel disease	Bloody diarrhoea
Psoriatic arthritis	Psoriasis	Skin plaques on extensor surfaces
		Nail dystrophy
Systemic Lupus Erythematosus	Photosensitivity	Rash on sun exposed skin
	Raynaud's phenomenon	Finger/toe colour changes
	Alopecia	Hair loss
	Serositis	Pleurisy, pericarditis, peritonitis
	Migraine	Migraine
	Anti-cardiolipin syndrome	Miscarriages, thromboses
Scleroderma	Raynaud's phenomenon	Finger/toe colour changes
	Oesophageal dysmotility	Difficulty swallowing or heartburn
	Malabsorption	Weight loss, diarrhoea

occurs. Patients in whom assessment for this is particularly relevant include patients who have suffered a fragility fracture, i.e. a fracture after falling from no more than standing, patients on systemic steroids or patients with known risk factors (SIGN 2003). Table 3.2 indicates the risk factors for osteoporosis. Chapter 20 covers assessment and management of osteoporosis in greater detail.

SCREENING FOR LOCOMOTOR PROBLEMS

THE GALS TOOL: GAIT, ARMS, LEGS, SPINE

One challenge facing clinicians in practice has been the development of a screening tool to rapidly identify whether a patient might have significant locomotor problems. It has long been common practice, faced with a new patient presenting with any symptoms, for clinicians to include some brief specific questions and examination to identify potential cardiac disease. Traditionally, no such screen was performed for the locomotor system. This had two effects: important locomotor problems were missed or ignored and more generally, the importance of the locomotor system to a patient's well being was under-estimated. This has been addressed by a group of clinicians who developed the GALS screen (Doherty et al 1992), a simple method of screening for locomotor problems. A normal GALS means significant locomotor problems are unlikely. An abnormal GALS means that there is a problem of some nature which requires further assessment. This problem could be musculoskeletal or neurological.

GALS is an acronym, standing for gait, arms, legs, spine. The screen begins with three questions:

1. Do you have any pain or stiffness in your muscles, joints or back?
2. Can you dress yourself completely without any difficulty?
3. Can you walk up and down stairs without any difficulty?

The screen continues with a physical assessment (Doherty et al 1992):

Gait

- Watch the patient standing, walking and turning, looking for symmetry, smoothness of movement, normal stride pattern and ability to turn quickly.

Table 3.2 Osteoporosis risk factors

NON-MODIFIABLE

Age	Especially each decade after the age of 60
Gender	Female sex at higher risk
Ethnicity	Caucasians at higher risk
Early menopause	
Family history of osteoporosis	Family history of kyphosis or low trauma fractures
Previous fragility fracture	
Secondary causes of osteoporosis	
Anorexia nervosa	Osteoporosis can result from low body mass index, causing a low oestrogen state; calcium and vitamin D deficiency also possible
Chronic liver disease	
Coeliac disease	
Hyperparathyroidisim	
Hypogonadism	
Inflammatory bowel disease	
Renal disease	
Rheumatoid arthritis	
Drugs	Corticosteroids Heparin Certain anti-convulsants, e.g. phenytoin
Modifiable risk factors	
Low body mass index	
Smoking	
Alcohol	
Exercise	Sedentary lifestyle and/or history of sedentary adolescence is associated with increased risk
Dietary calcium and Vitamin D intake	

Spine

- Inspect from behind: check for straight spine, normal paraspinal muscles, shoulder and gluteal muscle bulk, level iliac crests, no popliteal swelling, no hindfoot swelling or deformity.
- Inspect from the side: check for normal spinal curves. Ask the patient to touch their toes. Check for normal lumbar and hip flexion.
- Inspect from in front: ask the patient to tilt their head to bring their ear towards their shoulder on both sides. Check normal lateral cervical flexion.

Arms

- Ask the patient to put their hands behind their head with their elbows back. Check normal shoulder movements.
- Ask the patient to place both hands by their side with their elbows straight. Check full elbow extension
- Ask the patient to hold their hands out with palms down and fingers straight. Check no wrist or finger swelling or deformity.
- Ask the patient to turn both their hands over, so their palms face upwards. Check normal supination/pronation, normal palms.
- Ask the patient to make a tight fist. Check for normal fist formation.
- Ask the patient to place the tip of each finger on the tip of their thumb, in turn. Check normal fine precision and pinch grip.
- The examiner then squeezes across the second to fifth metacarpal head to test for tenderness suggestive of metacarpophalangeal (MCP) synovitis.

Legs

- With the patient standing, inspect from in front for normal lower limb appearances.
- Ask the patient to lie supine on the couch. Flex each hip and knee while holding the knee: check for normal knee flexion and for crepitus.
- Internally rotate each hip in flexion.
- Press on each patella for patellofemoral tenderness and palpate for an effusion.
- Squeeze across the metatarsal heads to check for tenderness due to metatarsophalangeal joint (MTP) disease.
- Inspect both soles for callosities.

Any abnormalities detected on the GALS screening examination would demand further evaluation by history and examination.

OUTLINE OF REGIONAL JOINT EXAMINATION

Regional examination of the musculoskeletal system is necessary if any abnormalities have been revealed by the history or the screening assessment (e.g. GALS). This is a more detailed examination and involves the examination of a group of joints, which are linked by function. There are five stages to examination of the joints:

1. Introduce the examination
2. Look at the joints
3. Feel the joint(s)
4. Move the joint(s)
5. Assess the function of the joint(s).

Introduction

It is very important to introduce the examination, explain what you are going to do, gain verbal consent to examine and ask the person to let you know if you cause them any pain or discomfort. To be sure not to miss any important clinical signs it is vital that the patient is relaxed and that they feel comfortable about being examined.

Look

Start with a visual inspection of the area at rest. Compare sides, looking for symmetry. Look for skin changes, muscle bulk, swelling in and around the joint, deformity and posture of the joint.

Feel

Feel the skin temperature with the back of your hand across the joint line. Assess any swelling for fluctuance and mobility. Hard bony swelling of osteoarthritis should be distinguished from the soft, boggy swelling of inflammatory arthritis. You should be able to elicit synovitis by the triad of warmth, swelling and tenderness.

Move

The full range of movement of the joint should be assessed. Compare sides. Both active and passive movement should be performed. The loss of active movement with full passive movement suggests a problem with the muscles, tendons or nerves rather than in the joints, or it may be an affect of pain in the joints. Joints may move further than expected – this is called hypermobility. Joint hypermobility is seen either as a localised condition in a single joint or a more generalised one. When seen in conjunction with musculoskeletal problems, it is recognised as a pathological condition and called hypermobility syndrome (uul-Kristensen et al 2007). A screen for hypermobility can be used e.g. Beighton (uul-Kristensen et al 2007).

Function

Make a functional assessment of the joint for example if there is limited elbow flexion can the person bring their hand to their mouth? In the lower limb function mainly involves gait, standing balance and the ability to rise from a sitting position.

Box 3.1 illustrates how these approaches might be put into practice using an examination of the hand and wrist as an example.

BOX 3.1   Examination of the hand and wrist

Introduce examination/gain consent

Inspect palms and back of hands for muscle wasting, skin and nail changes, nodes and deformities

Check for scars (e.g. carpal tunnel release)

Feel radial pulse, tendon thickening, bulk of thenar and hypothenar eminences

Assess median, ulnar and radial nerve sensation

Assess skin temperature

Squeeze metacarpophalageal joints (MCPJs)

Palpate swollen or painful joints, including wrists

Palpate for bony enlargement, nodules, cysts

Look and feel along ulnar border of the wrist (for signs of inflammation)

Assess full finger extension and full finger flexion (finger tuck)

Assess active and passive wrist flexion and extension

Assess median and ulnar nerve power

Assess function: grip and pinch, picking up small objects

Perform any special tests e.g. carpal tunnel syndrome, Phalen's test (Miedany et al 2008)

PRINCIPLES OF INVESTIGATIONS IN EVALUATING PATIENTS WITH RHEUMATIC DISEASES

The physical assessment of patients with rheumatological problems often includes performance of further investigations. A detailed description of such investigations is beyond the scope of this chapter. However, an outline of commonly performed tests, the indications for performing them and common abnormalities found are described. Greater detail will be provided, where relevant, elsewhere in the book.

BLOOD TESTS

Blood tests are usually performed, in the context of rheumatological disorders, where there is a suspicion of inflammatory, infective, neoplastic or metabolic disease. Common tests performed within the haematology laboratory are full blood count, Erythrocyte sedimentation rate (ESR) and clotting studies. Table 3.3 illustrates how blood tests can be used to detect abnormalities.

IMAGING

To complete the 'jigsaw' and arrive at a diagnosis, imaging is often undertaken. The gold standard for this is the plain radiograph. Plain radiographs can show the alignment of the bones, the joint space (indicating the thickness of the articular cartilage), the density of the bones, sometimes a joint effusion can be seen and intra-articular bodies may be seen.

More sophisticated imaging is also available such as ultrasound, magnetic resonance imaging (MRI) and computed tomography (CT). Ultrasound of joints is increasingly becoming used to assess joints for the existence of synovitis, which aids diagnosis and informs treatment decisions in inflammatory arthritis.

CONCLUSION

Successful clinical diagnosis and management of rheumatological problems in patients requires accurate history taking and examination. Simple screening questions (e.g. red flags) and physical tests (e.g. GALS) can help to establish where further clinical assessment is needed. Rheumatological conditions can present with multi-system and multi-joint involvement. An understanding of the importance of this can help to guide clinical questioning and assessments.

STUDY ACTIVITY

- Access the arc-funded Handbook on the Clinical Assessment of the Musculoskeletal System (which comes accompanied by a DVD on regional examination) (http://www.arc.org.uk/arthinfo/documents/6321.pdf) and practise the GALS on a colleague until you can remember the instructions.

ACKNOWLEDGEMENT

The chapter has used the framework of history taking suggested in the Arthritis Research Campaign's arc handbook of the clinical assessment of the musculoskeletal system, and Professor Paul Dieppe's original handbook for medical students (1991).

USEFUL WEBSITES

arc-funded handbook on the clinical assessment of the musculoskeletal system (accompanied by a DVD on regional examination) http://www.arc.org.uk/arthinfo/documents/6321.pdf/ (accessed March 2009).

Table 3.3 Blood tests		
BLOOD TEST	**COMMON ABNORMALITIES**	**EXAMPLES OF CONDITIONS ABNORMALITY FOUND IN**
Full blood count (FBC) includes: Haemoglobin (Hb)	Anaemia (low Hb)	Inflammatory diseases Deficiency states NSAID related bleeding
White cell count (WCC) Platelet count	High white cell count	Bacterial infection Inflammation
	Low white cell count	Certain anti-rheumatic drugs
	High platelet count	Inflammation Bleeding
	Low platelet count	Idiopathic autoimmune thrombocytopaenia
Erythrocyte Sedimentation rate (ESR)	Raised ESR	Inflammation Infections Malignancies
C reactive protein (CRP)	Raised CRP	As ESR (Quicker to change than ESR)

References and further reading

Doherty, M., Dacre, J., Dieppe, P., et al., 1992. The 'GALS' locomotor screen. Ann. Rheum. Dis. 51, 1165–1169.

Doherty, M., Woolf, A., 1999. Guidelines for rheumatology undergraduate core curriculum. EULAR standing committee on education and training. Ann. Rheum. Dis. 58 (3), 133–135.

Leerar, P.J., Boissonnault, W., Domholdt, E., et al., 2007. Documentation of red flags by physical therapists for patients with low back pain. J. Man. Manip. Ther. 15 (1), 42–49.

Miedany, Y., Ashour, S., Youssef, S., et al., 2008. Clinical diagnosis of carpal tunnel syndrome: old tests-new concepts. Joint, Bone, Spine: revue du rhumatisme 75 (4), 451–457.

SIGN, 2003. Management of osteoporosis. guideline 71. Scottish intercollegiate guidelines network. Edinburgh. Available from http://www.sign.ac.uk/guidelines/fulltext/71/index.html/ (accessed 24.01.09.).

Sizer Jr., P.B., Brismée, J.M., Cook, C., 2007. Medical screening for red flags in the diagnosis and management of musculoskeletal spine pain. Pain pract. official J. World Inst. pain 7 (1), 53–71.

uul-Kristensen, B., Røgind, H., Jensen, D.V., et al., 2007. Inter-examiner reproducibility of tests and criteria for generalized joint hypermobility and benign joint hypermobility syndrome. Rheumatology 46 (12), 1835–1841.

Chapter 4

The measurement of patient-reported outcome in the rheumatic diseases

Kirstie L. Haywood DPhil BSc (Hons) MCSP SRP Royal College of Nursing Research Institute, School of Health and Social Studies, University of Warwick, Coventry, UK

CHAPTER CONTENTS

KEY POINTS

- The measurement and communication of disease burden and the consequence of healthcare are essential components of healthcare. Patients have an important contribution to make to this process.
- Well-developed patient-reported outcome measures (PROMs) can provide a reliable, valid and clinically relevant resource for including the patient perspective in healthcare
- The effective incorporation of PROMs into routine practice requires training in the use and interpretation of PROMs and ongoing support to ensure the appropriate use of PROMs-related data. Further rigorous evaluation of the contribution of PROMs to routine practice is required
- Advances in technology, such as electronic data capture, may enhance the feasibility of PROM application, whilst the timely provision of scores may enhance the utility to routine practice. Demonstrating the cost effectiveness of incorporating PROMs into routine practice is essential to good practice and to attracting appropriate resources to support data collection

© 2010 Elsevier Ltd
DOI: 10.1016/B978-0-443-06934-5.00004-8

■ The application of well-developed PROMs in routine practice supports the identification of patients with the greatest needs, which in turn supports the provision of more timely and appropriate interventions to address those needs.

INTRODUCTION

Most modern healthcare systems embrace patient-centred care, entailing care that is responsive to the needs, preferences and values of the individual (Hibbard 2003). However, the experience of health and illness, and outcomes of healthcare desired by patients are multifaceted and often uniquely individual (Quest et al 2003, Ramsey 2002). Facilitating the patient to effectively communicate these values is an important part of patient-centred care. Although 'what matters' as an outcome of healthcare may differ between members of the healthcare team, the patient has a significant role to play (Ganz 2002, Haywood 2006, Hibbard 2003). Failure to include the patients' perspective may inadequately inform clinical decision-making, and provides a limited evaluation of healthcare. Whilst rheumatic diseases can affect survival, there is growing evidence demonstrating the significant negative impact on an individual's quality of life (e.g. Chorus et al 2003, Finlay & Coles 1995). A wide range of health care interventions in rheumatology are concerned with reducing the burden of disease and improving the patients' experience of ill-health, for example, alleviating pain and improving function, well-being or quality of life. Identifying the most important outcomes of care and the most appropriate methods of assessment is central to effective care delivery. Understanding patient-reported outcome, and the appropriate methods of measuring these outcomes, clearly has an important role to play in modern healthcare.

Across the rheumatic diseases, all therapeutic interventions require rigorous evaluation to provide an evidence-base for policy decision-making and clinical practice. This is of critical relevance to chronic conditions where treatment effects are often subtle and difficult to detect (Hobart et al 2004). Evaluation of healthcare can be used in several ways, for example:

● to determine the effectiveness of expensive, often long-term pharmaceutical and non-pharmaceutical interventions
● to determine the effectiveness of novel ways of providing healthcare, such as consultant therapists and nurse-led clinics
● to explore the marginal relative benefits of different healthcare interventions and methods of healthcare provision
● to determine the potential ecomonic implications of long-term therapies common to the rheumatic diseases
● to inform the equitable and appropriate allocation of health care resources for the treatment and management of patients with rheumatic disease.

This chapter will introduce the role of patient-reported outcome measures (PROMs) as an important mechanism to enhance patient participation in healthcare management and evaluation, with a particular focus on routine practice. Challenges to the use of PROMs are discussed. The chapter concludes by highlighting key areas for future debate and research into the effective use of PROMs of relevance to the rheumatology healthcare team.

MEASURING HEALTH

Health is a complex construct, the measurement of which should include issues of relevance to patients, healthcare professionals and providers. Measures of health outcome are often categorised as clinical or disease-focused, such as laboratory-based or radiographic assessment; or humanistic or patient-reported, such as health status and health-related quality of life (HRQL) (Ganz 2002, McHorney 2002). These two broad approaches to measurement provide wide ranging and complementary information, often of relevance to both patients and clinicians (Ganz 2002, McHorney 2002). Two classification frameworks are helpful for exploring the different concepts that can be measured: 1) the International Classification of Functioning, Disability and Health (ICF) (WHO 2001); and 2) Donabedian's Structure, Process and Outcome (Donabedian 1966).

INTERNATIONAL CLASSIFICATION OF FUNCTIONING, DISABILITY AND HEALTH

The revised International Classification of Functioning, Disability and Health (ICF) (Stucki et al 2007, WHO 2001) provides a useful framework for understanding disease impact and measuring the outcomes of healthcare. The central concept of 'functioning' has been broadened to embrace a biopsychosocial model of health, describing health in terms of biological, psychological, social and personal factors (Dagfinrud

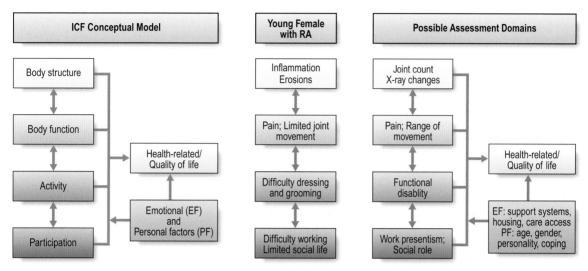

Figure 4.1 The International Classification of Function (ICF) Conceptual Model: illustrated with example of possible assessment domains for a woman with rheumatoid arthritis (RA).

et al 2005). Moreover, personal and environmental factors, acting as contextual facilitators or barriers, may further influence the impact of disease and its assessment (Dagfinrud et al 2005, Liang 2004).

The framework provides a dynamic and interactive model (Fig. 4.1), which complements traditional measures of 'body structure' and 'body function' (abnormalities or changes in bodily structure or function) with the broader assessment of 'activity' (abnormalities, changes or restrictions in an individual's interaction with the physical context or environment) and 'participation' (changes, limitations or restrictions in an individual's social context; involvement in a life situation, viewed from a societal perspective) (Wade & de Jong 2000).

Applying the relative burden of rheumatoid arthritis (RA) for a young female to the model (Fig. 4.1): RA may cause inflammation and joint damage in the small joints of the hand that can be detected by radiographic evaluation (body structure) and limitation in joint range of movement (body function). These changes may also further impact on an individual's ability to partake in particular activities, for example, dressing and personal grooming, or playing a musical instrument (activity), and subsequent ability to maintain their desired work role or to socialise with friends (participation). Patients experience the impact of disease as problems relating to their health status and quality of life, and it is usual for a patient to present at a clinic with problems associated with limitation in specific activities

or difficulties with participation, as outlined above. The combination of constructs reflects the person in his or her world (Van Echteld et al 2006), providing a systematic and comprehensive, more socially driven, approach to understanding the impact of ill-health (Wade & de Jong 2000).

The impact of ill-health, any associated assessment, and extent of information divulged by patients, may be further influenced by both environmental and/or personal factors, including the individual's relationship with members of the healthcare team. Health professionals are important facilitators in enhancing environmental factors for people with a rheumatic disease (Van Echteld et al 2006) through, for example, the provision of appliances to facilitate an individual's capacity for independence in dressing and grooming. Similarly, patients with ankylosing spondylitis (AS) identified family support as helpful (an environmental facilitator), whereas adverse weather was unhelpful (Van Echteld et al 2006). Personal factors include age, gender, coping mechanisms and personality, and are influenced by environmental factors, the level of social support, and individual factors including level of motivation, expectations for health and healthcare (Liang 2004).

The overall impact of these limitations may be captured within the broader concept of life quality – what do these limitations mean in terms of an individual's quality of life? Within the proposed framework, quality of life, or health-related quality of life, forms a separate assessment domain

---

BOX 4.1 Study activity: osteoporosis and the ICF framework

- Think of a patient with Osteoporosis.
- What are the presenting complaints of this patient when you review them in a clinic setting? How do these presenting features fit within the revised ICF framework?
- What aspects of disease burden do you normally measure in routine practice?
- How well does your routine assessment capture the wider impact of disease and healthcare from the patient perspective?
- What should or could be measured to capture the wider burden of disease?

(Wade & de Jong 2000). Standardisation of the ICF framework has supported the identification of key areas relevant to the wider understanding of 'function' (Stucki et al 2007, Van Echteld et al 2006), facilitated a better understanding and analysis of patient problems, and fostered communication between health professionals (Wade & de Jong 2000). In summary, the ICF provides a useful, conceptual model to guide appropriate assessment of what should be measured to capture the breadth of disease impact; it does not, however, direct how these health constructs, or domains, should be measured (Box 4.1).

STRUCTURE, PROCESS AND OUTCOME

Traditionally, the quality of health care has been assessed in terms of Donabedian's classic structure-process-outcome framework (Campbell et al 2000, Donabedian 1966, Mitchell & Lang 2004). Structure embraces the operational characteristics of a service, and includes patient, healthcare professional and organisational variables (Pringle & Doran 2003, Wade & de Jong 2000). Structure also considers the accessibility and relative quality of the many components of health care, for example, how accessible was care for an individual with a rheumatic disease? Process explores how the health care services work in relation to the nature and extent of the patients problem (Wade & de Jong 2000), and includes assessment of the appropriateness of care, location and timing. For example, did an individual with rheumatic disease receive care that was appropriate to their needs, at the right time, and in a suitable location? At the patient level, process measures may also include measures of disease process, such

as radiographic imaging, histological and biomedical markers (Bellamy 2005), and patient-reported measures of health status.

Measures of outcome reflect the overall aim of the healthcare service, and may include functional and clinical outcomes, or clinical targets. Although important, global outcome measures such as mortality and morbidity rates are generally irrelevant to a patient's experience and are generally unhelpful in communicating the broader impact of disease and success of healthcare (Clancy & Lawrence 2002). A necessary change of emphasis in assessment recognises the importance of measuring the quality of survival and the wider impact on an individual's health-related quality of life. From an individual perspective, important outcomes may assess if, for example, healthcare has minimised their experience of pain and fatigue, assisted the individual in maximising their participation in his/her chosen social setting or work environment, or reduced the distress and pain experienced by the patient's family and carers (Wade & de Jong 2000). Assessment that embraces the patient perspective has an important role to play in communicating their relative experience of disease and healthcare.

MEASURING HEALTH: THE PATIENTS' PERSPECTIVE

Challenges of including the patient's voice in the assessment process include identifying the most important outcomes and the most appropriate and acceptable methods of assessment (Fig. 4.2, Box 4.2).

PATIENT-REPORTED OUTCOME AND PROMs: DEFINITION

A patient reported outcome (PRO) has recently been defined as 'any report coming from patients about a health condition and its treatment' (Burke et al 2006). PRO assessment is therefore broad ranging, and includes health-related quality of life, needs assessment, treatment satisfaction and treatment adherence.

Well-developed, relevant and scientifically rigorous patient-reported measures or patient-reported outcome measures (PROMs) provide a measure of an individual's experiences and concerns in relation to their health, health care and quality of life (Fitzpatrick et al 1998, Ganz 2002). PROMs are largely self-completed questionnaires containing several questions,

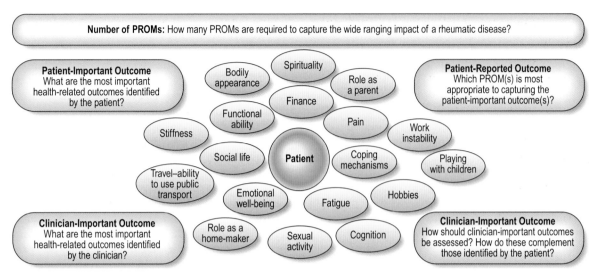

Figure 4.2 Identifying outcomes of importance and the most appropriate method of assessment.

BOX 4.2   Rheumatoid arthritis and patient important outcomes

■ Think of a patient with RA whom you have recently assessed.

■ What do you think are the most important outcomes of care for this patient?

■ How does the patient define the important outcomes of their care?

■ Are there any discrepancies between the important outcomes defined by yourself and the patient?

■ How would you assess and monitor those outcomes identified as being important by the patient?

---

or items, to reflect the broad nature of health-related concerns. They are available to measure a wide range of health-related concepts such as pain, physical disability, treatment side-effects, satisfaction or experience of health care, health care costs, and quality of life (McDowell 2006). Although variously referred to as measures of quality of life, health-related quality of life (HRQL), or health status, measures of health status often have a narrower focus, for example, the assessment of pain, fatigue and functional disability, than measures of HRQL, which may include a broader range of health-related domains, for example, emotional well-being and work disability. Measures of quality of life should capture all aspects of life, including non-health related issues.

PROM development has traditionally been dominated by clinical experts who, although knowledgeable,

cannot communicate the impact of ill-health and treatment in the same way as a patient (Fitzpatrick et al 1998). Furthermore, evidence of discrepant views between patients and health care providers in their assessment of important health outcomes (Hewlett 2003, Kessler & Ramsey 2002, Kvien & Heiberg 2003, Liang 2004) highlights the irrefutable need for simple and effective methods to enhance patient involvement in PROM development and evaluation. Application of the revised ICF framework has supported the comparative evaluation of available PROMs, and highlighted the often limited patient contribution to PROM development, the limited content of widely used PROMs, a lack of precision relating to the concepts assessed, and hence a limited ability to capture the broader concepts of patient participation (Van Echteld et al 2006). Where PROMs seek to communicate the patient voice, methods to ensure that patients reported outcomes embrace patient important outcomes are essential.

Once questions, or items, are generated to reflect a particular construct, such as fatigue, a measurement scale or set of response options are described for each item (Streiner & Norman 2003), such as a series of graded descriptive, or categorical, responses (i.e. no fatigue, mild, moderate, severe, very severe fatigue) with associated numerical values, or a horizontal visual analogue scale (VAS) with descriptive and numerical anchors (i.e. 0 'no fatigue' to 100 'extreme fatigue'). The associated numerical scores may then be combined, usually summed, to give a final score. The addition of numerical values does not guarantee that the distance between successive categories is the same, that is, continuous or interval level data, and the majority of measurement response scales produce categorical data on an ordinal level of measurement. However, under most circumstances, and unless score distribution is severely abnormal, data can be analysed as if continuous or interval level data (McDowell 2006, Streiner & Norman 2003).

Proxy completion of questionnaires where relatives or clinicians complete the measure on behalf of the individual can be an important source of information particularly in the case of children (Varni et al 2005), chronically debilitated or cognitively impaired patients (Neumann et al 2000). Discrepancies between a proxy measure of health and that reported by an individual have been observed. Discrepancies are often greater for non-observable constructs such as pain and depression, and less for more observable constructs such as physical ability (Ball et al 2001).

PATIENT–REPORTED OUTCOME MEASURES: TYPOLOGY

Garratt et al (2002) describe four broad categories of PROM: generic, domain-specific, condition or population-specific, and individualised.

Generic

Generic measures contain multiple concepts of health of relevance to both patients and the general population, supporting comparison of health between different patient groups, and between patient groups and the general population (Haywood 2006). Population-based normal values can be calculated for generic instruments which supports data interpretation from disease-specific groups (Ware 1997).

Two distinct classes of generic instrument can be described: health profiles and utility measures. Scores on different domains of health covered by a single health profile are presented separately to support data interpretation, therefore reflecting a clinical perspective. Sometimes an index or summary score may be generated, but proponents of profiles argue that measurement is most meaningful within separate domains (McDowell & Newell 1996). The Short-Form 36-item Health Survey (SF-36) (Ware 1997, Ware et al 2002) (www.sf-36.org) is a widely used example of a generic health profile both generally

and in patients with rheumatological or musculoskeletal conditions (Garratt et al 2002) (Table 4.1). The comparison of generic health status between members of the general population, and patients with RA or AS (matched for important factors such as age, gender, demographic, work and disease status) demonstrated that both patient groups had worse levels of physical (PCS) and mental (MCS) health when compared to the general population (Chorus et al 2003). When the two patient groups were compared, patients with RA reported worse levels of physical health, but better levels of mental health than patients with AS.

Utility measures incorporate the values and preferences for health outcome generated by the patient (direct weighting), reflecting the individual perspective, or the general population (indirect weighting), reflecting the societal perspective (Fitzpatrick et al 1998). Although utility measures usually include several domains of health, by providing numerical values for health states that use states of perfect health and death as reference values, utility measures can be used to generate single index values that combine health status with survival data – for example, to produce quality adjusted life years (QALYs). The EQ-5D is an example of a utility measure that incorporates indirect valuations of health states (EuroQolGroup 1990) (www.euroqol.org) (Table 4.1). Although widely used in the rheumatic diseases (Brazier et al 2004, Haywood et al 2002, Marra et al 2005), the EQ-5D has been criticised for having both limited item content and response options, and hence may be limited in detecting small, but important, changes in health in people with chronic ill-health (McDowell & Newell 1996), such as rheumatoid arthritis (Marra et al 2005) and ankylosing spondylitis (Haywood et al 2002).

Domain–specific PROMs

Measures may be specific to a health domain, such as fatigue, for example, the multi-dimensional fatigue inventory (MFI) (Smets et al 1995), or disease activity, for example, the Bath AS disease activity index (BASDAI) (Garrett et al 1994). Alternatively, they may be specific to a health problem, for example, the hospital anxiety and depression scale (HADS) (Zigmond & Snaith 1983) which is specific to depression and anxiety (Table 4.1), or a described function, for example, activities of daily living (McDowell 2006), such as the health assessment questionnaire (HAQ) (Bruce & Fries 2003, Fries et al 1980) (Table 4.1).

Table 4.1 Selected generic and specific patient-reported outcome measures (PROMs) of relevance to the rheumatic diseases

PROM (NUMBER OF ITEMS) (ASSOCIATED WEB-SITE WHERE AVAILABLE)	DEVELOPER	HEALTH DOMAINS (ITEMS)	RESPONSE SCALE	SCORE	ORIGIN	PURCHASE COST
Generic						
Short-form 36-item health survey (SF-36)$^\$$ version 2 (36) www.sf-36.org/	Ware 1997	8 domains Bodily pain (BP) (2), Vitality (V) (4), General Health (GH) (5), Mental Health (5), Physical functioning (10), Social functioning (2), Role-emotional (3), Role-physical (4)	Categorical: 3–6 options Recall: standard 4-weeks acute 1-week	Algorithm* Domain profile (0–100: 100 best health) Summary scores: Physical component summary (PCS), Mental component summary (MCS)	USA	Yes – see website
European quality of life questionnaire EuroQoL EQ-5D (5) www.euroqol.org/	EuroQoL Group,1990	EQ-5D 5 domains Anxiety/depression (1) Mobility (1) Pain/discomfort (1) Self-care (1) Usual activities (1) EQ-Thermometer (EQ-VAS) Global health (1)	EQ-5D Categorical: 3 options Recall: current health EQ-Thermometer 1x vertical VAS – current health	EQ-5D Domain profile: summation Utility index: (algorithm*) −0.59 to 1.00; 1.00 best health EQ-Thermometer VAS (0–100; 100 best health)	European	No – but register on website
Domain-specific Symptoms and disease activity						
Multi-dimensional Fatigue Inventory (MFI) (20)	Smett et al, 1995	5 domains General fatigue (4) Physical fatigue (4) Mental fatigue (4) Reduced motivation (4) Reduced activity (4)	Likert 7-point agreement scale: 'yes, that is true' to 'no, that is not true' Recall 'previous days'	Summation once items that are worded in positive/negative direction are corrected for. 5 domain scores	The Netherlands	No
Bath AS Disease Activity Index (BASDAI) (6) http://www.nass.co.uk/bath_indices.htm	Garrett et al 1994	1 domain AS-specific disease activity (6)	6 × 10cm horizontal VAS; descriptive anchors Recall: past week	Index: item summation Mean of items 5 and 6; mean of total score: 0–10 (0 no disease activity)	UK	No
Health problem						
Hospital Anxiety and Depression Scale (HADS) (14)	Zigmond Et Snaith 1983	2 domains: HADS-A Anxiety (7)	Categorical: 4 options: range 0 to 3. Descriptive terms vary according to item phrase (e.g., range from 'Most of the time' to 'Not at all').	Summation 2 domains: range 0 to 21, where higher scores represent greater levels of anxiety or depression. A total score is also reported by some authors.	USA	Yes – see NFER Nelson website To view HADS see SIGN website

(Continued)

Table 4.1 Continued

PROM (NUMBER OF ITEMS) (ASSOCIATED WEB-SITE WHERE AVAILABLE)	DEVELOPER	HEALTH DOMAINS (ITEMS)	RESPONSE SCALE	SCORE	ORIGIN	PURCHASE COST
http://shop.nfer-nelson.co.uk/icat/hospitalanxietyanddepress http://www.sign.ac.uk/guidelines/published/support/guideline57/hads.html		HADS-D Depression (7)	Recall 'past week'.			–
ADL/function Health Assessment Questionnaire (HAQ) (21) http://aramis.stanford.edu/HAQ.html http://www.mapi-research.fr/t_03_serv_dist_Cduse_haq.htm	Fries, 1980, Bruce & Fries 2003	Arthritis-specific function (core): 2 domains Disability (20), Discomfort (1)	Disability-categorical: 4 options Pain–1x 15cm VAS Recall: previous week	Disability 0-3; 0 best function Pain 0-3; 0 no pain	USA	No – see website
Condition-specific AS Quality of Life Questionnaire (ASQoL) (18) No website	Doward et al 2003	AS-specific HRQL (18)	Yes/No Recall: 'at the moment'	Index: 0-18; 0 best HRQL	UK, NL	No
Arthritis Impact Measurement Scale (AIMS) (45) See McDowell (2006)	Meenan et al 1980	Arthritis-specific HRQL 9 domains (total 45 items) Mobility (4), Physical activity (5), Dexterity (5), Household activity (7), Social activity (4), Activities of daily living (4), Pain (4), Depression (6), Anxiety (6)	Categorical: 2-6 options Recall: past month	Domain profile: item summation Normalisation procedure converts scores to 0-10 : 0 best health	USA	No
AIMS-2 (Core 57) See McDowell (2006)	Meenan et al 1992	Arthritis-specific HRQL Core 12 domains (total 57 items) Mobility level, Walking & Bending, Hand & Finger function, Arm function, Self-care tasks, Household tasks, Social activity, Social support, Pain – arthritis, Work, Tension/mood 44 additional items: satisfaction, impact on function, priorities for improvement	Categorical: 5 options Recall: past month	Domain profile: item summation Normalisation procedure converts scores to 0-10 : 0 best health	USA	No
Population-specific Quality of Life profile – Seniors Version No website	Raphael et al 1005	3 domains Being: physical (12), psychological (12), spiritual (12)	Categorical: 5 options Importance and enjoyment scores	Weighted summation 2-domain profile	Canada	No

Instrument	Author	Description	Response options / recall	Scoring	Country	Website
Paediatric Quality of Life Inventory (PedsQL) http://www.pedsql.org/conditions.html http://www.mapi-research.fr/t_03_serv_dist_Cduse_pedsql.htm	Varni et al 2005	Belonging: physical (12), social (12), community (12) Becoming: practical (13), leisure (13), growth (13) Core generic scale (range 15–23) Additional modules include: Arthritis; Family impact; Multidimensional Fatigue Scale; Pain questionnaire; Pain coping inventory; Rheumatology module	Categorical: Five options (0 'never a problem' to 4 'always a problem') Recall: standard past month; acute 10week	Index: −3.33 to +3.33 Items reverse scored, summed and linearly transformed to 0–100 for each domain: 100 best health Self or proxy completion	USA	See website
Specific to condition and domain						
Arthritis Self-Efficacy Scale (20) http://patienteducation.stanford.edu/research/searthritis.html	Lorig et al 1989	Pain (5), Function (9), Other symptoms (6) Developed for application in RA	Categorical: 10 options Recall 'present time'	Summation (score is the mean of the items)	USA	No – see website
Western Ontario and McMaster University Osteoarthritis Index (WOMAC) OA and function www.womac.org	Bellamy et al 1998	Osteoarthritis-related disability of the hip and knee. 3 domains Pain (5), Stiffness (2), Physical function (17)	Categorical: 5 options (0 none to 4 extreme) Recall: current health	Domain profile: item summation Pain 0–20; 0 no pain Stiffness 0–5; 0 non stiffness PF 0–68; 0 no physical limitation	Canada	No – see website
Individualised						
MACTAR-PET Interview completion	Tugwell et al 1987	Patients identify up to 15 preferences for improvement. Problems grouped: mobility & role activity; social interaction; appearance. 9 functional probes: mobility, self-care, leisure activities, communication, social interaction, role activities, emotional health, sleep and rest, appearance.	Problems ranked: 7-point Likert Scale for relative difficulty/severity/ frequency of each item. Importance of each item: 7-point importance scale (0–7)	Importance score multiplied relative difficulty/severity/ frequency score Results summed and divided by number of problems identified. Interview completion – requires up to 1-hour Score 0–49; higher scores greater perceived disability	Canada	No
PGI-AS No website	Haywood et al 2003	3 stage completion: 1: List important areas of life affected by AS (up to 5; plus 'All other areas of life affected by AS) 2: Severity of each area scored. 3: Points spent (total 10) to indicate priorities for improvement	Stage 2: 0–6 horizontal numerical scale with adjectival anchors Stage 3: allocate maximum of 10 points across all areas.	For each item listed in Stage 1 (Stage 2 score x Points spent in Stage 3): summation of each score/6. Multiply by 10. Self or interview completion Index score 0–100%; higher scores are better levels of health	UK	No; No website

*Further details on algorithms can be found in original publications

Condition or population-specific PROMs

Alternatively, measures may be specific to a particular condition or disease, for example, the arthritis impact measurement scale version 2 (AIMS2) is specific to people with arthritis and assesses physical, emotional and social well-being (Meenan et al 1992); or to a patient population, for example, the quality of life profile – seniors version (QLP-SV) (Raphael et al 1995) is specific to the assessment of quality of life in older people. Some measures may be specific to a population with additional modules that provide further disease or symptom specific information: for example, the paediatric quality of life inventory (PedsQL) (Varni et al 2005) has a core generic scale for the assessment of paediatric quality of life, with additional modules for fatigue (PedsQL multidimensional fatigue scale) and rheumatology-related problems (PedsQL rheumatology module pain and hurt scale) (Varni et al 2007). Numerous measures are specific to a condition and a health domain. For example, the arthritis self-efficacy scale (Lorig et al 1989) is specific to the assessment of self-efficacy in patients with rheumatoid arthritis, and the Western Ontario and McMaster university osteoarthritis index (WOMAC) is specific to the assessment of functional ability in lower limb osteoarthritis (Bellamy et al 1988) (Table 4.1).

Individualised

The majority of conventional PROMs are highly standardized questionnaires with a pre-determined set of items and response options. Although standardized questionnaires often have good measurement properties (Fitzpatrick et al 1998), they may omit issues of importance to individual patients, while containing items of little relevance to others. Measures that adopt a more individualised approach, such as the schedule for the evaluation of individual quality of life (SEIQoL) (McGee et al 1991) and the patient generated index (Martin et al 2007, Ruta et al 1994), support the incorporation an individual's problems and priorities in the assessment process. Evidence suggests that these measures have enhanced content validity in comparison to more standardized measures (Haywood et al 2003), and that patients' view them as more valid assessments of health (Neudert et al 2001).

Several individualised measures have encouraging evidence of required measurement properties following completion by patients with a range of rheumatic diseases including the disease repercussion profile (DRP) (RA) (Carr & Thompson 1994), the MACTAR-patient elicitation technique (MACTAR-PET) (RA) (Tugwell et al 1987), the personal impact health assessment questionnaire (PI HAQ) (RA) (Hewlett et al 2002) and the PGI (AS) (Haywood et al 2003) (Table 4.1).

The respondent burden associated with individualised measures is often greater than that observed for more standardized approaches, and several measures require interview administration. As a consequence, the application of individualised measures in clinical research is limited (Patel et al 2003). However, the enhanced content validity and relevance to patients suggests that individualised measures may have an important role to play in routine practice (Greenhalgh et al 2005, Marshall et al 2006) but to date there are no published trials that rigorously evaluate the role of individualised measures in this setting (Marshall et al 2006).

Condition-specific, scientifically rigorous PROMs that have involved patients in item generation have greater clinical relevance, are more acceptable to patients, and more responsive to change in health than generic measures (Wiebe et al 2003). However, the broad content of generic measures supports the identification of co-morbid features and unexpected treatment side-effects that may not be identified by specific measures. Furthermore, certain generic measures, such as the EQ-5D (EuroQoL Group 1990) and the SF-6D generated from the SF-36 version 2 (Ware et al 2002, Marra et al 2004, 2005), can inform economic evaluations of service delivery. The combination of generic and specific measures has been recommended in health outcome assessment (McDowell & Newell 1996), and together are an essential element in the development of evidence-based healthcare. Combined, the evidence supports determination of the absolute and comparative effectiveness of interventions, their marginal relative benefits, and the economic implications of long-term therapies. However, the optimal combination of measures has not been determined in a way that makes it easy to implement this recommendation across diverse patient groups. A fundamental consideration is the appropriateness of each measure to the proposed application.

PROMs: QUALITY ASSESSMENT

The measurement of patient-reported outcome in healthcare has enjoyed increasing attention over the last 25 years and as a result several hundred measures are now available. For many of the rheumatic diseases there is often a choice (Garratt et al 2002). However, the quality of PROMs varies widely, and guidance or consensus on selection is often lacking. The appropriate selection of an outcome measure should be guided by a wide range of measurement (reliability, validity, responsiveness to clinically important change, precision, interpretation) and practical issues (appropriateness, acceptability, feasibility). These concepts have been detailed by several authors (Fitzpatrick et al 1998, Haywood 2008, McDowell 2006), and are summarised in Tables 4.2 and 4.3.

The field of rheumatology benefits greatly from the work of Outcome Measures in Rheumatology and Clinical Trials (OMERACT: www.omeract.org). OMERACT recommend the application of a slightly different set of criteria, or 'filter', when assessing the appropriateness of PROM for application in defined settings (Bellamy 1999) (Tables 4.2, 4.3). The filter summarises measurement and practical properties under three headings: 1) Truth: is the measure truthful, does it measure what it purports to measure? Is the result unbiased and relevant? This concept relates to issues of face, content, construct and criterion validity; 2) Discrimination: does the measure discriminate between health states or situations that are of interest? The situations can be states at one time (for classification or prognosis) or states at different times (to measure change). The concept is related to issues of measurement reliability and responsiveness; and 3) Feasibility: can the measure be applied easily, given constraints of time, money, and interpretability? The concept of feasibility is an essential element in measurement selection.

It is essential that users are aware of these key properties to support appropriate selection, interpretation and communication of data generated. In selecting a PROM, the user must decide what exactly is required in terms of the proposed application, appropriateness to the patient (population) and setting, and the feasibility of application and scoring. In short, an appropriate balance between required detail, accuracy of assessment and the burden of collecting the information must be sought (McDowell 2006), as summarised in Table 4.4.

GUIDANCE FOR PROM SELECTION IN THE RHEUMATIC DISEASES

Working groups

Several resources now exist to support healthcare professionals in the selection and application of PROMs. OMERACT consists of several international working groups dedicated to improving measurement across the rheumatic diseases. In recent years a wider range of health professionals and patients have participated in the process, with a significant impact on the identification of patient-important outcomes. Using a data-driven, iterative consensus approach, core assessment domains have been recommended across a range of conditions including RA (Tugwell & Boers 1993), AS (van der Heijde et al 1997,1999), osteoarthritis (Bellamy et al 1997), osteoporosis (Sambrook 1997), systemic lupus erythematosus (Smolen et al 1999), systemic sclerosis (Merkel et al 2003) and fibromyalgia (Mease et al 2007) (Table 4.5).

For some groups associated outcome measures (for example, AS (van der Heijde et al 1997, van der Heijde et al 1999)) and guidance for the interpretation of improvement have been recommended (for example, AS (Anderson et al 2001, Van Tubergen et al 2003)). However, the majority of the initial recommendations did not involve patients in the identification of core domains. Recent patient involvement has raised the importance of including fatigue as a core patient-centred assessment domain (Kirwan & Hewlett 2007, Kirwan et al 2007). Moreover, significant developments in the measurement of health outcome in recent years suggest that core domains should be revisited, for example, the assessment of fatigue and quality of life in AS. Application of the revised ICF framework (Stucki et al 2007) and accessing the views of patients will be invaluable to further exploring the core concept of what should be measured in the rheumatic diseases.

Special interest groups within OMERACT have been established, including disease-specific groups such as the Assessment in AS (ASAS) group (www.asas-group.org), the Group for Research and Assessment of Psoriasis and Psoriatic Arthritis (GRAPPA) (www.grappanetwork.org/) (Gladman et al 2007), the OMERACT/OARSI initiative for osteoarthritis (www.oarsi.org/) (Pham et al 2003) and the fibromyalgia research and outcomes group (Mease et al 2007). Other special interest or task groups are listed on the OMERACT web-site and associated publications. There are additional task groups exploring concepts such as work productivity (Escorpizo et al 2007), assessing single joints (Giles et al 2007), biomarkers (Keeling et al 2007), imaging-related concepts, and the Effective Musculoskeletal Consumer (Kristjansson et al 2007). A focus is also provided for measurement specific concepts including assessment of the

Table 4.2 Criteria for selecting patient-reported outcome measures (PROMs): Measurement properties

CRITERION*	DEFINITION	EVALUATION
Reliability (OMERACT filter 'discrimination;)	Temporal stability-are the results stable over time?	Test-retest reliability assesses score temporal stability (correlation coefficient); scores should remain unchanged in stable patients
	Are the scores internally consistent? (multi-item measures only)	Internal consistency reliability evaluates the ability of items to measure a single underlying health domain (Cronbachs alpha). Reliability estimates >0.70 and 0.90 recommended for group and individual assessment respectively
Validity (OMERACT filter 'truth')	Does the PROM measure what it claims to measure?	
	Content validity – how well do items cover the important parts of health to be assessed?	Qualitative appraisal of item content.
	Face validity – what do the items appear to measure?	How were items generated? Role of clinicians, patients etc? Qualitative appraisal of item content. How were items generated? Role of clinicians, patients etc?
	Criterion validity – how well does the measure perform against a gold-standard measure of the same construct?	Quantitative evaluation-comparative evaluation (if gold-standard available)
	Construct validity	
	– does the PROM show convergence/divergence with appropriate variables?	Quantitative comparison with other variables (health, clinical, socio-demographic, service use) – e.g. what are the hypothesised and actual levels of correlation with other variables?
	– does the PROM show divergence between groups of patients?	Quantitative evidence of discriminative ability between defined patient (extreme) groups. For example, pain levels between active and non-active disease groups/general population.
	– is there evidence to support the hypothesised domain structure?	Internal construct validity (dimensionality)-statistical methods such as factor analysis
Responsiveness (OMERACT filter 'discrimination;)	Does the PROM detect change over time that matters to patients?	Change in health following an intervention or over time.
	(sometimes referred to as 'sensitivity to change')	Distribution-based assessment-relates score change to some measure of variability; e.g. Effect Size statistics. Anchor-based assessment-relationship between score change and external variable: e.g. patient's perception of change
Precision	How precisely do the PROM numerical values relate to the underlying spectrum of health, and discriminate between respondents in relation to their health?	Data quality and precision influenced by item coverage and response categories; where more than 20% of respondents have maximum bad or good health scores, score distribution indicates floor or ceiling effects respectively, and hence a lack of precision
	(sometimes referred to as 'sensitivity')	
Interpretability (included in OMERACT filter 'feasibility')	How interpretable are the scores?	Distribution-based – describe change over time and group differences that are likely to be clinically meaningful.
	How do the scores relate to meaningful or worthwhile change in health?	Anchor-based-relate score change or differences between groups to external variables to estimate 'Minimal Important Difference': e.g. patient or clinician perception of change

OMERACT headings (Bellamy 1999)
*Criterion headings informed by Fitzpatrick et al (1998) and Haywood (2007).

minimal clinical importance (MCI) and computerised adaptive testing (Chakravarty et al 2007). These groups often run assessment workshops linked to main rheumatology conferences.

Structured reviews

Clearly, selecting an appropriate PROM can be a time-consuming process. The growing availability of structured reviews of PROM performance

Table 4.3 Criteria for selecting patient-reported outcome measures (PROMs): practical properties

CRITERION*	DEFINITION	EVALUATION
Appropriateness		
	How well does the intended purpose of the PROM meet the intended application? Is it relevant?	For example, if the primary intent of the intervention is to reduce pain, pain should be an important component of a primary outcome measure
		If the patient has indicated that their ability to engage in paid employment is their most important outcome, how appropriate is the selected PROM to communicate this outcome?
Acceptability		
	Is the PROM acceptable to patients? How willing or capable of completing the PROM are the patients? Is it relevant?	Most readily assessed through completion/response rates, and missing values. Difficult to evaluate directly. Focus groups with patients are useful for exploring acceptability. Extensive involvement of patients during PROM development should improve acceptability.
Feasibility (OMERACT filter 'feasibility')		
	What time and resources are needed to collect, process and analyse the PROM?	Specific to the requirements of clinicians, researchers, and other staff.
		Is the PROM self-completed or does it require interview administration? How long does completion require? Is completion appropriate to the available setting?
		Are instructions for completion and scoring provided? Is special equipment, for example, computer completion, required or available for completion and scoring? How accessible is such equipment? How quickly can scores be generated? How are results presented to clinicians and/or patients? – for example, graphic representation of scores.
		If the scores are required for face-to-face discussion during the patient consultation, how quickly can the PROM be scored, analysed and fed-back to the healthcare professional and the patient?

*Criterion headings taken from Fitzpatrick et al (1998) and Haywood (2007)

in different patient populations of relevance to the rheumatic diseases, for example, low back pain (Bombardier 2000), knee-specific PROMs (Garratt et al 2004), ankylosing spondylitis (Haywood et al 2005), shoulder disability (Bot et al 2004) and the assessment of fatigue in RA (Hewlett et al 2007) can be useful assets to health practitioners seeking guidance for measurement selection.

Web-resources

In addition to the OMERACT related sites, a range of on-line resources exist to support the identification and selection of PROMs. For example, the Patient-Reported Health Instruments database hosted by the National Centre for Health Outcomes Development (NCHOD, PHI programme), Oxford University (http://phi.uhce.ox.ac.uk/), the patient-reported outcome and quality of life instruments database

(http://www.qolid.org/), the MAPI research institute (http://www.mapi-research.fr/index.htm) and the International Society for Quality of Life Research (http://www.isoqol.org/).

At the core of the PHI programme is a freely accessible website with a range of facilities, including a searchable bibliography, designed to support the identification, selection and application of PROMs. The website also provides summaries of published reviews of PROMs and evidence of expert consensus opinion across a growing range of disease and population-specific areas, including those of relevance to musculoskeletal practitioners. The PROQoLID and MAPI websites provide limited free access to a range of published PROMs, providing details of the developers, purpose, number of questions, and administration. Additional information can be accessed for a fee. Additional, selected websites of relevance to PROMs assessment are

Table 4.4 Assessing the appropriateness of a patient-reported outcome measure (PROM) to the proposed application	
QUESTION	WHAT SHOULD BE CONSIDERED?
What is the proposed application for the PROM?	In what setting is the PROM to be applied?-routine practice; clinical research; health policy; quality of care evaluation Will the data to be used to assess current disease state? Will the data be used to assess disease progress over time? Will the data be used to evaluate a programme of care? Are group level or individual level data required? Will the data be used to communicate the impact of healthcare to interested stakeholders? What outcomes are viewed as important indicators of care? Will the PROM be used to enhance patient involvement in the consultation process?
What patient characteristics will influence PROM selection?	Disease-specificity and co-morbidity Age – ability to self-complete; need for assistance; need for proxy completion. Level of disability – ability to self-complete; need for assistance; need for proxy completion Tolerance for completion – the relative length of PROM and associated respondent burden
What is the assessment time frame?	Will the assessment be cross-sectional, or longitudinal with multiple assessment points? What is the PROM recall period and how does this relate to the proposed application? Will the PROM be used to assess acute symptoms? This requires measurement that is responsive to clinically important change over relatively short time-frames Will the PROM be used to assess the long-term impact of a condition? The longer-term effects of disease impact requires measurement that is sensitive to small changes over relatively long time-frames
How complex/simple should the assessment be?	What detail is required? How broad ranging is the assessment provided? To whom will the results of the assessment be communicated? What is the important outcome to be communicated? How feasible is it to include the assessment of Body Structure, Body Function, Activity and Participation? What is the relevance of the proposed assessment to the clinical question? Is the data easily interpreted? For example, does the PROM produce a single index scores and/ or a profile score over several domains.
What facilities are required to support the assessment?	In what setting is the PROM to be applied? Clinic-based; trial-based completion; patient self-completion What support is required for PROM completion and scoring? For example, paper-based completion; electronic data capture and scoring; computer-based support etc. What is the associated cost of PROM completion, scoring, data feedback and administration support; plus computer support where appropriate. What facilities are required/available to support the real-time feedback of scores to inform shared clinical decision-making.

are available from the 'Links' page of the PHI Programme website (http://phi.uhce.ox.ac.uk/)

Individual PROMs

Many of the widely available PROMs have dedicated websites, as listed in Table 4.1. An up-dated list of these resources is available from the 'links' page of the PHI programme website (http://phi. uhce.ox.ac.uk/) (Box 4.3).

PROMs – APPLICATIONS

PROMs have been applied in research settings, including population-based health surveys and clinical trials, for several decades (Haywood 2006). However, over recent years there has been growing interest in the contribution to be made to routine practice settings. Application in routine practice will provide the focus of this section.

Table 4.5 OMERACT recommended core domains for rheumatoid arthritis, ankylosing spondylitis and osteoarthritis

SELECTED HEALTH DOMAINS	RA[a]	AS[b]	OA – HIP, KNEE AND HAND[c]
Acute phase reactants	core		
Analgesia count			optional
Biologic markers			optional
Fatigue	**	*	
Flares			optional
Functional ability/physical function	core	core	core
Global health status-patient	core	core	core
Global health status-physician	core		strongly recommended
Inflammation/stiffness		core	optional
Pain	core	core	core
Performance-based measures			optional
Quality of life		*	strongly recommended
Radiograph of joints/Imaging	core		core***
Spinal mobility		core	
Swollen joints	core		
Tender joints	core		
Time to surgery			optional
Utility			strongly recommended

References:
[a]Tugwell et al 1993
[b]Van der Heijde et al 1997
[c]Bellamy et al 1997.
*Not recommended due to novelty and uncertainty over measurement
**Not recommended in initial core set, but recent patient involvement suggests that fatigue should be considered a core domain
***Not recommended as routine in primary care

BOX 4.3   Study activity: identifying and selecting PROMs for a patient with osteoarthritis

A fifty-year old male long-distance lorry driver with moderate OA of the knee complains of pain and stiffness in his knees, and a difficulty getting in/out of the cab of his HGV. This is affecting his work: his knee pain increases during long drives and is finding it difficult to assist in loading/unloading the lorry. He is worried about the impact on his effectiveness at work.

The patient indicates that the most important outcomes of care are to reduce his pain and stiffness, particularly when driving for long periods, to improve his physical function so that he can get in/ out of his cab more readily. Ultimately, he hopes to improve his effectiveness at work.

- What core health outcomes will you include in your assessment?
- Which domains recommended by the OA OMERACT group will you assess?
- Will you include any additional outcomes to those recommended by the OA OMERACT group?
- How will you identify suitable PROMs for the assessment of the core domains?

ROUTINE PRACTICE

Enquiring about a patients' perception of health is a familiar part of the clinical encounter for most health professionals. Although medical care has historically concentrated on treating impairments to body structure and function, a patient's complaint is usually expressed in terms of their functional limitation and the wider impact on their ability to participate in society (Fig. 4.1). Increasingly, most clinicians recognise the importance of treating the patient as a whole, and not just treating the disease. Therefore, enquiring about the broader impact of disease, and identifying patient-important outcomes of care, is essential to patient-centred care (Fig. 4.2). Most simply, PROMs enable patients to report the impact of health problems and report the

course and outcome of interventions in accessible and meaningful ways.

Historically, clinicians have adopted a non-standardized approach to assessment, and although often helpful in developing a rapport between patient and clinician, it is unlikely that the information elicited is of benefit beyond the personal encounter (Morris et al 1998). Moreover, such non-standardized approaches have limited value in communicating the impact of health and associated healthcare, and in comparing health status between individuals. Members of the multidisciplinary healthcare team often establish individual relationships with patients, which provide the potential to elicit aspects of a patient's experience that may not necessarily be reported to other members of the team (Zebrack 2007). Standardized PROMs may provide a common language to facilitate communication between team members.

Three distinct applications of PROMs-related data of relevance to routine practice can be described (Fig. 4.3):

- the healthcare provider aggregates patient reported data at a group level to inform healthcare quality and service delivery

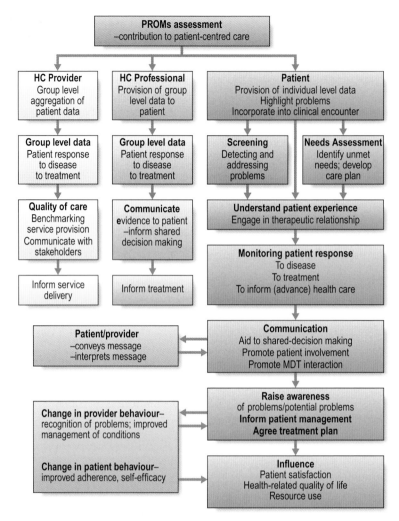

Figure 4.3 PROM application of relevance to routine practice: a cascade model.

- the healthcare professional shares group level data from clinical research with the patient to convey evidence of disease-burden and treatment effectiveness
- the patient completes the PROM in a routine practice setting, providing evidence of the impact of disease and associated healthcare.

Health care quality and service delivery

The assessment of health care quality has historically focused on the perspectives of the care-provider or healthcare organization, such as cost, length of stay and patient mortality, and within a chronic disease context few assessments have included the patient's experience of care (Groves & Wagner 2005). With the increasing culture of accountability, clinicians and patients are concerned that health care is both efficient and of high quality. At a managerial and policy level, measures of health outcome support the comparison of costs and benefits of competing health care programmes, where managers will seek to provide the best health care for the best price (Fig. 4.3). Rationing of healthcare is the inevitable consequence of limited resources, and the use of well-developed, responsive PROMs may provide beneficial information to support the distribution of healthcare resources (Haywood 2006, Department of Health 2008). Generic measures may be strategically important in health policy, particularly those that consider consumer needs and preferences, by supporting the comparison of health status and economic evaluation across population groups. For example, generic measures may support an evaluation of the relative health burden of people with OA on a waiting list for a total hip replacement versus those with RA waiting for access to hydrotherapy services.

Moreover, PROMs provide complementary evidence to more traditional measures of process and outcome, providing a more holistic assessment of the impact of service delivery. For example, aggregated data may assist the health care provider in identifying a common patient concern that requires, or suggests, a more systematic approach to health care provision (Fig. 4.3). Although limited empirical evidence for the performance of PROMs in quality of care evaluation exists (Appleby & Devlin 2004, Mitchell & Lang 2004), well-developed PROMs have the potential to provide reliable and valid group level data supporting the routine monitoring of patients health status for the purposes of quality assessment and, where appropriate, the comparative benchmarking of clinic performance (Appleby & Devlin 2004, Department of Health 2008) (Fig. 4.3). The simple format of most measures contributes to the acceptability and feasibility required for routine data collection, for example, measures may be self-completed in a clinic or ward setting (Haywood 2006).

Communicating the impact of disease and healthcare from group level data

With the advent of novel methods of service delivery, for example, consultant therapists, and new treatments for the rheumatic diseases with potentially toxic side-effects, patient acceptability and experience are an important determinant of overall effectiveness (Haywood 2006). Well-developed PROMs provide a powerful, quantifiable and standardized research tool, for use alongside more traditional methods of assessment, against which the effectiveness of health care interventions can be judged. Such measures have the potential to facilitate better research and to increase scientific knowledge about patient outcomes, and are increasingly accepted as valid measures of treatment effectiveness (Fitzpatrick et al 1998). Regulatory bodies, including the National Institute for Health and Clinical Excellence (NICE 2004) and the Federal Drug Administration (FDA) (Burke et al 2006), have provided guidance on the application of PROMs in support of treatment effectiveness. When applied in population-based surveys PROMs provide a important mechanism for assessing population and

community health status, illustrating the wide ranging burden of disease and the associated unmet needs. Guidance to support PROM selection for clinical research has been detailed by several authors (Burke et al 2006, Fitzpatrick et al 1998, Haywood 2006).

Where measured outcomes have increased relevance to routine practice, with demonstrated impact on patient outcome, this may facilitate the translation of knowledge into routine practice. Healthcare professionals may utilise group level PROM data from research to provide evidence of other patients' experience of the disease and associated healthcare. These data are expected to enable patients to develop a better understanding of the expected disease and healthcare impact in relation to the patient-reported variables, and hence to support shared decision-making (Fig. 4.3). Patient completion of PROMs in a routine practice setting may enhance their understanding and familiarity with such data.

Patient completion of PROMs in routine practice

Well-developed, standardized PROMs provide a systematic approach towards the elicitation, recording and monitoring of patient-generated information in routine practice (Figs. 4.3,4.4). Such data may inform health screening (Gilbody et al 2003, Higginson & Carr 2001, McHorney 2002), the identification of patient needs and preferences (Higginson & Carr 2001, McHorney 2002), contribute to shared decision-making, and the regular monitoring of disease impact (Higginson & Carr 2001, McHorney 2002, Skevington et al 2005), and ultimately inform and advance healthcare. Moreover, there is growing evidence that PROMs may further enhance communication between health professionals and individual patients (Fig. 4.4), and even influence a patients sense of well-being (Haywood et al 2006, Marshall et al 2006, Velikova et al 2004) (Fig. 4.3). The growing evidence in support of the role of PROMs suggests that they should be viewed as integral to routine practice, adding to and complementing the broad range of information captured from other sources, including traditional biomedical assessment, other members of the healthcare team, and family members.

Support for the potential contribution of PROMs to the consultation process stems from arguments that such measures play a diverse role in changing how health problems are viewed and managed by patients and their healthcare providers (Figs 4.3, 4.4). The introduction of PROMs may encourage patients

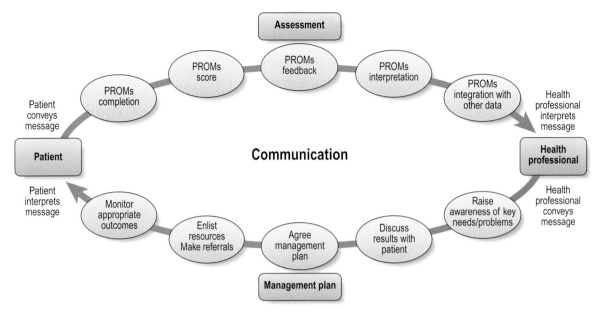

Figure 4.4 Using PROMs in routine practice.

to share health-related problems that concern them in addition to 'symptoms' elicited in traditional consultations. PROMs may also act as a trigger so that potential problems or concerns are raised earlier in the consultation process. Similarly, health professionals are stimulated to think outside of conventional limitations in identifying problems and selecting solutions jointly with patients. Especially in the context of chronic disease, PROMs may have a powerful role to play over time in facilitating shared, and timely, identification of goals and priorities between health professionals and patients faced with complex, evolving and multi-faceted problems (Marshall et al 2006).

However, as recently argued by several authors (Greenhalgh et al 2005, Haywood et al 2006, Marshall et al 2006), the evaluation of PROMs in routine practice settings needs to be far more thoughtfully designed to take account of the likely real world contribution of measures designed to enhance patient involvement. Until more appropriate evaluative studies have been conducted it is premature to reach definitive conclusions on the advantages of PROMs in routine practice. Highlighting the utility of PROMs in identifying the health needs, priorities and preferences of patients, whilst demonstrating the potential cost advantages from PROMs application by facilitating the provision of timely and appropriate interventions, may

ultimately provide the driving force for incorporating PROMs into routine clinical practice (Haywood et al 2008, Varni et al 2005).

Four key phases describing the decision-making process required when including PROMs application in routine practice can be described (Fig 4.5): 1) PROM selection; 2) the logistics of PROM application, scoring and feedback of data; 3) interpretation of results and associated action plan; and 4) longitudinal monitoring of care.

Selecting PROMs for use in routine practice

The clinical and patient perceived relevance of a PROM is central to PROM selection and application (Figs. 4.2, 4.5, Tables 4.2-4.4). PROMs should beneficially influence the care process by informing diagnosis and/or care planning. Selection therefore requires that they are appropriate to the primary clinical question. Similarly, the patient value placed on the outcome is central to understanding how ill-health or the outcomes of care affects their life: just because a PROM is completed by the patient, does not mean that it measures what is important to the patient. A wide range of constructs are necessary to explore the whole extent of a patient's experience of a chronic rheumatic disease (Fig. 4.2), and there are many available PROMs to address these constructs (Garratt et al 2002). Therefore, selecting those most

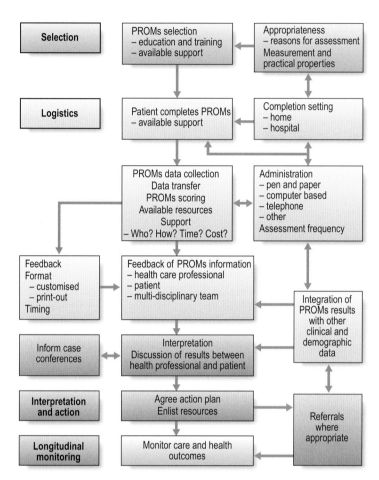

Figure 4.5 The decision-making process for PROM application in routine practice.

appropriate to the routine practice setting is crucial. Where the PROM supports the identification of 'what matters' to the patient it should contribute to the care process.

LOGISTICS OF APPLYING PROMs IN ROUTINE PRACTICE

Once the decision to include PROMs in routine practice has been made, attention to the logistics of collecting the required information is necessary to ensure that the application will serve the intended purpose. Two key issues should be considered (Fig. 4.5) (Bezjak 2007):

1. The method of administration and data collection
2. Support for data collection, scoring and feedback of data.

METHOD OF PROM ADMINISTRATION

Multiple methods for the administration and feedback of results from PROMs exist, including traditional pen and paper completion, and a growing range of methods supporting electronic data capture (Table 4.6). The choice of method should be informed by the reasons for PROM application, the rapidity with which results are required, the frequency with which assessments will occur, and available resources to support application, analysis and feedback of data. For example, if the application demands the immediate availability of scores to inform individual decision-making, some form of computer-based assessment is likely to be most appropriate. Similarly, if it is preferable for PROM results to be linked to other clinical and demographic data, a more sophisticated computer-based application may be preferred. Computer-based completion will also support integration of scores into the electronic record, more rapid aggregation of data, and customised feedback of data. Although pen and paper completion of PROMs is cheaper initially, such completion may be associated with increased financial and time costs in relation to scoring and feedback of data. The delayed and often limited presentation of results may also reduce data utility. Although the electronic capture of PROM information has start-up costs associated with the initial investment in soft and hard-ware, methods for data entry, data analysis and data feedback are integrated into the system and hence relative costs are reduced. However, continued technical support is essential.

The needs and disabilities of patients will inevitably inform administration modes. For example, patients with advanced RA may find it difficult to hold a fine pen, causing difficulties with self-completion of pen and paper formats or use of a palm-pilot/hand-held computer. Assistance may be required if pen and paper completion is the only available format. Alternatively, touch-screen technology may be more appropriate. It is rare for one system to accommodate the needs of all patients within routine practice and greater degrees of freedom in relation to the selected modes of administration are possible than within a research setting. It may be appropriate to combine modes to find the most feasible and most efficient for the encounter, to reduce burden and increase efficiency for patient and clinician. When pen-and-paper completion and computer-based completion are compared within the same setting, anecdotal evidence suggests that there is very little difference in terms of completion rates and level of acceptance, but scoring, analysis and feedback is easier following computer-based completion (Bezjak 2007).

The increasing availability of home computers supports the self-monitoring of disease via internet completion of PROMs, the results of which can be linked with disease self-management programmes (Van Stel et al 2007). The results may also be fed-back to members of the multidisciplinary team via email or dedicated web-pages, providing an efficient way to monitor active treatment. The real time feedback of information suggests that patients' needs can be addressed as and when they occur rather than at a pre-arranged clinic visit which may not coincide with, or be well-suited to, responding to symptoms and other quality of life issues (Donaldson 2007).

Support for data collection, scoring and feedback of data

The successful application of PROMs into routine practice requires appropriate support for both health professionals and patients. This support may relate to systems level support and the logistics of administration, or the personal support for both health professionals and patients.

Clinical practice varies widely, presenting many challenges for the application of PROMs. At a systems level, it is essential to explore how data collection fits in with the wider healthcare setting. That is, who supports it and how? Different modes of completion have different demands in relation to scoring and data feedback, and adequate investment is essential. For example, if the data are collected using pen and paper format, support to ensure that PROMs are scored and fed back in a timely manner to clinicians is required; without this support PROMs data may be left unused. If data are captured electronically, support to ensure that system failures are rapidly addressed is required.

The ability, knowledge and willingness of health professionals to incorporate PROMs into routine practice is critical to the relative success of PROMs as an intervention to enhance care (Haywood et al 2008, Jacobsen et al 2002). Familiar barriers to the incorporation of PROMs into routine practice include concern over the availability and appropriateness of questionnaires, patient disabilities, limited resources or time, limited knowledge, and limited guidance (Haywood et al 2008, Skevington et al 2005). There may also be an unwillingness to discuss certain items raised in PROMs, often because of the perceived lack of support or resources to address issues raised.

Although evidence from the oncology field suggests that the assessment of quality of life using PROMs does not add time to the clinical encounter (Velikova et al 2004), to reduce the perception of increased burden, the introduction of PROMs assessment may require some 'trade-off' with more traditional approaches to assessment being removed from assessment (Haywood et al 2008). Many clinicians lack knowledge and confidence in the use of PROMs, and to jettison familiar methods of assessment in favour of something new, irrespective of the evidence-base, requires significant support and guidance (Haywood 2006). Specific education provided via web-based facilities, support by the professional bodies and training courses have been highlighted as the most preferable routes to receive training and information (Haywood et al 2008). The clinical relevance of selected measures, supported by training and support to encourage a positive attitude to the usefulness of formal assessment should facilitate staff acceptance. Where more formal

Table 4.6 Modes of patient-reported outcome measure (PROM) administration		
ADMINISTRATION MODE	POSITIVES	NEGATIVES
Non-computer based completion		
Pen and paper	Mobile Simple Cheap to copy and integrate into practice Familiar	Potential high costs for data entry Potential delay in data feedback Limited presentation of scores
Computer-based completion		
Computer touch-screen	Independent completion Low administration demands Potential for cost-saving data collection Increasing familiarity Potential for rapid data transfer and scoring – supporting real time provision of scores Potential for integration with other data and with electronic record Attractive output features	Initial purchase cost Ongoing support essential – human resource cost Subject to regular hard-ware changes
Palm-pilot/ Personal digital assistant	As above	As above: Plus small display screen and small pen for entering response
Tablet-personal computer	As above: Plus large display screen	As above
Smart pen technology	As above: Plus easy to use – built-in scanner	As above
Voice-interactive technology	As above: Plus voice-interactivity reduces potential difficulties with pens or touch-screen data entry	As above
Telephone completion	Touch-pad completion Interview completion	
Internet completion		
Home-based computer – internet access	Independent completion Real-time collaboration Low administration demands Increasing familiarity Supports self-management	Data protection
Other		
Computer adaptive testing (CAT)	Reduced respondent burden. Increased precision of assessment	Not yet widely available

assessment becomes a regular part of assessment practice, supported by knowledgeable clinicians, patient acceptance is enhanced.

At the patient level, the concept of completing PROMs should be clearly introduced to support adherence. For example, explaining why they are being used, how they contribute to the therapeutic relationship, the frequency with which they will be completed, and how the results will be used. The logistics of, and available support for, PROM completion should also be discussed. The relevance, simplicity and appeal of the PROM will contribute to completion. Moreover, in order to accept the incorporation of more standardized PROM assessment into the care process, patients and clinicians need to experience any potential enhancement to their interactions (Haywood et al 2006).

Interpretation and action

For PROM-related information to successfully add to the armamentarium of information collected in routine practice, this information must be actionable. Although well-developed condition-specific or individualised measures are likely to have enhanced clinical relevance than generic measures, providing information that is more actionable, appropriate education and training in the application and interpretation of PROMs is required.

This perceived need for further training in the use of PROMs in routine practice has recently been confirmed in surveys of UK-based continence specialists (Haywood et al 2008) and GPs (Skevington et al 2005). Although guidance for score interpretation at a group level exists for some rheumatic diseases (for example, in AS (Anderson et al 2001, Van Tubergen et al 2003)), specific guidance for the interpretation of PROMs in rheumatology routine practice does not currently exist.

The presentation of PROM data provides a visual profile that raises key problems and highlights areas for concern. Rather than focusing on the aggregate score, clinicians should also explore the range of problems raised. The integration of clinical expertise with an understanding of PROM scores supports interpretation. Clinical intuition will often indicate when patients are not doing well, and well-developed PROMs may pick this up sooner than traditional measures (Fallowfield 2007). Information about PROM scores in particular clinical settings, and the 'normal pattern' of scores informed by condition or population-based values, should signal further action or referral. For example, various cut-points have been suggested for the Hospital Anxiety and Depression Score (HADS) to indicate levels of anxiety or depression (McDowell 2006). For each domain, a cut-point of 8/9 suggests mild anxiety or depression and 11/12 suggests severe anxiety or depression. The longitudinal monitoring of health supports the comparison of scores over time. Relating scores to additional clinical variables may further assist in decision-making. Where specific guidance for the interpretation of PROM score change is not available, evidence suggests that an acceptable starting point for the interpretation of a clinically important change in health is a score change of 10% or 10-point change on a 0-100 scale (Sloan et al 2005). Specific management guidelines related to score interpretation (Meadows et al 1998, Van Stel et al 2007, Varni et al 2005, Velikova et al 2004) and illustrations through the use of case vignettes, for example, of stable patients and patients whose health has deteriorated, may further assist this process (Velikova et al 2004) (Boxes 4.4, 4.5).

However, as with all methods of assessment, it is important to retain a healthy scepticism in relation to specific PROM scores: scores can be influenced by a range of contextual factors, including gender, age, race, ethnicity, completion format, setting, relationship with provider, and there is potential for wide variation at individual level. Application of PROMs at an individual level requires a trade-off between scientific precision and clinical usefulness, and critical thinking must be applied to all sources of information informing the health status of the individual. Exploring the performance of PROMs alongside other clinical variables is central to this.

Longitudinal monitoring

The routine application of PROMs recognises that not all health professionals will ask all patients all of the appropriate questions, all of the time, or in a way that patients will be able to answer (Ganiats 2007). Moreover, there is evidence that, without the use of PROMs, clinicians do not access information that is important to patients as well as they think they do (Fallowfield et al 2001). The routine application of PROMs supports the longitudinal monitoring of care and health outcomes (Figs. 4.3-4.5), providing information that is essential to the process of care. The longitudinal collection of individual data supports data interpretation over time.

The following box provides an illustration of the 'ideal' application of PROMs in a routine practice setting (Box 4.6).

CONCLUSION

The measurement of patient-reported outcome in the rheumatic diseases continues to evolve. Well-developed PROMs provide a major source of evidence of the patient experience to inform value judgements of both patients and members of the multi-disciplinary healthcare team (Patrick & Chiang 2000). They can inform routine practice, service delivery, and healthcare policy, while enhancing communication between patient and provider, leading to common understanding of the health problem, and agreed management solutions and outcomes; greater patient adherence and treatment satisfaction. Improved health status may then be achieved with advancing technology, electronic data capture of PROMs may enhance the feasibility of application, supporting the timely provision of scores and the clinical utility to routine practice. Moreover, information can be readily

BOX 4.4   Interpretation of PROM scores – profile of an 'unwell' patient

Subjective history:

- A 35-year-old man with ankylosing spondylitis
- Complains of low back pain radiating to his buttocks and posterior thighs and increasing reduction in spinal mobility. He reports low energy levels and is experiencing difficulty sleeping due to the low back pain and stiffness.
- He is experiencing increasing difficulties at work (he is a self-employed plumber) and has been forced to take several days sick leave.

PROM assessment (score presented graphically with cut-points highlighted):

- Functional ability: scores on the BASFI (6/10) suggest high levels of functional limitation.
- Disease activity: scores on the BASDAI (7/10) and pain VAS (9/10) suggest high levels of disease activity and pain respectively.
- HADS scores (9) suggest mild levels of anxiety and depression.
- General health status-profile: SF-36. The most significant limitations are in physical function, vitality (fatigue), role-physical (possibly work), role-emotional and bodily pain (all below population mean value). Low scores on the role-emotional suggest moderate levels of emotional distress.
- The patient reports multiple symptoms – fatigue, pain, stiffness and disturbed sleep. There are financial problems linked to his difficulties at to work. He is feeling anxious about the financial impact on his family of not being able to work.

Actions taken:

- PROM scores assessed alongside other assessments.
- Pain and stiffness have been identified as major problems. Symptomatic drugs have been adjusted.
- Referrals have been made to physiotherapy to further assist with pain control and to support an exercise programme to enhance physical functioning.
- Referrals have been made to occupational therapy to assist with possible work modifications and work pacing.
- The levels of fatigue have been noted and will be re-assessed at the follow-up assessment.
- The emotional distress experienced by the patient was not reported in the annotation. This will be closely monitored and referrals made where appropriate.

BOX 4.5   Interpretation of PROM scores – profile of a 'well' patient

Subjective history:

- A 54-year-old man with stable ankylosing spondylitis
- No particular complaints reported.
- Still working full-time as a teacher.

PROM assessment (score presented graphically with cut-points highlighted):

- Functional ability: low scores on the BASFI (2/10) suggest mild functional limitation.
- Disease activity: low scores on the BASDAI (2/10) and pain VAS (1/10) suggest low levels of disease activity and pain respectively.
- General health status-profile: SF-36. High scores on all domains suggesting good general health. All scores are above the population mean.
- Scores on symptom scales are generally low with only minor problems noted on pain and fatigue scales – but these are unlikely to be of clinical significance
- HADS shows low scores – no emotional distress.

Actions taken:

- PROM scores assessed alongside other assessments.
- No major problems identified.
- No major problems reported by the patient.
- Continue with usual care and routine monitoring.

distributed between members of the multidisciplinary team, fostering information flow between different care providers and supporting the continuity of care. Demonstrating the cost effectiveness of incorporating PROM assessment into routine practice is essential to good practice, and to attracting the necessary resources to support more efficient data capture (Haywood et al 2008).

Members of the multidisciplinary team should be engaged in the development, selection and use of PROMs in routine practice. This will require training and support to foster the necessary change in assessment culture. It is essential that opportunities for further development of consensus around core sets, responder criteria, PROM development and selection are identified, and that patients and members of the wider multidisciplinary team contribute fully to this process. Further evaluation of the

---

BOX 4.6   Application of PROMs in routine practice: an illustration

PROM selection

■ The choice of PROM has been selected in advance and flagged in the appointment system so that the patient receives the appropriate PROM on arrival at the clinic.

PROM completion

■ The patient self-completes the PROM in the waiting area using a touch-screen computer tablet. Data are immediately fed to a central server.

PROM scoring

■ Data are analysed and fed-back to clinician (and patient) in time for the clinical appointment.

PROM feedback

■ Data are integrated with other clinical and demographic results and a customised presentation is provided.
■ Interpretation of PROM scores is supported by the provision of condition-specific and norm-based values. Cut-points (points at which scores significantly higher/lower than the norm) are highlighted on the print-out.

PROM interpretation and action plan

■ Scores suggestive of health-related problems are discussed between clinician and patients and a plan of action is agreed.
■ Referral to other health professionals is made where appropriate.
■ Data are also fed-back to other team members and used in a planned case-conference.

Monitoring

■ Patient-important outcomes are monitored longitudinally.

---

contribution of PROMs to routine practice is required that takes into account the roles of different members of the multidisciplinary team.

In summary patient-centred care and patient participation in decisions about health and healthcare are important goals of healthcare. Patient-reported outcome measures have the potential to enhance patient participation and patient-provider collaboration, providing information that is reliable, valid and of relevance to a range of stakeholders, thus supporting patient choice. However, challenges exist with regards to the selection, application and performance of PROMs, particularly in a routine practice setting. These challenges must be addressed if PROMs are to be more widely accepted as key sources of evidence of the impact of ill-health and treatment effectiveness, and a mechanism to enhance patient participation in routine practice.

References and further reading

Anderson, J., Baron, G., van der Heijde, D., et al., 2001. Ankylosing Spondylitis Assessment Group preliminary definition of short-term improvement in Ankylosing Spondylitis. Arthritis Rheum. 44, 1876–1886.

Appleby, J., Devlin, N., 2004. Measuring Success in the NHS. Using Patient-Assessed Health Outcomes to Manage the Performance of Healthcare Providers. King's Fund, London.

Ball, A.E., Russell, E.M., Seymour, D.G., et al., 2001. Problems in using health survey questionnaires in older patients with physical disabilities. Can proxies be used to complete the SF-36? Gerontology 47 (6), 334–340.

Bellamy, N., Kirwan, J., Boers, M., et al., 1997. Recommendations for a core set of outcome measures for future phase III clinical trials in knee, hip, and hand osteoarthritis.Consensus development at OMERACT III. J. Rheumatol. 24, 799–802.

Bellamy, N., 2005. Science of assessment. Ann. Rheum. Dis. 64 (Suppl 2), ii42–ii45.

Bellamy, N., Buchanan, W., Goldsmith, C., et al., 1988. Validation Study of WOMAC: a health status instrument for measuring clinically important patient relevant outcomes to antirheumatic drug therapy in patients with osteoarthritis of the hip or knee. J. Rheumatol. 15, 1833–1840.

Bellamy, N., 1999. Clinimetric concepts in outcome assessment: the OMERACT filter. J. Rheumatol. 26 (4), 948–950.

Bezjak, A., 2007. Logistics of Collecting Patient-Reported Outcomes (PROS) in Clinical Practice: an overview. Conference on Patient Reported Outcomes in Clinical Practice. International Society for Quality of Life Research. Budapest, Hungary, Proceedings, p13-14. 2007

Bombardier, C., 2000. Outcome assessments in the evaluation of treatment of spinal disorders. Spine 25, 3097–3103.

Bot, S.D.M., Terwee, C.B., Van der Windt, D.A.W.M., et al., 2004. Clinimetric evaluation of shoulder disability questionnaires: a systematic review of the literature. Ann. Rheum. Dis. 63, 335–341.

Brazier, J., Roberts, J., Tsuchiya, A., et al., 2004. A comparison of the EQ-5D and SF-6D across seven patient groups. Health Econ. 13, 873–884.

Bruce, B., Fries, J.F., 2003. The Stanford Health Assessment Questionnaire: a review of its history, issues, progress, and documentation J. Rheumatol. 30, 167–178.

Burke, L., Stifano, T., Dawisha, S., 2006. Guidance for Industry – Patient-Reported Outcome Measures : Use in Medical Product Development to Support Labelling Claims. U.S Department of Health and Human Sciences, Rockville, MD Food and Drug Administration.

Campbell, S.M., Roland, M.O., Buetow, S.A., 2000. Defining quality of care. Soc. Sci. Med. 51 (11), 1611–1625.

Carr, A.J., Thompson, P.W., 1994. Towards a measure of patient-perceived handicap in rheumatoid arthritis. Br. J. Rheumatol. 33, 378–382.

Chakravarty, E.F., Bjorner, J.B., Fries, J.F., 2007. Improving patient reported outcomes using item response theory and computerized adaptive testing. J. Rheumatol. 34 (6), 1426–1431.

Chorus, A.M., Miedema, H.S., Boonen, A., et al., 2003. Quality of life and work in patients with rheumatoid arthritis and ankylosing spondylitis of working age. Ann. Rheum. Dis. 62, 1178–1184.

Clancy, C.M., Lawrence, W., 2002. Is outcomes research on cancer ready for prime time? Med. Care 40, III92–III100.

Dagfinrud, H., Kjeken, I., Mowinckel, P., et al., 2005. Impact of functional impairment in ankylosing spondylitis: impairment, activity limitation, and participation restrictions J. Rheumatol. 32 (3), 516–523.

Donabedian, A., 1966. Evaluating the quality of medical care. Milbank Q. 44 (Suppl.), 166–206.

Donaldson, M., 2007. A non-visit approach to use of PROS in Oncology practice. Conference on Patient Reported Outcomes in Clinical Practice. International Society for Quality of Life Research. Budapest, Hungary, Proceedings, p14-15.

EuroQol-Group, 1990. EuroQol – A New Facility For The Measurement Of Health-Related Quality Of Life. The EuroQol Group. Health Policy 16, 199–208.

Escorpizo, R., Bombardier, C., Boonen., et al., 2007. Worker productivity outcome measures in arthritis J. Rheumatol. 34 (6), 1372–1380.

Fallowfield, L., Ratcliffe, D., Jenkins, V., et al., 2001. Psychiatric morbidity and its recognition by doctors in patients with cancer. Brit. J. Cancer 20 84 (8), 1011–1015.

Fallowfield, L., 2007. Training healthcare professionals in communication about PROS in clinical practice. Conference on Patient Reported Outcomes in Clinical Practice. International Society for Quality of Life Research. Budapest, Hungary, Proceedings, p15-16.

Finlay, A.Y., Coles, E.C., 1995. The effect of severe psoriasis on the quality of life of 369 patients. Brit. J. Dermatol. 132 (2), 236–244.

Fitzpatrick, R., Davey, C., Buxton, M. J., et al., 1998. Evaluating Patient-Based Outcome Measures for use in Clinical Trials. Health Technol. Assess. 2, I–Iv 1-74.

Fries, J.F., Spitz, P., Kraines, R.G., et al., 1980. Measurement of patient outcome in arthritis. Arthritis Rheum. 23, 137–145.

Ganz, P.A., 2002. What Outcomes Matter To Patients: A Physician-Researcher Point Of View. Med. Care 40 (III), I11–I119.

Ganiats, T., 2007. Content for PROS used in Clinical Practice: the clinician perspective. Conference on Patient Reported Outcomes in Clinical Practice. International Society for Quality of Life Research. Budapest, Hungary, Proceedings, p12-13.

Garratt, A., Schmidt, L., Mackintosh, A., et al., 2002. Quality of life measurement: bibliographic study of patient assessed health outcome measures. Brit. Med. J. 324, 1417–1421.

Garratt, A.M., Brealey, S., Gillespie, W.J., et al., 2004. Patient-assessed health instruments for the knee: a structured review. Rheumatology (Oxford) 43 (11), 1414–1423.

Garrett, S., Jenkinson, T., Kennedy, L., et al., 1994. A new approach to defining disease status in ankylosing spondylitis: The Bath ankylosing spondylitis disease activity index. J. Rheumatol. 21, 2286–2291.

Gilbody, S.M., Whitty, P.M., Grimshaw, J.M., et al., 2003. Improving the detection and management of depression in primary care. Qual. Saf. Health Care 12 (2), 149–155.

Giles, J.T., Mease, P., Boers, M., et al., 2007. Assessing single joints in arthritis clinical trials. J. Rheumatol. 34 (3), 641–647.

Gladman, D.D., Mease, P.J., Strand, V., et al., 2007. Consensus on a core set of domains for psoriatic arthritis. J. Rheumatol. 34 (5), 1167–1170.

Greenhalgh, J., Long, A.F., Flynn, R., 2005. The use of patient reported outcome measures in routine clinical practice: Lack of impact or lack of theory? Soc. Sci. Med. 60, 833–843.

Groves, T., Wagner, E.H., 2005. High quality care for people with chronic diseases. Brit. Med. J. 330, 609–610.

Haywood K.L., Garratt A.M., Carrivick, S.E., et al., 2009. Continence specialists use of quality of life information in routine practice: A national survey of practitioners. Quality of Life Research. May 18(4), 423-433.

Haywood, K.L., Garratt, A.M., Dziedzic, K., Dawes, P.T., 2002. Generic measures of health-related quality of life in ankylosing spondylitis: reliability, validity and responsiveness. Rheumatology (Oxford) 41 (12), 1380–1387.

Haywood, K.L., Garratt, A.M., Dziedzic, K., et al., 2003. Patient centered assessment of ankylosing spondylitis-specific health related quality of life: evaluation of the Patient Generated Index. J. Rheumatol. 30 (4), 764–773.

Haywood, K.L., Garratt, A.M., Dawes, P.T., 2005. Patient-assessed health in ankylosing spondylitis: a structured review. Rheumatology (Oxford) 44 (5), 577–586.

Haywood, K.L., 2006. Patient-reported outcome I: measuring what matters in musculoskeletal care. Musculoskeletal Care 4 (4), 187–203.

Haywood, K., Marshall, S., Fitzpatrick, R., 2006. Patient participation in the consultation process: a structured review of intervention strategies. Patient Educ. Couns. 63 (1-2), 12–23.

Haywood, K.L., Garratt, A. M., Carrivick, S., et al., 2008. Continence specialists use of

quality of life information in routine practice: a national survey of practitioners. Qual. Life Res. in press.

Hewlett, S., Smith, A.P., Kirwan, J.R., 2002. Measuring the meaning of disability in rheumatoid arthritis: the Personal Impact Health Assessment Questionnaire (PI HAQ). Ann. Rheum. Dis. 61 (11), 986–993.

Hewlett, S.A., 2003. Patients and clinicians have different perspectives on outcomes in arthritis. J. Rheumatol. 30, 877–879.

Hibbard, J.H., 2003. Engaging healthcare consumers to improve the quality of care. Med. Care 41, I-61–I-70.

Higginson, I.J., Carr, A.J., 2001. Measuring quality of life: Using quality of life measures in the clinical setting. Brit. Med. J. 322, 1297–1300.

Hobart, J.C., Riazi, A., Lamping, D.L., et al., 2004. Improving the evaluation of therapeutic interventions in multiple sclerosis: development of a patient-based measure of outcome. Health Technol. Assess. 8 (9), 1–48.

Jacobsen, P.B., Davis, K., Cella, D., 2002. Assessing quality of life in research and clinical practice. Oncology (Williston Park) 16 (9 Suppl 10), 133–139.

Keeling, S.O., Landewe, R., van der Heijde, D., et al., 2007. Testing of the preliminary OMERACT validation criteria for a biomarker to be regarded as reflecting structural damage endpoints in rheumatoid arthritis clinical trials: the example of C-reactive protein. J. Rheumatol. 34 (3), 623–633.

Kessler, L., Ramsey, S.D., 2002. The outcomes of the cancer outcomes research symposium: a commentary. Med. Care 40 (III), 104–108.

Kirwan, J.R., Hewlett, S., 2007. Patient perspective: reasons and methods for measuring fatigue in

rheumatoid arthritis. J. Rheumatol. 34 (5), 1171–1173.

Kirwan, J.R., Minnock, P., Adebajo, A., et al., 2007. Patient perspective: fatigue as a recommended patient centered outcome measure in rheumatoid arthritis. J. Rheumatol. 34 (5), 1174–1177.

Kristjansson, E., Tugwell, P.S., Wilson, A.J., et al., 2007. Development of the effective musculoskeletal consumer scale. J. Rheumatol. 34 (6), 1392–1400.

Kvien, T.K., Heiberg, T., 2003. Patient perspective in outcome assessments–perceptions or something more? J. Rheumatol. 30, 873–876.

Liang, M.H., 2004. Pushing the limits of patient-oriented outcome measurements in the search for disease modifying treatments for osteoarthritis. J. Rheumatol. 70, 61–65.

Lorig, K., Chastain, R.L., Ung, E., et al., 1989. Development and evaluation of a scale to measure perceived self-efficacy in people with arthritis. Arthritis Rheum. 32 (1), 37–44.

Marra, C.A., Esdaile, J.M., Guh, D., et al., 2004. A comparison of four indirect methods of assessing utility values in rheumatoid arthritis. Med. Care 42 (11), 1125–1131.

Marra, C.A., Woolcott, J.C., Kopec, J.A., et al., 2005. A comparison of generic, indirect utility measures (the HUI2, HUI3, SF-6D, and the EQ-5D) and disease-specific instruments (the RAQoL and the HAQ) in rheumatoid arthritis. Soc. Sci. Med. 60 (7), 1571–1582.

Marshall, S., Haywood, K., Fitzpatrick, R., 2006. Impact of patient-reported outcome measures on routine practice: A structured review. J. Eval. Clin. Pract. 12 (5), 559–568.

Martin, F., Camfield, L., Rodham, K., et al., 2007. Twelve years' experience with the Patient Generated Index (PGI) of quality of life: a graded structured review. Qual. Life Res. 16 (4), 705–715.

McDowell, I., 2006. Measuring Health: A Guide to Rating Scales and Questionnaires, third ed. Oxford University Press, New York.

McDowell, I., Newell, C., 1996. Measuring Health: A Guide to Rating Scales and Questionnaires, second ed. Oxford University Press, New York.

McGee, H.M., O'Boyle, C.A., Hickey, A., et al., 1991. Assessing the quality of life of the individual: the SEIQoL with a healthy and a gastroenterology unit population. Psychol. Med. 21 (3), 749–759.

McHorney, C.A., 2002. The potential clinical value of quality-of-life information response to Martin. Med. Care 40 (III), 56–62.

Meadows, K.A., Rogers, D., Greene, T., 1998. Attitudes to the use of health outcome questionnaires in the routine care of patients with diabetes: a survey of general practitioners and practice nurses. Brit. J. Gen. Pract. 48 (434), 1555–1559.

Mease, P., Arnold, L.M., Bennett, R., et al., 2007. Fibromyalgia syndrome. J. Rheumatol. 34 (6), 1415–1425.

Meenan, R.F., Mason, J.H., Anderson, J.J., et al., 1992. AIMS2. The content and properties of a revised and expanded arthritis impact measurement scales health status questionnaire. Arthritis Rheum. 35 (1), 1–10.

Merkel, P.A., Clements, P.J., Reveille, J.D., et al., 2003. Current status of outcome measure development for clinical trials in systemic sclerosis. J. Rheumatol. 30 (7), 1630–1647 Report from OMERACT 6.

Mitchell, P.H., Lang, N.M., 2004. Framing the problem of measuring and improving healthcare quality: has the quality health outcomes model been useful? Med. Care 42 (II), 4–11.

Morris, J., Perez, D., McNoe, B., 1998. The use of quality of life data in clinical practice. Qual. Life Res. 7, 85–91.

Neudert, C., Wasner, M., Borasio, G.D., 2001. Patients' assessment of quality of life instruments: a randomised study of SIP, SF-36 and SEIQoL-DW in patients with amyotrophic lateral sclerosis. J. Neurol. Sci. 191, 103–109.

Neumann, P.J., Araki, S.S., Gutterman, E.M., 2000. The use of proxy respondents in studies of older adults: lessons, challenges, and opportunities. J. Am. Geriatr. Soc. 48 (12), 1646–1654.

NICE, 2004. Guide to the Methods of Technological Appraisal. National Institute of Health and Clinical Excellence, London.

Patel, K., Veenstra, D., Patrick, D., 2003. A review of selected patient-generated outcome measures and their application in clinical trials. Value Health 6, 595–603.

Patrick, D.L., Chiang, Y.P., 2000. Measurement of health outcomes in treatment effectiveness evaluations: conceptual and methodological challenges. Med. Care 38 (III), 4–25.

Pham, T., Van Der Heijde, D., Lassere, M., et al., 2003. Outcome variables for osteoarthritis clinical trials: The OMERACT-OARSI set of responder criteria. J. Rheumatol. 30 (7), 1648–1654.

Pringle, D., Doran, D., 2003. Patient Outcomes as an Accountability. In: Doran, D.M. (Ed.), Nursing-Sensitive Outcomes. State of the Science. Jones and Bartlett Publishers, London, pp. 1–26.

Quest, E., Aanerud, G.J., Kaarud, S., et al., 2003. Patients' perspective. J. Rheumatol. 30 (4), 884–885.

Ramsey, S., 2002. What is cancer outcomes research? A diversity of perspectives for an emerging field. Med. Care 40 (Suppl. 6), III-1–III-2.

Raphael, D., Smith, T.F., Brown, I., et al., 1995. Development and properties of the short and brief versions of the Quality of Life Profile - Seniors Version. International Journal of Health Sciences 6, 161–168.

Rose, M., Bezjak, A., 2009. Logistics of collecting patient-reported outcomes (PROS) in clinical practice: An overview and practical examples. Qual. Life Res. Feb. 18(1), 125–136. Epub 2009 Jan 20.

Ruta, D., Garratt, A.M., Leng, M., et al., 1994. A new approach to the measurement of quality of life. The Patient-Generated Index. Med. Care 32 (11), 1109–1126.

Sambrook, P., 1997. Guidelines for osteoporosis trials. J. Rheumatol. 24, 1234–1236.

Skevington, S.M., Day, R., Chisholm, A., et al., 2005. How much do doctors use quality of life information in primary care? Testing the trans-theoretical model of behaviour change. Qual. Life Res. 14, 911–922.

Sloan, J.A., Cella, D., Hays, R.D., 2005. Clinical significance of patient-reported questionnaire data: another step toward consensus. J. Clin. Epidemiol. 58 (12), 1217–1219.

Smets, E.M., Garssen, M., et al., 1995. The Multidimensional Fatigue Inventory (MFI) psychometric qualities of an instrument to assess fatigue. J. Psychosom. Res. 39 (3), 315–325.

Smolen, J., Strand, V., Cardiel, M., et al., 1999. Randomized clinical trials and longitudinal observational studies in systemic lupus erythematosus: consensus on a preliminary core set of outcome domains. J. Rheumatol. 26 (2), 504–507.

Streiner, D., Norman, G., 2003. Health Measurement Scales: A Practical Guide To Their Development And Use 3rd edn. Oxford Medical Publications, Oxford.

Stucki, G., Boonen, A., Tugwell, P., et al., 2007. The World Health Organisation International Classification of Functioning, Disability and Health: a conceptual model and interface for the OMERACT process. J. Rheumatol. 34 (3), 600–606.

Tugwell, P., Bombardier, C., Buchanan, W.W., et al., 1987. The MACTAR patient preference disability questionnaire -an individualized functional priority approach for assessing improvement in physical disability in clinical trials in rheumatoid arthritis. J. Rheumatol. 14, 446–451.

Tugwell, P., Boers, M., 1993. Developing consensus on preliminary core efficacy endpoints for rheumatoid arthritis clinical trials. OMERACT committee. J. Rheumatol. 20 (3), 555–556.

Van der Heijde, D., Bellamy, N., Calin, A., et al., 1997. Preliminary core sets for endpoints in ankylosing spondylitis. Assessments in ankylosing spondylitis working group. J. Rheumatol. 24 (11), 2225–2229.

Van der Heijde, D., Van der Linden, S., Dougados, M., et al., 1999. Ankylosing spondylitis: plenary discussion and results of voting on selection of domains and some specific instruments. J. Rheumatol. 26 (4), 1003–1005.

Van Echteld, I., Cieza, A., Boonen, A., et al., 2006. Identification of the most common problems by patients with ankylosing spondylitis using the international classification of functioning, disability and health. J. Rheumatol. 33 (12), 2475–2483.

Van Stel, H.F., Van der Meer, V., Bakker, M.J., et al., 2007. Internet based self-monitoring in adults with asthma using the asthma control questionnaire. Conference on patient reported outcomes in clinical practice. International Society for Quality of Life Research. Budapest, Hungary. Proceedings: Abstract 133.

van Tubergen, A., van der Heijde, D., Anderson, J., et al., 2003. Comparison of statistically derived ASAS improvement criteria for ankylosing spondylitis with clinically relevant improvement according to an expert panel. Ann. Rheum. Dis. 62 (3), 215–221.

Varni, J.W., Burwinkle, T.M., Lane, M.M., 2005. Health-related quality of life measurement in pediatric clinical practice: an appraisal and precept for future research and application. Health Qual. Life Outcomes 16 (3), 34.

Varni, J.W., Burwinkle, T.M., Limbers, C.A., et al., 2007. The PedsQL as a patient-reported outcome in children and adolescents with fibromyalgia: an analysis of OMERACT domains. Health Qual. Life Outcomes 12 (5), 9.

Velikova, G., Booth, L., Smith, A.B., et al., 2004. Measuring Quality of Life in routine oncology practice improves communication and patient well-being: A Randomized Controlled Trial. J. Clin. Oncol. 22, 714–724.

Wade, D.T., de Jong, B.A., 2000. Recent advances in rehabilitation. Brit. Med. J. 320 (7246), 1385–1388.

Ware, J., 1997. SF-36 Health Survey. Manual Interpretation Guide. Minrod Press.

Ware, J.E., Kosinski, M., Dewey, J.E., 2002. How to Score Version Two of the SF-36 Health Survey (Standard and Acute Forms). Quality Metric Inc, Lincoln, RI.

WHO, 2001. International Classification of functioning, disability and health. World Health Organisation, ICF. Geneva.

WHOQol Group, 1994. The Development Of The World Health Organisation Quality of Life Assessment Instrument (The WHOQol). In: Orley, J., Kuyken, W. (Eds.) Quality of Life Assessment: International Perspectives. Springer-Verlag, Berlin, pp. 41–47.

Wiebe, S., Guyatt, G., Weaver, B., et al., 2003. Comparative responsiveness of generic and specific quality-of-life instruments. J. Clin. Epidemiol. 56, 50–52.

Zebrack, B., 2007. The use and utility of patient-reported outcomes: reflections from a cancer survivor and research scientist. Conference on Patient Reported Outcomes in Clinical Practice. International Society for Quality of Life Research. Budapest, Hungary. Proceedings: p10-11.

Zigmond, A.S., Snaith, R.P., 1983. The Hospital Anxiety and Depression Scale. Acta Psychiat. Scand. 67, 361–370.

Chapter 5

Applying the biopsychosocial model to the management of rheumatic disease

Sarah Ryan RGN PhD MSc BSc FRCN Staffordshire Rheumatology Centre, Haywood Hospital, Stoke on Trent NHS Primary Care Trust, Stoke on Trent, UK

Alison Carr PhD Nottingham University, City Hospital, Nottingham, UK

CHAPTER CONTENTS

KEY POINTS

- Living with a rheumatological condition has the potential to impact on physical, psychological and social function.
- Adopting a biopsychosocial approach can provide a framework to identify the impact of illness.
- Chronic pain is a multifaceted experience with sensory, affective and cognitive components.
- Psychological models help to explain health behaviour.
- Understanding health behaviour can enhance adherence with treatment and improve outcome.

INTRODUCTION

Living with a chronic condition, such as rheumatoid arthritis (RA), impacts all functional domains. Health professionals help patients develop coping skills to minimise the condition's effects on physical and psychological wellbeing. To do this effectively health professionals must understand why and how people adopt or reject certain health behaviours. By utilising the biopsychosocial model of care, illness impact on physical, psychological and social aspects of function is addressed and a wider range of therapeutic options offered that have meaning and relevance to the individual.

This chapter is divided into four sections addressing: the biopsychosocial model; the impact of arthritis; pain; and social cognition models that help explain health behaviour.

SECTION 1: THE BIOPSYCHOSOCIAL MODEL AND ITS IMPORTANCE IN ARTHRITIS MANAGEMENT

Recognition that understanding patient's beliefs, feelings, thoughts and health behaviour is necessary to aid our understanding of the patient's condition has led to a move from a disease model to a biopsychosocial model of care, which acknowledges the importance of psychological and social factors as well as the physical impact of living with arthritis. For example, physical impact can include symptoms of pain, stiffness and fatigue. Psychological effects may include feelings of frustration, low mood and give rise to concerns about the future, whilst social implications can include concerns about work, role within the family and continuing to engage in valued leisure activities.

Adopting a biopsychosocial approach to care has increased the range of therapeutic options for patients. Cognitive behavioural therapy (CBT), which aims to identify and change maladaptive patterns of thought and behaviour, is of benefit in patients with RA. In newly diagnosed RA patients, CBT improves a patient's sense of control regarding their condition and prevents development of negative illness perceptions (Sharpe et al 2003). CBT is also useful for patients with depression (Parker et al 2003).

Other psychological interventions involve improving confidence in carrying out specific behaviours, i.e. self efficacy, which will be discussed in Section 4. If a person believes they can play an active role in managing some of the impact of their condition, through employing strategies such as pacing, goal setting and exercise, they are more likely to do so than a patient with little or no such confidence. Active self-management is associated with higher levels of adherence. Even if the intended goal is not achieved, the process of striving for it leads to better outcomes (Jerant 2005).

Involving significant others in care management can also have a positive effect on outcomes. If the family is unaware why an individual is encouraged to pace their activities, this may be perceived as 'laziness' and lead to family conflict. Spouses of patients attending an education programme to increase their knowledge of RA experienced a change in their perceptions towards the condition, which were largely negative before the programme (Phelan et al 1994). The importance of the family on outcome was illustrated in a study of the benefits of behavioural interventions to minimise pain in patients with RA. Intervention incorporating family support was more effective in reducing pain than the intervention with the family alone (Radojenic et al 1992). Adopting a biopsychosocial model of care ensures all factors influencing a patient's ability to manage and cope with their condition can be identified and, where possible, addressed.

SECTION 2: THE IMPACT OF RHEUMATOLOGICAL CONDITIONS

Patients are individuals with a life history, beliefs, standards and expectations (Bendor 1999). RA cannot be considered solely in terms of its physical consequences. The potential psychological, social and economic impact must be considered.

WORK

Work disability can occur early in arthritis (Fex et al 1998). People with a musculoskeletal condition are more likely to stop working if they:

- are older
- are female
- have fewer years in education
- have pain and co-morbidity
- have limitations in function.

(Yelin 1995)

Cox (2004), focusing on the needs of newly diagnosed RA patients, found that being able to continue working was a major concern: 'The only question I could think of, is the question I really want answering - am I going to get back to work full-time?'. A National Rheumatoid Arthritis Society (2003) survey showed 54% of participants attributed not being in full-time work to RA and 30% of employed participants worked part-time because of RA. Mancuso et al (2000) found those seemingly successfully employed still faced major challenges, made major adaptations in order to stay at work and still perceived their jobs to be in jeopardy.

Early intervention through liaison with employers, consideration of alternative ways of working, work place assessment and if necessary retraining is important to keep patients at work (see Ch. 9: Occupational therapy). Vocational issues that may need considering are shown in Box 5.1.

LEISURE

Engaging in a specific leisure activity will be influenced by the individual's level of motivation, and the belief participation can be done to a reasonable standard. The physical and psychological impact of arthritis, such as pain, reduced muscle strength, fatigue and reduced self esteem, may hinder both the desire and ability to partake in leisure. Many difficulties are faced participating in leisure (Fex et al 1998, Hakkinen et al 2003, Wikstrom et al 2005). Inaccessible facilities, lack of transport, absence of support or negative attitudes from others may all impact negatively on leisure (Specht et al 2002).

MOOD

Depression in RA is 2–3 times higher than in the general population (Dickens & Creed 2001). Data from baseline co-morbidity levels in over 7,000 patients starting biologic treatments found 19% had a formal diagnosis of depression at any one time (Hyrich et al 2006).

Depression in RA is linked to:

- pain
- functional disability:
- work disability
- poor adherence to treatment
- lack of social support
- low confidence in the ability to manage symptoms
- high daily stresses

(Dickens & Creed 2001, Lowe et al 2004, Sheehy et al. 2006).

If depression is suspected it must be assessed and treated. It is not acceptable to acknowledge it is associated with RA and not treat it. In Stoke-on-Trent in the UK, a combined liaison psychiatry clinic run by a liaison psychiatrist and a rheumatology nurse consultant assesses for mental health problems and advises on appropriate treatment. For depression this involves anti-depressants and/or CBT.

SOCIAL SUPPORT

Interpersonal relationships contribute to physical, psychological and social state wellbeing. Through our social support systems we validate beliefs, emotions, action and seek information and advice. Core activities carried out within social networks include:

- Instrumental activities–cooking, cleaning, financial management and shopping.
- Nurturing activities–making family arrangements, maintaining family ties, looking after family members and listening to others.

Ryan et al (2003) demonstrated that patients wanted to remain active in both domains. Aspects of social support enhancing control perceptions include:

- remaining active in family activities
- receiving ongoing support from family members (and not just at the time of increased activity such as a 'flare' of the condition)
- achieving a balance between support needs and support provision.

Many inflammatory conditions are characterised by unpredictability regarding symptom occurrence, treatment efficacy and overall prognosis. Different levels of support will be required from health professionals related to patients' identified needs (Box 5.2).

BOX 5.1   Vocational issues (Gordon et al 1997)

- Flexible hours
- Self paced activities
- Shortened working weeks
- Working at home
- Rest/work schedule
- Equipment and modifications to aid employment
- Work space design and adaptation of the work environment

BOX 5.2   Support that health professionals can provide

- Cognitive-discussing the individual's thoughts about the situation
- Affective-exploring the emotions connected to the situation
- Instrumental-e.g. arranging for a home assessment and OT to evaluate and discuss problems in situ
- Informational-providing advice on how to manage a specific symptom, such as pain.

SEXUALITY AND BODY IMAGE

Sexuality is an individual self-concept expressed as feelings, attitude, beliefs and behaviour (RCN 2000). RA features which impact negatively on sexuality and body image include joint pain and stiffness, fatigue, low mood, physical changes and treatment visibility, including splints (Hill et al 2003). Patients indicate they would like the opportunity to discuss sexuality concerns with healthcare professionals (Hill et al 2003) but due to a lack of privacy, time, knowledge and skills, this often does not occur. Many types of arthritis extensively affect people's lives. Living with chronic pain considerably contributes to this.

SECTION 3: PAIN

Pain is an unpleasant sensory and emotional experience associated with actual or potential tissue damage, or described in terms of such damage (International Association for the Study of Pain (IASP) 1994). It is a common symptom across rheumatic conditions. It is a unique, subjective and unverifiable person experience (Turk & Melzack 1992). Acute pain is often transient and the source of pain is identifiable and treatable, e.g. active synovitis of the knee. Chronic pain is an ongoing experience associated with a plethora of other symptoms including anxiety, depression and sleep disturbance.

Patients with RA cite pain as their most important symptom (Minnock et al, 2003). Pain is associated with impaired quality of life, depression and disability in both RA and OA (Spranglers et al 2000). Chronic pain in fibromyalgia results in reduced physical activities, increased mood symptoms, withdrawal from the workplace and increased use of health care services (Hughes et al 2006). When helping patients manage their pain, a biopsychosocial model aids fully comprehending the pain experience and enables planning care that is meaningful for the patient.

PAIN MECHANISMS

The 'specificity theory' attributed to Descartes in 1664 reflects early understanding of pain mechanisms. In this model, skin pain receptors are activated by a painful stimulus and messages conveyed to the brain enabling action to be taken, e.g. removing the hand from a fire. Pain is purely a physical phenomenon with a direct relationship between the amount of stimulation (damage) to nociceptors

and pain experienced. But this does not explain the variation in pain experience for a given stimulus or injury. Why do some patients take longer to recover from whiplash than others? Why does pain persist beyond the time of tissue healing?

Melzack and Wall's gate control theory of pain (1965) revolutionised understanding of pain mechanisms (Fig. 5.1). This demonstrated that the transmission of pain messages could be modulated within the spinal cord via descending messages from the brain (our cognitions and emotions) or altered by activating another source of sensory receptor (e.g. exercise to release endorphins).

PAIN RECEPTORS

Sensory receptors are situated in the tissues of the skin, synovium of joints and arterial walls. These are activated by various stimuli including:

- mechanical changes: increased synovial fluid in the joint cavity and proliferation of the inflamed synovial tissues causes pain by distension and stretching of the capsule
- temperature changes
- inflammatory changes: the release of prostaglandin, bradykinin, histamine and serotonin.

Peripheral sensory nerves transmit signals from the peripheries to the central nervous system enabling stimulus identification. Alpha delta fibres (thin and myelinated) transmit the sharp pain of an acute injury and slower C-fibres (unmyelinated) produce the dull aching pain of a more persistent problem or the burning quality of neuropathic pain (McCabe 2004).

Sensory nerves deliver information from the peripheries to the dorsal horn where they terminate.

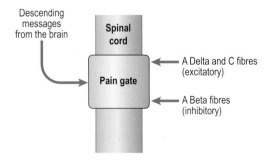

Figure 5.1 A simplified diagram of the gate control theory of pain.

This information is then interpreted by transmission cells (T-cells) transmitting information to the local reflex circuits and the brain. When the Alpha delta and C fibres are stimulated T cells are activated resulting in the substantia gelatinosa (SG) being suppressed so that the 'pain gate' opens and messages pass to the brain to be perceived as pain. When large fibres become activated (Alpha beta) they suppress T cell activity and close the gate. Alpha beta fibres transmit the sensation of touch. Acupuncture and electrical nerve stimulation work on the same principle and excite large fibre activity. Nerve impulses descending from the brain can also operate 'the gate'.

CASE STUDY 5.1   POSSIBLE PAIN PATHWAYS IN A CASE STUDY OF A PATIENT WITH RA (BASED ON AN EXAMPLE BY McCABE 2004)

Mrs Jones is a 44-year-old women diagnosed with RA 5 years ago. She works as a legal assistant in a busy law firm. She has had to take time off which is worrying her. Mrs Jones is married with no children. Over the last 3 months she has experienced more early morning stiffness (from 30 minutes to 2 hours) and has pain and inflammation in both wrists and her right knee. Mrs Jones describes her pain as 'burning and tender to touch'. The pain disturbs her sleep and she has difficulty with mobility.

Peripheral mechanisms

The inflammatory process (demonstrated by swelling, pain and stiffness) has generated peripheral sensitization. Reporting burning pain indicates activation of the C fibres or changes in the dorsal horn resulting in central sensitization. Problems with mobility may be due to changes in knee intra–articular pressure.

Central mechanisms

Generalised tenderness indicates a lowering of the Alpha beta fibre threshold and may have been induced by the duration of symptoms. Changes in proprioception due to knee swelling may create a mismatch in the motor and sensory systems. This mechanism has been proposed as an explanation for the perception of stiffness in RA (Haigh et al 2003). Other factors that may influence Mrs Jones' pain are her lack of sleep and work concerns.

PERIPHERAL AND CENTRAL SENSITIZATION

The gate theory of pain is portrayed as a hard-wired system but we know this is not the case (McCabe 2004). If persistent stimulation occurs the Alpha delta and C fibres will be activated by weak non-noxious stimuli (Devor & Seltzer 1999). This sensitization occurs in the peripheries due to tissue damage or release of chemical inflammatory mediators (e.g. substance P) into the skin from damaged C fibres and the increase in the activity of calcium channels within the spinal cord. The presence of allodynia (pain from a non noxious stimuli) and hyperalgesia (increased response to a painful stimulus) can occur due to a lowering in the Alpha beta threshold so that pain now becomes a painful stimulus (McCabe 2004).

Pain is affected by many physical, psychological and social factors. Effective pain control using a variety of approaches is thus essential in biopsychosocial management of arthritis. These approaches are discussed in subsequent chapters.

SECTION 4: HEALTH BEHAVIOUR, COPING AND CONCORDANCE

Health behaviour refers to the ways in which people with arthritis perceive, understand and manage their condition. Understanding factors affecting health behaviours, coping and concordance helps maximise effective biopsychosocial management. Influences on health behaviours include:

- demographic factors, e.g. age, gender, culture, socio-economic
- social and environmental factors: e.g. access to care and societal attitudes to illness and treatment
- personal factors, e.g. personality, emotions and cognitions.

There are several psychological models, known as social cognition models, developed to predict and explain health behaviour. The most commonly used are:

- Health belief model (HBM)
- Health locus of control (HLC)
- Social cognitive theory
- Theory of planned behaviour (TPB)
- Self-regulatory model (SRM)

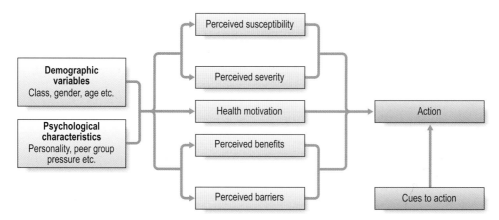

Figure 5.2 The health belief model (adapted from Abraham and Sheeran 2005).

THE HEALTH BELIEF MODEL

This model is based on two aspects of health behaviour (Fig. 5.2):

1. The perception of threats to health based on an estimation of perceived susceptibility to illness and severity of illness consequences.
2. An evaluation of the behaviour required to avoid/ reduce these threats including the benefits, efficacy and costs of engaging in health behaviours.

Cues to action can trigger performance of health behaviours if the underlying beliefs about threat perception and behavioural evaluation are favourable (Becker et al 1977).

   Take, for example, a patient whose RA is affecting ability to work. They believe that without some form of drug treatment they will become progressively disabled (high threat). They know there are several treatment options. Despite concerns about medications (costs) they believe some are very effective (benefits). Media reports of a new wonder treatment for RA may prompt them to seek treatment (cues to action).

   The HBM has been used as a basis for the Beliefs about Medicine Questionnaire (Horne et al 1999). This focuses on the perceived threat of illness and medication and the consequences of taking or not taking medication. It has been used to explain/ predict adherence to medication. For example, if arthritis pain is perceived as severe and medication is perceived as effective and relatively safe, patients are more likely to take it to manage their pain (Horne, Mitchell, Weinman, 2001 personal communication).

HEALTH LOCUS OF CONTROL

The Health Locus of Control model is based on Rotter's Social Learning Theory (Rotter 1954). It proposes that health behaviours are predicted by the extent to which an individual believes they can perform the behaviour and that it will be effective. Individuals with an internal locus of control (LOC) are more likely to take action to manage their symptoms than an individual with more external LOC who believes their symptoms are a result of chance and looks to other sources, such as the doctor, to manage their symptoms. However, this model has been tested in a wide range of therapeutic areas with conflicting results.

   The most widely used measure is the Multiple Health Locus of Control (MHLC) Scale (Wallston et al 1978), evaluating beliefs about health behaviours in general, and the variance in results might relate to individuals holding different beliefs depending on the situation. For example, an individual might have a high internal LOC for weight loss (i.e. they believe they are responsible and have the ability to reduce their weight) but a high external LOC for managing their arthritis, believing this is the doctor's responsibility. Ryan et al (2003) found that within a medical consultation, contrary to the HLC model, an external LOC increased the patient's perceived control over their ability to live with their arthritis. This may be because patients view their condition as too unpredictable and mutifacted to manage without external professional support and view the consultation as a partnership where their issues could be voiced and management appropriate to their needs provided.

In an attempt to make the HLC a stronger predictor of health behaviour it has been adapted to include: the value the individual places on their health and the extent to which an individual is confident in carrying out behaviours they believe will be effective. In other words, for an individual to engage in health behaviour, such as exercise, they need to value their health, believe they are responsible for it, be confident they can exercise and believe exercise will be effective.

SOCIAL COGNITIVE THEORY

In this model health behaviour is seen as the result of three sets of beliefs:

1. Beliefs that there are consequences to threats or events that occur without personal involvement or action (situational-outcome expectancies). This involves an evaluation of the health risk and individual's perception of their susceptibility to that risk.
2. Beliefs that behaviour will result in specific outcomes (action-outcome expectancies).
3. Beliefs that behaviours are within the individual's control and they have the ability to perform the behaviour (self-efficacy).

Self-efficacy (SE) has a direct effect on behaviour: an individual's beliefs that he/she can perform a behaviour predict performance of it. It can also influence intention to perform a behaviour. Studies have demonstrated individuals intend to perform behaviours they are confident they can achieve (Bandura 1992, Schwarzer 1992).

Self-efficacy has been widely applied in arthritis to:

1. Explain health behaviours: a high SE for medication and exercise improves adherence to medicines and leads to participation in exercise.
2. Understand the relationship between physical and psychological factors e.g. a higher SE is related to less pain, joint stiffness and fatigue, improved function and better mood.
3. As a basis for interventions to help patients manage or cope with their arthritis.

Questionnaire measures of self-efficacy include the

- Generalised Self-Efficacy Scale (GSES) (Barlow et al 1996): measures belief in ability across a range of situations and is not specific to musculoskeletal pain.
- Arthritis Self-Efficacy Scale (Barlow et al 1997): assesses self-efficacy in people with arthritis and has three subscales: belief in ability to control pain, function and other symptoms.
- Rheumatoid Arthritis Self-Efficacy Scale (RASE) (Hewlett et al 2001): evaluates individuals' beliefs in their ability to perform specific health behaviours rather than their actual ability or their outcome expectancy.

THEORY OF PLANNED BEHAVIOUR

The Theory of Planned Behaviour (TPB) is an extension of the Theory of Reasoned Action (TRA) (Fishbein & Ajzen 1975, Ajzen & Fishbein 1980). Both models are based on the premise that individuals make logical, reasoned decisions to engage in specific behaviours by evaluating the information available to them. The performance of a behaviour is determined by the individual's intention to engage in it (influenced by the value the individual places on the behaviour, the ease with which it can be performed and the views of significant others) and the perception that the behaviour is within his/her control. In RA a TPB model based on attitudes, social support, self efficacy and intention was moderately successful in predicting and explaining self management of arthritis (Strating et al 2006). Whilst no validated questionnaires are available, a comprehensive guide to developing measures of TPB components is given in Ajzen (1991). A challenge in TPB measurement is the difficulty in conceptualising and capturing attitudes.

THE SELF–REGULATORY MODEL AND ILLNESS BELIEFS

The Self-Regulatory model (SRM) (Leventhal et al 1997) describes how biological, psychological and social factors interact to influence how individuals perceive their symptoms and illness and the health behaviours they subsequently adopt (Fig. 5.3). These perceptions, or illness representations, are a set of beliefs, emotions and disease experiences which individuals use to evaluate information about their disease and to regulate their subsequent behaviour. The SRM differs from the other social cognition models in placing equal importance on the emotional reaction to health threats.

Studies of people's illness representations have identified five categories of illness beliefs:

- Symptoms/identity (recognising the symptoms as associated with illness)

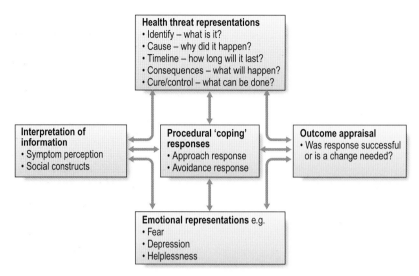

Figure 5.3 The self-regulatory model (adapted from Hobro et al 2004).

- Timeline (beliefs about how long the illness will last)
- Consequences (beliefs about the outcome of the illness)
- Control/cure (beliefs about the extent to which the illness can be treated/controlled and the role of the individual in managing the illness)
- Causes (beliefs about the causes of illness).

The illness perceptions questionnaire (IPQ) (Weinman et al 1996) was originally developed to quantify these. It has been used to understand patients' responses to illness and predict or explain treatment adherence. It has since been revised to improve its psychometric properties (Moss-Morris et al 2002) and consists of eight categories:

- symptoms/identity
- timeline acute/chronic
- timeline cyclical
- consequences
- personal control
- treatment control
- emotional representations (emotional responses to the illness)
- coherence (the extent to which patients understand or comprehend illness).

In addition to use in research, it could be used in practice to identify misperceptions of treatment/illness or lack of understanding affecting adherence to treatment/lifestyle advice that might be addressed through educational interventions.

COMMONALITIES BETWEEN THE SOCIAL COGNITION MODELS (SCMs)

Whilst there are many similarities between these, the main differences are the underlying psychological theory. There are specific patient-completed questionnaires available to capture each construct and they can be, and often are, used in combination. However, this is not always helpful. For example, in a study of patients with either OA or RA self-efficacy, but not locus of control, was associated with health status in patients with RA, whilst in patients with OA, locus of control was a better predictor of health status (Cross et al 2006). It is unclear how findings can be meaningfully interpreted in a clinical setting. Moreover, interventions aimed at changing behaviour (such as promoting exercise, increasing medication adherence) may draw on several SCMs. The most commonly applied theories are Social Cognitive Theory and the Health Belief Model, with increasing interest in the Self-Regulatory Model.

HEALTH BEHAVIOURS (COPING, CONCORDANCE, HEALTH BELIEFS)

Coping

Coping is the ability to generate and maintain psychological well-being despite living with a serious condition (Folkman 1997) and is linked to better psychological adjustment outcomes (Smith et al 1997).

People with arthritis live with the physical, social and economic consequences of the disease over long periods and may have to cope with uncertainty about long term outcome as well as unpredictability of recurrent fluctuations in disease activity. How people with RA cope has been shown to influence current and long-term psychological and physical adjustment (Burckhardt et al 1997, Smith & Wallston 1992, Smith et al 1997, Zautra & Manne 1992).

Coping behaviours have been extensively studied in chronic disease and are typically classified as active (good) coping strategies, such as information-seeking and self management, and passive (bad) coping strategies, such as catastrophising and wishful thinking. In arthritis studies, effective coping has been equated with perceived control over arthritis and its impact on daily life (Felton & Revenson 1984) and with self efficacy for pain and other arthritis symptoms (Keefe et al 1997, Lefebvre et al 1999). Coping behaviours are influenced by the individual's appraisal of the threat and the coping options available. Whilst it is assumed that active coping behaviours are more effective in helping patients adapt to and manage their condition, there is more evidence to support ineffectiveness of passive coping.

Questionnaires which identify coping strategies:

- Ways of coping scale (Folkman & Lazarus 1988): a 42-item questionnaire assessing three coping domains: emotion-focused coping, problem-focused coping and the seeking of social support (Felton & Revenson 1984).
- Coping strategies questionnaire (Rosenstiel & Keefe 1983): a 44-item questionnaire with seven subscales and two effectiveness items assessing pain coping strategies. Subscales are grouped into Active (coping self-statements, diverting attention, ignoring pain sensations, interesting activity level and reinterpreting the pain sensation) and Passive coping (catastrophising praying and hoping)
- Arthritis Helplessness Index (Nicassio et al 1985): a 15-item disease-specific measure of coping measuring perceptions of ability to control arthritis.
- London Coping with Rheumatoid Arthritis scale (Newman et al 1990): has 36 coping strategy items assessing frequency of use. Results are used to identify and group individuals with similar coping patterns rather than pre-defining if each coping strategy alone is helpful or unhelpful.

Concordance

Concordance describes a partnership between the health professional and patient in which both work together to agree optimal treatment based on a balance of treatment risks and benefits and compatibility with the patient's goals and preferences. Concordance is increasingly used instead of 'compliance' which is viewed as excluding patients from being equal partners in treatment decisions. It is unclear how frequently concordance occurs in clinical practice. It is limited by many factors including:

- Difficulties interpreting information about relative risks and benefits of treatment (for both health professionals and patients)
- Lack of training for health professionals in achieving concordance
- Lack of time and resources
- Some patients do not want an active role in treatment decision making.

Treatment decisions based on concordance may increase effective use of treatment.

Between 30–70% of patients take their medication according to the prescribed regimen (Conrad 1985, Donovan & Blake 1992, Hill et al 2001, Viller et al 1999). Figures are similar for non-pharmacological interventions such as exercise (O'Reilly et al 1999). Factors influencing how patients use treatments are complex and often independent of age, gender or disease severity (Kraag et al 1994, Rejeski et al 1997). They include:

- patients' beliefs about disease and treatments
- patients' expectations of treatment
- use of alternative healthcare (e.g. complementary therapies)
- interpretation of the risks of treatment
- the quality of the relationship between patient and doctor
- patients' knowledge and understanding of treatment
- treatment factors such as the complexity of the regimen e.g. adherence with weekly bisphosphonates in osteoporosis is higher than with daily bisphosphonates (Carr et al 2006).

Patient health beliefs about disease and treatment

Many patients with RA and OA do not initially interpret their symptoms as evidence of disease but instead attribute them to stress, or more commonly, normalise them in terms of their age and activities (Goodwin et al 1999, Hampson 1994, Sakalys 1997). Even where patients interpret their symptoms as evidence of underlying disease, their family, friends and even health professionals may not. In a study of newly referred patients with RA, more than 50% reported that family, friends or doctors had normalised, minimised or disbelieved their symptoms (Sakalys 1997).

RA patients' beliefs have been associated with medication use (Neame & Hammond 2005). In general, patients perform cost–benefit analyses on their prescribed medication (Donovan 1991) and are more likely to take this when their perception of the necessity for medication (effectiveness and the perceived consequences of untreated illness) outweighs concerns about it (side-effects, addiction and development of tolerance) (Horne & Weinman 1999, Neame & Hammond 2005). Sixty percent of patients with RA report fear of side-effects is a major factor influencing their decisions to alter dose or frequency (Donovan & Blake 1992). Patients often allow themselves a 'trial of treatment' during which they adhere to the treatment regimen, evaluating its effectiveness against their beliefs and expectations (Donovan & Blake 1992). Where outcome does not meet expectations, they may be more likely to change regimen or stop treatment.

THE CLINICAL CONSULTATION

High levels of non-adherence may occur if interventions have not addressed underlying health and treatment beliefs driving patient behaviour. It would be useful within the clinical consultation if patients' beliefs about illness and treatment are elicited, their expectations of treatment are identified and realistic treatment goals negotiated (Carr & Donovan 1998, Horne 1999). A consultation guide has been developed based on the evidence for factors influencing adherence (Daltroy 1993) but its effectiveness in promoting adherence or concordance has not been evaluated (Box 5.3).

Concordance, i.e. an equal partnership between patient and health professional in which treatment goals are negotiated on the basis of patient preference and priorities, is promoted by addressing these.

Questionnaires for assessing adherence and concordance

Whilst useful in identifying how patients take their medicines (de Klerk et al 1999), their usefulness in

---

> **BOX 5.3   Stepwise model of a consultation to improve adherence (from Daltroy 1993)**
>
> Step 1 The patient is encouraged to express all concerns
> Step 2 The patients' concerns are discussed
> Step 3 Doctor and patient share their models (beliefs) of disease and symptoms
> Step 4 Doctor and patient share their goals for treatment
> Step 5 Treatment goals are agreed and priorities are set
> Step 6 Doctor and patient share their models (beliefs) of treatment
> Step 7 Potential barriers to adherence are identified
> Step 8 Plans are made to overcome these
> Step 9 The doctor provides written information on disease and the treatment regimen, annotated with individual patients' detail/concerns

---

> **STUDY ACTIVITIES**
>
> - Take a case history from a patient with a rheumatological condition and identity its psychological and social impact using a biopsychosocial approach.
> - Using the gate control theory of pain, record how you would explain to a patient how their thoughts can affect their perception of pain.
> - After reading section 4, list the factors that may influence whether a patient will engage in a specific health behaviour, such as exercise.

---

promoting adherence is limited because they provide little information about why patients take their medications in this way, or why they choose not to follow their prescribed treatment regimen at all. Established, validated questionnaires that elicit some of the health beliefs underlying adherence can be used to identify misperceptions and reasons for non-adherence. These include the IPQ and IPQ-R (Moss-Morris et al 2002, Weinman et al 1996) and the Beliefs about Medication Questionnaire (Horne et al 1999).

Understanding theories of health behaviour and factors influencing coping and concordance enhance effectiveness of treatment and planning and delivering effective patient education.

CONCLUSION

The ways in which people with arthritis perceive, understand and manage their condition, how active they are, which treatments they use, whether and how they take their prescribed medication and how they cope with the symptoms of their arthritis, are influenced by a complex interaction of many factors. By increasing the health professional's knowledge in this area a relationship based on concordance principles can be introduced into clinical care and patients will be able to cope more effectively with the physical, psychological and social impact of their condition.

References and further reading

Abraham, C., Sheeran, P., 2005. The health belief model. In: Conner, M., Norman, P. (Eds.) Predicting Health Behaviour. Open University Press, Milton Keynes, pp. 28–80.

Ajzen, A., Fishbein, M., 1980. Understanding Attitudes and Predicting Social Behaviour. Prentice-Hall, Englewood Cliffs, NJ.

Ajzen, I., 1991. The theory of planned behaviour. Organ. Behav. Hum. Dec. Process. 50, 179–211.

Bandura, A., 1992. Self-efficacy mechanism in psychobiologic functioning. In: Schwarzer, R. (Ed.), Self-efficacy: Thought control of action. Hemisphere, Washington DC, pp. 335–394.

Barlow, J.H., Williams, B., Wright, C., 1996. The generalised self-efficacy scale in people with arthritis. Arthritis. Care Res. 9 (3), 189–196.

Barlow, J.H., Williams, B., Wright, CC., 1997. The reliability and validity of the arthritis self-efficacy scale in a UK context. Psychol. Health Med. 2 (1), 3–17.

Becker, M.H., Haefner, D.P., Kasl, S.V., et al., 1977. Selected psychosocial models and correlates of individual health-related behaviours. Med. Care 15, 27–46.

Bendor, R., 1999. Arthritis and I. Ann. Intern. Med. 131 (2), 150–152.

Burckhardt, C., Clark, S., O'Reilly, S., Bennett, R., 1997. Pain coping strategies of women with fibromyalgia: Relationship to pain, fatigue and quality of life. J. Musculoskelet. Pain 5 (3), 5–21.

Carr, A.J., Donovan, J.L., 1998. Why doctors and patients disagree. Br.J. Rheumatol. 37, 1–6.

Carr, A.J., Thompson, P.W., Cooper, C., 2006. Factors associated with adherence and persistence to bisphosphonate therapy in osteoporosis: a cross-sectional survey. Osteoporos. Int. 17 (11), 1638–1644.

Conrad, P., 1985. The meaning of medications: another look at compliance. Soc. Sci. Med. 20, 29–37.

Cox, M., 2004. The development of a user led clinical service for newly diagnosed RA patients. Musculoskel. Care 2 (4), 229–239.

Cross, M., March, L., Lapsley, H., et al., 2006. Patient self-efficacy and health locus of control: relationships with health status and arthritis-related expenditure. Rheumatology 45 (1), 92–96.

Daltroy, L.H., 1993. Doctor patient communication in rheumatological disorders. Bailliere's Clin. Rheumatol. 7, 221–239.

De Klerk, E., van der Heijde, D., van der Tempel, H., et al., 1999. Development of a questionnaire to investigate patient compliance with antirheumatic drug therapy. J. Rheumatol. 26, 2635–2641.

Devor, M., Seltzer, Z., 1999. Pathophysiology of damaged nerves in relation to chronic pain. In: Wall, P.D., Melzack, R. (Eds.) Textbook of Pain, fourth ed. Churchill Livingstone, Edinburgh, pp. 129–163.

Dickens, C., Creed, F., 2001. The burden of depression in patients with RA. Rheumatology 40, 1327–1330.

Donovan, J., 1991. Patient education and the consultation: the importance of lay beliefs. Ann. Rheum. Dis. 50, 418–421.

Donovan, J.C.L., Blake, D.R., 1992. Patient non-compliance: deviance or reasoned decision-making. Soc. Sci. Med. 34, 507–513.

Felton, B.J., Revenson, T.A., 1984. Coping with chronic illness: a study of illness controllability and the influence of coping strategies on psychological adjustment. J. Counsel. Clin. Psychol. 52, 343–353.

Fex, E., Larson, B.M., Nived, K., et al., 1998. Effect of arthritis on work status and social and leisure time activities in patients followed 8 years from onset. J. Rheumatol. 25 (1), 44–50.

Fishbein, M., Ajzen, I., 1975. Belief, Attitude, Intention and Behaviour. John Wiley & Sons, New York.

Folkman, S., 1997. Positive psychological states and coping with severe stress. Soc. Sci. Med. 45 (8), 1207–1221.

Folkman, S., Lazarus, R.S., 1988. Manual of the Ways of Coping Questionnaire. Consulting Psychologists Press, Paolo Alto, CA.

Goodwin, J.S., Black, S.A., Satish, S., 1999. Aging versus disease: the opinions of older black, hispanic and non-hispanic white Americans about the causes and treatment of common medical conditions. J. Am. Geriatric Soc. 47, 973–979.

Gordon, P.A., Stoelb, M., Chiriboga, J., 1997. The vocational implication of two common rheumatic diseases. J. Rehabil. 63 (1), 15–19.

Haigh, R.C., McCabe, C.S., Halligan, P., Blake, D.R., 2003. Joint stiffness in a phantom limb: Evidence of central nervous system involvement in rheumatoid arthritis. Rheumatology 42, 888–892.

Hakkinen, A., Hannonen, P.J., Nyman, K., et al., 2003. Aerobic and neuromuscular performance capacity of physically active females with early or long term rheumatoid arthritis compared to matched healthy women. Scand. J. Rheumatol. 31, 345–350.

Hampson, S.E., Glasgow, R.E., Zeiss, A.M., 1994. Personal models of osteoarthritis and their relation to self-management and quality of life. J. Behav. Med. 17, 143–158.

Hewlett, S., Cockshott, Z., Kirwan, J., et al., 2001. Development and validation of a self-efficacy scale for use in British patients with rheumatoid arthritis (RASE). Rheumatology 40 (11), 1221–1230.

Hill, J., Bird, H., Johnson, S., 2001. Effect of patient education on adherence to drug treatment for rheumatoid arthritis: A randomised controlled trial. Ann. Rheum. Dis. 60, 869–875.

Hill, J., Bird, H., Thorpe, R., 2003. Effects of rheumatoid arthritis on sexual activity and relationships. Rheumatology 42, 280–286.

Hobro, N., Weinman, J., Hankins, J., 2004. Using the self-regulatory model to cluster chronic pain patients: the first step towards identifying relevant treatments. Pain 108, 276–283.

Horne, R., 1999. Patients' beliefs about treatment: The hidden determinant of treatment outcome. J. Psychosom. Res. 47, 491–495.

Horne, R., Weinman, J., 1999. Patients' beliefs about prescribed medicines and their role in adherence to treatment in chronic physical illness. J. Psychosom. Res. 47, 555–567.

Horne, R., Weinman, J., Hankins, M., 1999. The Beliefs about Medicines Questionnaire: the development and evaluation of a new method for assessing the cognitive representation of medication. Psychol. Health 14, 1–24.

Hughes, G., Martinez, C., Myon, E., et al., 2006. The impact of a diagnosis on fibromyalgia on health care resource use by primary care patients in the UK. Arthritis. Rheum. 54 (1), 177–182.

Hyrich, K., Symmons, D., Watson, K., et al., 2006. Baseline co-morbidity rates levels in biologic and standard DMARD treated patients with RA: results from a national register. Ann. Rheum. Dis. 65, 895–898.

International Association for the Study of Pain (IASP), 1994. Classification of chronic pain. Description of chronic pain syndromes and definitions of pain terms, second ed. IASP, Seattle.

Jerant, A.F., von Friederichs-Fitzwater, M.M., Moore, M., 2005. Patients' perceived barriers to active self management of chronic conditions. Patient Educ. Couns. 57, 300–307.

Katz, P.P., Yelin, E.H., 2004. Activity loss and the onset of depressive symptoms; do some activities matter more than others. Arthrit. Rheum. 44, 1194–1202.

Keefe, F.J., Kashikar-Zuck, S., Robinson, E., et al., 1997. Pain coping strategies that predict patients' and spouses' ratings of patients' self-efficacy. Pain 73 (2), 191–199.

Kraag, G.R., Gordon, D.A., Menard, H.A., et al., 1994. Patient compliance with tenoxicam in family practice. Clin. Ther. 16, 581–593.

Lefebvre, J.C., Keefe, F.J., Affleck, G., et al., 1999. The relationship of arthritis self-efficacy to daily pain, daily mood and daily pain coping in rheumatoid arthritis patients. Pain 80 (1-2), 425–435.

Leventhal, H., Benyamini, Y., Brownlee, S., et al., 1997. Illness representations: Theoretical foundations. In: Petrie, K.J., Weinman, J.A. (Eds.) Perceptions of Health and Illness. Harwood, The Netherlands.

Lowe, B., Willand, L., Eich, W., et al., 2004. Psychiatric comorbidity and work disability in patients with inflammatory diseases. Psychosom. Med. 66, 395–402.

McCabe, C.S., 2004. Pain mechanisms and the rheumatic diseases. Musculoskel Care 2 (2), 75–89.

Mancuso, C.A., Paget, S.A., Charlson, M.E., 2000. Adaptations made by RA patients to continue working. Arthritis. Care Res. 13 (2), 89–99.

Melzack, R., Wall, P.D., 1965. Pain mechanisms: A new theory. Science 150, 971–979.

Minnock, P., Fitzgerald, O., Bresnihan, B., 2003. Women with established RA perceive pain as the predominant impairment in health status. Rheumatology 42, 995–1000.

Moss-Morris, R., Weinman, J., Petrie, K.J., et al., 2002. The revised Illness Perceptions Questionnaire (IPQ-r). Psychol. Health 17, 1–16.

National Rheumatoid Arthritis Society, April 2003. The National

Rheumatoid Arthritis Society Survey. NRAS, Berkshire.

Neame, R., Hammond, A., 2005. Beliefs about medications: a questionnaire survey of people with rheumatoid arthritis. Rheumatology 44, 762–767.

Newman, S., Fitzpatrick, R., Lamb, R., et al., 1990. Patterns of coping in RA. Psychol. Health 4, 187–200.

Nicassio, P.M., Wallston, K.A., Callahan, L.F., et al., 1985. The measurement of helplessness in RA: the development of the arthritis helplessness index. J. Rheumatol. 12, 462–467.

O'Reilly, S., Muir, K., Doherty, M., 1999. Effectiveness of home exercise on pain and disability from osteoarthritis of the knee: a randomised controlled trial. Ann. Rheum. Dis. 58, 15–19.

Parker, J.C., Smarr, K.L., Slaughter, J. R., et al., 2003. Management of depression in rheumatoid arthritis: a combined pharmacologic and cognitive behavioural approach. Arthritis. Rheum. 49, 766–777.

Phelan, M., Campbell, A., Byrne, J., et al., 1994. The effect of an education programme on the perception of arthritis by spouses of patients with rheumatoid arthritis. Scand. J. Rheumatol. 74 (Suppl).

Radojenic, V., Nicassio, P.M., Weisman, M.H., 1992. Behavioural interventions with and without family support for rheumatoid arthritis. Behav. Ther. 23, 13–30.

Rejeski, W.J., Brawley, L.R., Ettinger, W., et al., 1997. Compliance to exercise therapy in older participants with knee osteoarthritis: implications for treating disability. Med. Sci. Sport. Exerc. 29, 977–985.

Rosenstiel, A.K., Keefe, F.J., 1983. The use of coping strategies in chronic low back pain patients: relationship to patient characteristics and current adjustment. Pain 17 (1), 33–44.

Rotter, J.B., 1954. Social Learning and Clinical Psychology. Englewood Cliffs, NJ.

Royal College of Nursing (RCN), 2000. Sexuality and Sexual Health in Nursing practice. Royal College of Nursing, London.

Ryan, S., Hassell, A., Dawes, P., et al., 2003. Control perceptions in patients with rheumatoid arthritis: the role of social support. Musculoskel Care 1 (2), 108–118.

Sakalys, J.A., 1997. Illness behaviour in rheumatoid arthritis. Arthritis Care Res. 10, 229–237.

Schwarzer, R., 1992. Self-efficacy in the adoption and maintenance of health behaviours: Theoretical approaches and a new model. In: Schwarzer, R. (Ed.), Self-efficacy: thought control of action. Hemisphere, Washington DC, pp. 217–241.

Sharpe, L., Sensky, T., Timberlake, N., et al., 2003. Long-term efficacy of a cognitive behavioural treatment from a randomised controlled trial for patients recently diagnosed with rheumatoid arthritis. Rheumatology 42, 435–441.

Sheehy, C., Murphy, E., Barry, M., 2006. Depression in RA-underscoring the problem. Rheumatology 45, 1325–1327.

Smith, C., Wallston, K., 1992. Adaptation in patients with chronic rheumatoid arthritis: Application of a general model. Health Psychol. 11 (3), 151–162.

Smith, C., Wallston, K., Dwyer, K., et al., 1997. Beyond good and bad coping: A multidimensional examination of copping with pain in persons with rheumatoid arthritis. Ann. Behav. Med. 19 (1), 1–11.

Specht, J., King, G., Brown, E., et al., 2002. The importance of leisure in the lives of persons with cognitive physical disability. Am. J. Occup. Ther. 56 (4), 436–445.

Spranglers, M.A., de Regt, E.B., Andries, F., et al., 2000. What chronic conditions are associated with better or poorer quality of life. J. Clin. Epidemiol. 53 (9), 895–907.

Strating, M., van Schurr, W., Suurmeijer, T., 2006. Contribution of partner support in self-management of rheumatoid arthritis patients. An application of the theory of planned behaviour. J. Behav. Med. 29 (1), 51–60.

Turk, D.C., Melzack, R., 1992. Handbook of Pain Assessment. Guildford, New York.

Viller, F., Guillemin, F., Briancon, S., et al., 1999. Compliance to drug treatment of patients with RA : a 3 year longitudinal study. J. Rheumatol. 26, 2114–2122.

Wallston, K.A., Wallston, B.S., DeVellis, R., 1978. Development of multidimensional health locus of control (MHLC) scales. Health Educ. Monogr. 6, 160–170.

Weinman, J., Petrie, K.J., Moss-Morris, R., et al., 1996. The Illness Perception questionnaire: a new method for assessing cognitive representation of illness. Psychol. Health 11, 114–129.

Wikstrom, I., Jacobsson, L.T.H., Arvidsson, B., 2005. How people with rheumatoid arthritis perceive leisure activities: a qualitative study. Musculoskel Care 3 (2), 74–84.

Yelin, E., 1995. Musculoskeletal conditions and employment. Arthritis. Care Res. 8 (4), 311–317.

Zautra, A., Manne, S., 1992. Coping with rheumatoid arthritis: A review of a decade of research. Ann. Behav. Med. 14, 31–39.

Chapter 6

Patient education and self management

Alison Hammond PhD MSc BSc(Hons) DipCOT FCOT Centre for Rehabilitation and Human Performance Research, University of Salford, Greater Manchester and Derby City General Hospital, Derby Hospitals NHS, Foundation Trust, Derby, UK

Karin Niedermann MPH BScPT Institute of Physiotherapy, University of Applied Sciences, Winterthur and Department of Rheumatology, University Hospital Zurich, Switzerland

CONTENTS

KEY POINTS

- Patient education should be based on a needs analysis and tailored to individual needs.
- Patient education should aim to influence not only knowledge, but also behaviour and health status.

© 2010 Elsevier Ltd
DOI: 10.1016/B978-0-443-06934-5.00006-1

- Patient education should be planned and have a sound theoretical base, applying health psychology and educational theory to practice.
- Patient education should strengthen self-efficacy and teach self-management skills effectively, allowing adequate practise with feedback.
- Patient education should be evaluated using measures appropriate to the planned outcomes.

INTRODUCTION

Patient education is an essential additive intervention in the care of people with rheumatic diseases. Therapists' professional codes of conduct emphasise the importance of ensuring patients are provided with adequate information to gain informed consent and enable informed choices about treatment. However, patient education goes beyond just providing information: targeting behaviour, beliefs and attitudes. It may be provided both formally and informally. In either case it should be planned and goal oriented, based on an assessment. Interventions should adopt theoretical models and not only apply educational and counselling methods but a psycho-educational approach. The goal of patient education is self-management, i.e. the patient is empowered and able to take responsibility for the day-to-day management of the illness. Patients are considered as partners in the whole education process.

DEFINING PATIENT EDUCATION

Patient education is any combination of planned and organized learning experiences designed to facilitate voluntary adoption of behaviour and/or beliefs conducive to health (Burckhardt et al 1994).

This definition points out the main issues of patient education: interventions ought to be *planned* just as in any other therapeutic intervention. This requires assessment of patients' educational needs, definition of educational goals, clear plans and procedures for achieving these and (re)evaluation. Targets may be attitudes, beliefs, motivation and *behaviour*. A basic knowledge and understanding of the disease and possible interventions is helpful, but knowledge does not necessarily lead to changes in attitudes and behaviour. A systematic approach should be used as knowledge, attitudes, values, emotions and behaviours influence each other. The

Table 6.1 Summary of patient education approaches

APPROACH	EDUCATIONAL METHODS	EXAMPLE
Educational	Information	Using a teaching approach, e.g. short lectures, explanations, written information.
Counselling	Counselling	Communication approach, specifically adapted to and reinforcing individual's motivation
Psycho-educational	Cognitive behavioral interventions Motivational interviewing	Assessing and enabling changes in beliefs and attitudes; problem solving; skills training; goal-setting and contracting; home programmes.

patient's decision for behavioural change is always *voluntary* – the health professionals' task is to provide effective interventions and optimal learning situations. A summary of patient education approaches is provided in Table 6.1.

AIMS OF PATIENT EDUCATION

The aims of patient education are directed at:
- facilitating informed consent
- improving understanding about the condition and its management (cognitive change)
- supporting awareness (knowledge, risks), motivation (attitudes, social influence, self-efficacy) and emotional adjustment
- enabling behavioural changes and self-management
- maintaining, and if possible improving, health or at least slowing deterioration
- enabling adequate and appropriate use of the health care system
- reducing health care costs.

SELF-MANAGEMENT

Self-management is the 'individual's ability to manage the symptoms, treatment, physical and psychosocial consequences and life style changes inherent in living with a chronic condition' (Barlow et al 2002, Newman et al 2004). This implies several important points:

- Patients need problem solving abilities, decision making techniques and confidence in their self-management ability.
- Partnership is needed between patients and health care professionals (HCPs). HCPs provide appropriate medical and therapeutic recommendations to patients and then enable them to learn relevant skills and strategies in a concordant relationship.
- Patients take responsibility for day-to-day management of their illness.

EMPOWERMENT

Empowerment is a relatively new term in the context of care but is an important aim in relation to self-management. It's the precondition for and consequence of self-management ability. Empowered patients are able to develop and strengthen their own (health) competencies, such as the appropriate knowledge, attitudes and skills needed to cope with the disease in their own life context (Virtanen et al 2007).

DEVELOPING PATIENT EDUCATION INTERVENTIONS: A 7-STEP APPROACH

Taal et al (1996) suggested a 7-step approach for the development, conduct and evaluation of patient education (Box 6.1). This structure is applied in this chapter.

STEP 1: ANALYSE THE PROBLEMS

It has consistently been demonstrated that effective interventions ought to be tailored to the needs of the individual patient. Before developing a patient education intervention, a careful and thorough analysis of the patient's health behaviour in relation to his/ her health problem is needed. This analysis aims to understand possible determinants for the patient's coping and self-management abilities.

> **BOX 6.1   7-step approach to development of patient education (after Taal et al 1997)**
>
> Step 1: Analyse the problem
> Step 2: Make use of (a) theoretical model(s)
> Step 3: Influence knowledge, behaviour and health status
> Step 4: Teach effective self-management skills
> Step 5: Strengthen self-efficacy appraisals and use effective methods of teaching self-management skills
> Step 6: Involvement of people from the person's social environment
> Step 7: Proper evaluation of intervention effectiveness.

Coping with a chronic disease is a lifelong and daily challenge. Disease acceptance and coping with a chronic disease is an interaction between person and disease. It matters which life aspects are important to an individual and how the disease interferes in the patient's life. Limitations in physical ability might be a huge problem for one individual, whereas another person perceives the impact on social networks, e.g. loss of friends, as much more important.

Important factors influencing health behaviour and coping are:

- demographic factors, such as age, gender, socio-economic status and the illness itself
- social factors such as: cultural background; attitudes of family, friends and peers; and societal attitudes to illness and treatment
- environmental factors (availability and access to care)
- personal factors such as personality, beliefs, attitudes and emotions.

There is evidence that individual beliefs and attitudes are better predictors of patients' abilities to cope with the illness than disease severity, age or gender (Buchi et al 1998) (Fig. 6.1).

Beliefs or cognitions: sense of coherence, health locus of control, self–efficacy

Sense of coherence (SOC) is considered as an adaptive dispositional orientation (i.e. within the personality) that enables coping with adverse experience (Antonovsky 1979, 1990, Eriksson & Lindstrom 2006). SOC integrates the meaningfulness,

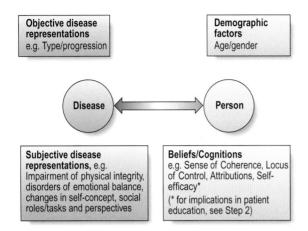

Figure 6.1 The relationship between demographic, disease-related and personality factors.

comprehensibility and manageability of a situation or disease. The more a person is able to understand and integrate (comprehensibility), to handle (manageability) and to make sense (meaningfulness) of an experience or disease, the greater the individual's potential to successfully cope with the situation or the disease. As it is a personality trait it is more likely to be a predictor of behaviour than a factor to influence in interventions. High SOC is associated with perceived good health and predictive of positive health outcomes (Eriksson & Lindstrom 2005).

Health locus of control (HLC)(Rotter 1954) differentiates between whether people attribute an outcome to their own abilities or actions and, as such, is under their personal (internal) control (e.g. I did not exercise enough today because I was not in the mood, or did not put in enough effort) or whether an outcome is independent of one's actions (external control), attributing it to fate or chance (e.g. bad weather, no time, no social support). Findings related to HLC predicting health behaviour are weak and inconsistent (Wallston 1992) (see Ch. 5, Section 4).

Self-efficacy theory is considered as one of the most powerful determinants of behaviour (Bandura 1977). The confidence a person has to successfully execute a specific behaviour or task in the future, i.e. (self)-efficacy expectation, and the person's belief that the desired behaviour has a positive effect, i.e. outcome expectation, determine the initiation of the process to perform a behaviour, to expend effort and to continue to do so when difficulties are arising (Bandura 1990). (See Ch. 5, Section 4).

Self-efficacy refers to perceived ability in specific domains of activities. It is a specific state, although

a variety and range of positive mastery experiences may lead to a general sense of self-efficacy (Bandura 1977). A patient with rheumatoid arthritis (RA) might very well have high self-efficacy to follow a drug prescription correctly but low self-efficacy for using joint protection methods correctly.

Patients with chronic diseases who demonstrate high self-efficacy have a better prediction for rehabilitation outcome (Hammond et al 1999). In people with RA, higher self-efficacy has been shown to be associated with better ability to cope with their disease, as well as with better current (Taal et al 1996) and future (2 and 5 year) health status (Brekke et al 2001, 2003).

Motivation and goal setting

Adopting health behaviours is 'unfortunately' not just a logical, rational decision-making process solely dependent on information. Rather it depends on complex interactions, including attitudes to illness, expectations of health, previous experiences of the illness and social pressure (Price 2008).

Motivation for behavioural change is determined by cognitions, emotions and intentions and is central for applying what has been learned. The distinction between approach (success-related) and avoidance (failure-related) motivation is fundamental in explaining human behaviour (Elliot et al 2001). Important factors for effective goals are that they should be:

- personal goals: i.e. achievable goals, oriented towards the person succeeding rather than failing
- 100% within the person's control for goal achievement (see locus of control and self-efficacy)
- attractive and emotionally positively loaded (e.g. fun to do)

(Emmons 1992, Siegert & Taylor 2004).

Compliance, adherence and concordance

In the past, there was much focus on patient's *compliance* with treatment. The term compliance denotes following a prescribed regimen, indicating a more passive patient role. This is an inappropriate term in therapy as we work collaboratively with clients. Adherence suggests a more equitable role in which the patient participates in goal-setting and treatment with shared responsibility for outcome (Agras 1989) and probably reflects well the tenacity patients with chronic disease need to maintain behavioral adjustments over their life (-time) (Haynes et al 2002, Price 2008). In relation to medication-taking the term concordance is now commonplace. It refers to the interactional decision-making process in agreeing a management plan between patient and health professional. Partnership may optimise therapy and health gains and discordance is resolved through compromise or agreeing to disagree (Treharne et al 2006). "Concordance" is likely to become a more common term in therapy practice in future.

Adherence to treatment

Non-adherence is considered as one of the main barriers to the effectiveness of treatment interventions (Carr 2001). The following factors are important determinants of adherence:

- Positive belief regarding the necessity for an intervention
- Positive perceived benefit of the intervention
- No concerns regarding possible side effects: this is true for medication (Neame & Hammond 2005), as well as for non-pharmacological interventions such as wearing wrist working splints (Agnew 1995, Veehof et al 2008). Symptom seriousness was an important factor for adherence, whereas concerns about splints reducing function were reasons for stopping wear (Veehof et al 2008)
- Positive interaction with health professionals: patients generally appreciate an equal dialogue with health professionals (Lempp et al 2006). It has been shown that physician-patient communication can positively or negatively influence health outcomes and effectiveness of health care delivery (Teutsch 2003)
- Readiness to change (see Step 2, the Transtheoretical model)
- Confidence in having the necessary skills (self-efficacy): the confidence in one's ability to perform a given behaviour is strongly related to one's actual ability to perform that behaviour (Bandura 1977). For example, self-efficacy was found to be the only determinant for medication compliance (Brus et al 1999). People in the process of behavioural change generally move from lower to higher self-efficacy (Keefe et al 2000)
- Family support (see social support)
- Access to and previous perceptions and experiences of the health system, often related to culture and socio-economic status (Garcia Popa-Lisseanu et al 2005).

Social support

Family and friends form a social network that may be a source for social support. However, this may be perceived as positive or problematic, contributing to decreased or increased depression respectively in people with RA. Size and perceived availability of social network contribute to reducing negative affective reactions of patients with RA (Fitzpatrick et al 1988). Support is problematic when it is not needed or desired or when it does not meet the recipient's needs. Both, positive and problematic support were demonstrated to be associated with coping and depression with arthritis (Revenson et al 1991) and lack of sympathy and understanding from the social network contributes to fatigue (Riemsma et al 1998). Positive and negative social support has the same effects on men and women, but effective social support strategies differ between men and women (Kraaimaat et al 1995). For women, it is their perceived degree of emotional support, whilst for men it is the number of friends that significantly contributes to support.

There are inconsistent findings as to whether family members should participate in self-management education programmes. There are studies reporting no effects (van Lankveld et al 2004) or even negative effects on self-efficacy and fatigue (Riemsma et al 2003a,b). Positive effects have also been identified, such as high levels of satisfaction with social support and positive quality of life outcomes (Minnock et al 2003), quality of marital status and pain severity (Waltz et al 1998).

STEP 2: MAKE USE OF A THEORETICAL MODEL

As with other therapeutic interventions, patient education must be planned and goal oriented, thus including assessment, intervention and evaluation. What are the aims of the new patient education programme you want to develop and thus what elements should be included? Which components have been demonstrated to work successfully in changing patients' attitudes, beliefs and behaviour? There is a wide range of theories and models to guide practitioners in designing effective and efficient patient education interventions.

Several models and theories are commonly used in patient education.

- Health belief model, including the concept of pros and cons

- The Theory of Planned Behaviour
- Social Cognitive Theory
- The Transtheoretical Model.

The Health Belief Model

The Health Belief Model (HBM) (Becker et al 1977) (see Ch. 5) is one of the oldest models but still provides an important framework for designing theory-based interventions, though newer models and their components seem to better explain the complexity of behaviour (and behaviour changes) (Fig. 6.2).

The implications for patient education are:

- perceived severity of disease: provide accurate information
- perceived susceptibility to disease and consequences: evaluate risk behaviours
- expected benefits: emphasise and reinforce the pros (i.e. benefits, e.g. less pain, better well-being)
- perceived barriers for changing behaviour: discuss and reduce cons (i.e. costs, e.g. effort, time, access)
- cues to action (the external and internal factors triggering behaviour): use these to frame educational messages (e.g. social support, potential rewards, pain (or no pain) after exercising)

Low perceived susceptibility may reduce motivation. There is some evidence that increasing worries created by information (e.g. mass media campaigns, information booklets) can help to change (self-reported) health behaviour (Sogaard & Fonnebo 1992).

The Theory of Reasoned Action and Theory of Planned Behaviour

The Theory of Reasoned Action (Fishbein & Ajzen 1975) and the Theory of Planned Behaviour (Ajzen 1985) (see Ch. 5) also consider intention and perceived control as other important determinants for health behaviour. Intention towards a behaviour is shaped by the person's attitudes and subjective norm (expectancies of social environment) which act as pros and cons towards a behaviour. Perceived control emerged from work on locus of control and perceived self-efficacy and it was assumed that intention and perceived control interact.

The implications for patient education are:

- Consider attitudes: reinforce the advantages of the target behaviour and address barriers.
- Develop strategies for improving control over environmental factors (i.e. problem solving strategies): e.g. time constraints, weather conditions.
- Take into account social environment and influences.

Social Cognitive Theory

Self-efficacy (Bandura 1977, 1990) is a central concept in social cognitive theory and is acquired by direct experience, vicarious experience (role modelling), verbal persuasion and reinterpretation of physiological signals. Action-oriented

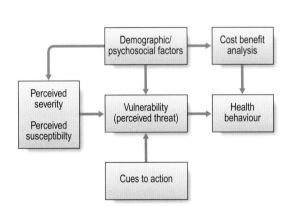

Figure 6.2 The health belief model.

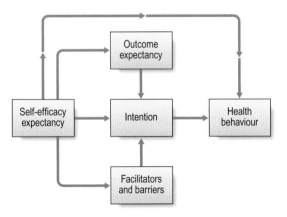

Figure 6.3 Social cognitive theory or self-efficacy.

interventions in occupational and physiotherapy provide unique possibilities to acquire self-efficacy. Direct experience is the most powerful strategy. Success leads to success (see Chs. 5 & 6, Steps 1 & 5) (Fig. 6.3).

The implications for patient education are:

- Include as many practical sessions as possible for practising the behaviour (direct experience).
- Use group settings, in which peers perform the same behaviour (role modeling).
- Discuss 'homework', i.e. goals patients set to make changes and the pros and cons regarding these behaviours (verbal persuasion).
- Help people perceive the difference between disease symptoms and, for example, the normal effects of exercising (re-interpretation of physiological signals).

The Transtheoretical Model

The development of the Transtheoretical Model (TTM) (Prochaska et al 1992) was an important step to better understand behavioural change, demonstrating that individuals cycle through a series of five stages of readiness to change when modifying health behaviours.

In the pre-contemplation and contemplation stages there is no or little problem awareness and thus no intention to change in the future (i.e. the next 3–6 months). In the preparation stage taking action is planned for the near future (i.e. within a month). In the action stage activities are performed to modify behaviour, experiences or the environment and in the maintenance stage the new behaviour is consolidated and integrated into daily life (i.e. it is performed regularly over at least 6 months). Behaviour change takes time and regression, i.e. relapse into previous behaviours, is the rule rather than the exception, visualised by the spiral pattern of the TTM (Fig. 6.4).

The second key construct relates to the processes of change, i.e. the strategies that are important when moving from one stage to the next. In the lower stages (1–3) cognitive and affective strategies are important, whereas in the upper stages (4 and 5) behavioural processes are most important. The TTM states that lower stages of change are associated with lower levels of self-efficacy, in which the cons are more important than the pros. In contrast, in the upper stages behaviour performance

is associated with higher levels of self-efficacy and pros outweigh cons.

The implications for patient education are:

- acknowledge that not all people are ready for change and even if ready, not all are in the same stage of change, which requires individualised interventions tailored to the stages where people are
- people who fail to participate may be in stages 1 and 2, thus provision of (more) information, addressing increasing motivation and reinforcing pros is important, rather than advice about what and how to do things
- in stage 3, provide action plans and practical advice, addressing self-efficacy and cons
- in stage 4, support action and self-efficacy by diaries, cues to action and rewards
- in stage 5, address relapse prevention: identify risk situations and prepare to re-start the plan
- be aware of the long-term perspective of behavioural changes.

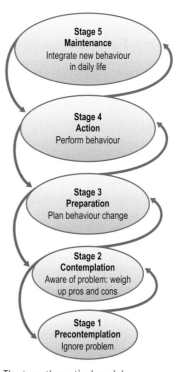

Figure 6.4 The transtheoretical model.

Adult Learning – the learning process

Health professionals have the responsibility to fully explore the patient's situation and tailor interventions based on personal needs, anticipate patients' difficulties in following recommendations and communicate in a way that is effective (Stone 1979). Learning, i.e. gathering knowledge and skills, is not automatic and has to be enhanced by teaching and methodological choices. Favourable learning situations involve several learning processes. Learning processes do not occur in isolation but in combination (Berlinger et al 2006).

Learning as a self-directed process
Self-directedness (Fig. 6.5) is:

- a precondition for every (internal) learning process. Learning consists of self-regulative components and lies within the responsibility and abilities of the learning person.
- a learning goal. To become self-directed in learning is strongly associated with self-efficacy.
- a strategy for teaching. The 'teacher' acts as a coach and provides only as much support and external guidance as necessary.

Learning as an active process
- The learning person must be involved actively. Acquiring knowledge and linking it to existing cognitive structures involves mental performance. Intrinsic motivation, or at least internal regulation, is necessary.

Learning as a situational process
- Successful learning is linked to the individual's context, pre-knowledge, experiences and beliefs.

Learning as a constructive process
- Learning is constructing. New knowledge and skills form new structures in the brain, interpreting and cross-linking with former structures (pre-knowledge, experiences, beliefs) and existing concepts' structures. Use of former experiences, analogies and training situations that are similar to 'real life' are helpful.

Learning as an emotional process
- Learning, i.e. the construction process of building new structures and concepts, is a highly emotional process, guided by the limbic system. A positive and relaxed atmosphere and relationship with the therapist or within the group increases attention and memory storage.

Learning as a social and interactive process
- When learning with others, new knowledge structures are compared and adjusted, questioned or confirmed and finally consolidated. Group education may provide such additional positive effects.

Learning as a goal–oriented process
- Learning is enhanced by clear realistic goals. Interventions and learning procedures are planned based on the learning goals. After agreement between client and therapist, the client can take control and responsibility for the learning process.

Implications for patient education from a learning point of view

People may have one or more learning styles: activists prefer learning through doing; theorists prefer reading and discussion; pragmatists prefer to act and see what they learn from it; reflectors prefer to consider before acting (Honey & Mumford 1992). Adapt teaching to best suit the person's preferred learning style. In group education, a mix of approaches, particularly a practical, task-focussed approach, is more likely to be effective than solely talks and discussion.

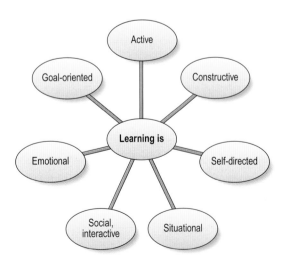

Figure 6.5 Adult learning processes. After Berlinger et al 2006, with permission of H.E.P Verlag AG.

STEP 3: INFLUENCE KNOWLEDGE, BEHAVIOUR AND HEALTH STATUS

Effective patient education enables understanding about the condition and health care, coping, changing health behaviours to self-manage effectively, improving or maintaining health status and reducing health costs. It requires effective teaching and learning strategies. Information giving is an important part, but not all of patient education. Solely providing information does not necessarily mean a person learns or changes. Patient education tailored to the person's needs is more effective (Lorish et al 1985).

Identifying needs

First, assess and prioritise aspect/s of education to focus on:

- cognitive change – improving relevant knowledge and understanding.
- affective or attitudinal change – e.g. the motivation (or readiness) to learn, to change and the confidence to do so.
- psychomotor and behavioural change – the physical and cognitive skills and the habits and routines to make recommended changes enough to make a difference.

Patient education needs are not just informational needs. For example, five people with RA attended occupational therapy and physiotherapy and were given information about joint protection and home exercises. At follow-up, they are honest and tell you they have either not tried or are doing little. Are they all "unmotivated, uncompliant" patients? Asking them why, can identify that their reasons may differ (Table 6.2). In practice, different approaches may then be relevant to enable change.

What do people want to learn?

Patient education interventions should be based on identifying target group's needs (Lorig & Visser 1994). Priorities must be set about what to teach in the time available. Better to teach fewer things well than many badly. Written information can supplement lower priority topics. Determine:

- the potential knowledge and behaviours to teach which, based on published evidence, are most important in affecting health status
- then which are the most likely to change, given the time available or how much is realistically needed to enable change (Lorig et al 2001).

Information needs of an individual can be assessed formally using the Educational Needs Assessment Tool, which identifies the importance of 39 items in seven domains (managing pain, movement, managing feelings, arthritis process, treatment, self-help and support) and is available for rheumatoid arthritis, osteoarthritis, systemic lupus erythematosus, ankylosing spondylitis and

Table 6.2 Examples of educational needs and patient education actions

EDUCATIONAL NEED	ACTION
Not understanding need to use, e.g. exercise/ joint protection (cognitive need).	Assess readiness to learn. Improve quality of information giving; recheck understanding and recall.
Knowing why and how but not wanting to (attitudinal need).	Assess importance of and readiness to change. Explore illness, health and exercise beliefs – any attitudinal barriers? E.g. exercise is ineffective; joint protection irrelevant at this disease stage; other strategies (e.g. diet, herbal remedies) are more effective. Consider psychological strategies (e.g. active listening, counselling, motivational interviewing) to discuss barriers and beliefs.
Knowing why, how and want to but lacks confidence (attitudinal need).	Explore self-efficacy for behaviour; assess confidence in and readiness to change. Start at simple, achievable levels building gradually. Goal-setting, collaborative action plans and regular review improve confidence step-by-step. Group programmes provide opportunity to see others succeed (modelling).
Wants to but experiencing pain when trying. Observation/ discussion identify performing incorrectly (psychomotor need).	Teach correct techniques step-by-step again, allow adequate practice, with feedback, to improve skill. Check over several sessions.
Knowing why, how and want to but not making time (behaviour need).	Habit change helped by discussing: daily and weekly routines; identify possible barriers, collaborative problem solving, discuss times and practice routines. Goal-setting, action plans and review.

connective tissue disease (Hardware et al 2004, Hill et al 2004).

Informally, negotiating multiple behavioural changes may be helped by agenda setting. After gaining rapport, initial data, and open-endedly asking about the person's information needs, an agenda-setting chart may help identify options. This visually displays their topics of interest or concern and you can then add what you commonly offer (Fig. 6.6). If concerns or topics outside your practice are raised, actively listen and acknowledge these. Concerns may prevent the person gaining education benefits. Explain if you cannot personally address some issue/s and ask if there is action they need to take, referral elsewhere is needed or if airing the concern was sufficient today. Continue identifying topics of interest, allowing time to reflect and discuss options. ("What do you think? How do you feel about any of these?"). Adopt a 'curious state of mind' to identify their priorities: "Which of these do you feel most ready to think about changing?" (Rollnick et al 1999).

To plan group programmes, topics can be identified by: surveys with larger numbers of people (items should be generated initially with patients to ensure it is not health professional driven); matrix assessments (e.g. 15–20 people, a variation of the Delphi process), in which the group write individual needs first, then the number interested in each topic is identified and a consensus gained of higher and lower priorities; focus groups (6–12 people) led by a person unfamiliar to the group, to identify

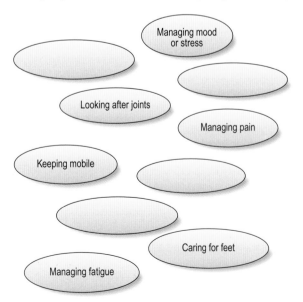

Figure 6.6 Example of an agenda setting chart.

Managing mood or stress

Looking after joints

Managing pain

Keeping mobile

Caring for feet

Managing fatigue

concepts; or individual un- or semi-structured interviews (Lorig et al 2001). If the programme will be used widely, the opinions of many people are needed to ensure representativeness.

A survey of people with rheumatoid, inflammatory and psoriatic arthritis (n = 365, disease duration 10.5 (SD 8.5) years; 36% < 5 years) identified: most (70–75%) were 'very interested' in learning more about joint protection, keeping mobile, maintaining independence and managing the disease themselves; two thirds (60–69%) about arthritis, its potential future effects and treatment, managing pain, fatigue and mood, and communicating with health professionals; and half (50–55%) about diet, complementary therapies and claiming benefits. There were no significant differences between people with more or less than 5 years disease duration or diagnostic groups (Hammond & Badcock 2002). This helped structure content and priorities within a health-professional-led modular education programme (Hammond et al 2008). The lay-led Arthritis Self-Management Programme is also based on detailed needs assessment (Lorig et al 1985).

Information giving – cognitive change

As well as what to teach we need to consider how to teach it. The majority of people (70%) prefer a patient-centred approach respecting their views, but 30% prefer a biomedical approach demonstrating authority (Swenson et al 2006). Patients' preferred approach should be determined. Better outcomes are associated with a patient-centred approach. Patients want: clear explanations (oral and written); to lead discussions and ask questions; be listened to and understood; and to remain in control of their condition, which paradoxically can include refusing interventions even when recognising their importance (Ward et al 2007).

Some information giving is factual, e.g. what is arthritis, how does exercise affect joints. But much focuses on helping people change, e.g. why, what, when and how to….for example, exercise. Giving information, talking about action and telling people what to do, rather than asking what they want first and identifying if they are ready to learn, may undermine autonomy (personal freedom) and lead to resistance. This may be apparent though for example, reluctance, arguing, defensiveness, objecting, denial or not following advice. Good consulting enables the person to express their fears about change, without feeling judged or pressurised into action (Rollnick et al 1999).

Information giving is best as information exchange. Useful questions in a patient-centred approach are:

- Would you like to know more about…?
- How much do you know about…?
- Would you like to know how…?

These help elicit readiness to learn. Use open-ended questions to probe for responses, as almost half of people are reluctant to ask questions even if wanting more information (Ley 1988). If they do not want information (pre-contemplation) and are resistive, explore why. Confirm you appreciate change is difficult, they have other demands in life and there are barriers to change. Identify barriers to readiness (see Table 6.2 for examples) and address these. People also have a choice not to learn or to change.

If they are ready, practical considerations are:

- realise information will be interpreted in terms of their illness perceptions (see Ch. 11). Finding out these helps adjust your explanation.
- check understanding by asking questions regularly, or prompting the person to paraphrase explanations. For example, asking 'I'm not sure if I have explained that enough for you (or quite right)' often this prompts people to say 'I think you mean..' You can then tease out aspects needing further clarification.
- appreciate recall is often poor. The more information presented, the poorer the recall. Keep it simple. Recall is generally not related to educational level or age but is affected by anxiety during and quality of education provided.

Recall of verbal information can be improved by many strategies. (For examples see Box 6.2). Written information should be provided to reinforce verbal information (Box 6.3).

In one-to-one education, adapt teaching to best suit the person's preferred learning style(s). In group education, a mix of approaches, particularly a practical, task-focused approach, is more effective than talks and discussion. Much of our therapy includes teaching skills (e.g. exercise, joint protection). The more the practical component, with feedback on performance, the better.

Enabling attitudinal changes

Readiness to change (see the Transtheoretical model) and self-efficacy (see Social Cognition theory) influence willingness to make behavioural changes. Such changes require perceiving importance of change,

confidence to do so and these influence readiness to make specific behaviour changes (Rollnick et al 1999). Discussion should promote behaviour change-talk to help identify the pros and cons of change

---

BOX 6.2   Strategies to enhance recall

- Tell important information first (primacy effects).
- Stress the most important parts.
- Simplification-use non-technical words (e.g. bend not flex). Explain technical terms when necessary (e.g. inflammation). Keep explanations short. Use short sentences. Keep to a few key messages each session.
- Explicit categorisation – structure information to "tell them what you are going to tell them, tell them, and tell them what you told them." Summarise pre- and post- each topic, and at the beginning and end of the session overall. This helps people encode information more readily.
- Repetition – ensure key facts are repeated by paraphrasing, and asking the person to repeat back or paraphrase what learnt.
- Use specific rather than general statements, e.g. rather than "you need to regularly exercise to keep fit," state "you are aiming to exercise or be physically active five times a week for 30 minutes in total a day getting yourself a little out of breath. We can discuss what you believe is achievable to get started". Then mutually determine this (e.g. walking 5 minutes a day for 3 days this week).

BOX 6.3   Tips for good written communication

- Use everyday language
- Avoid instructions without giving a brief explanation
- Short sentences
- Active and present tenses
- Small blocks of text. Use clear headings to separate
- Question and answer format if possible
- Font size at least 12 point
- Avoid excess use of upper case
- Include plenty of 'white space' (large margins, spaces between paragraphs)
- Use diagrams and pictures. Photographs are better than line drawings if possible.
Department of Health (2003)

Table 6.3 Three topics to encourage behaviour change talk (after Rollnick et al 1999)

IMPORTANCE: WHY?	CONFIDENCE: HOW?	READINESS: WHEN?
Is it worthwhile? How will it benefit me? Why should I? What will change as a result? At what costs? Will it make a difference? What could happen if I don't do it?	Can I do it? How will I do it? How will I cope with doing it?	Shall I do it now? What about other priorities?

and work through any ambivalence towards changing (Table 6.3).

Motivational interviewing is a technique for helping people explore their motivations for making changes, based on a collaborative process of listening, exploring values and concerns and guiding to make decisions, respecting autonomy to choose whether to change or not (Rollnick et al 2008). There is a growing body of evidence that it promotes self-management in chronic diseases but has been little evaluated in rheumatic diseases as yet (Shannon & Hillsden 2007). Short training courses are available and texts by Rollnick et al (1999 & 2008) provide practical examples of applying techniques in practice.

STEP 4: TEACH EFFECTIVE SELF-MANAGEMENT SKILLS

Effective skills include exercise, relaxation, joint protection, strategies for coping with pain and stress, communicating effectively with health professionals, problem-solving, and goal-setting. Learning these new skills demands a lot of effort and takes much training time (Taal et al 1996). The content of programmes should be evidence-based using effective evidence-based teaching techniques. People should not just be provided with information (verbally and in written form) but the skills themselves need adequate practice with feedback during education sessions. There should be a structured approach to encouraging people to practice skills sufficiently (Taal et al 1996). Materials and equipment to enable this should be supplied as far

as possible to reduce barriers to home practice, and feedback and review provided. The person also needs to know when to apply the skill appropriately. Some techniques are recommended for use permanently (e.g. joint protection) but others vary with health status (e.g. relaxation). The person also needs to know how to modify self-management methods to suit changing needs. This decision-making process also needs discussion.

STEP 5: STRENGTHEN SELF-EFFICACY APPRAISALS AND USE EFFECTIVE METHODS OF TEACHING SELF-MANAGEMENT SKILLS

As the person shifts from precontemplation to contemplation and preparation, a structured approach to strengthening self-efficacy, teaching self-management skills and changing habits and routines is needed.

Strengthening self-efficacy

Social cognitive theory highlights self-efficacy (confidence) is key to enabling behavioural change (Bandura 1977). It can be improved through:

- Performance accomplishments: gaining skills step-by-step, starting within the person's ability, gradually increasing complexity and difficulty as the person improves. Sufficient practice at home enables this. Using goal-setting in contracts combined with feedback is very effective (Taal et al 1996).
- Vicarious experience or Modelling: seeing others like oneself achieve is a powerful promoter of confidence ('If they can do it, so could I').The more alike people are, the more effective is the modeling force. In group programmes, ensure at least two people of similar ages or the same gender are within a group.
- Reinterpreting physiological signals: for example, explaining that aches are a natural consequence of exercise and not a sign of arthritis worsening.
- Persuasion: e.g. to try alternatives. This is most commonly used, but less effective than the above strategies.

Applying these approaches within education programmes increases use of exercise, relaxation, cognitive symptom and fatigue management, and joint protection (Barlow et al 1998, Hammond et al 2008, Lorig et al 1985, Taal et al 1996).

Effective teaching

Effective teaching requires forward planning to enable effective information and skills learning. The environment should be comfortable, with appropriate temperature and lighting, free of distracting noise, and comfortable seating. Careful consideration should be given to audio-visual aids. For group programmes, whilst powerpoint is 'professional' it may take time to set up correctly. Many patients are not familiar with teaching and training environments. It can convey a more 'formal' atmosphere, promoting people watching the screen rather than the therapist and each other. A pre-prepared flip-chart is cheaper and less formal. Group comments can be added to spare sheets and it is easily updated as teaching topics change. Careful attention is needed to vary tone of voice. Particularly if a standard programme is being followed, key points and concepts must be taught as stated but not simply 'read out'. A personalised approach should be taken.

Developing psychomotor skills requires people to form schemas or movement patterns in their minds (Schmidt & Lee 2005). Mackway-Jones and Walker (1999) recommend six stages for teaching:

1. Layout: plan for sufficient space, ensure no obstacles. Check patient(s) can see clearly. Furniture, equipment or people may need to be moved (Fig. 6.7).
2. Equipment: ensure all required is to hand, the therapist is totally familiar with its use. Anything not immediately required should be placed to one side to avoid distraction.
3. Initial orientation: explain why the skill (self-management behaviour) is performed, its relevance to the person, the objectives of the teaching session and how the person will be participating.
4. Skills teaching: a four-part approach can be used:
   - Demonstrate the whole skill at normal speed *without* commentary. This provides a clear picture of what is to be learnt without distraction. The therapist must be confident in demonstrating the skill.
   - Demonstrate the skill *with* commentary: breaking it down-step-by-step. Use clear, short instructions to avoid information overload.
   - Demonstrate the skill whilst asking the person to provide a commentary: if they are confident in doing so, let them describe each step first before you do it. If not, start/continue each step as a prompt. Errors need correcting, but allow a few seconds for self-correction. If not, prompt a re-think or tell the answer if struggling. If in a group, ask the whole group.
   - Person demonstrates the skill with commentary. Provide feedback to confirm if correct or prompt identifying errors (allowing a few seconds as above).

This means the person will have seen three demonstrations and heard two descriptions before doing it themselves. In a group situation, the last two stages can be shared amongst the group members (working in pairs or threes) with each person trying the skill in turn (see Fig. 6.8). This is much less 'threatening' than talking through the skill in front of the whole group and provides further opportunity for modelling. Watching less skilled "demonstrators" allows opportunities to problem-solve when others make mistakes.

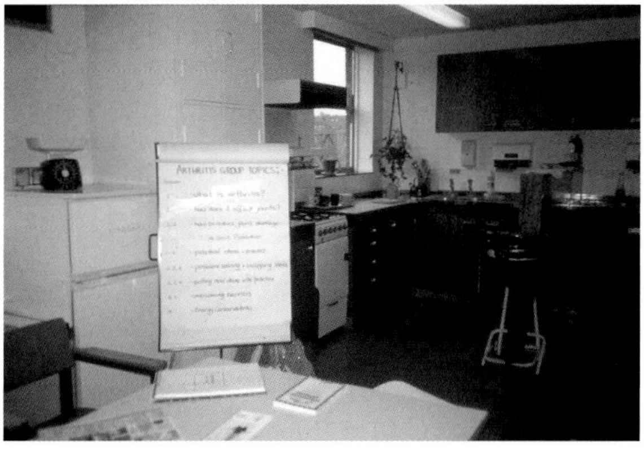

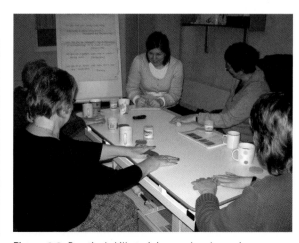

Figure 6.7 Group education programme.

Figure 6.8 Practical skills training – a hand exercise group.

5. Practice: once successfully completed, allow sufficient time for practice. This may need to be done at home, so strategies to promote home practice are needed (see below). Skills in teaching sessions should become progressively more complex and varied, as skills are better learnt through varied than repetitive practice (Schmidt & Lee 2005). This will also help people generalize skills to other settings. Mental practice using motor imagery also speeds up skills learning.

6. Closure: Once the skill is successfully completed, allow time for final questions or discussing difficulties. Summarise key points. End by ensuring the person knows follow-up actions to take.

Behavioural approaches and goal-setting

Change is the person's responsibility. But there can be barriers to changing behaviour, including not having (making) the time, and forgetting. Once the person knows how to perform a specific skill, regular practice is needed to consolidate skill and develop new habits and routines. Teaching people how to set long and short-term goals and action plans helps promote this. Long term goals are what they wish to achieve from the education. Short-term are the steps to achieve this. Short-term goals should state: what, how much, when, how often and the time frame. Getting people to write goals down, and/or say aloud in a group what they intend to do, increases the likelihood they will fulfill them. Goals should be what the person wants to do, not what the therapist expects them to do. An example of applying behavioural approaches in education can be found in Chapter 10.

STEP 6: THE INVOLVEMENT OF PEOPLE FROM THE PERSON'S SOCIAL ENVIRONMENT

Using self-management effectively will be helped by support from significant others. As discussed above, there is conflicting evidence for the effectiveness of including significant others in education programmes. Keefe et al (1996) identified people attending a group OA programme with their spouse did better than those attending without a spouse in terms of improved pain and disability. However, Riemsma et al (2003a) in a trial with people with RA found that those in a spouse-attended group fared worse than those attending non-spouse attended groups. Post-education interviews identified those attending groups without spouses felt more able to discuss their problems openly without fear of upsetting those close to them. Having significant others attend is thus not always helpful. But encouraging their involvement through asking patients to share information materials with relatives and getting them to assist in practice is important. This allows the person to decide on the degree of involving relatives, as not all are supportive. Providing a carers-only education meeting is also beneficial.

STEP 7: PROPER EVALUATION OF INTERVENTION EFFECTIVENESS

Outcomes most relevant to the aims of the intervention provided should be selected.

- Knowledge: There are several valid, reliable RA specific instruments testing domains of: symptoms, tests, drug therapy, joint protection, energy conservation and exercise: the RA Patient Knowledge Questionnaire (Hill et al 1991); the ACREU RA Knowledge Questionnaire (Lineker et al 1997); the Patient Knowledge Questionnaire (Hennell et al 2004). There are multiple choice instruments for use in ankylosing spondylitis (Lubrano et al 1998a) and psoriatic arthritis (Lubrano et al 1998b).

- Belief in ability to manage the disease: Two self-efficacy measures are widely used. A UK validated version of the Arthritis Self-Efficacy Scale for confidence to manage pain and other symptoms (Barlow et al 1997a) and the RA Self Efficacy scale evaluating belief in potential for initiating 28 self-management behaviours (relaxation, relationships, function, leisure activities, exercise, sleep, medication and fatigue) (Hewlett et al 2001).

- Perceived control: The Rheumatology Attitudes Index measures degree of feeling in control of arthritis (Callahan et al 1988).

- Mood: the Positive and Negative Affect Scale identifies improved or lowered mood states (Watson et al 1988), in contrast to clinical depression and anxiety.

- Adherence with health behaviours: use of cognitive symptom management (e.g. relaxation, distraction) and exercise can be measured using self-report scales (Lorig et al 1996).

- Pain and fatigue: can be measured using a 100mm visual analogue scale (VAS). Care must be taken selecting appropriate question wording, anchor points, time scale and ensuring the VAS measures 100mm when photocopied. Typical questions are: 'over the last week, in general how has your pain/fatigue been?' with anchor points of 'no pain/fatigue' to 'pain/fatigue as bad as it could be.' Some find these difficult to complete because of fluctuating symptoms. More detailed pain and fatigue assessments are available (see Ch. 4).

- Health status: Two measures are widely used. The Multidimensional Health Assessment Questionnaire (MDHAQ) includes the modified HAQ measuring functional ability (8 items); 100mm pain and fatigue VASs (pain/fatigue no problem to a major problem); a 100 mm VAS of perceived health (very bad to very well); self-reported duration of early morning stiffness (minutes); psychological distress; and a modified Rheumatology Attitudes Index including items related to medications (Pincus et al 2005). The Arthritis Impact Measurement Scales 2 (AIMS2) includes sub-scales evaluating upper and lower limb function, activities of daily living, pain and psychosocial status, as well as satisfaction with health (Meenan et al 1992).

- Overall impact: the Health Education Impact Questionnaire measures 8 areas of: health behaviour; engagement; emotional well-being; self monitoring; attitudes; skill acquisition; social support; and health service navigation (Osborne et al 2007).

Further generic and disease specific arthritis measures are described and reviewed in Katz (2003), Lorig et al (1996) and in Chapter 4.

EVIDENCE FOR PATIENT EDUCATION INTERVENTIONS

Effectiveness depends on the quality and type of education provided.

ONE-TO-ONE WRITTEN AND VERBAL INFORMATION GIVING

Individual education is the commonest provided in practice. Surprisingly, there is relatively little evidence for effectiveness in arthritis. Written information has been evaluated in several studies. Barlow et al (1997b, Barlow & Wright 1998) conducted a randomised controlled trial (n = 108) evaluating the **arc** (Arthritis Research Campaign) RA booklet with people with established RA (15 years duration). Knowledge about arthritis and treatment, mood, reassurance and coping significantly improved. Walker et al (2007) tested the additional effect of a mind map in people with RA alongside the **arc** RA booklet (n = 363; 13 years duration). Knowledge significantly improved but those with low literacy (15% of participants) did not. Good quality written information is important but those functionally illiterate need good quality, structured verbal information giving.

The evidence for effectiveness of individual verbal education is less clear. A trial (n = 150) comparing receiving a booklet on RA, treatment, and self-management methods with 1 hour of individualised instruction from a therapist plus the booklet found both groups significantly improved knowledge in comparison to usual care only, suggesting additional individual education was redundant (Maggs et al 1996). However, attitudinal (eg self-efficacy) and behavioural changes were not evaluated.

There are few studies of education provided during routine appointments. Riemsma et al (1997) randomised people with established RA (n = 216; average 13 years duration) to three groups: (1) usual care (i.e. information giving during routine appointments as necessary from a rheumatology nurse); (2) usual care plus an arthritis self-help book; and (3) structured one-to-one education based on the provided self-help book during routine appointments. Nurses in the latter group received training in education, goal-setting and progress review. All groups improved similarly, suggesting structured behavioural education was no more effective than "ad hoc" information giving. However, nurses providing structured education reported difficulty applying it in routine practice due to time constraints. Hill et al (2001) compared structured 1:1 education (7×30 minute sessions), provided by a rheumatology nurse using a self-efficacy approach, about RA, drug treatment and self-management, with routine out-patient care (i.e. ad hoc information giving) (n = 100; disease duration 12 years). Significant improvements occurred in knowledge and drug therapy concordance in the education group but not health status. Attitudinal and health behaviour change were not evaluated. Sufficient time for education is needed to be effective. Further studies of individualised education are needed to identify the most effective and cost-effective methods, particularly to enable health behaviour changes.

GROUP EDUCATION

Riemsma et al (2003b) reviewed group patient education trials from 1966–1998 for people with RA specifically. Education had small but significant effects on disability, joint counts, patients' global assessment and psychological status (anxiety and depression) at 3 months, but not 12 months. Few studies conducted longer-term follow-ups. They further compared:

- information only interventions (e.g. information giving, persuasion, booklets)
- counselling (e.g. enhancing social support, discussion of problems) and
- behavioural interventions (e.g. skills practice with feedback, goal-setting, home programmes with review).

Only behavioural interventions showed significant effects. Other reviews have identified longer-term benefits result from behavioural patient education in RA, improving pain, functional ability and tender joint counts (Hirano et al 1994, Superio-Cabuslay et al 1996).

HEALTH PROFESSIONAL LED GROUP PROGRAMMES

Recently, trials of health-professional led cognitive-behavioural therapy (CBT) approach group education have shown mixed results. For example, a five session programme (12.5 hours) of relaxation, psychological coping, managing pain and mood using CBT approaches, with didactic teaching about RA, medication, joint protection and thermotherapy was compared to usual care (n = 79; RA duration 13 years; 7 facilitators) (Kirwan et al 2005). Patient knowledge improved, but at 8 months no significant differences in pain, self-efficacy, mood or health status occurred.

An eight session programme (52 hours) teaching active coping strategies, diet, relaxation and exercise using CBT approaches with didactic teaching about RA and medication was compared to usual care (n = 208; RA duration 13 years; 10 facilitators) (Giraudet-le Quintrec et al 2007). At 1 year, knowledge and helplessness improved but not health behaviours or health status.

A nine session modular programme (22.5 hours) using CBT approaches including joint protection, exercise, managing fatigue, mood and pain with information about RA and medication was compared to a five session (10 hour) programme teaching similar content but not using CBT approaches (n = 167; disease duration 7 years) (Hammond et al 2008). At one year, the modular programme led to significant improvements in pain, self efficacy, use of health behaviours and health status. As well as applying CBT approaches, reflection about the personal need for change was encouraged. Modules were led by one facilitator to promote continuity discussing about the personal impact of arthritis and change. Small group practice actively promoted modelling (Hammond 2003). How programmes are taught matters.

LAY-LED GROUP ARTHRITIS EDUCATION PROGRAMMES

Substantial research has been undertaken evaluating the Arthritis Self-Management Programme (ASMP). This 15 hour programme uses CBT approaches and is equally effective delivered by trained lay leaders as health professionals (Lorig et al 1986), improves self-efficacy, health behaviours and health status for at least 4 years and reduces health care costs (Lorig et al 1993) and is effective in the UK (Barlow et al 1998). The full 15 hour programme is significantly more effective than shortened versions (Lorig et al 1998) and than a generic chronic disease self-management programme (Lorig et al 2005). A mail delivered and an internet delivered version of the ASMP have been tested, with similar results to the small group programme (Lorig et al 2004, 2008).

Most ASMP studies have been with community recruited volunteers, who may be particularly motivated. Is it effective when delivered to people recruited from primary care? A UK study (n = 812) recruited people with hip or knee OA (average age 68 years) from 74 GP Practices. A third did not attend. At 1 year, the ASMP reduced anxiety and increased self-efficacy for symptom management but did not affect health status or health care use (Buszewicz et al 2006). A US study (n = 187) of people with either RA, OA or fibromyalgia recruited from primary care identified at 4 months there was no difference between ASMP and control groups for any health status or satisfaction measures (Solomon et al 2002). The authors suggest that primary care participants may be more representative of people with arthritis and thus evidence from studies with volunteers is not necessarily generalisable. Nevertheless, for volunteers it is effective.

On average, ASMP participants in community trials are 70 years old, with 15 years disease duration and 72% have OA (Bruce et al 2007). Is the ASMP equally effective in OA, RA and fibromyalgia? The recent internet-based ASMP trial identified it was significantly effective in OA in improving pain, fatigue, disability, self-efficacy, self-reported health and reducing distress. In RA it was significantly effective in improving pain and self-reported health. It was not effective in fibromyalgia (Lorig et al 2008).

Trials of patient education in other conditions have similarly shown marked differences in outcomes. Further research is needed to identify what are effective patient education processes, who benefits most from such group programmes and what strategies maintain changes longer-term.

CONCLUSION

Brady et al (2000) recommended all team members help people with arthritis in perceiving that self-management is valuable. Regular encouragement is needed to help people commence using a variety of self-management methods and ongoing support is needed to help maintain it. If group programmes are available, repeated offers to refer should be given. People may not initially wish to attend, but may want to do so in the future. People may be at different stages of change for different strategies and their use of methods will wax and wane as their arthritis and life events vary over time. Patient education is a long-term process not just a one-off event.

STUDY ACTIVITIES

1. Reflect on a one-to-one education session that you have either recently observed or have yourself provided.
   - What were the good points of the session - what went well?
   - What did not go so well? Why was this?
   - What were the aims of this intervention?
   - Were the needs of the patient identified and if so were these satisfied? What feedback was obtained?
   - How effective do you think the session was in terms of addressing the aims? How can you tell?
   - How do you think it might be improved in the future?
2. Select a patient needs assessment tool from those described within this chapter. Obtain a copy and use this with a patient. Afterwards, discuss with the person how helpful (or not) using the assessment has been.
3. Using the information on practical skills teaching provided, design a short teaching session for a common skill you teach your patients. Try this with a client. Reflect on whether this has improved your practice.

USEFUL WEBSITES

http://www.dh.gov.uk/en/Publicationsandstatistics/Publications/PublicationsPolicyAndGuidance/DH_4070141 "Toolkit for Producing Patient Information." – guidance on how to produce written information for patients. (accessed March 2009).
www.motivationalinterviewing.org Information on techniques and training resources. (accessed March 2009).

http://www.crd.unimelb.edu.au/heiq/ Information about the Health Education Impact Questionnaire. (accessed March 2009).
http://www.patienteducation.stanford.edu/programs/asmp.html Arthritis self-Management Programme website (includes access to relevant programme evaluation questionnaires). (accessed March 2009).

References and further reading

Agnew, P.J., Maas, F., 1995. Compliance in wearing wrist working splints. J. Occup. Ther. J. Res. 15 (3), 165–180.

Agras, W.S., 1989. Understanding compliance with the medical regimen: the scope of the problem and a theoretical perspective. Arthritis Care Res. 2 (3), S2–S7.

Ajzen, I., 1985. From intentions to actions: A theory of planned behavior. In: Action Control: From Cognitions To Behaviour. Hogrefe & Huber, Seattle WA, pp. 11–39.

Antonovsky, A., 1979. Health, Stress and Coping. Jossey-Bass, San Francisco.

Antonovsky, A., 1990. Personality and health: testing the sense of coherence model. In: Friedman, H.S. (ed.), Personality and Disease. Wiley, New York, pp. 155–177.

Bandura, A., 1977. Self-efficacy: towards a unifying theory of behaviour change. Psychol. Rev. 84, 191–215.

Bandura, A., 1990. Self-regulation of motivation through anticipatory and self-reactive mechanisms. Nebr. Symp. Motiv. 38, 69–164.

Barlow, J.H., Williams, B., Wright, C.C., 1997a. The reliability and validity of the arthritis self-efficacy scale in a UK context. Psychol. Health Med. 2, 3–17.

Barlow, J.H., Pennington, J.C., Bishop, P.E., 1997b. Patient education leaflets for people with rheumatoid arthritis: a controlled study. Psychol. Health Med. 2 (3), 221–235.

Barlow, J.H., Wright, C.C., 1998. Knowledge in patients with rheumatoid arthritis: a longer-term follow-up of a randomized controlled trial of patient education leaflets. Br. J. Rheumatol. 37, 373–376.

Barlow, J.H., Turner, A.P., Wright, C.C., 1998. Long-term outcomes of an arthritis self-management programme. Br. J. Rheumatol. 37, 1315–1319.

Barlow, J., Wright, C., Sheasby, J., et al., 2002. Self-management approaches for people with chronic conditions: a review. Patient Educ. Couns. 48, 177–187.

Becker, M.H., Haefner, D.P., Kasl, S.V., et al., 1977. Selected psychosocial models and correlates of individual health-related behaviors. Med. Care 15 (Suppl. 5), 27–46.

Berlinger, D., Birri, T., Zumsteg, B., 2006. Didactic principles for effective practice. In: From Practice to Practice, From Learning to Teaching (in German). aeb series, Bern, Switzerland, pp. 96–100.

Brady, T.J., Sniezek, J.E., Conn, D. L., 2000. Enhancing patient self-management in clinical practice. Bull. Rheum. Dis. 49 (7), 1–4.

Brekke, M., Hjortdahl, P., Kvien, T.K., 2001. Self-efficacy and health status in rheumatoid arthritis: a two-year longitudinal observational study. Rheumatology 40 (4), 387–392.

Brekke, M., Hjortdahl, P., Kvien, T. K., 2003. Changes in self-efficacy and health status over 5 years: a longitudinal observational study of 306 patients with rheumatoid arthritis. Arthritis Rheum. 49 (3), 342–348.

Bruce, B., Lorig, K., Laurent, D., 2007. Participation in patient self-management programs. Arthritis Rheum. 57 (5), 851–854.

Brus, H., van de Laar, M., Taal, E., et al., 1999. Determinants of compliance with medication in patients with rheumatoid arthritis: the importance of self-efficacy expectations. Patient Educ. Couns. 36 (1), 57–64.

Buchi, S., Sensky, T., Sharpe, L., et al., 1998. Graphic representation of illness: a novel method of measuring patients' perceptions of the impact of illness. Psychother. Psychosom. 67 (4–5), 222–225.

Burckhardt, C.S., Lorig, K., Moncur, C., et al., 1994. Arthritis and musculoskeletal patient education standards. Arthritis Found. Arthritis Care Res. 7, 1–4.

Buszewicz, M., Rait, G., Griffin, M., et al., 2006. Self management of arthritis in primary care: a randomised controlled trial. Br. Med. J. 333 (7574), 879–883.

Callahan, L.F., Brooks, R.F., Pincus, T., 1988. Further analysis of learned helplessness in arthritis using a "Rheumatology Attitudes Index." J. Rheumatol. 15, 418–426.

Carr, A., 2001. Barriers to the effectiveness of any intervention in OA. Best Pract. Res. Clin. Rheumatol. 15 (4), 645–656.

Department of Health, 2003. Toolkit for producing patient information, V2.0 http://www.dh.gov.uk/en/Publicationsandstatistics/Publications/

PublicationsPolicyAndGuidance/DH_4070141 (accessed 27.11.08).

Elliot, A.J., Chirkov, V.I., Kim, Y., et al., 2001. A cross-cultural analysis of avoidance (relative to approach) personal goals. Psychol. Sci. 12 (6), 505–510.

Emmons, R.A., 1992. Abstract versus concrete goals: personal striving level, physical illness, and psychological well-being. J. Pers. Soc. Psychol. 62 (2), 292–300.

Eriksson, M., Lindstrom, B., 2005. Validity of Antonovsky's sense of coherence scale: a systematic review. J. Epidemiol. Community Health 59 (6), 460–466.

Eriksson, M., Lindstrom, B., 2006. Antonovsky's sense of coherence scale and the relation with health: a systematic review. J. Epidemiol. Community Health 60 (5), 376–381.

Fishbein, M., Ajzen, I., 1975. Belief, Attitude, Intention and Behaviour. An Introduction to Theory and Research. Addison-Wesley, Reading, MA.

Fitzpatrick, R., Newman, S., Lamb, R., et al., 1988. Social relationships and psychological well-being in rheumatoid arthritis. Soc. Sci. Med. 27 (4), 399–403.

Garcia Popa-Lisseanu, M.G., Greisinger, A., Richardson, M., et al., 2005. Determinants of treatment adherence in ethnically diverse, economically disadvantaged patients with rheumatic disease. J. Rheumatol. 32 (5), 913–919.

Giraudet-LeQuintrec, J.-S., Mayoux-Benhamou, A., Ravaud, P., et al., 2007. Effect of a collective educational program for patients with rheumatoid arthritis: a prospective 12-month randomised controlled trial.. J. Rheumatol. 34 (8), 1684–1691.

Hammond, A., Lincoln, N., Sutcliffe, L., 1999. A crossover trial evaluating an educational-behavioural joint protection programme for people with rheumatoid arthritis. Patient Educ. Couns. 40, 1044–1051.

Hammond, A., Badcock, L., 2002. Improving education about arthritis: identifying the educational needs of people with chronic inflammatory arthritis. Rheumatology 41 (Suppl. 1) 87(216).

Hammond, A., 2003. Patient education: helping people change. Musculoskeletal Care 1 (2), 84–97.

Hammond, A., Bryan, J., Hardy, A., 2008. Effects of a modular behavioural arthritis education programme: a pragmatic parallel-group randomised controlled trial. Rheumatology 47 (11), 1712–1718.

Hardware, B., Lacey, E.A., Shewan, J., 2004. Towards the development of a tool to assess educational needs in patients with arthritis. Clin. Eff. Nurs. 8 (2), 111–117.

Haynes, R.B., McDonald, H.P., Garg, A.X., 2002. Helping patients follow prescribed treatment: clinical applications. JAMA 288 (22), 2880–2883.

Hennell, S.L., Brownsell, C., Dawson, J.K., 2004. Development, validation and use of a patient knowledge questionnaire (PKQ) for patients with early rheumatoid arthritis. Rheumatology 43, 467–471.

Hewlett, S., Cockshott, Z., Kirwan, J., et al., 2001. Development and validation of a self-efficacy scale for use with British patients with Rheumatoid Arthritis (RASE). Rheumatology 40, 1221–1230.

Hill, J., Bird, H.A., Hopkins, R., 1991. The development and use of a patient knowledge questionnaire. Br. J. Rheumatol. 30, 45–49.

Hill, J., Bird, H., Johnson, S., 2001. Effect of patient education on adherence to drug treatment for rheumatoid arthritis: a randomised controlled trial. Ann. Rheum. Dis. 60, 869–875.

Hill, J., Tennant, A., Adebajo, A., 2004. Further development of an educational needs tool (ENAT) for patients with rheumatoid arthritis. Arthritis Rheum. 50 (Suppl. 9), 616.

Hirano, P.C., Laurent, D.D., Lorig, K., 1994. Arthritis patient education studies: 1987–1991: a review of the literature. Patient Educ. Couns. 24, 9–54.

Honey, P., Mumford, A., 1992. The Manual of Learning Styles. Berkshire, Honey, Ardingly House.

Katz, P. (Ed.), 2003. Patient outcomes in rheumatology. Arthritis Care Res. 49 (S5) S1–S244.

Keefe, F.J., Caldwell, D.S., Baucom, D., et al., 1996. Spouse-assisted coping skills training in the management of osteoarthritic knee pain.. Arthritis Care Res. 9 (4), 279–291.

Keefe, F.J., Lefebvre, J.C., Kerns, R. D., et al., 2000. Understanding the adoption of arthritis self-management: stages of change profiles among arthritis patients. Pain 87 (3), 303–313.

Kirwan, J.R., Hewlett, S., Cockshott, Z., et al., 2005. Clinical and psychological outcomes of patient education in rheumatoid arthritis.. Musculoskelet. Care 3 (1), 1–16.

Kraaimaat, F.W., Van Dam-Baggen, R. M., Bijlsma, J.W., 1995. Association of social support and the spouse's reaction with psychological distress in male and female patients with rheumatoid arthritis. J. Rheum. 22 (4), 644–648.

Lempp, H., Scott, D.L., Kingsley, G.H., 2006. Patients' views on the quality of health care for rheumatoid arthritis. Rheumatology 45 (12), 1522–1528.

Ley, P., 1988. Communicating with Patients: improving communication, satisfaction and compliance. Chapman and Hall, London.

Lineker, S.C., Badley, E.M., Hughes, E. A., et al., 1997. Development of an instrument to measure knowledge in individuals with rheumatoid arthritis: the ACREU rheumatoid arthritis knowledge questionnaire. J. Rheum. 24, 647–653.

Lorig, K., Chastain, R., Ung, E., et al., 1985. Development and evaluation of a scale to measure perceived self efficacy in people with arthritis. Arthritis Rheum. 23, 37–44.

Lorig, K., Feigenbaum, P., Regan, C., et al., 1986. A comparison of lay-taught and professional – led self-management courses. J. Rheum. 13, 763–767.

Lorig, K., Mazonson, P.D., Holman, H.R., 1993. Evidence suggesting that health education for self-management in patients with chronic arthritis has sustained health benefits while reducing health care costs. Arthritis Rheum. 36 (4), 439–446.

Lorig, K., Visser, A., 1994. Arthritis patient education standards: a model for the future. Patient Educ. Couns. 24, 3–7.

Lorig, K., Stewart, A., Ritter, P., et al., 1996. Outcome Measures for Health Education and other Health care Interventions. Sage, Thousand Oaks, CA, USA.

Lorig, K., Gonzalez, V.M., Laurent, D., et al., 1998. Arthritis self-management variations : three studies. Arthritis Care Res. 11 (6), 448–455.

Lorig, K., et al., 2001. Patient Education: A Practical Approach, third ed. Sage, London.

Lorig, K., Ritter, P.L., Laurent, D., et al., 2004. Long-term randomized controlled trials of tailored-print and small-group arthritis self-management interventions. Med. Care 42 (4), 346–354.

Lorig, K.R., Ritter, P.L., Laurent, D. D., et al., 2008. The internet-based arthritis self-management program: a one-year randomized trial for patients with arthritis or fibromyalgia. Arthritis Rheum. 59 (7), 1009–1017 0004-3591.

Lorig, K., Ritter, P.L., Plant, K., 2005. A disease-specific self-help program compared with a generalized chronic disease self-help program for arthritis patients. Arthritis Care Res. 53 (6), 950–957.

Lorish, C.D., Parker, J., Brown, S., 1985. Effective patient education: a quasi-experimental study comparing an individualised strategy with a routinised strategy. Arthritis Rheum. 28, 1289–1297.

Lubrano, E., Helliwell, P., Parson, W., et al., 1998a. Patient education in psoriatic arthritis: a cross-sectional study on knowledge by a validated self-administered questionnaire. J. Rheum. 25 (8), 1560–1565.

Lubrano, E., Helliwell, P., Moreno, P., et al., 1998b. The assessment of knowledge in ankylosing spondylitis patients by a self-administered questionnaire. Br. J. Rheumatol. 37, 437–441.

Mackway-Jones K., Walker, M., 1999. Pocket guide to Teaching for Medical Instructors. BMJ Books, London.

Maggs, F.M., Jubb, R.W., Kemm, J. R., 1996. Single blind randomized controlled trial of an educational booklet for patients with chronic arthritis. Br. J. Rheumatol. 35, 775–777.

Meenan, R.F., Mason, J.H., Anderson, J.J., et al., 1992. AIMS2: the content and properties of a revised and expanded Arthritis Impact Measurement Scales health status questionnaire. Arthritis Rheum. 35, 1–10.

Minnock, P., Fitzgerald, O., Bresnihan, B., 2003. Quality of life, social support, and knowledge of disease in women with rheumatoid arthritis. Arthritis Rheum. 49 (2), 221–227.

Neame, R., Hammond, A., 2005. Beliefs about medications: a questionnaire survey of people with rheumatoid arthritis. Rheumatology 44 (6), 762–767.

Newman, S., Steed, L., Mulligan, K., 2004. Self-management interventions for chronic illness. Lancet 364 (9444), 1523–1537.

Osborne, R.H., Elsworth, G.R., Whitfield, K., 2007. The Health Education Impact Questionnaire (heiQ): An outcomes and evaluation measure for patient education and self-management interventions for people with

chronic conditions. Patient Educ. Couns. 66 (2), 192–201.

Pincus, T., Yazici, Y., Bergman, M., 2005. Development of a multidimensional health assessment questionnaire (MDHAQ) for the infrastructure of standard clinical care. Clin. Exp. Rheum. 23 (5, Suppl. 39), S19–S28.

Price, P., 2008. Education, psychology and 'compliance'. Diabetes Metab. Res. Rev. 24 (Suppl.1), S101–S105.

Prochaska, J.O., DiClemente, C.C., Norcross, J.C., 1992. In search of how people change. Applications to addictive behaviors. Am. Psychol. 47 (9), 1102–1114.

Revenson, T.A., Schiaffino, K.M., Majerovitz, S.D., et al., 1991. Social support as a double-edged sword: the relation of positive and problematic support to depression among rheumatoid arthritis patients. Soc. Sci. Med. 33 (7), 807–813.

Riemsma, R.P., Tall, E., Brus, H.L., et al., 1997. Coordinated individual education with an arthritis passport for patients with rheumatoid arthritis. Arthritis Care Res. 10 (4), 238–249.

Riemsma, R., Rasker, J., Taal, E., et al., 1998. Fatigue in rheumatoid arthritis: the role of self-efficacy and problematic social support. Br. J. Rheumatol. 37 (10), 1042–1046.

Riemsma, R., Taal, E., Rasker, J., 2003a. Group education for patients with rheumatoid arthritis and their partners. Arthritis Rheum. 49 (4), 556–566.

Riemsma, R.P., Kirwan, J., Rasker, J., et al., 2003b. Patient education for adults with rheumatoid arthritis. Cochrane Database of Syst. Rev. (2) CD003688.

Rollnick, S., Mason, P., Butler, C., 1999. Health Behaviour Change: A Guide for Practitioners. Churchill Livingstone, Edinburgh.

Rollnick, S., Miller, W.R., Butler, C.C., 2008. Motivational Interviewing in Health Care: Helping Patients

Change Behaviour. Guilford Press, New York.

Rotter, J.B., 1954. Social Learning and Clinical Psychology. Englewood Cliffs, NJ.

Schmidt, R.A., Lee, T., 2005. Motor Control and Learning: A Behavioural Emphasis, fourth ed. Human Kinetics Europe Ltd.

Shannon, R., Hillsden, M., 2007. Motivational interviewing in musculoskeletal care. Musculoskelet. Care 5 (4), 206–215.

Siegert, R.J., Taylor, W.J., 2004. Theoretical aspects of goal-setting and motivation in rehabilitation. Disability Rehabil. 26 (1), 1–8.

Sogaard, A.J., Fonnebo, V., 1992. Self-reported change in health behaviour after a mass media-based health education campaign. Scand. J. Psychol. 33 (2), 125–134.

Solomon, D., Warsi, A., Brown-Stevenson, T., et al., 2002. Does self-management education benefit all populations with arthritis? A randomised controlled trial in a primary care physician network. J. Rheum. 29 (2), 362–368.

Stone, G.C., 1979. Patient compliance and the role of the expert. J. Soc. Issues 5, 34–59.

Superio-Cabuslay, E., Ward, M.M., Lorig, K., 1996. Patient education interventions in osteoarthritis and rheumatoid arthritis. A meta-analysis comparison with non-steroidal anti-inflammatory drug treatment. Arthritis Care and Res. 9, 292–301.

Swenson, S.L., Zettler, P., Lo, B., 2006. 'She gave it her best shot right away': patient experiences of biomedical and patient-centered communication.. Patient Educ. Couns. 61 (2), 200–211.

Taal, E., Rasker, J.J., Wiegman, O., 1996. Patient Education and self-Management in the Rheumatic Diseases: a self-efficacy approach. Arthritis Care Res. 9 (3), 229–238.

Teutsch, C., 2003. Patient-doctor communication. Med. Clin. North Am. 87 (5), 1115–1145.

Treharne, G.J., Lyons, A.C., Hale, E. D., et al., 2006. 'Compliance' is futile but is 'concordance' between rheumatology patients and health professionals attainable? Rheumatology 45 (1), 1–5.

van Lankveld, W., van Helmond, T., Naring, G., et al., 2004. Partner participation in cognitive-behavioral self-management group treatment for patients with rheumatoid arthritis. J. Rheum. 31 (9), 1738–1745.

Veehof, M.M., Taal, E., Willems, M. J., 2008. Determinants of the use of wrist working splints in rheumatoid arthritis. Arthritis Rheum. 59 (4), 531–536.

Virtanen, H., Leino-Kilpi, H., Salantera, S., 2007. Empowering discourse in patient education. Patient Educ. Couns. 66 (2), 140–146.

Walker, D., Adebajo, A., Heslop, P., et al., 2007. Patient education in rheumatoid arthritis: the effectiveness of the ARC booklet and the mind map. Rheumatology 46, 1593–1596.

Wallston, K., 1992. Hocus-pocus, the focus isn't strictly on locus: Rotter's social learning theory modified for health. Cognit. Ther. Res. 16, 183–199.

Waltz, M., Kriegel, W., van't Pad Bosch, P., 1998. The social environment and health in rheumatoid arthritis: marital quality predicts individual variability in pain severity. Arthritis Care Res. 11 (5), 356–374.

Ward, V., Hill, J., Hale, C., et al., 2007. Patient priorities of care in rheumatology out-patient clinics: a qualitative study. Musculoskelet. Care 5 (4), 216–228.

Watson, D., Clark, L.A., Tellegen, A., 1988. Development and validation of brief measures of positive and negative affect: the PANAS scales. J. Pers. Soc. Psychol. 54 (6), 1063–1070.

Chapter 7

The principles of therapeutic exercise and physical activity

Mike V. Hurley PhD MCSP Rehabilitation Research Unit, Kings College London, Dulwich Community Hospital, London, UK

Lindsay M. Bearne PhD MSc MCSP School of Biomedical and Health Sciences, Kings College London, London, UK

CHAPTER CONTENTS

KEY POINTS

- Physical activity is essential for muscle, joint, general physical, psychological and social health, function and well-being
- Muscle sensorimotor dysfunction may cause or exacerbate joint pain, damage or impaired functioning
- Formal and informal exercise and physical activity can improve and maintain muscle function, safely
- Integrated exercise and self-management rehabilitation programmes challenge erroneous health beliefs, give people active coping strategies and enhance self-efficacy, self-esteem and social interaction
- Simple practical advice about lifestyle change can help improve management of chronic rheumatic conditions, but burdensome lifestyle changes are unpopular and require motivation and reinforcement to facilitate implementation.

INTRODUCTION

This chapter provides a brief overview of the importance of muscle, exercise and physical activity in the aetiology and management of common rheumatic conditions, such as osteoarthritis, rheumatoid arthritis, ankylosing spondylitis, juvenile idiopathic arthritis, and others. It also gives practical advice on how to help people begin and continue regular exercise. Exercises for individuals with specific conditions can be found within the chapters following.

JOINTS = MOVEMENT

The reason for having a joint is to enable us to move and so function. Joints were made to move, if we do not move our joints stiffen, our muscles get weaker, we tire sooner and control of movement is poorer. All of these can contribute to pain, disability and increase the risk of developing acute and chronic ill-health (diabetes, heart disease, high blood pressure, depression, obesity). Physical activity is any movement produced by skeletal muscles that expends energy (Caspersen et al 1985). Exercise is a subcategory of physical activity defined as the planned, structured and repetitive movement, to maintain or improve physical fitness (e.g. cardiovascular fitness, muscle strength and endurance, flexibility and body composition) and psychological well being (ACSM 2006). Remaining physically activity is vital for everyone and benefits our muscles, joints, general physical (respiratory, cardiovascular health), psychological (self-confidence, self-esteem,) and social (independence, social interaction) well-being.

THE IMPORTANCE OF MUSCLE

Until relatively recently little consideration had been given to the importance of muscles in rheumatic conditions, most interest concentrated on what was happening inside the joint. However, synovial joints are comprised of intra-articular (bone cartilage, capsule, etc) and extra-articular structures (muscles, ligaments, nerves). If any articular structure is dysfunctional normal joint functioning will be compromised, leading to joint damage, pain and disability (Hurley 1999).

To appreciate the importance of muscle we need to appreciate its sensorimotor functions. Some muscle functions are obvious, others are less obvious but just as important. The most obvious function of muscle is to contract and effect controlled movement. Controlled antagonistic muscle activity enables functional stability so that we are mobile yet stable - we can stand upright, walk, stabilise our upper arms so our hands can perform dexterous movements. This control depends on accurate proprioceptive sensory information much of which arises from muscle receptors (muscle spindles and golgi tendon organs) that informs us about our body position, movement and loading. Without this sensory information we would not be able to produce controlled movement and over time uncontrolled, clumsy, jarring movement results in damage, so our muscles are vital for joint protection.

If, due to natural ageing processes, reduced activity, injury or rheumatic disease, muscles become deconditioned (weak, easily fatigued, proprioception impaired, movement poorly controlled) then neuromuscular protective mechanisms that protect our joints will be compromised. Over time this can result in damage to cartilage and subchrondral bone, pain and disability. Importantly, this means muscle sensorimotor dysfunction may be a cause of joint damage rather than simply a consequence of it (Hurley 1999). Therefore, maintaining well conditioned muscles may enable us to maintain healthy joints, or ameliorate some of the effects of joint damage.

BENEFITS OF EXERCISE

Muscle's involvement in arthritis is good news, because of all the structures that comprise our joints, muscle is the tissue we can manipulate most easily through exercise and physical activity. When physical activity levels exceed the habitual load on our physiological or anatomical systems, our bodies adapt to accommodate the increased load-the 'overload principle'. Exercise can increase strength, endurance and motor control, reducing pain and disability and minimising joint damage.

RANGE OF MOVEMENT

Movement is vital for joint health and function as it maintains the length of soft tissues (joint capsule, ligaments, tendons, muscles), washes synovial fluid across the avascular articular cartilage bringing nutrients and removing waste, stimulates repair and reduces joint effusion (Buckwalter 1995). Therefore joints must be moved through their full range of movement (ROM) frequently to avoid soft tissues shortening, cartilage atrophying and articulating bones fusing. Maintaining joint mobility is important for everybody, but even more so for people with rheumatic conditions who are at increased risk of loss of joint mobility and consequent stiffness, pain, muscle weakness and functional limitations (Zochling et al 2006).

Movement can be maintained and regained by performing slow, controlled and sustained stretches at the end of ROM (Dagfinrud et al 2005). The amount of stretching done depends on how 'irritable' a joint is - how easily pain and effusion are provoked and if the stretching regimen has just begun. These should be performed in three to four sets of 5–10 stretches, two to three times a day (30–120 stretches in total) with each stretch held for 10–30 seconds without 'bouncing' (Fig. 7.1). This may cause mild discomfort, but should not cause pain.

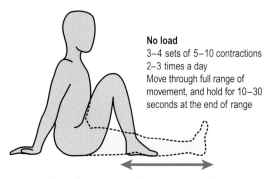

No load
3–4 sets of 5–10 contractions
2–3 times a day
Move through full range of
movement, and hold for 10–30
seconds at the end of range

Figure 7.1 To maintain or regain joint range of movement.

MUSCLE FUNCTION

Inactivity leads to muscle weakness and increased fatigability. Fortunately, muscle has considerable ability to adapt to the loads and stresses placed on it. Specific rehabilitation regimens use the overload principle to improve muscle function. Using the load someone can lift only once through a certain range, called the 1 repetition maximum (1RM), as the reference load (Fig. 7.2) such regimens can:

- increase maximal strength requires that muscles must work against very high resistances. Performing three to eight contractions, using a load that is 60–85% of the 1RM, two to three times a day can lead to 'hypertrophic' strengthening within a week enabling people to lift this weight more easily, increasing their 1RM. Greater loads will then be required to maintain the same strengthening stimulus (Fig. 7.3).
- increased power or explosive force production requires performing fewer contractions (5–10 sets of 5–10 contractions) using lighter loads (30–60% of their 1RM) two to three times a day, i.e. 50–300 contractions each day (Fig. 7.4).
- improve endurance so that contractions can be sustained for longer requires performing many contractions (10 sets of 10–20 contractions) against low resistance (0–30% of the 1RM) 5–10 times a day, i.e. 500–2000 (Fig. 7.5)
- improve controlled movement which requires frequent practice of specific activities so that muscle activity patterns that make up a movement become automatic, performed without much conscious thought.

FUNCTION

While we can address many specific aspects of muscle dysfunction with exercise regimens our ultimate aim is to help people maintain, regain and

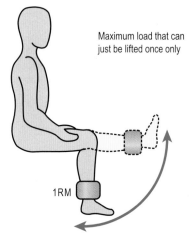

Maximum load that can
just be lifted once only

1RM

Figure 7.2 The heaviest load a person can lift through a range of movement once only – the 'one repetition maximal, 1RM'.

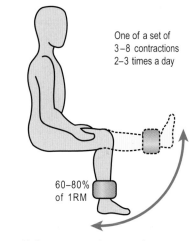

One of a set of
3–8 contractions
2–3 times a day

60–80%
of 1RM

Figure 7.3 To improve muscle strength.

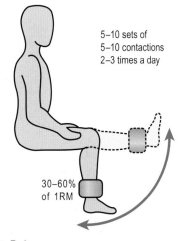

5–10 sets of
5–10 contactions
2–3 times a day

30–60%
of 1RM

Figure 7.4 To improve power.

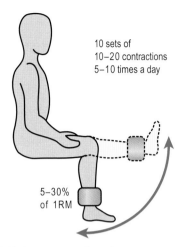

10 sets of
10–20 contractions
5–10 times a day

5–30%
of 1RM

Figure 7.5 To improve muscle endurance.

maximise functioning. Most people with rheumatic conditions want a level of muscle function that will enable them to perform their daily activities, as easily and comfortably as possible. Activities of daily living require a combination of strength, endurance and control, so exercise regimens that address muscle dysfunction must address these deficits. However, people also need to perform the activities that address their function deficits with functional activities such as sit-to-stand, steps-ups, stair climbing and balance (Fig. 7.6). These allow people to appreciate the relevance of exercise in the carry-over to easier performance of activities of daily living, maintenance of functional independence and their active involvement in their management.

Progression of exercise is achieved by 'overloading' the tissues and pushing the limits of an individual's current capabilities, for example increasing resistance, making the activity more challenging (lowering the height of a chair for sit-to-stand, increasing the height of the step for step-ups) or increasing the number of repetitions. Continuing to exercise at a given level will maintain strength, endurance, fitness and functioning at that level. However, once exercise is stopped, the stimulus for adaptation is removed and people regress. Consequently, doing less will result in regression and loss of muscle strength, endurance and control.

FORMAL REHABILITATION PROGRAMMES

Typically, exercise-based rehabilitation is carried out in hospital out-patient departments. These regimens take various forms, but predominantly involve land-based exercises supervised by health-care professionals (usually physiotherapists, occupational therapists, exercise therapists) who devise an individualised exercise programme to address each patient's needs and goals, using the overload principle to increase muscle strength, endurance, joint flexibility and function. This is performed individually or in groups and supplemented with a home exercise regimen. After they have completed the regimen (usually between one and six sessions) they are discharged with advice to continue exercising, follow-up is rare (Walsh & Hurley 2005).

Reviews of research regimens demonstrate that exercise is safe and effective for people with a wide range of rheumatic conditions (Brosseau et al 2004, de Jong & Vlieland 2005, Devos-Comby et al 2006, Fransen et al 2002, Hurley 2003, Klepper 2003, Minor 1999, Munneke et al 2005, Pelland et al 2004, Pendleton et al 2000, Roddy et al 2005, Stenström & Minor 2003, van Baar et al 1999, van Tulder et al 2002).

However, often these research regimens bear little resemblance to the clinical management as they tend to be prolonged, complex regimens that require supervised use of sophisticated equipment so people become reliant on therapists. Once supervised rehabilitation stops, people's motivation to exercise wanes, exercise ceases and the benefits are lost. To sustain benefits, patients must continue to participate in regular exercise. Given the size of the population, the chronic, long-term nature of rheumatic conditions and limited resources, the clinical applicability of many exercise regimens is limited. Clinically practicable regimens have been developed that are more likely to be deliverable to large numbers of people (Bearne et al 2002, Ettinger et al 1997, Hay et al 2006, Hurley et al 2007, McCarthy et al 2004, Thomas et al 2002).

Hydrotherapy employs water-based exercises that utilises the warmth and buoyancy of water to relax muscles and reduce the weight-bearing load and stress on our legs and trunk, but also uses water to assist and resist movement to help us exercise more effectively (Cochrane et al 2005, Epps et al 2005, Foley et al 2003, Fransen et al 2007, Green et al 1993, Patrick et al 2001, Takken et al 2003, Verhagen et al 1997, 2004). Hydrotherapy is very popular with people but requires dedicated facilities and therapists which makes it very expensive. Given the limited healthcare budgets and the large number of people with rheumatic conditions only a small minority of people will ever receive a brief, one-off course of hydrotherapy. Increasingly

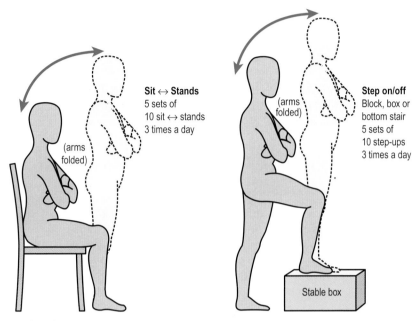

Figure 7.6 To improve function.

local community pools are organising 'aquatherapy' classes that provide more people with the opportunity to participate in controlled water-based exercise classes, supervised by experienced therapists at moderate cost (Cochrane et al 2005). If aquatherapy classes are not available recreational swimming and exercising gently in a local pool is an excellent way to keep stiff painful joints moving.

Tai Chi and Yoga are other less traditional ways of exercising that are popular and widely available and early small trials have found them to be effective (Ernst 2006, Fransen et al 2007), but not everyone wants to participate in these types of activities. It makes no difference where people exercise whether they exercise alone at home, in a leisure centre or join an exercise class (Ashworth et al 2005), so personal preferences can be accommodated. Although people are often reluctant to exercise in groups the additional benefit of group exercise classes is the peer support and motivating reinforcement fellow participants provide, the facilities and social interaction all of which encourages commitment to long-term exercise.

SAFETY

The first rule of any healthcare intervention is 'do no harm'. Physical activity and exercise is contraindicated in very few people-those with advanced, serious, unstable medical conditions, and those with very deformed and unstable joints. Theoretical fears that exercise and physical activity exacerbates inflammatory rheumatic conditions (Blake et al 1989, Merry et al 1991) have not been supported by evidence. In fact in people with mild to moderate rheumatic disease exercise improves aerobic fitness, muscle strength, pain and disability following exercise programs without exacerbating symptoms, radiological damage or disease activity (Bearne et al 2002, Brosseau et al 2005, Ekdahl & Broman 1992, Minor 1999, Munneke et al 2005, Nordemar et al 1981, Stenstrom et al 1991, 1993, van den Ende et al 1998, Zochling et al 2006). It is important that physical activity and exercise is sensibly planned and not overambitious, any new activity should be started slowly, increased gradually and performed moderately (see Patient Information Sheet 7.1). As a rough guide people are exercising moderately when they can do an activity and still hold a conversation but cannot sing (the informal 'talk test') and vigorously when they cannot talk while doing an activity (Meldrum 2003).

People may have concerns about the safety of exercise, which need to be discussed to allay fear and anxiety. Initially, supervised exercise may be required in order to reassure people that exercise is safe and encourage them to exercise. People with severe joint malalignment might be discouraged from undertaking strenuous strengthening exercises (Brouwer et al 2007) but should still be counselled to be physically active with precautions such as little and often, using a walking stick, etc. But it should be emphasised that for the vast majority of people sensibly planned physical activity and exercise is not harmful and the benefits of physical activity far outweigh the risks of inactivity.

INFORMAL EXERCISE AND PHYSICAL ACTIVITY

Fitting something else into a busy life is difficult. Moreover, notions of 'going for the burn' and 'no pain no gain' are incorrect, misguided, off-putting and potentially dangerous. If people perceive exercise as a damaging, burdensome chore, requiring 'blood, sweat and tears', expert instruction and supervision, and access to expensive, sophisticated, user-unfriendly equipment and facilities, they are unlikely to commence and continue exercising.

There's no denying that acquiring health benefits from exercise does require effort, will-power and determination, but it does not require long bouts of exhausting, strenuous exercise, joining a gym or use of equipment. Since exercise is a subcategory of physical activity, our usual daily physical activities-walking, gardening, shopping, housework, occupational and leisure activities, a day out, etc – can all be regarded as 'informal' exercise that have health benefits (ACSM 2006, Fletcher et al 2001, NICE 2006, Pate et al 1995). The workload incurred during common daily physical activities can be expressed as metabolic equivalent (MET) of lying quietly doing nothing, e.g. lying = 1.0 (referent value), shopping = 4.2 (Fletcher et al 2001).

To attain health benefits, people need to accumulate 30 minutes of physical activity on most days of the week. This could, for example, be achieved by one 30-minute brisk walk, or accumulated during two 15-minute walks, or three 10-minute walks. Additional benefits are gained from doing activities for longer or at higher intensity, and as health benefits acquired from physical activity are 'dose-related', within reason, the more people do the better.

Walking is a very safe, simple and beneficial physical activity that doesn't require specialist equipment or facilities. People can easily begin to exercise by increasing the amount they walk-walking rather than driving, getting off a bus earlier and walking the last bit. Almost anything that gets you up, active and out is good. More 'formal' exercise (e.g. cycling, swimming, yoga, Tai Chi or exercise classes) are excellent, but require extra effort, equipment, facilities and sometimes supervision which may be unavailable. People need to find something that they want to do that is comfortable, enjoyable, affordable and available, and find ways to integrate it into their lifestyle (NICE, 2006).

PSYCHOSOCIAL EFFECTS OF PHYSICAL ACTIVITY AND EXERCISE

Illness does not take place in a biological vacuum. People are not just affected by the biological or anatomical disruption caused by a pathology, they are also affected by their and other people's psychological and emotional reaction to illness and many other social, and environmental factors (Hurley et al 2003, Main & Watson 2002, Turk 1996) (see Chs 5 & 11). People with rheumatic conditions are often elderly, have been inactive for some time, are unfit and have co-morbidities (e.g. respiratory, cardiovascular). While many people intuitively understand that movement is good for joints, they are concerned and confused by their experience that activity often causes joint pain and rest eases it. They interpret pain as signalling activity-induced joint damage, assume that rest prevents damage and promotes healing, and surmise that reducing physical activity will prolong the life of their joints and begin to avoid activities. These 'fear-avoidance' beliefs and behaviours lead to people becoming less active with all the attendant problems and consequences of inactivity (Dekker et al 1992).

The traditional 'biomedical model' of ill-health takes little account of health beliefs, but aims to 'cure' the underlying pathology using medical or surgical interventions, the patient is a passive recipient of these interventions. The 'biopsychosocial model' of ill-health (Main & Watson 2002, Turk 1996) is described in detail in Chapter 5. This model accepts there is often a biological cause of ill-health and symptoms. It takes a holistic approach to the assessment and treatment of rheumatic conditions and places much more importance on the influence of people's health beliefs, understandings, experiences, emotions and social environment on their reaction to their health problems, their ability to cope with and adjust to living with the consequences of chronic ill-health. People's attitudes and beliefs about their health, how they cope with ill-health and their confidence in their ability to do what they need to determines their reaction to ill-health and their ability to exercise.

Attitudes and beliefs about the cause and prognosis of ill-health and effective treatment are major determinants of illness behaviour and willingness to exercise and undertake physical activity. People who 'catastrophise' and believe their ill-health to be inevitable, incurable and untreatable, will feel demoralised, anxious and helpless and their self-confidence is undermined (Main & Watson 2002, Turk 1996, Turner et al 2000). Coping strategies are efforts people make to minimize the effects of ill-health. People who employ passive coping strategies (e.g. resting, avoiding activities, relinquishing responsibility for pain control to others) have worse pain and function than people who use active coping strategies (e.g. remaining physically active, diverting attention) and avoid catastrophising (Keefe et al 1996). The coping strategies employed are based on people's beliefs and past experiences. Self-efficacy is a person's confidence in their ability to perform tasks like taking exercise (Bandura 1977). People with high self-efficacy are less anxious, less depressed and report less pain, are more physically active and more willing to attempt and persevere with exercise programmes than people with low self-efficacy (McAuley 1992, McAuley et al 1993).

Crucially, psychosocial traits are not set in stone, they can be altered for better or worse by positive and negative experiences (Main & Watson 2002, Turk 1996). This malleability presents opportunities to promote exercise and physical activity. Patient education and self-management interventions successfully challenge erroneous ill-health beliefs (Bodenheimer et al 2002, Coulter & Ellins 2007, Holman & Lorig 1997, Newman et al 2004, Superuio-Cabuslay et al 1996, Warsi et al 2003) about physical activity. For example informing people that rheumatic conditions are not untreatable, that pain-related activity does not signal joint damage, that movement is good for joints, inactivity is bad, how they could easily become more active, and reassure them about what they can (not) do. They also help people re-evaluate their problems, reduce anxiety, catastrophising and fear-avoidance behaviours and give people active strategies enabling them to help themselves.

INTEGRATED REHABILITATION PROGRAMMES

The most effective chronic ill-health management regimens integrate exercise with patient education on healthy life-styles, self management of disease and coping strategies (Griffiths et al 2007, Hurley et al 2007). Such programmes maximise the benefits from both physical and educational approaches, challenging erroneous health beliefs and inappropriate behaviour. The positive mastery experienced following successful completion of a simple, practical exercise regimen that people can perform themselves without exacerbating symptoms gives tangible, meaningful improvements (Hurley et al 2007). Such regimes enhance self-efficacy and provide active coping strategies (exercise/physical activity) that enable people to help themselves, reducing helplessness, disability and social isolation. The danger is that unsuccessful, negative experiences (for example involvement in complex exercise regimens, requiring expensive, specialized equipment, facilities and supervision) undermine self-efficacy, encourage passive coping strategies and dependency on others.

GETTING PEOPLE TO BEGIN AND CONTINUE EXERCISING

This section gives some practical advice about helping people begin and continue to exercise regularly. This may be best given during a supervised rehabilitation programme, reinforced with written information and regular follow-up.

GETTING GOING

People who are not normally active should be advised to begin with gentle non-weightbearing joint range of movement exercises (sitting on a bed, settee or the floor slowly bend and straighten their knees) (Fig. 7.1) or low impact activities such as a gentle walk (see Patient Information Sheet 7.2). They should assess how far they can walk before the onset of pain, set a target well within this distance, walk little and often within this distance, at a comfortable pace, resting frequently, using a walking stick if needed and training shoes or shoes with viscoelastic soles or insoles to reduce impact forces (Whittle 1999).

People often begin to experience pain after doing an activity for a short time, but continue to do the task until it is completed or pain becomes so bad they have to rest. This can reinforce negative feelings and worries about the association between physical activity and pain and joint damage. It can be helped by teaching people 'rest-activity cycling', where physical activity is interspersed with rest or less strenuous activities (pacing) (see Ch.10). People are encouraged to recognise how long it takes for them to begin to feel tired or experience mild discomfort, told to take a short rest at this point before returning to the task and take another break if pain starts to increase again or finish the task another time. Implementing simple relaxation techniques can also help reduce tension and anxiety (see Ch.11). Although rest-activity cycling may seem inconvenient and time consuming, people will find that by implementing it the time spent being active will gradually increase, activities will get easier and they will incur less pain.

To avoid 'woolly' plans being forgotten people should construct a very specific 'action plan' of achievable, personally meaningful goals. These might be simple 'functional' common activities of daily living such as walking to the shops, climbing a flight of stairs or doing the housework. The action plan should state exactly what activities they are going to do, when, where and how, and should be placed where it will be seen often (on a fridge door). Telling other people what they are trying to do can elicit peer support and turning intention into action (Mazzuca & Weinberger 1998).

People should always be nudging the boundaries of their capabilities, so that over days, weeks or months, if necessary, the frequency and intensity of exercises and activities is increased, for example by increasing the distance walked a little each time, walking more often and a little brisker. Monitoring progress highlights progress and goal-attainment, which is a powerful motivator for continued adherence. Once a goal has been achieved this achievement should be appreciated and rewarded. Then a slightly more challenging target can be set to push the boundaries of their capabilities a little further. If a goal proves too difficult a less ambitious target should be set to avoid disillusionment and undermining self-confidence and esteem. Once people have reached a level of physical activity that suits them, maintaining that level will maintain the gains they have achieved, dropping below this results in regression.

KEEPING GOING

Long term participation in regular exercise is disappointing; more than 50% of people stop exercising within 1 year (see Patient Information Sheet 7.3). This probably reflects the time and effort required for exercise which competes with work, family and leisure commitments, their attitudes and beliefs about exercise, family and social support and networks, and the many other priorities and problems in people's lives. Long term adherence to exercise can be improved by enhancing self-efficacy which improves patient adherence with exercise programs (McAuley 1992, McAuley et al 1993, Rejeski et al 1998). Sustaining long–term adherence requires regular follow-up, and reinforcement of healthcare messages is usually required to re-motivate people. Unfortunately, given finite healthcare resources the large patient population and the chronic nature of benign rheumatic conditions, supervised exercise and regular follow-up is logistically difficult. Finding ways in which people maximise self-management and self-motivation are essential, for example people need to remind themselves of the health benefits of physical activity; exercise should be seen as a necessity not a chore; the dangers of inactivity should be understood; improvements that simple activities can bring should be experienced; and the support of family and friends should be encouraged.

Inevitably, people will experience times when they don't, won't or can't exercise, because of pain, other commitments, inclement weather or they are too tired. Identifying potential barriers to exercise and planning ways of overcoming them can help. If a joint is painful they could rest until this subsides. If the weather's bad, exercise indoors, take a walk where it's sheltered or maybe rest for a day. It is important that a legitimate reason doesn't become an excuse, so when the pain subsides, enthusiasm returns or the weather cheers up, unless people resume their previous level of activity, joint stiffness, pain, muscle weakness and disability will get worse.

CONCLUSION

In summary, muscle and movement are essential for joint health. Unfortunately, erroneous health beliefs (of the patient and health care practitioner) and poor patient management can be a barrier to exercise. As a consequence unchallenged inappropriate health beliefs lead to health behaviours that can exacerbate the problems associated with chronic rheumatic conditions. Exercise is very safe for most people, and common physical activities are an excellent way of people gaining health benefits associated with 'formal' exercise regimens. One of the best ways of increasing participation in regular physical activity is by participation in integrated exercise and self-management rehabilitation programmes. These enable people to appreciate, through experience, how a simple exercise programme is safe, reduces pain and improves function. In addition, these programmes use the more holistic biopsychosocial model of healthcare to challenge erroneous health beliefs, giving people active coping strategies and enhancing important psychosocial factors such as self-efficacy, self-esteem and social interaction. Ultimately, however, people need to appreciate that the benefits of simple physical activity far out-weigh the time and effort incurred.

References and further reading

ACSM, , 2006. American College of Sports Medicine's guidelines for exercise testing and prescription. Williams and Wilkins, Lippencott. Philadelphia, USA

Ashworth, N.L., Chad, K.E., Harrison, E.L., et al., 2005. Home versus center based physical activity programs in older adults. Cochrane Database Syst. Rev. CD004017.

Bandura, A., 1977. Self-efficacy: towards a unifying theory of behavior change. Psychol. Rev. 84, 191–215.

Bearne, L.M., Scott, D.L., Hurley, M.V., 2002. Exercise can reverse quadriceps sensorimotor dysfunction that is associated with rheumatoid arthritis without exacerbating disease activity. Rheumatology 41, 157–166.

Blake, D.R., Merry, P., Unsworth, J., et al., 1989. Hypoxic-reperfusion injury in the inflamed human joint. Lancet, 289–293.

Bodenheimer, T., Lorig, K., Holman, H., et al., 2002. Patient self-management of chronic disease in primary care. J. Am. Med. Assoc. 288, 2469–2475.

Brosseau, L., Pelland, L., Wells, G., et al., 2004. Efficacy of aerobic exercises for osteoarthritis (part II): a meta-analysis. Phys. Ther. Rev. 9, 125–145.

Brosseau, L., Wells, G.A., Tugwell, P., et al., 2005. Ottawa panel evidence-based clinical practice guidelines for therapeutic exercises and manual therapy in the management of osteoarthritis. Phys. Ther. 85, 907–911.

Brouwer, G.M., Van Tol, A.W., Bergink, A.P., et al., 2007. Association between valgus and varus alignment and the development and progression of radiographic osteoarthritis of the knee. Arthritis Rheum. 56, 1204–1211.

Buckwalter, J.A., 1995. Osteoarthritis and articular cartilage use, disuse, and abuse: experimental studies. J. Rheumatol. 43 (Suppl.), 13–15.

Caspersen, C.J., Powell, K.E., Christenson, G.M., 1985. Physical activity, exercise and physical fitness: definitions and distributions for health -related research. Public Health Rep. 100, 126–146.

Cochrane, T., Davey, R.C., Matthes Edwards, S.M., 2005. Randomised controlled trial of the cost-effectiveness of water-based therapy for lower limb osteoarthritis. Health Technol. Assess. 9, 1–130.

Coulter, A., Ellins, J., 2007. Effectiveness of strategies for informing, educating, and involving patients. Br. Med. J. 335, 24–27.

Dagfinrud, H., Kvien, T.K., Hagen, K. B., 2005. The Cochrane review of physiotherapy interventions for ankylosing spondylitis. J. Rheumatol. 32, 1899–1906.

de Jong, Z., Vlieland, T.P., 2005. Safety of exercise in patients with rheumatoid arthritis. Curr. Opin. Rheumatol. 17, 177–182.

Dekker, J., Bott, B., van der Woude, L. H.V., et al., 1992. Pain and disability in osteoarthritis: a review of biobehavioral mechanisms. J. Behav. Med. 15, 189–214.

Devos-Comby, L., Cronan, T., Roesch, S.C., 2006. Do exercise and self-management interventions benefit patients with osteoarthritis of the knee? A meta-analytic review. J. Rheumatol. 33, 744–756.

Ekdahl, C., Broman, G., 1992. Muscle strength, endurance and aerobic capacity in rheumatoid arthritis: a comparative study with healthy subjects. Ann. Rheum. Dis. 51, 35–40.

Epps, H., Ginnelly, L., Utley, M., et al., 2005. Is hydrotherapy cost-effective? A randomised controlled trial of combined hydrotherapy programmes compared with physiotherapy land techniques in children with juvenile idiopathic arthritis. Health Technol. Assess. 9.

Ernst, E., 2006. Complementary or alternative therapies for osteoarthritis. Nat. Clin. Pract. Rheumatol. 2, 74–80.

Ettinger, W.H., Burns, R., Messier, S.P., et al., 1997. A randomised control trial comparing aerobic exercise and resistance exercise with a health education program in older adults with knee osteoarthritis. J. Am. Med. Assoc. 277, 25–31.

Fletcher, G.F., Balady, G.J., Amsterdam, E.A., et al., 2001. Exercise standards for testing and training: a statement for healthcare professionals from the American Heart Association. Circulation 104, 1694–1740.

Foley, A., Halbert, J., Hewitt, T., et al., 2003. Does hydrotherapy improve strength and physical function in patients with osteoarthritis – a randomised controlled trial comparing a gym based and a hydrotherapy based strengthening programme? Ann. Rheum. Dis. 62, 1162–1167.

Fransen, M., McConnell, S., Bell, M., 2002. Therapeutic exercise for people with OA of the hip and knee: a systematic review. J. Rheumatol. 29, 1737–1745.

Fransen, M., Nairn, L., Winstanley, J., et al., 2007. Physical activity for osteoarthritis management: a randomized controlled clinical trial evaluating hydrotherapy or Tai Chi classes. Arthritis Care Res. 57, 407–414.

Green, J., McKenna, F., Redfern, E., et al., 1993. Home exercises are as effective as outpatient hydrotherapy for osteoarthritis of the hip. Rheumatology 32, 812–815.

Griffiths, C., Foster, G., Ramsay, J., et al., 2007. How effective are expert patient (lay led) education programmes for chronic disease? Br. Med. J. 334, 1254–1256.

Hay, E.M., Foster, N.E., Thomas, E., et al., 2006. Effectiveness of community physiotherapy and enhanced pharmacy review for knee pain in people aged over 55 presenting to primary care: pragmatic randomised trial. Br. Med. J. 333, 995–998.

Holman, H.R., Lorig, K.R., 1997. Patient education: essential to good health care for patients with chronic arthritis. Arthritis Rheum. 40, 1371–1373.

Hurley, M.V., 1999. The role of muscle weakness in the pathogenesis of osteoarthritis. Rheum. Dis. Clin. North Am. 25, 283–298.

Hurley, M.V., 2003. Muscle dysfunction and effective rehabilitation of knee osteoarthritis: what we know and what we need to find out. Arthritis Rheum. 49, 444–452.

Hurley, M.V., Mitchell, H.L., Walsh, N., 2003. In osteoarthritis, the psychosocial benefits of exercise are as important as physiological improvements. Exerc. Sports Sci. Rev. 31, 138–143.

Hurley, M.V., Walsh, N.E., Mitchell, H.L., et al., 2007. Clinical effectiveness of "ESCAPE–knee pain" a rehabilitation programme for chronic knee pain: a cluster randomised trial. Arthritis Rheum. 57, 1211–1219.

Keefe, F.J., Kashikar-Zuck, S., Opiteck, J., et al., 1996. Pain in arthritis and musculoskeletal disorders: the role of coping skills training and exercise interventions. J. Ortho. Sports Phys. Ther. 24, 279–290.

Klepper, S.E., 2003. Exercise and fitness in children with arthritis: evidence of benefits for exercise and physical activity. Arthritis Care Res. 49, 435–443.

Main, C., Watson, P., 2002. Psychological aspects of pain. Man. Ther. 4, 203–215.

Mazzuca, S., Weinberger, M., 1998. Social support. In: Brandt, K.D., Doherty, M., Lohmander, L. (Eds.), Osteoarthritis. Oxford University Press, Oxford, pp. 331–338.

McAuley, E., 1992. The role of efficacy cognitions in the prediction of exercise behavior in middle-aged adults. J. Behav. Med. 15, 65–88.

McAuley, E., Lox, C., Duncan, T.E., 1993. Long-term maintenance of exercise, self-efficacy and physiological change in older adults. J. Gerontol. (Psycholo. Sci.) 48, 218–224.

McCarthy, C.J., Mills, P.M., Pullen, R., et al., 2004. Supplementing a home exercise programme with a class-based exercise programme is more effective than home exercise alone in the treatment of knee osteoarthritis. Rheumatology 43, 880–886.

Meldrum, D.A.N., 2003. Lets get physical-exercise guidelines for cardiac patients. Perspect. Cardiol., 29–33.

Merry, P., Williams, R., Cox, N., et al., 1991. Comparative intra-articular pressure dynamics in joints with acute traumatic and chronic inflammatory effusions: potential implications for hypoxic-reperfusion injury. Ann. Rheum. Dis. 50, 917–920.

Minor, M.A., 1999. Exercise in the treatment of osteoarthritis. Rheum. Dis. Clin. North Am. 25, 397–415.

Munneke, M., de Jone, B.A., Zwinderman, A.H., et al., 2005. Effect of a high-intensity weight-bearing exercise program on radiologic damage progression of the large joints in subgroups of patients with rheumatoid arthritis. Arthritis Care Res. 53, 410–417.

Newman, P.S., Steed, L., Mulligan, K., 2004. Self-management interventions for chronic illness. The Lancet 364, 1523.

NICE, 2006. Four commonly used methods to increase physical activity: brief interventions in primary care, exercise referral schemes, pedometers and community- based exercise programmes for walking and cycling. National Institute for Health and Clinical Excellence, London http://www.nice.org.uk/ (accessed January 2009).

Nordemar, R., Ekblom, B., Zachrisson., et al., 1981. Physical training in rheumatoid arthritis: a controlled long- term study. Scand. J. Rheumatol. 10, 17–30.

Pate, R.R., Pratt, M., Blair, S.N., et al., 1995. Physical activity and public health. A recommendation from the centers for disease control and prevention and the American College of Sports Medicine. J. Am. Med. Assoc. 273, 402–407.

Patrick, D.L., Ramsey, S.D., Spencer, A.C., et al., 2001. Economic evaluation of aquatic exercise for persons with osteoarthritis. Med. Care 39, 413–424.

Pelland, L., Brosseau, L., Wells, G., et al., 2004. Efficacy of strengthening exercises for osteoarthritis (part I): a meta analysis. Phys. Ther. Rev. 9, 77–108.

Pendleton, A., Arden, N., Dougados, M., et al., 2000. EULAR recommendations for the management of knee osteoarthritis: report of a task force of the Standing Committee for International Clinical Studies Including Therapeutic Trials (ESCISIT). Ann. Rheum. Dis. 59, 936–944.

Rejeski, W.J., Ettigner, W.H., Martin, K., et al., 1998. Treating disability in knee osteoarthritis with exercise: a central role for self-efficacy and pain. Arthritis Care Res. 11, 94–101.

Roddy, E., Zhang, W., Doherty, M., 2005. Aerobic walking or strengthening exercise for osteoarthritis of the knee? A systematic review. Ann. Rheum. Dis. 64, 544–548.

Stenstrom, C., Lindell, B., Swanberg, P., et al., 1991. Intensive dynamic training in water for rheumatoid arthritis functional class II: a long term study or effects. Scand. J. Rheumatol. 20, 358–365.

Stenstrom, C.H., 1993. Dynamic Therapeutic Exercise in Rheumatoid Arthritis. Karolinska Institute, Stockholm.

Stenström, C.H., Minor, M.A., 2003. Evidence for the benefit of aerobic and strengthening exercise in rheumatoid arthritis. Arthritis Care Res. 49, 428–434.

Superuio-Cabuslay, E., Ward, M.M., Lorig, K.R., 1996. Patient education interventions in osteoarthritis and rheumatoid arthritis: a meta-analytic comparison with nonsteroidal antiinflammatory drug treatment. Arthritis Care Res. 9, 292–301.

Takken, T., van der Net, J., Kuis, W., et al., 2003. Aquatic fitness training for children with juvenile idiopathic arthritis. Rheumatology 42, 1408–1414.

Thomas, K.S., Muir, K.R., Docherty, M., et al., 2002. Home based exercise programme for knee pain and knee osteoarthritis: randomised controlled trial. Br. Med. J. 325, 752–756.

Turk, D.C., 1996. Biopsychosocial perspectives on chronic pain. In: Gatchel, R.J., Turk, D.C. (Eds.), Psychological Approaches to Pain Management: A Practitioner's Handbook. Guildford Press, New York, pp. 3–32.

Turner, J.A., Jensen, M.P., Romano, J.M., 2000. Do beliefs, coping and catastrophizing independently predict functioning in patients with chronic pain? Pain 85, 115–125.

van Baar, M.E., Assendelft, W.J.J., Dekker, J., et al., 1999. Effectiveness of exercise therapy in patients with osteoarthritis of the hip and knee. A systematic review of randomised clinical trials. Arthritis Rheum. 42, 1361–1369.

van den Ende, C.H.M., Vliet Vlieland, T.P.M., Munneke, M.W., et al., 1998. Dynamic exercise therapy in rheumatic arthritis: a systematic review. Br. J. Rheumatol. 37, 677–687.

van Tulder, M., Malmivaara, A., Esmail, R., et al., 2002. Exercise therapy for low back pain. A systematic review within the framework of the Cochrane Collaboration Back review Group. Spine 25, 2784–2796.

Verhagen, A.P., Bierma-Zeinstra, S.M.A., Cardoso, J.R., et al., 2004. Balneotherapy for rheumatoid arthritis. Cochrane Database Syst. Rev.

Verhagen, A.P., de Vet, H.C.W., de Bie, R.A., et al., 1997. Taking Baths: the efficacy of balneotherapy in patients with arthritis. A systematic review. J. Rheumatol. 24, 1964–1971.

Walsh, N.E., Hurley, M.V., 2005. Management of knee osteoarthritis in physiotherapy outpatient departments in Great Britain and Northern Ireland. Rheumatology 44 (Suppl. 1), 383.

Warsi, A., LaValley, M.P., Wang, P.S., et al., 2003. Arthritis self-management education programs: a meta-analysis of the effect on pain and disability. Arthritis Rheum. 48, 2207–2213.

Whittle, M., 1999. Generation and attenuation of transient impulsive forces beneath the foot: a review. Gait Posture 10, 264–275.

Zochling, J., van der Heijde, D., Dougados, M., et al., 2006. Current evidence for the management of ankylosing spondylitis: a systematic literature review for the ASAS/EULAR management recommendations in ankylosing spondylitis. Ann. Rheum. Dis. 65, 423–432.

PATIENT INFORMATION SHEET 7.1

EXERCISING SAFELY

Controlled physical activity/exercise has many health benefits and few dangers, and very few people are too old or infirm to benefit, but remember the following:

- Always ensure you are stable and safe when exercising
- Start a new exercise/activity slowly and cautiously
- Progress slowly, gradually increasing the time, frequency and intensity of exercising
- Work hard within your capabilities but near your maximum

- Exercise moderately – that's when you can hold a conversation while doing an activity
- Exercise is not a cure for rheumatic diseases. There are likely to be fluctuations in pain levels; during times of increased pain, reduce your activity until the pain subsides
- If an activity causes prolonged pain, discomfort or swelling lasting more than a couple of days or wakes you at night, rest for a couple of days
- As the pain settles resume exercising gently, gradually building up the exercises as before but leaving out activities that caused pain or adding them cautiously
- Blood, sweat and tears are NOT essential – or desirable

PATIENT INFORMATION SHEET 7.2

GET GOING

- Set simple, challenging, but realistic, achievable goals
- Pursue them in a very focused way
- Plan exactly what, when, where and how you will achieve your goals
- Write an action plan to remind you how you intend to achieve your goals
- Put your action plan where you will see it often and stick to it
- Monitor your progress, e.g. circle the days on a calendar when you've exercised and aim to cover it with circles

- If you can't achieve a goal make it easier
- When you achieve your goal, tell everybody, reward yourself
- When you have achieved a goal, revise your goals and action plan, setting more challenging goals to improve further or maintain the improvement.

PATIENT INFORMATION SHEET 7.3

KEEP GOING

- Starting to exercise is the hardest thing
- Get support of family and friends
- Monitor yourself-keeping account of what you have done reminds you to do it and charts your improvement
- Reward yourself when you achieve a goal
- Believe in yourself and your ability to be active – think about the simple things you have achieved when you thought you could not
- Believe exercise will help you and think about the difference the things you have achieved have made to your life
- Exercise for the right reasons because it helps, you want to and you enjoy it – it is not a sentence
- Find something you like to do or you will not continue it
- Think about how to overcome barriers
- Plan for relapse – when the going gets tough decide how you can 'tough' it out and get back to exercising again.

Chapter 8

Physical therapies: treatment options in rheumatology

Lindsay M. Bearne PhD MSc MCSP School of Biomedical and Health Sciences, Kings College London, London, UK

Michael V. Hurley PhD MCSP Rehabilitation Research Unit, Kings College London, Dulwich Community Hospital, London, UK

CHAPTER CONTENTS

KEY POINTS

- Physical therapies aim to control pain, minimise joint stiffness and limit joint damage with the least adverse treatment effects
- There is some evidence that TENS, thermotherapy and acupuncture can relieve pain in some rheumatic conditions but insufficient evidence for the efficacy of many electrotherapy interventions and manual therapy

- Physical therapies are safe and popular with powerful placebo effects and are useful in the overall management of rheumatic conditions.

INTRODUCTION

Physical therapies are non-pharmalogical treatments which are widely used by therapists in the management of rheumatic diseases. This chapter briefly reviews the role of physical therapies (electrophysical agents (EPA), thermotherapy and cryotherapy, manual therapy and acupuncture) in common rheumatic conditions and discusses the current evidence and recommendations for clinical practice for these therapies.

THE AIMS OF PHYSICAL THERAPIES IN RHEUMATIC DISEASES

It is important our assessment and management of patients with rheumatic disease is holistic. This means therapists should consider the person with the rheumatic condition rather than the structure (e.g. synovial joint) or the pathological process (e.g. rheumatoid arthritis) prior to selecting any therapy. This holistic perspective has been conceptualised as the biopyschosocial model (see Chs 5 & 11) and suggests there is far more than just the pathology or structure which has an impact on the outcome of the disease. Therefore, a detailed subjective and objective patient assessment, which includes psychosocial factors (Kendall 1997) and health related quality of life, should be obtained (Ch. 4) and a collaborative

© 2010 Elsevier Ltd
DOI: 10.1016/B978-0-443-06934-5.00008-5

process used to develop realistic, achievable, measurable patient orientated goals. As all patients with rheumatic disease are different, starting from a different baseline and with different needs, the physiological and psychological impact of each physical therapy should be considered on an individual basis.

When considered in a biopyschosocial context, physical therapies predominantly address the 'bio' aspect and aim to control pain, minimise joint stiffness, limit joint damage with the least adverse treatment effects. However, if applied judiciously physical therapies help maximise function and health-related quality of life.

ELECTROPHYSICAL AGENTS

Electrophysical agents (EPA) are used by healthcare practitioners to relieve pain, improve muscle function and reduce inflammation. An underlying premise of all EPAs is that applying an external energy source can beneficially alter physiological processes. In the management of rheumatic disease, electrical stimulation, low level laser therapy, ultrasound therapy and short wave diathermy are most frequently used.

SENSORY STIMULATION FOR PAIN RELIEF

Sensory stimulation means applying electrical stimulation with the intention of increasing the afferent nerve input. This effects a change at the spinal or supraspinal level of the neurological system (centrally), which can be used to alter pain perception. The rationale for this treatment is provided by the pain gate theory (Melzack & Wall 1965). This theory proposes that pain perception is regulated by a 'gate' at the level of the dorsal column of the spinal cord, which may be opened or closed by means of other inputs from peripheral nerves or the central nervous system (see Ch. 5). Essentially, electrical stimulation is aimed at modifying the peripheral input (stimulation of the A beta mechanoreceptor fibres at the skin) which inhibits nociceptor activity of C and A delta fibres (at the posterior horn) thus changing the level of excitability of the central components of the neurological system, e.g. central nociceptive transmission cells, wide dynamic range neurons (Robertson et al 2006).

Additionally, electrical stimulation is responsible for releasing chemical mediators (e.g. encephalins), which have a morphine type inhibitory effect on the C- fibre (nociceptor) system. Furthermore, activation of the A delta fibres may provoke impulses in the mid brain which inhibit the neurons at the original site via stimulation of the descending inhibitory pathways (Galea 2002). Thus, by changing the sensory input the perception of pain may be altered but not the underlying cause of the pain.

TRANSCUTANEOUS ELECTRICAL NERVE STIMULATION

Transcutaneous electrical nerve stimulation (TENS) is an easily applied, non-invasive modality with relatively few contraindications (Fox & Sharp 2007, Robertson et al 2006) which can be readily adopted as a pain management strategy for patients with rheumatic conditions. Small battery operated TENS machines deliver an electrical impulse via surface skin electrodes (Fig. 8.1). Five parameters can be adjusted to achieve most effective pain relief – waveform, pulse duration and frequency, intensity and electrode position. Therapeutic methods of applying TENS are categorized into conventional, 'acupuncture-like', burst, brief intense and modulation (Watson 2007). Selection is based on the underlying condition, severity and duration of symptoms (Brosseau et al 2004) (Table 8.1). Recent meta-analyses of six randomised controlled trials (RCT) involving 268 patients with lower limb osteoarthritis (OA) suggest all modes of TENS improve pain, but not range of movement, function or strength regardless of the treatment protocol (Brosseau et al 2004). In patients with knee OA, longer courses of treatment (>4 weeks) and greater intensity protocols (high burst or low frequency) may produce greatest pain relief (Osiri et al 2000). In people with inflammatory disease, acupuncture-like TENS reduces pain and increases muscle power,

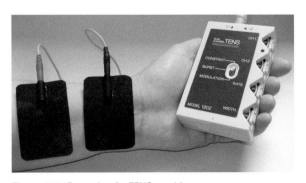

Figure 8.1 Example of a TENS machine.

whilst conventional TENS improves self reported disease activity but not pain (Brosseau et al 2003a).

Clinical guidelines recommend acupuncture-like TENS for improving pain, oedema and power in patients with RA, (Brosseau et al 2004) as a relatively safe adjunct therapy for the relief of pain in patients with OA (Philadelphia Panel 2001) and for osteoporotic (OP) patients with intractable pain especially those with chronic low back pain and recent vertebral factures (Chartered Society of Physiotherapy 1999).

INTERFERENTIAL THERAPY

Interferential therapy (IFT) is an alternative method of sensory nerve stimulation, which applies two alternating currents of slightly different frequencies (kHz) at right angles to each other in a continuous stream. Theoretically, where the currents intersect an area of maximum stimulation is produced. However, as the spread of the current reduces the intensity in deep tissues the superimposed current may be less effective than immediately under electrodes and therefore may not achieve the desired therapeutic response (Robertson et al 2006). Clinically, medium frequency currents are applied which pass through the skin more comfortably than a typical low frequency current (due to skin resistance). At the intersection of the currents a beat frequency produces an effect similar to a low frequency current (Fig. 8.2). Using appropriate frequencies, sensory nerve

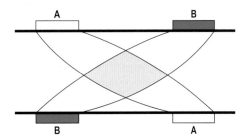

Current 'A' is at 4000 Hz and current 'B' is at 3900 Hz
Interference current (beat frequency) generated in the
central zone at the difference between input currents
which would be 100 Hz

Figure 8.2 Diagrammatic representation of interferential current (Watson 2000).

Table 8.1 Possible therapeutic methods and parameters for applying TENS (adapted with permission from www.electrotherapy.org)

PROTOCOL	DEFINITION	POSSIBLE PAIN RELIEF MECHANISMS	TREATMENT PARAMETERS
Conventional	High frequency 90–130 Hz Pulse width $<$100 μs	Pain relief via pain gate mechanism	Treatment time: at least 30 minutes but as long as needed Intensity: definitely there but comfortable Limited carry over effect
Acupuncture	Low frequency -2–5Hz Pulse width $>$200 μs	Pain relief via opioid mechanism	Treatment time: at least 30 minutes but as long as needed Intensity: definite/strong sensation Positive carry over effect
Burst	Low frequency 10 Hz Burst impulses – 2–3 per second	Pain relief via all pain mechanisms	Treatment time: at least 30 minutes but as long as needed Intensity: definite/strong sensation
Brief intense	High frequency $>$80 Hz Pulse width $>$150 μs	Pain relief via pain gate mechanism	Treatment time: 15–30 minutes Intensity: close to tolerance Indication: to achieve rapid pain relief
Modulation	All characteristics are varied throughout application	All pain relief mechanisms may be stimulated	Treatment time: at least 30 minutes but as long as needed Intensity: strong/definitely there but comfortable Indication: suitable for long term use as modulation diminishes the accommodation effects of the sensory nerves to a 'regular' stimulation pattern

stimulation can be achieved, activating the pain gate mechanism (between 80–130Hz) and opioid mechanisms (<10Hz) associated with pain relief.

Evidence for the effectiveness of IFT in rheumatic disease is limited but it may reduce pain in patients with psoriatic arthritis (Walker et al 2006) and when combined with ultrasound may reduce pain and improve sleep in patients with fibromyalgia (Almeida et al 2003). However, due to the size of the apparatus, application of IFT is limited to use within the healthcare setting and therefore encourages reliance on healthcare practitioners rather than promoting self-management. Whilst there is some evidence to support the efficacy of sensory stimulation for pain relief no studies directly compare the clinical effectiveness of TENS and IFT. Without evidence of superior efficacy of one form of sensory stimulation, the small, battery operated TENS machine offers a relatively safe, inexpensive, easily self administered method of symptom control in patients with rheumatic diseases.

MOTOR STIMULATION OF INNERVATED MUSCLE

Motor stimulation is the production of a muscle contraction by electrical stimulation of the motor nerves. It is used for; increasing muscle strength and endurance, re-education of motor control, oedema reduction, increasing joint and soft tissue mobility and altering muscle structure and function (trophic changes). Therapeutically it can be used as a sole treatment, (Bircan et al 2002) superimposed over an active muscle contraction (Strojnik 1998) or as an adjunct to an exercise regimen (Fitzgerald et al 2003).

Gradual onset short duration pulses may be selected at frequencies between 30-100 Hz with on-off times and rate of ramping (progression) varying with clinical considerations. The number of repetitions is defined by the training response required and the amplitude is set at maximum individual tolerance. A two second pulse, followed by four second rest with a one second ramp, mimics physiological muscle contraction although the complexity of normal muscle group activity cannot be simulated (Robertson et al 2006).

In patients with rheumatoid arthritis (RA) with secondary disuse atrophy of the first dorsal interosseous of the hand, muscle stimulation improves hand function, strength and fatigue resistance of the first dorsal interosseus muscle (Oldham & Stanley 1989). Similarly, functional performance and quadriceps muscle torque improved by 10% in people with OA knee following muscle stimulation (Talbot et al 2003).

Whilst not included in any clinical guidelines for patients with rheumatic disease, motor stimulation should be considered as an adjunctive therapy for patients with gross muscle weakness secondary to rheumatic disease. However, the high amplitude needed to evoke a muscle contraction can be uncomfortable and may diminish patient compliance with the treatment.

LOW LEVEL LASER THERAPY

Low level laser therapy (LLLT) utilises a pencil-like beam of electromagnetic waves of a single frequency and defined wavelength to promote tissue healing and pain relief in a broad spectrum of soft tissue injuries and diseases. The effects of LLLT are not thermal but photochemical reactions in cells, termed *photobioactivation*. LLLT produces its physiological and therapeutic effects by applying enough energy to disturb local electron orbits, initiate chemical change, disrupt molecular bonds and produce free radicals at the cell membrane to control the inflammatory response, promote healing and pain relief (Box 8.1) (Robertson et al 2006, Watson 2000).

In patients with rheumatic disease the evidence for the use of LLLT is mixed. In patients with OA, LLLT is ineffective for pain relief (Brosseau et al 2005). However, LLLT is recommended in clinical practice guidelines for patients with RA as it improves pain and morning stiffness, but not function, range of

---

BOX 8.1   The potential photobioactivation effects of low level laser therapy

Altered cell proliferation
Activation & proliferation of fibroblasts
Altered cell motility
Alteration of cell membrane potentials
Activation of phagocytes
Stimulation of angiogenesis
Stimulation of immune responses
Alteration of action potentials
Increased cellular metabolism
Altered prostaglandin production
Stimulation of macrophages
Altered endogenous opioid production
Stimulation of mast cell degranulation

movement, joint tenderness or swelling (Brosseau et al 2004).

ULTRASOUND THERAPY

In the management of rheumatic diseases, ultrasound therapy (US) is commonly used as an adjunctive therapy for its proposed effects on inflammation as well as for pain relief. It uses sound waves at very high frequencies (0.5-5 MHz) to produce mechanical vibration within the tissues. If applied in high doses absorption of US results in heating, which decreases pain and fluid viscosity, increases metabolic rate and blood flow (thermal effects) (Nussbaum 1997). At lower doses of US or following pulsed US non thermal, mechanical effects such as stable cavitation (formation of gas bubbles in tissues), standing waves (reflected waves superimposed on incident waves) and acoustic streaming (fluid movement which exerts pressure changes on a cell) occur (Maxwell 1992) which cause membrane distortion, increased permeability, increased nutrient transfer and facilitation of tissue repair (Mortimer & Dyson 1988). When applied to acutely inflamed tissues it encourages the inflammatory process to progress to the proliferation stage (Watson 2000).

Whilst there is evidence to support the physiological effects of US in laboratory or animal studies, (Mortimer & Dyson 1988) evidence for its clinical effectiveness in people with rheumatic conditions is limited (Brosseau et al 2004, Zhang et al 2007) and it is only recommended for those with arthritis of the hand (Casimiro et al 2002, Welch et al 2001). Moreover, a recent review concludes US may only be effective for people with carpal tunnel syndrome and those with calcific tendonitis of the shoulder (Roberston & Baker 2001) despite being a frequently used electrophysical modality in musculoskeletal conditions (Kitchen & Partridge 1996).

SHORT WAVE THERAPY

Short wave diathermy (SWD) produces its physiological and therapeutic effects by rapidly alternating electrical and magnetic currents at short wave frequencies (27.12 MHz). Continuous SWD is applied to tissues either inductively (metal cable, covered in insulating rubber, which is wrapped around the part to be treated) or capacitively (plate or malleable electrodes placed next to the area to be treated), usually for 20–30 minutes. It increases skin temperature by 3-7°C, muscle temperature by 2-6°C (Robertson et al 2006) and intra-articular heating has also been demonstrated (Oosterveld et al 1992).

Pulsed short wave diathermy (PSWD) or pulsed electromagnetic energy (PEME) is an intermittent oscillating high frequency (27.12 MHz) output. The mean power depends on the peak (pulse) power, duration and frequency of the pulse. As a thermal effect is only produced with outputs above 7 Watts, the non thermal physiological effects of PSWD are postulated to occur due to agitation of ions, molecules, membranes and perhaps cells which accelerates membrane transport, phagocytic, and enzymatic activity (Kitchen & Partridge 1992, Low 1995, Robertson et al 2006).

Brief, high intensity bursts of electromagnetic energy:

- increase the number and activity of cells in the injured region
- improve re-absorption of haematoma
- reduce oedema
- increase the rate of fibrin deposition
- increase collagen deposition and organisation
- increase nerve growth and repair (Robertson et al 2006).

Whilst based on reasonable biophysical evidence (Hill et al 2002), the evidence for the clinical effective of short wave therapy is mixed and some studies report no improvement of pain, stiffness or disability in patients with lower limb OA following PSWD (Callaghan et al 2000, Klaber Moffett et al 1996, Laufer et al 2005, Thamsborg et al 2005) whilst others conclude pulsed SWD may be beneficial (Van Nguyen & Marks 2002) after lengthy courses of treatment (Jan et al 2006). There is no evidence to suggest SWD may be beneficial for people with RA and it is not included in guidelines for the management of any rheumatic conditions.

ACUPUNCTURE

Acupuncture literally means 'needle piercing' – the practice of inserting very fine needles into the skin to stimulate specific anatomic points in the body (called acupoints or acupuncture points) for therapeutic purposes (Fig. 8.3). Heat, pressure, friction, suction, or impulses of electromagnetic energy may be used to stimulate the points.

Acupuncture is one of the more popular complementary interventions for arthritis (Ernst 1997)

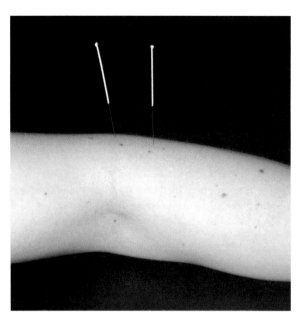

Figure 8.3 Acupuncture treatment.

and it is gaining acceptance and utilization within western healthcare systems as a form of pain relief (Tindle et al 2005) where its effects are explained through the pain gate theory (Melzack & Wall 1965) and stimulation of the release of neurochemicals in the central nervous system (Cheung & Pomeranz 1979). In its traditional form (as a component of traditional Chinese medicine) acupuncture points are stimulated to balance the movement of energy (qi) in the body along energy channels (meridians) to restore health and the production of acupuncture analgaesia is explained via neural, humeral and biomagnetic mechanisms (Cao 2002).

Acupuncture is used by many physiotherapists, often within the NHS, and the Acupuncture Association of Chartered Physiotherapists is a recognised special interest group within the profession. Many doctors have also been trained in acupuncture, and there is a group of practitioners who have trained in acupuncture and who mainly work privately, sometimes also prescribing Chinese herbs (see Ch. 14).

Acupuncture needles can of course cause injuries, (for example, accidental penetration of the lung, which causes a pneumothorax or collapsed lung), but in the hands of a trained practitioner acupuncture is very safe (White et al 2001). The only contraindications are in patients who have an undiagnosed bleeding disorder, or a fear of needles.

There is no evidence that acupuncture interacts with other treatments.

There is growing evidence that acupuncture is beneficial for pain management in peripheral joint osteoarthritis. A systematic review of 18 randomized controlled trials (RCTs) of acupuncture and electroacupuncture and a meta-analysis of data from three studies suggests acupuncture relieves pain in peripheral joint OA compared with sham acupuncture (Kwon et al 2006). This is supported by a recent systematic review and meta–analysis of eight RCTs which concurs that acupuncture is superior to sham acupuncture or usual care and suggests the effect size is comparable to that of nonsteroidal anitiinflammatory drugs (NSAIDs) whilst having fewer side effects (White et al 2007). However, the addition of acupuncture to a course of advice and exercise for osteoarthritis of the knee provided no further improvement in function and pain (Foster et al 2007) and whilst the National Institute of Health and Clinical Excellence recommended acupuncture for low back pain, their osteoarthritis guidelines do not (NICE 2008, 2009).

In patients with RA acupuncture does not alter pain, medication use or disease activity (Casimiro et al 2002). In patients with fibromyalgia, the evidence of effectiveness is mixed (Berman et al 1999, Mayhew & Ernst 2007, Sim & Adams 2002); some studies report short-lived, small beneficial effects (Deluze et al 1993, Guo & Jia 2005, Martin et al 2006) and others report no positive effects of acupuncture (Assefi et al 2005, Sprott 1998). Consequently, acupuncture is only recommended for short-term pain control in peripheral joint OA (Kwon et al 2006, White et al 2007) and in osteoporosis (Chartered Society of Physiotherapy 1999) but not in fibromyalgia (Mayhew & Ernst 2007) or RA (Casimiro et al 2005).

THERMOTHERAPY AND CRYOTHERAPY

Thermotherapy (the therapeutic application of a heating agent) and cryotherapy (the therapeutic application of a cooling agent) are widely used treatments to reduce pain, oedema and muscle spasm, improve tissue healing and facilitate range of motion and function. Clinically, superficial heating can be achieved by conductive methods, such as heat pads or paraffin wax baths, by radiation such as infra red light therapy and by convection, such as sauna or steam room (Hicks & Gerber 1992).

Heating of the deeper tissues can be achieved by short wave diathermy (electromagnetic energy) and high doses of ultrasound therapy, which are discussed earlier in this chapter. Cryotherapy includes the use of ice packs and ice baths, commercially available gel packs or sprays and massage with ice over acupuncture points or painful areas.

Prior to application of either therapy, skin testing to establish normal cutaneous sensation is recommended as both heat and cold therapy have a measurable effect on surface and intra-articular temperature of joints, skin micro-circulation and core temperature (Oosterveld et al 1992) and patients with abnormal cutaneous sensation (e.g. diabetic neuropathy) are at risk of damage (Fox & Sharp 2007).

Thermotherapy and cryotherapy produce analgaesia via the pain gate theory (Melzack & Wall 1965) and reduce muscle spasm. However, thermotherapy increases tissue temperature, blood flow, metabolism and connective tissue extensibility, whilst cryptherapy decreases tissue blood flow by initially causing vasoconstriction followed by vasodilatation (the 'hunting reflex'), reducing tissue metabolism, oxygen utilization, inflammation and connective tissue extensibility (Box 8.2). Whilst there are differences in physiological responses, both therapies can be used in patients with rheumatic conditions and patient preference as well as physiological response should be considered when selecting which therapy to use.

Despite being used for years as a safe and effective symptomatic treatment of rheumatic conditions, systematic reviews of thermotherapy and cryotherapy highlight a lack of good quality research (Brosseau et al 2003b). In patients with RA, hot or cold therapy has no effect on pain, swelling, ROM, strength or function (Dellhag et al 1992, Ivey et al 1994, Kirk & Kersley 1968, Rembe 1970); whereas ice massage improves pain, joint mobility and function in patients with knee OA (Yurtkuran & Kocagil 1999) and ice packs reduce swelling (Hecht et al 1983) and improve range of movement (Lin 2003) but may not relieve symptoms in painful peripheral joint conditions (Clarke et al 1999). Similarly, short-term application of hot packs are not useful in peripheral joint osteoarthritis (Hecht et al 1983) but may control pain and improve disability if applied for longer periods to patients with acute non specific low back pain (Nadler et al 2003a, 2003b).

Based on some evidence and anecdotal reports of effectiveness, thermotherapy and cryotherapy are useful palliative self management therapies for rheumatic patients and should be included in

---

BOX 8.2   The physiological changes in response to heat and cold therapy

	CRYOTHERAPY	THERMOTHERAPY
Pain	↓	↓
Muscle spasm	↓	↓
Metabolism	↓	↑
Blood flow	↓	↑
Inflammation	↓	↑
Oedema	↓	↑
Connective tissue extensibility	↓	↑

---

the management of patients with RA (Brosseau et al 2004), OA (Brosseau et al 2004, NICE 2008, Zhang et al 2007) and osteoporosis (Chartered Society of Physiotherapy 1999).

MANUAL THERAPY

Manual therapy is the skilled application of passive movement to a joint either within ('mobilisation') or beyond its active range of movement ('manipulation'). This includes oscillatory techniques, high velocity low amplitude thrust techniques, sustained stretching and muscle energy techniques. Manual therapy can be applied to joints, muscles or nerves and the aims of treatment include pain reduction, increasing range and quality of joint movement, improving nerve mobility, increasing muscle length and restoring normal function. There are three paradigms for its therapeutic effects; physiological, biomechanical or physical, and psychological (Fig. 8.4).

The physiological effects of manual therapy include the reduction of pain via the pain gate theory (Melzack & Wall 1965) and stimulation of the descending inhibitory tracts. Indirectly, manual therapy can reduce pain via inhibition of muscle spasm which reduces tension on the periarticular structures, lowering intraarticular pressure, or reduces nociceptor activity (Zuzman 1986).

The biomechanical effects of manual therapy include altering tissue extensibility and fluid dynamics thus facilitating repair and remodelling. Temporary increases in tissue extensibility following manual therapy occur through the mechanisms of creep (tissue lengthening following application of a constant force or load) and preconditioning

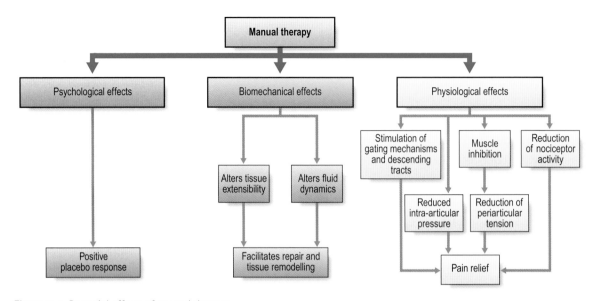

Figure 8.4 Potential effects of manual therapy.

(elongation following repeated loading) (Panjabi & White 2001). More permanent length changes need sufficient force, which are achieved in spinal manual therapy (Harms & Bader 1997), to produce microtrauma which elongates collagenous tissues (Threlkeld 1992). Repetitive movement of inflamed joints alters fluid dynamics, reducing intra articular pressure (Jayson & Dixon 1996, Levick 1979, Nade & Newbold 1983), increasing the rate of synovial blood flow and synovial fluid clearance (James et al 1994) thus improving range and movement quality.

The psychological effects of manual therapy or any therapy which has direct physical contact, such as massage, produces a response to the 'laying on of hands'. This placebo response (a response produced by a mechanism with incidental ingredients or components which have no remedial effect for the disorder but result in a positive effect of treatment) is enhanced by 'learned expectancy' (previous experience of a stimuli establishes an habitual direction of response) and the therapeutic benefits of the patient – therapist interaction and relationship (Roche 2002).

Manual therapies are commonly used interventions regardless of reported non vascular and vascular side effects (Ernst 2007). Whilst mobilisations (movement to a joint within its physiological range of movement) are not associated with serious complications, manipulations (high velocity low amplitude trust techniques applied beyond active joint range of movement) can have severe adverse reactions. Spinal manipulation, particularly when performed on the cervical spine, is

associated with mild to moderate adverse effects (30-61% of all patients) and can result in serious complications such as vertebrobasilar artery dissection followed by stroke (Ernst 2007, Taylor & Kerry 2005). Consequently, premanipulative testing protocols attempt to identify patients at risk of vertebrobasilar artery insufficiency (Magarey et al 2004) although the effectiveness of this screening has yet to be established. All guidelines contraindicate the use of manipulation in patients with RA due to the risk of joint instability particularly in the upper cervical spine (Neva et al 2006) and caution should be exercised when considering the use of manipulation in other inflammatory rheumatic conditions.

Whilst there is some evidence of the effectiveness of manual therapy in the treatment of acute and sub acute spinal pain (Bronfort et al 2004, Ferreira et al 2006, UK BEAM trial team 2004) in patients with peripheral joint disease manual therapy is often combined with other therapies which makes the relative contribution of each therapy difficult to determine (Deyle et al 2005). In patients with OA knee, a combination of manual therapy and exercise improves function and pain more than exercise (Deyle et al 2005). In patients with hip OA manual therapy improves pain, range of movement and function more than exercise alone (Hoeksma et al 2004). Those patients with the severest x-ray changes respond least to manual therapy although baseline levels of function, pain and range of movement do not predict treatment response (Hoeksma et al 2005). Consequently, evidence-based practice guidelines recommend the use of manual therapy combined with exercise for the reduction of pain in peripheral joint osteoarthritis (Brosseau et al 2005, NICE 2008).

MASSAGE

Massage has been used to reduce pain and oedema, increase circulation, improve muscle tone and enhance joint flexibility for years. Its effect may be explained by the pain gate theory (Melzack & Wall 1965) but it is also likely to have a placebo response similar to other manual therapies.

Evidence of its efficacy in rheumatic patients is limited; a course of massage improves function and pain in patients with OA knee (Perlman et al 2006) and pain and quality of life in patients with fibromyalgia (Brattberg 1999) although it is ineffective in patients with neck pain (Ezzo et al 2007). However, a systematic review of nine studies suggests massage is beneficial in patients with sub acute and chronic non-specific low back pain especially when combined with exercise and education but it was no better than manipulation and inferior to TENS for back pain relief (Furlan et al 2003). Whilst massage is not often recommended in clinical guidelines, as it has high patient satisfaction and low adverse effects it is a viable adjunct to therapy for patients with rheumatic disease.

CONCLUSION

Physical therapies are often used in the management of rheumatic conditions to relieve pain and improve function. Within the biopsychosocial model of health, physical therapies influence the 'bio' element of this framework but, if self administered, may enhance an individual's ability to cope with their condition, thus improving their quality of life. Whilst there is some evidence for their efficacy (whether they work under ideal, controlled circumstances), evidence to support their clinical effectiveness (whether they work in usual clinical practice) remains weak.

There is some evidence that thermotherapy, TENS, and acupuncture can relieve pain in some rheumatic conditions but insufficient evidence for the efficacy of many electrotherapy interventions and manual therapy. However, insufficient evidence of effectiveness should not be interpreted as 'ineffective' – it also indicates an absence of evidence. Therefore clinical decisions should be made following a thorough assessment of an individual's symptoms and treatment based on the available good quality evidence (basic principles and clinical effectiveness), practice guidelines, clinical experience and patient preference (Jones 1995) until a sufficient body of good quality studies are completed to unequivocally direct the use of physical therapies in the management of rheumatic disease.

STUDY ACTIVITIES

- Review the current guidelines for the management of rheumatoid arthritis (RA) on the NICE website (http://guidance.nice.org.uk) and consider which physical modalities may be included in an evidence based treatment programme for a patient with moderate, well controlled RA.
- Access the 'electrotherapy on the web – an educational resource' website (www.electrotherapy.org) and review the theories and evidence underpinning the use of transcutaneous electrical nerve stimulation (TENS). Consider how you would explain these concepts to a patient who is using TENS for pain relief, within the biopyschosocial framework.

USEFUL WEBSITES

www.electrotherapy.org/ accessed January 2009.
www.macpweb.org accessed January 2009.
www.csp.org.uk accessed January 2009.

References and further reading

Almeida, T.F., Roizenblatt, S., Benedito- Silva, A.A., et al., 2003. The effect of combined therapy (ultrasound and interferential current) on pain and sleep in fibromyalgia. Pain 104 (3), 665–672.

Assefi, N., Sherman, K., Jacobsen, C., et al., 2005. A randomised clinical trial of acupuncture compared with sham acupuncture in fibromyalgia. Ann. Intern. Med. 143, 10–21.

Berman, B.M., Ezzo, J., Hadhazy, V., et al., 1999. Is acupuncture effective in the treatment of fibromyalgia? J. Fam. Pract. 48 (3), 213–218.

Bircan, C., Senocak, O., Peker, O., et al., 2002. Efficacy of two forms of electrical stimulation in increasing quadriceps strength: a randomised controlled trial. Adv. Clin. Rehabil. 16 (2), 194–199.

Brattberg, G., 1999. Connective tissue massage in the treatment of fibromyalgia. Eur. J. Pain. 3 (3), 235–244.

Bronfort, G.H.M., Evans, R.L., Bouter, L.M., 2004. Efficacy of spinal manipulation and mobilization for low back pain and neck pain: a systematic review and best evidence synthesis. J. Spine. 4 (3), 335–356.

Brosseau, L., Judd, M.G., Marchand, S., et al., 2003a. Transcutaneous electrical nerve stimulation (TENS) for the treatment of rheumatoid arthritis in the hand. Cochrane. Database. Syst. Rev. 3 (CD004377).

Brosseau, L., Wells, G.A., Tugwell, P., et al., 2004. Ottawa panel evidence based clinical practice guidelines for electrotherapy and themotherapy interventions in the management of rheumatoid arthritis. Phys. Ther. 8 (11), 1016–1143.

Brosseau, L., Wells, G.A., Tugwell, P., et al., 2005. Ottawa panel evidence-based clinical practice guidelines for therapeutic exercises and manual therapy in the management of osteoarthritis. Phys. Ther. 85 (9), 907–971.

Brosseau, L., Yonge, K.A., Robinson, V., et al., 2003b. Thermotherapy for treatment of osteoarthritis. Cochrane. Database. Syst. Rev. 4, 1–8.

Callaghan, M.J., Whittaker, P.A., Grimes, S., 2000. An evaluation of pulsed shortwave on knee osteoarthritis using radioleucoscintigraphy: a pragmatic randomised, double blind controlled trial. Joint. Bone. Spine. 72, 150–155.

Cao, X. 2002. Scientific bases of acupuncture analgesia. Acupuncture Electrotherapy Research, 27(1):1-14.

Casimiro, L., Barnsley, L., Brosseau, L., et al., 2005. Acupuncture and electroacupuncture for the treatment of rheumatoid arthritis. Cochrane. Database. Syst. Rev. 4, 1–16 (CD003788).

Casimiro, L., Brosseau, L., Robinson, V., et al., 2002. Therapeutic ultrasound for the treatment of rheumatoid arthritis. Cochrane. Database. Syst. Rev. 3 (CD003787).

Chartered Society of Physiotherapy. 1999. Physiotherapy guidelines for the management of osteoporosis. London, Chartered Society of Physiotherapy

Cheung, R.S., Pomeranz, B.P., 1979. Electroacupuncture analgesia could be mediated by at least two pain-relieving mechanisms; endorphin and non-endorphin systems. Life. Sci. 25 (23), 1957–1962.

Clarke, G.R., Willis, L.A., Stenner, L., et al., 1999. Evaluation of Physiotherapy in the treatment of osteoarthritis of the knee. Rheumatol. Rehabil. 13, 190–197.

Dellhag, B., Wollersjö, I., Bjelle, A., 1992. Effect of active hand exercise and wax bath treatment in rheumatoid arthritis patients. Arthritis. Care. Res. 5 (2), 87–92.

Deluze, C., Bosia, L., Zirbs, A., et al., 1993. Electroacupuncture in fibromyalgia: results of a randomised controlled trial. Br. Med. J. 306, 393.

Deyle, G.D., Allison, S.C., Matekel, R.L., et al., 2005. Physical therapy treatment effectiveness for osteoarthritis of the knee: a randomized comparison of supervised clinical exercise and manual therapy procedures versus a home exercise program. Phys. Ther. 85 (12), 1301–1317.

Ernst, E., 1997. Acupuncture as a symptomatic treatment of osteoarthritis. A systematic review. Scand. J. Rheumatol. 26 (6), 444–447.

Ernst, E., 2007. Adverse effects of spinal manipulation: a systematic review. J. R. Soc. Med. 100 (7), 330–338.

Ezzo, J.H.B.G., Gross, A.R., Myers, C.D., et al., 2007. Cervical Overview Group. Massage for mechanical neck disorders: a systematic review. Spine 32 (3), 353–362.

Ferreira, P.H., Ferreira, M.L., Maher, C.G., et al., 2006. A specific stabilisation exercise for spinal and pelvic pain: A systematic review. Aust. J. Physiother. 52, 79–88.

Fitzgerald, G.K., Piva, S.R., Irrgang, J.J., 2003. A modified neuromuscular electrical stimulation protocol for quadriceps strength training following anterior cruciate ligament reconstruction. J. Orthop. Sports. Phys. Ther. 33 (9), 492–501.

Foster, N.E., Thomas, E., Barlas, P., et al., 2007. Acupuncture as an adjunct to exercise based physiotherapy for osteoarthritis of the knee: randomised controlled trial. Br. Med. J. 335 (Sep).

Fox, J., Sharp, T., 2007. Practical Electrotherapy - a guide to safe application. Elsevier, London.

Furlan, A.D., Brosseau, L., Imamura, M., et al., 2003. Massage for low back pain (Cochrane review). Cochrane. Libr. (2).

Galea, M., 2002. Neuroanatomy of the nocioceptive system. In: Baxter, G.D. (Ed.), Pain: a Textbook of Pain for Therapists. Harcourt publishers, Edinburgh, pp. 13–41.

Guo, X., Jia, J., 2005. Comparison of therapeutic effects on fibromyalgia syndrome between dermal-neurological electric stimulation and electric acupuncture. Chin. J. Clin. Rehabil. 9, 171–173.

Harms, M.C., Bader, D.L., 1997. Variability of forces applied by experienced therapists during spinal mobilisation. Clin. Biomech. 12 (6), 393–399.

Hecht, P.J., Backmann, S., Booth, R.E., et al., 1983. Effects of thermal therapy on rehabilitation after total knee arthroplasty: a prospective randomised study. Clin. Orthop. Relat. Res. 178, 198–201.

Hicks, J.E., Gerber, L.H., et al., 1992. Rehabilitation of patients with osteoarthritis. In: Moskiwitz, R.W., Howell, D.S., Goldberg, V.M. (Eds.) Osteoarthritis: Diagnosis Medical and Surgical Management. WB Saunders Co, pp. 427–464.

Hill, J., Lewis, M., Mills, P., 2002. Pulsed short wave diathermy effects on human fibroblast proliferation. Arch. Phys. Med. Rehabil. 83, 832–836.

Hoeksma, H.L., Dekker, J., Ronday, H.K., et al., 2005. Manual therapy in osteoarthritis of the hip: outcome of subgroup analysis. Rheumatology 44, 461–464.

Hoeksma, H.L., Dekker, J., Ronday, H.K., et al., 2004. Comparison of manual therapy and exercise therapy in osteoarthritis of the hip: a randomised clinical trial. Arthritis. Rheum. 51 (5), 722–729.

Ivey, M., Johnston, R.V., Uchida, T., 1994. Cryotherapy for postoperative pain relief following knee arthroplasty. J. Arthroplasty. 9 (3), 285–290.

James, M.L., Cleland, L.G., Gaffney, R.D., et al., 1994. The effect of exercise on 99mTc-DTPA clearance from knees with effusions. J. Rheumatol. 21, 501–504.

Jan, M.H., Chai, H.M., Wang, C.L., et al., 2006. Effects of repetitive shortwave diathermy for reducing synovitis in patients with knee osteoarthritis: an ultrasonographic study. Phys. Ther. 86 (2), 236–244.

Jayson, M.I., Dixon, A.S.J., 1996. Intra articular pressure in rheumatoid arthritis of the knee: Pressure changes during joint use. Ann. Rheum. Dis. 29, 401–408.

Jones, M., 1995. Clinical reasoning and pain. Man. Ther. 1, 17–24.

Kendall, N.S. (1997). Guide to assessing psycho-social yellow flags in acute low back pain: risk factors for long term disability and work loss Wellington, New Zealand: Accident and Compensation commission of New Zealand and the National Health Committee

Kirk, J.A., Kersley, G.D., 1968. Heat and cold in the physical treatment of rheumatoid arthritis of the knee: A controlled clinical trial. Ann. Phys. Med. Rehabil. 9 (7), 270–274.

Kitchen, S., Partridge, C., 1996. A survey to examine clinical use of ultrasound, shortwave diathermy and laser in England. Br. J. Ther. Rehabil. 3 (12), 644–650.

Kitchen, S., Partridge, C., 1992. Review of shortwave diathermy continuous and pulsed patterns. Physiotherapy 78, 243–252.

Klaber Moffett, J., Richardson, P., Frost, H., et al., 1996. Placebo controlled, double blind trial to evaluate the effectiveness of pulse short wave therapy for osteoarthritic hip and knee pain. Pain 167, 121–127.

Kwon, Y.D., Pittler, P.H., Ernst, E., 2006. Acupuncture for peripheral joint osteoarthritis. A systematic review and meta-analysis. Rheumatology 45 (11), 1331–1337.

Laufer, Y., Zilberman, R., Porat, R., 2005. Effect of pulsed shortwave diathermy on pain and function of subjects with osteoarthritis of the knee: a placebo controlled, double blind clinical trial. Clin. Rehabil. 19, 255–263.

Levick, J.R., 1979. An investigation into the validity of subatmospheric pressure recordings from synovial fluid and their dependence on joint angle. J. Physiol. 289, 55–67.

Lin, Y.H., 2003. Effects of thermal therapy in improving the passive range of knee motion: comparison of cold and superficial heat applications. Clin. Rehabil. 17 (6), 618–623.

Low, J., 1995. Dosage of some pulsed short wave diathermy trials. Physiotherapy 81, 611–616.

Magarey, M.E., Rebbeck, T., Coughlan, B., et al., 2004. Pre-manipulative testing of the cervical spine review, revision and new clinical guidelines. Man. Ther. 9 (2), 95–108.

Martin, D., Sletten, C., Williams, B., et al., 2006. Improvement in fibromyalgia symptoms with acupuncture; results of a randomised controlled trial. Mayo. Clin. Proc. 81, 749–757.

Maxwell, L., 1992. Therapeutic ultrasound: its effects on the cellular and molecular mechanisms of inflammation and repair. Physiotherapy 78 (6), 421–426.

Mayhew, E., Ernst, E., 2007. Acupuncture for fibromyalgia-a systematic review of randomised clinical trials. Rheumatology 46, 801–804.

Melzack, R., Wall, P.D., 1965. Pain mechanisms: a new theory. Science 150, 971–979.

Mortimer, A.J., Dyson, M., 1988. The effect of therapeutic ultrasound on calcium uptake in fibroblasts. Ultrasound. Med. Biol. 14 (6), 499–506.

Nade, S., Newbold, P.J., 1983. Factors determining the level and changes in intra articular pressure in the knee joint of the dog. Am. J. Physiol. 338, 21–36.

Nadler, S.F., Steiner, D.J., Erasala, G.N., et al., 2003a. Continuous low-level heat wrap therapy for treating acute non specific low back pain. Arch. Phys. Med. Rehabil. 84 (3), 329–334.

Nadler, S.F., Steiner, D.J., Petty, S.R., et al., 2003b. Overnight use of continuous low-level heat wrap therapy for relief of low back pain. Arch. Phys. Med. Rehabil. 84 (3), 335–342.

Neva, M.H., Hakkinen, A., Makinen, H., et al., 2006. High prevalence of asymptomatic cervical spine subluxation in patients with rheumatoid arthritis waiting for orthopaedic surgery. Ann. Rheum. Dis. 65 (7), 884–888.

NICE, 2008. National Institute for Health and Clinical Excellence. Osteoarthritis: national clinical guideline for care and management in adults. London: NICE www.nice.org.uk/CG059 www.nice.org.uk/CG059.

NICE, 2009. National Institute for Health and Clinical Excellence. The early management of persistent non specific low back pain. May 2009. London: NICE www.nice.org.uk/CG in press.

Nussbaum, E.L., 1997. Ultrasound to heat or not to heat: that is the question. Phys. Ther. Rev. 2, 59–72.

Oldham, J.A., Stanley, J.K., 1989. Rehabilitation of atrophied muscle in the rheumatoid arthritic hand: a comparison of two methods of electrical stimulation. J. Hand. Surg. 14 (3), 294–297.

Oosterveld, F.G.J., Rasker, J.J., Jacobs, J.W.G., et al., 1992. The effect of local heat and cold therapy on the intra articular and skin surface temperature of the knee. Arthritis. Rheum. 35, 146–151.

Osiri, M., Welch, V., Brosseau, L., et al., 2000. Transcutaneous electrical nerve stimulation for knee osteoarthritis. Cochrane. Database. Syst. Rev. 4 (CD002823).

Panjabi, M.M., White, A.A., 2001. Biomechanics in the musculoskeletal system. Churchill Livingstone, New York.

Perlman, A.L., Sabrina, A., Williams, A.-L., et al., 2006. Massage therapy for osteoarthritis of the knee. A randomised controlled trial. Arch. Intern. Med. 166, 2533–2538.

Philadelphia Panel, 2001. Philadelphia Panel evidence-based clinical practice guidelines on selected rehabilitation interventions for knee pain. Phys. Ther. 81 (10), 1675–1700.

Rembe, E.C., 1970. Use of cryotherapy on the postsurgical rheumatoid hand. Phys. Ther. 50 (1), 19–23.

Robertson, V., Ward, A., Low, J., Reed, A., 2006. Electrotherapy Explained. Principles and Practice, 7th edn. Elsevier, London.

Robertson, V.J., Baker, K.G., 2001. A review of therapeutic ultrasound: effectiveness studies. Phys. Ther. 81 (7), 1339–1350.

Roche, P., 2002. Placebo and patient care. In: Gifford, L. (Ed.), Topical issues in Pain; Placebo and nocebo, pain management, muscles and pain, Vol. 4. CNS Press Limited, Falmouth, pp. 19–41.

Sim, J., Adams, N., 2002. Systematic review of randomized controlled trials of nonpharmacological interventions for fibromyalgia. Clin. J. Pain. 18 (5), 324–336.

Sprott, H., 1998. Efficiency of acupuncture in patients with fibromyalgia. Clin. Bull. Myofacial Ther. 3, 37–43.

Strojnik, V., 1998. The effects of superimposed electrical stimulation of the quadriceps muscles on performance in different motor tasks. J. Sports. Med. Phys. Fitness. 38 (3), 194–200.

Talbot, L.A., Gaines, J.M., Ling, S.M., et al., 2003. A home-based protocol of electrical muscle stimulation for quadriceps muscle strength in older adults with osteoarthritis of the knee. Br. J. Rheumatol. 30 (7), 1571–1578.

Taylor, A.J., Kerry, R., 2005. Neck pain and headache as a result of internal carotid artery dissection: implications for manual therapists. Man. Ther. 10 (1), 73–77.

Thamsborg, G., Florescu, A., Oturai, P., et al., 2005. Treatment of knee osteoarthritis with pulsed electromagnetic fields: a randomized, double-blind, placebo-controlled study. Osteoarthritis. Cartilage. 13 (7), 575–581.

Threlkeld, A.J., 1992. The effects of manual therapy on connective tissue. Phys. Ther. 72 (12), 893–902.

Tindle, H.A., Davis, R.B., Phillips, R.S., et al., 2005. Trends in use of complementary and alternative medicine by US adults: 1997-2002. Altern. Ther. Health. Med. 11 (1), 42–49.

UK BEAM trial team, 2004. United Kingdom back pain exercise and manipulation (UK BEAM) randomised trial: effectiveness of physical treatments for back pain in primary care Dec 11. Br. Med. J. 329 (7479), 1377.

Van Nguyen, J., Marks, R., 2002. Pulsed magnetic fields for treating osteoarthritis. Physiotherapy 88, 458–470.

Walker, U.A., Uhl, M., Weiner, S.M., et al., 2006. Analgesic and disease modifying effects of interferential current in psoriatic arthritis. Rheumatol. Int. 10, 904–907.

Watson, T. 2007. Electrotherapy on the web-an educational resource Accessed 2009 www.electrotherapy.org/

Watson, T., 2000. The role of electrotherapy in contemporary physiotherapy practice. Man. Ther. 5 (3), 132–141.

Welch, V.B.L., Peterson, J., Shea, B., et al., 2001. Therapeutic ultrasound for osteoarthritis of the knee. Cochrane. Database. Syst. Rev. 3 (CD003132).

White, A., Hayhoe, S., Hart, A., et al., 2001. Adverse events following acupuncture: prospective survey of 32 000 consultations with doctors and physiotherapists. Br. Med. J. 323 (7311), 485–486.

White, A., Foster, N.E., Cummings, M., et al., 2007. Acupuncture treatment for chronic knee pain: a systematic review. Rheumatology 46 (March), 384–390.

Yurtkuran, M., Kocagil, T., 1999. Electroacupuncture and ice massage: comparison treatment for osteoarthritis of the knee. Am. J. Acupunct. 27, 133–140.

Zhang, W., Doherty, M., Leeb, B.F., et al., 2007. EULAR evidence based recommendations for the management of hand osteoarthritis: report of a Task Force of the EULAR Standing Committee for International Clinical Studies Including Therapeutics (ESCISIT). Ann. Rheum. Dis. 66 (3), 377–388.

Zuzman, M., 1986. Spinal manipulative therapy: review of some proposed mechanisms, and a new hypothesis. Aust. J. Physiother. 32 (2), 89–99.

Chapter 9

Occupational therapy: treatment options in rheumatology

Lynne Goodacre PhD Dip COT University of Central Lancashire, Preston, UK

Janet E. Harkess BSc OT Whytemans Brae Hospital, Kirkcaldy, UK

CHAPTER CONTENTS

KEY POINTS

- The role of the occupational therapist in rheumatology is to: improve a person's ability to perform daily tasks and valued life roles; facilitate successful adaptation to disruption in lifestyle, prevent loss of function and improve or maintain psychological status
- With its focus on occupational performance the link between biological, psychological, social factors and activity is central to OT interventions which are characterized by a patient centred approach
- Interventions are informed by the use of accurate and timely assessment to identify areas of activity limitation of relevance to the individual
- Some of the main approaches used by occupational therapists focus on improving occupational performance by:
  - using alternative methods of doing an activity
  - using assistive devices (i.e. assistive technology)
  - adapting the built environment.
- Occupational therapists play a central role in enabling people with rheumatic diseases to remain in employment for as long as possible.

© 2010 Elsevier Ltd
DOI: 10.1016/B978-0-443-06934-5.00009-7

INTRODUCTION

Occupational therapy aims to help a person with a rheumatic disease be who they want to be and do the things they want to do, need to do or are expected to do (Law et al 2005). The role of the occupational therapist in rheumatology is to: improve a person's ability to perform daily tasks and valued life roles; facilitate successful adaptation to disruption in lifestyle, prevent loss of function and improve or maintain psychological status (College of Occupational Therapists 2003). This is achieved by promoting health and well being through occupation across the life course. This chapter will explore some of the primary interventions used by occupational therapists to achieve this aim focusing on key occupational roles.

THE IMPACT OF RHEUMATOID ARTHRITIS ON OCCUPATIONAL PERFORMANCE

Longitudinal cohort studies of people with rheumatoid arthritis (RA) highlight its significant impact in terms of activity limitation with up to 49% of participants experiencing moderate disability after 10 years (Symmons & Silman 2006, Wolfe 2000). Whilst the model of progressive disability suggests that this occurs as a consequence of disease over time, recent work has questioned this linear model. Some evidence suggests that most disability occurs in the first 3 years of diagnosis whilst the work by Wolfe suggests that, on an individual basis, the impact of RA on activity limitation may be more variable and chaotic and less linear (Wolfe 2000). Routine assessment of activity is important therefore to identify early when activity limitation starts to occur in a person's illness trajectory.

Many studies provide insights into the significant challenges faced by people living with rheumatic diseases in terms of its impact on all areas of activity. Longitudinal studies suggest that over a five year period people with RA can lose the ability to undertake 10% of the activities they value (Katz 1995). Approximately one-third of people with RA report stopping work within 3 years of being diagnosed (Young et al 2000) and leisure activities are also affected profoundly. Fex et al 1998 found that 75% of the 106 patients in their study had to alter leisure time activities and 50% were not satisfied with their recreation.

OCCUPATIONAL THERAPY MANAGEMENT

Factors including age, stage of disease, life context, personal priorities, beliefs and culture all influence a person's illness experience and the specific challenges they face. There is therefore no standard approach to the occupational therapy management of a person with a rheumatic disease. Emphasis is placed on conducting accurate and timely assessment to identify areas of activity limitation of relevance to the individual.

Theoretical models underpinning occupational therapy such as the Canadian Model of Occupational Performance (Canadian Association of Occupational Therapists 1997) (Fig. 9.1), the Person Environment Occupational Performance Model (Christiansen et al 2005), the Model of Human Occupation (Kielhofner 2002) and the newer Kawa model (Iwama 2006) are aligned closely to the biopsychosocial model described in chapter 5. With its focus on occupational performance the link between biological, psychological, social factors and activity is central to OT interventions which are characterised by a patient centred approach.

THE EVIDENCE BASE

There is a growing body of evidence relating to the efficacy of occupational therapy interventions which allows therapists, clinicians and managers as well as the service user to make informed decisions about the best treatment options and design their interventions and services accordingly. Steultjens et al (2004) found varying degrees of evidence for the effectiveness of occupational therapy (Table 9.1), most of which is derived from work undertaken with people with inflammatory arthritis. Some areas of practice, such as work and leisure, remain under evaluated and further research is required in these areas.

ASSESSMENT OF ACTIVITY LIMITATION

Assessment is fundamental to the planning of interventions and the evaluation of their efficacy. The focus of assessments used by occupational therapists is on identifying areas of activity limitation defined by the World Health Organization (WHO) as difficulties an individual may have in executing

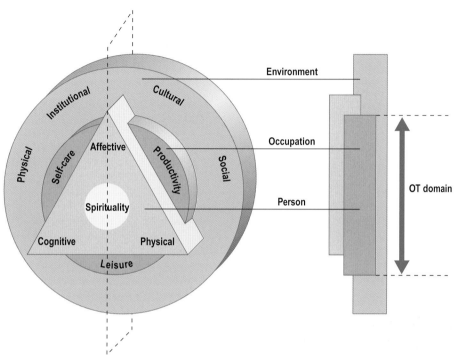

Figure 9.1 The Canadian Occupational Performance Model. Reproduced from The Canadian Model of Occupational Performance and Engagement. In: Townsend E, Polatajko H (2007) Enabling Occupation II: Advancing an Occupational Therapy Vision for Health, Well-being & Justice through Occupation. CAOT Publications ACE, Ottawa, ON p. 23 with permission of CAOT Publications ACE.

activity (WHO 2001). Assessment of activity limitation can broadly be categorised as the use of standardized assessments and the use of structured interviews.

THE INITIAL INTERVIEW

Occupational therapy interventions are based upon information gathered in the structured initial interview. Therapists use this interview to gain background information about the person and explore the context of their lives, e.g. family and social support, employment, hobbies and interests, type of housing, current use of assistive devices and adaptations, benefits, self-management and coping strategies as well as relevant information about their impairment and the treatment they are receiving. This process information may also be supplemented with standard assessments or a structured interview exploring specific areas of activity in detail. This identifies specific areas of activity limitation to inform treatment planning.

STANDARDIZED ASSESSMENT

Standardized assessments of activity limitation are used extensively in research and clinical contexts to:

- Inform treatment planning
- Provide base line information
- Monitor disease progression
- Assess the efficacy of clinical interventions.

Many of the quality of life assessments used in rheumatology incorporate subscales for activities of daily living alongside measures of psychological well-being and symptoms. For example, the Arthritis Impact Measurement Scale 2 (AIMS2) has subscales assessing physical activity, dexterity, household activity, social activities and activities of daily living (Meenan et al 1992). Some measures focus specifically on activity limitation and have been developed for use with a number of different rheumatic diseases e.g. the Disability Index of the Health Assessment Questionnaire (HAQ) (Fries et al 1980). Others are disease specific, such as the Bath

Table 9.1 Evidence for the most commonly reported occupational therapy treatments for rheumatoid arthritis

TREATMENT OPTIONS	NO. OF STUDIES PUBLISHED	AUTHOR(S) OF HIGHEST QUALITY ARTICLES	TYPE AND QUALITY OF STUDY	EVIDENCE
Comprehensive occupational therapy	2	Helewa et al (1991)	High quality RCT	Home based occupational therapy demonstrated statistically significant effect on functional ability.
		Hammond et al (2004)	High quality RCT	6-week session OT programme improves self-management
Training of motor function (hand exercises)	8	Hoenig et al (1993)	High quality RCT	No evidence
		O'Brien et al (2006)	High quality RCT	Home strengthening exercises are more effective than stretches or advice alone
Joint protection and Energy Conservation (see Ch. 10 for references)	8	Hammond et al (1999) Hammond et al (2001)	High quality RCT High quality RCT	Strong evidence that joint protection leads to an improvement in functional ability
Advice/instruction about assistive devices. In Treatment options to avoid	2	Hass et al (1997)	Low quality CCT	Insufficient data to determine outcomes
		Nordenskiold (1994)	High quality OD	Significant improvement in pain
Provision of splints	16	Nordenskiold (1990)	Sufficient quality OD	Significant reduction of pain in wearing working splints in both studies
(see Ch. 12)		Pagnotta et al (1998)	Sufficient quality OD	Significant reduction of pain in wearing working splints in both studies
Provision of working splints		Stern et al (1996)	Low quality RCT	Significant improvement in function over a week
		Tijhaus et al (1998)	High Quality RCT	No difference in pain grip strength or ROM between 2 types of working splints
Provision of resting splints		Feinberg (1992)	Low quality CCT	Significant decline in dexterity
		Callinan et al (1996)	Low quality RCT	Significant improvement in pain wearing a resting splint over 4 weeks
		Adams et al (2008)	High quality RCT	Resting splints should not be used as a routine treatment of patients with early RA.
Swan neck deformity		Ter Schegget et al (1997)	High Quality RCT	No significant difference in grip strength or range of movement
Boutonnière splint		Palchik et al (1990)	Low quality RCT	Significant improvement in grip strength when wearing splint 24 hours for 6 weeks

Key: OD = observational design RCT = randomised controlled trial CCT = case control studies

Ankylosing Spondylitis Functional Index (Calin et al 1994).

Whilst some assessments, such as the HAQ, cover a broad range of activities others focus on specific domains of activity, e.g. The Rheumatoid Arthritis Work Instability Scale (Gilworth et al 2003) or the Parenting Disability Indices (Katz et al 2003). These may be used as an additional assessment when more detailed information is required about a specific area of activity limitation. Other measures focus on activity limitation associated with specific regions of the body, such as the Oxford Hip Score (Dawson et al 1996) or The Disabilities of the Arm Shoulder and Hand (Hudak et al 1996).

Standardized assessments have been evaluated extensively to ensure that they are valid, (measuring what they claim to measure), reliable (are as accurate as possible) and sensitive to change (able to detect change when change has occurred). Many of the measures described above are self-complete questionnaires comprising a range of predefined activities against which a person rates the level of difficulty they experience when completing each activity. However some assessment may include observation or assessment of a person completing specific activities. Others incorporate an element of measurement such as grip strength or range of movement, e.g. The Jebsen Test of Hand Function (Jebsen et al 1969). Whilst standardized measures have demonstrated efficacy in clinical and research contexts one of the criticisms of their use in a clinical context is their inability to capture activities which are important to clients (Hewlett 2003).

A recent development has been the patient generated index which enables each person to identify areas of activity limitation of greatest concern to them. Two examples relevant to activity limitation are the MACTAR Patient Preference Disability Questionnaire (Tugwell et al 1987) and the Canadian Occupational Performance Measure (COPM) (Law et al 1990, 2005). The COPM is informed by a semi-structured interview during which people are asked to identify areas of activity limitation and rank them in order of importance. For the top five activities, they rate their current performance of the activity and satisfaction with their current performance. These activities inform the treatment programme and the person is reassessed to evaluate the efficacy of the intervention. The COPM is congruent with a person centred approach and does not constrain the activities a client can identify (see Ch. 4 for further information on patient reported outcome measures).

SEMI-STRUCTURED INTERVIEWS

Whilst the use of standardized assessments is encouraged as a basis for assessment many therapists, in a clinical context, continue to use a semi-structured interview format exploring a wide range of areas of activity. Such interviews are often formulated on a departmental basis. However, this in-depth information cannot be used as an accurate measure against which treatment outcomes can be assessed. Therefore increasingly therapists are using a combination of initial interview and standardized measures to inform their interventions

PROMOTING INDEPENDENCE IN KEY ACTIVITIES

This section explores some of the main areas of activity limitation experienced by people with rheumatic diseases and provides insights into the ways in which such limitations can be reduced. The use of joint protection, energy conservation, orthotics and psychological support are addressed in other chapters but are inherent to maintaining independence.

THE IMPACT OF RHEUMATIC DISEASES ON SELF CARE AND HOUSEHOLD ACTIVITIES

The loss of ability to perform activities of daily living is one of the most documented consequences of rheumatic diseases (Symmons & Silman 2006, Wolfe 2000). Sokka et al (2003) demonstrated that patients with rheumatoid arthritis have a 7-fold risk of functional disability in self care activities as measured by the HAQ compared to the normal population.

OCCUPATIONAL THERAPY INTERVENTIONS

The strongest evidence in rheumatology occupational therapy is also informed by the impact of interventions on activities of daily living (Hammond et al 1999, 2001, Helewa et al 1991). Some of the main approaches used by occupational therapists focus on improving occupational performance by:

- using alternative methods of doing an activity
- using assistive devices (i.e. assistive technology)
- adapting the built environment.

Using alternative methods

The development of skills in joint protection and energy conservation is one of the main occupational therapy interventions to maintain levels of activity and is described in chapter 10.

Using assistive devices

People with arthritis are one of the largest user groups of assistive devices (Rogers & Holmes 1992). These are used to:

- increase or maintain functional ability
- reduce pain experienced when doing a task
- reduce the energy required to complete a task
- reduce the stress placed on joints during activity
- increase the safety with which a task is completed
- support carers in undertaking specific activities.

Devices are usually provided on a permanent basis but, in some instances, may only be required for a short period, e.g. post joint replacement surgery. Studies suggest that up to a third of devices

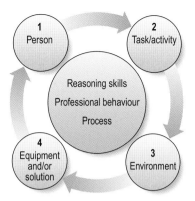

Figure 9.2 Key factors to consider when assessing for assistive technology (adapted from the Trusted Assessor Framework Winchcombe & Ballinger 2005).

provided remain unused (Scherer 2002). A number of factors contribute to non-use, such as changes in the person's condition, the impact of comorbidities, lack of involvement in the assessment process, inadequacy of the device, embarrassment and a preference for person assistance (Wielandt & Strong 2000). Therefore, careful assessment is required considering factors relevant to:

- the person- identifying the specific difficulties they are experiencing, their priorities and product preferences and specific impairment issues influencing product choice
- the task - identifying specific activity components and actions needed to complete the task
- the environment - features influencing product choice such as dimensions, circulation space and whether the equipment will be used in more than one environment
- equipment/solution – features of specific products influencing choice (Fig. 9.2).

(Winchcombe & Ballinger 2005)

The majority of large devices, such as bath lifts, are supplied via statutory services. Depending on where a person lives, smaller items may have to be purchased privately. As designers and manufacturers are starting to accommodate the needs of a wide range of users in product design more mainstream household products and appliances are becoming increasingly accessible and easy to use for people with arthritis.

Adapting the environment

In some circumstances it is necessary to carry out minor adaptations or more extensive building work within the person's home or work place. Common

---

BOX 9.1   Additional resources related to assistive devices and adaptations

- Disabled Living Foundation: provides information and advice about assistive devices and a wide range of fact sheets can be downloaded from their website. The DLF also produces DLF Data the main national database for assistive devices.
- Assist UK leads a national network of demonstration centres across the country that provide impartial information and advice on AT and inclusive design.
- Research Institute for Consume Affairs (RICAbility) produce a variety of consumer reports related to a range of consumer products including: Easier Living; Ins and outs of bathing; Making your kitchen easier to use; Choosing a vacuum cleaner that's easier to use; Choosing a washing machine that's easier to use; Choosing an iron that's easier to use; Choosing an electric kettle that's easier to use; Motoring and arthritis
- Arthritis Care provides a range of leaflets and online information. Titles include Independent Living and Arthritis. Working with Arthritis and Home Sweet Home.
- Arthritis Research Campaign publishes a range of leaflets: Looking after your Joints when you have Arthritis and Gardening and Arthritis.
- National Rheumatoid Arthritis Society provides information and advice relating to lifestyle issues. Publications include: Rheumatoid arthritis and computing; I Want to Work. A Self-Help Guide for People with Rheumatoid Arthritis; When an Employee has Rheumatoid Arthritis: An Employers Guide and I Want to Work, Report from the 2007 Work Survey.

Note: website addresses can be found at the end of the chapter.

---

adaptations for people with rheumatic diseases include the installation of level access showers, stairlifts and the creation of easier access into the home. Such work can be undertaken through statutory services or people may choose to fund such work privately.

As people develop an understanding of the problems associated with living with arthritis they often make changes to their home environment when undertaking renovation work. For example, installing lever taps, easier door handles and locks, raising electric sockets, designing easily accessible and energy saving kitchens, raising toilet height and installing a downstairs toilet (see Box 9.1 and Fig. 9.3).

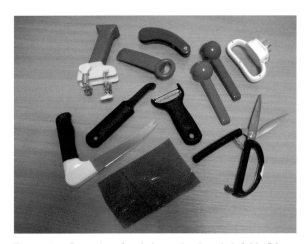

Figure 9.3 Examples of assistive technology helpful in RA.

THE IMPACT OF RHEUMATIC DISEASES ON FAMILY ROLES

Studies exploring impact on parenting roles consistently identify the challenges faced with different aspects of childcare (Backman et al 2007, Grant 2001, Katz et al 2003). These studies highlight practical problems and also the psychological consequences of being unable to fulfil perceived parenting roles. Whilst attention has focused on the experiences of women with RA, recent studies have also explored the experiences of women with ankylosing spondylitis (AS), systemic lupus erythematosus (SLE) and juvenile idiopathic arthritis (Backman et al 2007). Problems are also experienced by men undertaking fathering roles and by men and women in relation to grandparenting roles (Barlow et al 1999). A survey of 231 women with RA identified that greater parenting disability was associated with poorer general function, more pain and fatigue, more parenting stress and greater psychological distress (Katz 2003).

ASSESSMENT

Few standardized assessments of parenting disability exist. One example is the Parenting Disability Index (Katz 2003). Assessment may take place when problems arise, but also therapists can work with mothers during pregnancy to help prepare for the arrival of their child, advise on the purchase of appropriate childcare equipment, put in place the necessary practical support and advise on fatigue management.

INTERVENTIONS

Practical problems, especially with regard to caring for babies and younger children, are experienced in all aspects of childcare such as holding, lifting, carrying, bathing and changing, dressing and feeding. For women with RA these problems can be exacerbated in the early months of motherhood by an increase in their disease activity. Careful selection of products can help to reduce the problems experienced. There is a wide variation in the design and usability of prams, car seats, cots and feeding equipment and guiding parents to think about such features as weight, size, design of controls, fastenings, switches and general ease of use when selecting products can save a great deal of money.

As children grow, parents with arthritis may experience problems in taking part in the wider aspects of the child's life such as school or club activities, family outings and holidays. Studies exploring parenting with rheumatic conditions highlight the emotional consequences associated with being unable to fulfil such activities (Backman et al 2007, Grant 2001, Katz et al 2003). Psychological support is therefore an important aspect of working with parents. This may be provided by the therapist but also facilitated through referral to a voluntary sector organisation such as Arthritis Care, The Disabled Parents Network or the National Rheumatoid Arthritis Society (Box 9.2).

THE IMPACT OF RHEUMATIC DISEASES ON EMPLOYMENT

Despite medical advances (Bejarano et al 2008, Puolakka et al 2004) the incidence of work disability in rheumatoid arthritis is still significant (Eberhardt et al 2007, Young et al 2000). The National Rheumatoid Arthritis Society (NRAS) 'I want to work' survey (2007) reported that only 54.8% of respondents were in employment - nearly 30% less than the Government's 80% target of employment for all working age adults (Department of Work and Pensions (DWP) 2007). Of those not in employment, 28.4% had given up work within 1 year and 59% were work disabled within 6 years of diagnosis. Other rheumatic diseases, such as systemic lupus erythematosus, have even higher levels of work disability with rates of 47% at diagnosis (Yelin et al 2004).These figures pose a challenge to both clinicians and policy makers with the increased emphasis

---

BOX 9.2   Additional resources for parenting with arthritis

- The Disabled Parents Network –provides information, advice and support to disabled parents
- Arthritis Care – website has a section on Living with Arthritis - parenting with disability
- Research Institute for Consumer Affairs (RICAbility) produce a range of consumer reports for disabled parents on childcare products including: pushchairs, highchairs, baby carriers, bottle warmers and sterilisers; safety gates
- National Rheumatoid Arthritis Society (NRAS)- website has a section on pregnancy which provides a range of information on aspects of pregnancy, childbirth and childcare including: My Experience of Pregnancy, Birth and Caring for a Small Baby whilst coping with Rheumatoid Arthritis: a members story, Coping with your Baby when you have Rheumatoid Arthritis and Handy Tips
- Arthritis Research Campaign produces a booklet: Pregnancy and Arthritis

Note: website addresses can be found at the end of the chapter.

BOX 9.3   Questions to ask in a work interview

- Patients details, e.g. name, address, date of birth
- Current medication and other therapies
- Specific joint symptoms, fatigue or other medical issues affecting work performance
- Abilities and routines at home/leisure
- Educational background including any qualifications
- Past employment history and occupational interests/aptitudes
- Current employment details (job title, employers details, hours of work, shift pattern, breaks, previous and current sick leave, financial status - current pay, e.g. full/half pay and disability/or Employment Support Allowance (formerly Incapacity Benefit) etc
- Does the person have an occupational health provider? – take details
- Preparing for work and method of travel
- Psychosocial information – interpersonal relationships, job importance and satisfaction, amount of autonomy, perceived stress etc., job values, job goals
- Job demands, job concerns and limitations.

---

on keeping people in work and extending working life beyond the current retirement age of 65.

The personal costs of unemployment from decreased quality of life and social exclusion are enormous but the socioeconomic costs are also great. The DWP report forecasted in 2007 that in 2007-2008 429,000 people with musculoskeletal diseases would claim £1.429 billion via the Employment and Support Allowance (ESA). Prognostic factors for work disability in rheumatoid arthritis include higher HAQ scores, lower educational status, older age, and manual work (Eberhardt et al 2007).

VOCATIONAL REHABILITATION

Employment issues in rheumatic diseases must therefore be addressed as early as possible (Frank and Chamberlain 2001, Nordmark et al 2006). The College of Occupational Therapy (COT) Specialist Section on Work clearly identifies the role and opportunities for occupational therapists to be involved in vocational rehabilitation (COT 2007) and this is expanded upon in the Work Matters Booklet (COT 2007). The NRAS I want to work Survey (NRAS 2007) also identified the need for more occupational therapists to be trained to provide work rehabilitation.

Work screening

Given the potential for people to experience work related problems at an early stage in their disease it is vital that work related problems are detected early and dealt with by an appropriate individual, e.g. an occupational therapist, other health professional or employment advisor. Work instability is used to describe a mismatch between a person's functional capacity and the demands of their job (Gilworth et al 2003). The Rheumatoid Work Instability Scale (RA- WIS) (Gilworth et al 2003) is a validated screening tool developed to detect, measure and prioritise people's work instability.

Work interview

If work problems are identified a specific work interview can be undertaken. Cynkin et al (1990) describe a potential structure for a work interview as does Melvin (1998). Box 9.3 suggests some of the information the therapist should collect.

Standardized semi-structured work interviews such as the Worker Role Interview (WRI) are also available (Velozo et al 1999).

STANDARDIZED ASSESSMENT TOOLS

Various assessment tools are available and are listed in the Work Matters booklet (COT 2007).

In some instances the work interview may identify the need to carry out a more detailed assessment to determine work abilities. This can be done through a detailed job analysis (Joss 2007) using a mix of analysis tools, e.g. the Valpar Profile Analysis Guide (Valpar International Corporation 2007a) in combination with the Revised Handbook for Analyzing Jobs (US Department of Labor 1991).

A Functional Capacity Evaluation (FCE) is an all-encompassing term to describe the physical assessment of an individual's ability to perform work-related activity (American Occupational Therapy Association 2008). Work samples such as the VALPAR Work Samples (Valpar International Corporation 2007b) are criterion referenced standardized work simulated assessments which are analysed using the methods time management (MTM) industrial performance standards. A worksite assessment is valuable for environmental, ergonomic and job demands assessment and to gain an impression of psychosocial and interpersonal issues at work. Evaluating employment interventions is essential to ensure ongoing work stability. Once a person leaves employment it is much more difficult for them to reenter it.

INTERVENTIONS: THE EVIDENCE

There has been little high quality research carried out demonstrating the positive effects of occupational therapy alone in improving work outcomes in rheumatic diseases. A small RCT (n = 28) by Macedo et al (2007) found that, at 6-month follow-up, comprehensive occupational therapy significantly improved functional ability, pain, work satisfaction and reduced work instability in rheumatoid arthritis, although there were no differences in number of days work missed or work performance.

A systematic review of vocational rehabilitation carried by de Buck et al (2002) identified six multidisciplinary rehabilitation programs, five of which showed a marked positive effect of work rehabilitation on work status (work disability, sick leave, job modification, paid occupation, retraining). Proof of benefit was limited due to limitations and differences in methodologies and none were randomized controlled trials. Allaire et al (2003) carried out a randomized controlled trial (RCT) demonstrating that people receiving vocational rehabilitation stayed in work longer compared to the control group receiving written advice only. The intervention was delivered by experienced rehabilitation counselors. It consisted of two 1.5-hour sessions with three components: job accommodation,

> **BOX 9.4   Interventions applicable in work rehabilitation**
>
> - Joint protection techniques
> - Fatigue management techniques
> - Flexible working, home working, reduced hours, graded return, modification of duties, using a support worker
> - Work hardening
> - Equipment, ergonomic/environmental adaptations and orthotics
> - Education – impact of disease on work, prognosis, work abilities, legislation DDA health and safety
> - Liaison with government and local employment schemes such as Pathways to Work Condition Management programmes
> - Advice on Retraining or gaining educational qualifications
> - Reports with recommendations for employers, employment advisors, insurance companies
> - Expert witness for tribunals
> - Advocacy – liaison with colleagues employers, employment advisors, etc
> - Self-advocacy training /modeling/ job coaching
> - Post-work counselling.

vocational counseling and guidance, and education and self-advocacy.

De Buck et al (2004) conducted a RCT evaluating patient and occupational physician satisfaction with a multidisciplinary job retention vocational rehabilitation programme for patients with rheumatic diseases. The team included an occupational therapist. The individualized programme addressed job accommodation issues, promotion of self-efficacy, changes in medication, exercise, functional training and psychological interventions. Patients were most satisfied with the interpersonal approach and knowledge gained and least satisfied with waiting times for the final work report and application of advice. Unfortunately, the programme did not impact on work status.

The extent of work rehabilitation needed varies considerably between patients. Verbal or written advice may be all that is required. For example, explaining employees' and employers' rights and responsibilities under the Disability Discrimination Act (1995), issuing a copy of the Working Horizons booklets (Arthritis Care 2006) or 'I want to work': guide for people with arthritis/employers (NRAS 2007). More complex interventions may be required and these are described in Box 9.4.

THE IMPACT OF RHEUMATIC DISEASES ON COMMUNITY, SOCIAL AND CIVIC LIFE

The International Classification of Function Disability and Health (WHO 2001) lists community life, recreation and leisure, play, religion and spirituality, human rights and political life and citizenship as areas included in community, social and civic life.

Rheumatic diseases have a significant impact on people's lifestyles including their leisure time and participation in community life (Fex et al 1998, Wikstrom et al 2006, Yelin et al 1987). As well as having lower rates of functional ability and lower rates of employment, people with arthritis also experience reductions in their leisure activities. Fex et al (1998) in a longitudinal survey found that 75% of people with rheumatoid arthritis had to change their leisure activities and 50% were unsatisfied with their recreation. Wikstrom et al (2006) identified that newly diagnosed RA patients performed significantly fewer leisure activities but did not have less interest in them. Predictors for low performance in leisure activities are lower education, higher age and higher HAQ score (Fries et al 1980). Loss of valued activities, including leisure, is correlated with poorer psychological status (Katz & Yelin 1994).

The term 'leisure' is hard to define by task alone. One person's social or leisure activity may be another person's paid employment, for example playing football or jewellery making. Leisure here is used to describe those activities not generally involving self-maintenance or paid employment.

OCCUPATIONAL THERAPY AND LEISURE

Occupational therapists have traditionally included the area of social participation and leisure in patient assessment. However, the political climate, the predominantly physical nature of rheumatic diseases and time constraints have led to less focus on these areas compared to self care employment and household activities. Turner et al (2000) found occupational therapists working in physical disability spent less time in assessing leisure areas compared to those working in psychosocial settings. This is alarming in view of the high incidence of psychosocial issues affecting those with rheumatic diseases.

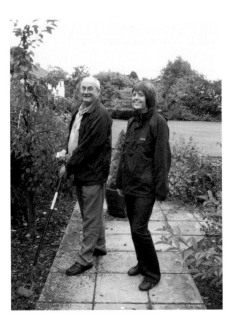

Figure 9.4 Gardening using adapted equipment.

Leisure assessment

The occupational therapy initial interview helps identify which leisure activities the person is involved in and how important they are in relation to other activities and roles. The COPM categorises leisure into three areas: quiet recreation, active recreation and socialisation. The UK Modified Interest Checklist (Heasman & Brewer 2008) is based on the Model of Human Occupation and gathers information on a client's strength of interest and engagement in 74 activities in the past, present and future and can be used with adolescents or adults.

Leisure interventions

Joint protection, fatigue management, assistive technology, adaptations and orthotics all help to improve performance in leisure activities. Some patients may benefit from new or increased leisure activities, including aerobic exercise activities (Plasqui 2008) to assist in pain management and improve physical and psychological wellbeing. Rheumatology occupational therapy/rehabilitation assistants have a valuable role in enabling the person to achieve their leisure goals whether it be at home or in the wider community (Fig. 9.4).

CONCLUSION

The focus of occupational therapy interventions on the promotion and maintenance of independence in all areas of activity is central to the management of people with rheumatic diseases. People make sense of an illness experience not only in terms of how it makes them feel but also the impact that it has on their life. Whilst the onset of a rheumatic disease requires a person to reassess their understanding of their body in terms of how it feels and what it is capable of doing, many people manage to lead active and fulfilling lives. This is achieved through a process of learning relevant strategies and skills to manage their impairment and maximize their independence. This enables them to *be* and do the things they want to do, need to do or are expected to do within the context of their impairment.

STUDY ACTIVITIES

1. Develop your understanding of people's experience of living with rheumatoid arthritis.
   - Visit the rheumatoid arthritis section of healthtalkonline (www.healthtalkonline.org) and listen to the views and experiences which are being shared in this resource. A great deal of valuable information is provided on this site but listen specifically to the sections relating to occupational therapy, work, parenting and childcare and personal life and changes at home.
2. Develop your understanding of how the design of products can influence the ease with which they can be used.
   - Think about some of the products that you use in your daily life and find difficult to use. Choose one which would also be used by a person with arthritis and think about:
   - Why is it difficult to use?
   - How could be it made easier to use?

   - Do some market research. Find as many examples of the product as possible on the internet, in magazines and shops and compare features such as shape, size, weight, ease of use, portability, controls. Also have a look at some of the sites highlighted in this chapter and find examples of assistive technologies which may be easier to use. Summarise your findings and thinking about the needs of a person with arthritis to identify the product which you feel would be the easiest for them to use and justify your choice.
3. Developing your understanding of the impact of RA on employment
   - Visit the NRAS website (www.rheumatoid.org.uk) and read the two publications: 'I want to work – a self help guide for people with rheumatoid arthritis' and 'When an employee has rheumatoid arthritis - a guide for employers.'

USEFUL WEBSITES

Research Institute for Consumer Affairs (Ricability)
   www.ricability.org.uk
Arthritis Care
http://www.arthritiscare.org.uk
National Rheumatoid Arthritis Society
http://www.rheumatoid.org.uk
The Arthritis Research Campaign (arc)
http://www.arc.org.uk

Disabled Parents Network
http://www.disabledparentsnetwork.org.uk
Disabled Living Foundation
www.dlf.org.uk
Assist UK
www.assist-uk.org.

References and further reading

Adams, J., Burridge, J., Mullee, M., et al., 2008. The clinical effectiveness of static resting splints in early rheumatoid arthritis: a randomized controlled. Rheumatology 47 (10), 1548–1553.

Allaire, S., Li, W., La Valley, M., 2003. Reduction of job loss in persons with rheumatic diseases receiving vocational rehabilitation: a randomized controlled trial. Arthritis Rheum. 48 (11), 3212–3218.

American Association of Occupational Therapy www.aota.org/Consumers/WhatisOT/WI/Facts/35117.aspx. Accessed 13/10/08.

Arthritis Care, , 2006. Working Horizons (2nd edn) (booklet). Arthritis Care, London.

Backman, C., Del Fabro Smith, L., Smith, S., et al., 2007. 'Sometimes I can, sometimes I can't': the influence of arthritis on mothers' habits OTJR: occup. Participation Health 27; Supplement 1: 775–785.

Barlow, J., Cullen, L.A., Foster, N.E., et al., 1999. Does arthritis influence perceived ability to fulfil a parenting role? Perceptions of mothers, fathers and grandparents. Patient Educ. Couns. 37 (2), 141–151.

Bejarano, V., Quinn, M., Philip, G., et al., 2008. Effect of the early use of the anti-tumor necrosis factor adalimumab on the prevention of job loss in patients with early rheumatoid arthritis. Arthritis Care Res. 59 (10), 1467–1474.

Calin, A., Garrett, S., Whitelock, H., et al., 1994. A new approach to defining functional ability in ankylosing spondylitis: the development of the Bath Ankylosing Spondylitis Functional index. J. Rheumatol. 21 (12), 2281–2285.

Callinan, N.J., Mathiowetz, V., 1996. Soft versus hard resting hand splints in rheumatoid arthritis: pain relief, preference, and compliance. Am. J. Occup. Ther. 50, 347–353.

Canadian Association of Occupational Therapists, 1997. Enabling Occupation: An occupational therapy perspective. CAOT Publications, Ottawa, ON.

Christiansen, C.H., Baum, C.M., Bass-Haugen, J., 2005. Occupational Therapy: Performance, Participation, and Well-being, third ed. SLACK, Thorofare, NJ.

College of Occupational Therapists, 2007. Occupational Therapy in Vocational Rehabilitation: A Brief Guide to Current Practice in the UK. College of Occupational Therapists, London.

College of Occupational Therapists, 2007. Work Matters: Vocational Navigation for Occupational Therapy Staff. College of Occupational Therapists and National Inclusion Programme, London.

College of Occupational Therapists, 2003. Occupational Therapy Clinical Guidelines for Rheumatology. College of Occupational Therapists, London.

Cynkin, S., Robinson, A.M., 1990. Occupational Therapy and Activities Health: Toward Health through Activities, second ed. Little Brown Book Company, Boston.

Dawson, J., Fitzpatrick, R., Carr, A., et al., 1996. Questionnaire on the perceptions of patients about total hip replacement. J. Bone Joint Surg. 78-B, 185–190.

De Buck, P., Schoones, J., Allaire, S., et al., 2002. Vocational rehabilitation in patients with chronic rheumatic diseases: A systematic literature review. Semin. Arthritis Rheum. 32 (3), 196–203.

De Buck, P.D.M., Breedveld, J., van der Giesen, F.J., et al., 2004. A multidisciplinary job retention vocational rehabilitation programme for patients with chronic rheumatic diseases: patients' and occupational physicians' satisfaction. Ann. Rheum. Dis. 63 (5), 562–568.

Disability Discrimination Act, 1995. (c. 50), ISBN 0105450952 HMSO, London.

Department of Work and Pensions, 2005. Five Year Strategy: Opportunity and Security Throughout Life. DWP Publications, The Stationery Office, Norwich.

Eberhardt, K., Larsson, B., Nived, K., et al., 2007. Work disability in rheumatoid arthritis-development over 15 years and evaluation of predictive factors over time. J. Rheumatol. 34 (3), 481–487.

Feinberg, J., 1992. Effect of the arthritis health professional on compliance with use of resting hand splints by patients with rheumatoid arthritis. Arthritis Care Res. 5 (1), 17–23.

Fex, E., Larsson, B.M., Nived, K., et al., 1998. Effect of rheumatoid arthritis on work status and social and leisure time activities in patients followed 8 years from onset. J. Rheumatol. 25 (1), 44–50.

Frank, A., Chamberlain, M., 2001. Keeping our patients at work: implications for the management of those with rheumatoid arthritis and musculoskeletal conditions. Rheumatology 40 (11), 1201–1205.

Fries, J., Spitz, P., Kraines, R., et al., 1980. Measurement of patient outcome in arthritis. Arthritis Rheum. 23 (2), 137–145.

Gilworth, G., Chamberlain, M.A., Harvey, A., et al., 2003. Development of a work instability scale for rheumatoid arthritis. Arthritis Care Res. 49 (3), 349–354.

Grant, M., 2001. Mothers with arthritis, child care and occupational therapy: insight through case studies. Br. J. Occup Ther 64 (7), 322–329.

Hammond, A., Lincoln, N., Sutcliffe, L., 1999. A crossover trial evaluating an educational-behavioural joint protection programme for people with rheumatoid arthritis. Patient Educ. Couns. 37 (1), 19–32.

Hammond, A., Freeman, K., 2001. One year outcomes of a randomised controlled trial of an educational-behavioural joint protection programme for people with rheumatoid arthritis. Rheumatology 40 (9), 1044–1051.

Hammond, A., Young, A., Kidao, R., 2004. A randomised controlled trial of occupational therapy for people with early rheumatoid arthritis. Ann. Rheum. Dis. 63 (1), 23–30.

Hass, U., Brodin, H., Andersson, A., et al., 1997. Assistive technology selection: a study of participation of users with rheumatoid arthritis. IEEE Trans. Rehabil. Eng. 5, 263–275.

Heasman, D., Brewer, P., 2008. The UK Modified Interest Checklist www.moho.uic.edu accessed 3.2.09

Helewa, A., Goldsmith, C.H., 1991. Effects of occupational therapy home service on patients with rheumatoid arthritis. Lancet 337, 1453–1457.

Hewlett, S., 2003. Patients and clinicians have different perspectives on outcomes in arthritis. J. Rheumatol. 30 (4), 877–879.

Hoenig, H., Groff, G., Pratt, K., et al., 1993. A randomized controlled trial of home exercise on the rheumatoid hand.. J. Rheumatol. 20, 785–789.

Hudak, P., Amadio, P., Bombardier, C., 1996. Development of an upper extremity outcome measure: the DASH (disabilities of the arm, shoulder and hand) The Upper Extremity Collaborative Group (UECG). Am. J. Ind. Med. 29 (6), 602–608.

Iwama, M., 2006. The Kawa Model. Culturally Relevant Occupational Therapy. Churchill Livingstone, Edinburgh.

Jebsen, R., Taylor, N., Trieschmann, R., et al., 1969. An objective and standardized test of hand function. Arch. Phys. Med. Rehabil. 50 (6), 311–319.

Joss, M., 2007. The Importance of Job Analysis in Occupational Therapy. Br. J. Occup. Ther. 70 (7), 301–303.

Katz, P., Yelin, EH., 1994. Life activities of persons with rheumatoid arthritis with and without depressive symptoms. Arthritis Care Res. 7 (2), 69–77.

Katz, P., 1995. The impact of rheumatoid arthritis on life activities. Arthritis Care Res. 8 (4), 272–278.

Katz, P., Pasch, L., Wong, B., 2003. Development of an instrument to measure disability in parenting activity among women with rheumatoid arthritis. Arthritis Care Res. 48 (4), 935–943.

Kielhofner, G., 2002. A Model of Human Occupation: Theory and application, third ed. Lippincott, Williams & Wilkins, Baltimore.

Law, M., Baptiste, S., McColl, M.A., et al., 1990. The canadian occupational performance measure: an outcome measure for occupational therapy. Can. J. Occup. Ther. 57 (2), 82–87.

Law, M., Baptiste, S., Carswell, A., et al., 2005. Canadian Occupational Performance Measure, fourth ed. CAOT Publications, Ottawa, ON.

Macedo, A.M., Oakley, S., Panayi, G.S., et al., 2007. Functional and work outcomes improve in RA patients who receive timely comprehensive occupational therapy. ACR Annu. Meet. http://www.rheumatology .org/annual/07wrapup.asp abstract 338. Accessed 13.1.09.

Madill, H., Townsend, E., Schultz, P., 1989. Implementing a health promotion strategy in occupational therapy education and practice. Can J. Occup. Ther. 56 (2), 67–72.

Meenan, R.F., Mason, J.H., Anderson, J.J., et al., 1992. AIMS 2: the content and properties of a revised and expanded Arthritis Impact Measurement Scales health status questionnaire. Arthritis Rheum. 35 (1), 1–10.

Melvin, J., Jensen, G., 1998. Rheumatologic Rehabilitation Series: Vol 1 Assessment and Management. American Occupational Therapy Association, Bethesda, MD.

National Rheumatoid Arthritis Society, 2007. I Want to Work: a self-help guide for people with Rheumatoid Arthritis. National Rheumatoid Arthritis Society, Berkshire.

National Rheumatoid Arthritis Society, 2007. I Want to Work: Employment and Rheumatoid Arthritis. A National Survey. National Rheumatoid Arthritis Society, High Wycombe.

Nordenskiold, U., 1990. Elastic wrist orthoses: reduction of pain and increase in grip force for women with rheumatoid arthritis. Arthritis Care Res. 3, 158–162.

Nordenskiold, U., 1994. Evaluation of assistive devices after a course in joint protection. Int. J. Technol. Assess. Health Care 10, 293–304.

Nordmark, B., Blomqvist, P., Andersson, B., et al., 2006. A 2-year follow up of work capacity in early rheumatoid arthritis: a study of multidisciplinary team care with emphasis on vocational support. Scand. J. Rheumatol. 35 (1), 7–14.

O'Brien, A.V., Jones, P., Mullis, R., et al., 2006. Conservative hand therapy treatments in rheumatoid arthritis. A randomised controlled trial. Rheumatology 45 (5), 577–583.

Pagnotta, A., Baron, M., Korner-Bitensky, N., 1998. The effect of a static wrist orthosis on hand function in individuals with rheumatoid arthritis. J. Rheumatol. 25, 879–885.

Palchik, N.S., Mitchell, D.M., Gilbert, N.L., et al., 1990. Non- surgical management of the boutonniere deformity. Arthritis Care Res. 3, 227–232.

Plasqui, G., 2008. The role of physical activity in rheumatoid arthritis. Physiol. Behav. 94 (2), 270–275.

Puolakka, K., Kautiainen, H., Möttönen, T., et al., 2004. Impact of initial aggressive drug treatment with a combination of disease-modifying anti-rheumatic drugs on the development of work disability in early rheumatoid arthritis: a five-year randomized follow-up trial. Arthritis Rheum. 50 (1), 55–62.

Rogers, J., Holmes, D., 1992. Assistive technology device use in patients with rheumatic disease: a literature review. Am. J. Occup. Ther. 46 (2), 120–127.

Scherer, M., 2002. The change in emphasis from people to person: introduction to the special issue on assistive technology. Disabil. Rehabil. 24 (1,2,3), 1–4.

Sokka, T., Krishnan, E., Hakkinen, A., et al., 2003. Functional disability in rheumatoid arthritis patients compared with a community population in Finland. Arthritis Rheum. 48 (1), 59–63.

Stern, E.B., Ytterberg, S.R., Krug, H.E., Mahowald, M.L., 1996. Finger dexterity and hand function: effect of three commercial wrist extensor orthoses on patients with rheumatoid arthritis. Arthritis Care Res. 9 (3), 197–205.

Steultjens, E.M.J., Dekker, J., Bouter, L.M., et al., 2004. Occupational therapy for rheumatoid arthritis. Cochrane Database of Systematic Reviews Issue 1 Art. No.: CD003114. DOI: 10.1002/14651858.CD003114. pub2.

Symmons, D., Silman, A. , 2006. Aspects of early arthritis. What determines the evolution of early undifferentiated arthritis and rheumatoid arthritis? An update from the Norfolk Arthritis Register. Curr. Opin. Rheumatol. 19 (2), 204–231.

Ter Schegget, M.J., Knipping, A.A., 1997. The swan-neck splint in rheumatoid arthritis. Ned Tijdschr. Ergotherapie 25, 172–182.

Tijhuis, G.J., Vlieland, T.P.M., Zwinderman, A.H., et al., 1998. A comparison of the Futuro wrist orthosis with a synthetic ThermoLyn Orthosis:utility and clinical effectiveness. Arthritis Care Res. 11 (3), 217–222.

Turner, H., Chapman, S., McSherry, A., et al., 2000. Leisure assessment in occupational therapy: an exploratory study. Occup. Ther. Health Care 12, 73–85.

Tugwell, P., Bombardier, C., Buchanan, W., et al., 1987. The MACTAR Patient Preference Disability Questionnaire: an individualised functional priority approach for assessing improvement in clinical trials in rheumatoid arthritis.. J. Rheumatol. 14, 446–451.

US Department of Labor Employment and Training Administration, 1991. The Revised Handbook for Analysing Jobs. Jist Works, Indianapolis.

Valpar International Corporation, 2007a. Valpar Profile Analysis Guide. Valpar International Corporation Tucson, Arizona.

Valpar International Corporation, 2007b. Valpar Component Work Samples. Valpar International Corporation Tucson, Arizona.

Velozo, C., Kielhofner, G., Gern, A., et al., 1999. Worker role interview: toward validation of a psychosocial work-related measure. J. Occup. Rehabil. 9 (3), 153–168.

Wielandt, T., Strong, J., 2000. Compliance with prescribed adaptive equipment: a literature review. Br. J. Occup. Ther. 63 (2), 65–75.

Winchcombe, M., Ballinger, C., 2005. A Competence Framework for Trusted Assessors. Assist UK.

Wikstrom, I., Book, C., Jacobsson, L.T.H., 2006. Difficulties in performing leisure activities among persons with newly diagnosed rheumatoid arthritis: a prospective, controlled study.. Rheumatology 45 (9), 1162–1166.

Wolfe, F., 2000. A reappraisal of HAQ disability in rheumatoid arthritis. Arthritis Rheum. 43 (12), 2751–2761.

World Health Organisation, , 2001. International Classification of Functioning Disability and Health. WHO, Geneva www.who.int.

Yelin, E., Trupin, L., Katz, P., 2004. Presentation: Work disability and SLE: Incidence and correlates. New York, NY: 7th International Congress on Systemic Lupus Erythematosus and Related Conditions: Session on long-term outcome: heart and vessels May 9-13 Abstract 23A www.medscape.com. Accessed 15/08/08.

Yelin, E., Lubeck, D., Holman, H., et al., 1987. The impact of rheumatoid arthritis and osteoarthritis: the activities of patients with rheumatoid arthritis and osteoarthritis compared to controls. J. Rheumatol. 14 (4), 710–717.

Young, A., Dixey, J., Cox, N., et al., 2000. How does functional disability in early rheumatoid arthritis (RA) affect patients and their lives? Results of 5 years of follow-up in 732 patients from the early RA Study (ERAS). Rheumatology 39 (6), 603–611.

Chapter 10

Joint protection and fatigue management

Alison Hammond PhD MSc BSc(Hons) DipCOT FCOT Centre for Health, Sport and Rehabilitation Research, University of Salford, Greater Manchester and Royal Derby Hospital, Derby Hospitals NHS Foundation Trust, Derby, UK

CHAPTER CONTENTS

KEY POINTS

- Joint protection and fatigue management should be an essential component of therapy
- Effective approaches should be used including educational, cognitive and behavioural approaches
- Enabling self management is the responsibility of the whole team.

INTRODUCTION

Joint protection and fatigue management address the priority concerns of people with arthritis: pain, fatigue and hand and finger function (Heiburg & Kvien 2002, Hewlett et al 2005). Joint protection underlies all rehabilitation of people whose joints are at risk from arthritis (Cordery & Rocchi 1998), yet fatigue management is often inadequately addressed (Hewlett et al 2005). To be effective, both require people with arthritis changing habits and routines. Teaching facts can be done quickly but enabling long-term behavioural change requires greater input. This chapter discusses what joint protection and fatigue management strategies are, practical applications, evidence for effectiveness, how to help people change and outcome measures.

DOI: 10.1016/B978-0-443-06934-5.00010-3

JOINT PROTECTION

Joint protection developed from understanding pathophysiology of joint diseases, joint biomechanics, forces applied during activity and how these contribute to the development of deformity (Brattstrom 1987, Chamberlain et al 1984, Cordery 1965, Cordery & Rocchi 1998, Melvin 1989). The aims of joint protection in inflammatory arthritis are to:

- reduce pain, during activity and at rest, resulting from pressure on nociceptive endings in joint capsules from inflammation and mechanical forces on joint
- reduce forces on joints: internal (i.e. from muscular compressive forces e.g. during strong grip) or external (i.e. forces applied to joints whilst carrying or pulling/pushing objects)
- help preserve joint integrity and reduce risk of development and/or progression of deformities
- reduce fatigue, by reducing effort required for activity performance
- improve or maintain function.

  For people with osteoarthritis (OA) the aims are to:

- reduce loading on articular cartilage and subchondral bone,
- strengthen muscle support
- improve shock absorbing capabilities of joints (Cordery & Rocchi 1998).

Joint protection is an active coping strategy to improve daily tasks and role performance helping reduce frustration arising from difficulties with these, enhance perceptions of control and improve psychological status (Hammond et al 1999). Much of joint protection literature focuses on hand problems in rheumatoid arthritis (RA), so this is explored in detail in this chapter but strategies are similarly applicable in other conditions and for other joints.

PATHOPHYSIOLOGY OF HAND DEFORMITIES AND BIOMECHANICAL BASIS OF JOINT PROTECTION

Considering why deformities develop with RA helps in understanding how joint protection may contribute to preserving joint integrity. Deformities develop due to a combination of persistent synovitis disrupting joint structures and both normal and abnormal forces passing over joints (Adams et al 2005, Flatt 1995). In the longer-term, disruptions to bony architecture from erosions and osteophytes can further alter joint mechanics at any joint.

The wrist

The ulnar side is an early inflammation site. Triangular fibrocartilage disruption allows the proximal carpal row to rotate ulnarward. The distal row compensates by sliding radially, producing a radially deviating wrist. Laxity of the radio-ulnar ligament permits rotation of the radius and ulna, with the ulnar styloid becoming more prominent. Extensor carpi ulnaris can become displaced volarly, passing beneath the wrist joint axis, exerting a flexor pull. This, combined with wrist ligament laxity, and the natural volar incline of the distal radius, increases risk of wrist volar subluxation.

The metacarpophalangeal (MCP) joints

Persistent synovitis can weaken MCP collateral ligaments, volar plates and dorsal hoods leading to joint instability. The finger extensors can then slip volarly and ulnarly, increasingly acting as weak flexors. Normal MCP joint features contribute to ulnar deviation once joint structure is disrupted. These include: the flexor tendons approach the index and middle fingers from an ulnar direction exerting a significant ulnar torque; the metacarpal head anatomically predisposes to tendons slipping ulnarward; and the ulnar interossii exert a stronger pull than the radial (see Fig. 16.3 Ch 16).

The interphalangeal (IP) joints

Persistent synovitis can disrupt positioning of the extensor tendon central slip and lateral bands allowing Boutonniere deformity to develop. MCP joint inflammation can cause protective spasms in the interossii causing MCP flexion during finger extension (the intrinsic plus position), contributing to Boutonniere and swan-neck deformity development (see Fig. 16.4 Ch 16).

JOINT PROTECTION AND THE HANDS

Anatomical disruptions, combined with normal daily hand use patterns, can promote deformity. Power grip requires MCP ulnar deviation, especially in the 4th and 5th fingers. During lifting, external pressures in a volar or longitudinal direction increase strain on weakened wrist ligaments. Strong pinch grips increase intrinsic muscle pull promoting imbalance at the IP joints. Hand joint protection in RA thus focuses on changing movement patterns to limit: strong grips, twisting movements and sustained grips at the MCPs (reducing MCP ulnar forces); lifting heavy objects and sustained wrist radial positioning (reducing wrist volar and radial forces); and tight, prolonged key, tripod and pinch grips (reducing volar and ulnar forces on the MCP and IP joints).

In the early stages, many with RA are all too aware of hand function problems: dropping items, weaker grip, reduced dexterity and frustration from activities taking longer and being more painful. However, early signs of RA can be subtle (see Fig. 10.1). Whilst swelling may be noticeable, many do not notice a more prominent ulnar styloid, slight wrist radial deviation and 5th MCP ulnar deviation, early correctable finger deformities, nor gradual loss of movement. In early RA average losses are 20° wrist extension, 30° wrist flexion, 15° MCP flexion and only 40% of normal power and pinch grip strength (Hammond et al 2000). A third can develop hand deformities by two years (Eberhardt et al 1990). This suggests joint protection and hand exercises should be provided early and effectively to limit decline (Fig. 16.4 Ch 16).

JOINT PROTECTION PRINCIPLES

Principles taught are shown in Box 10.1 and in Chapter 16 (Box 16.4). Focus on priority messages in plain English. For example, for the hands:

- Spread the load of what you lift (e.g. use two hands)
- Use stronger, larger joints

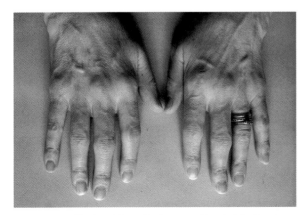

Figure 10.1 The hand in early rheumatoid arthritis showing swelling of the metacarpophalangeal joints and proximal interphalangeal joints. With permission from: Goldenburg DL 2003 Clinical features of rheumatoid arthritis. In: Hochberg MC et al (eds.) Rheumatology 3rd edn, Elsevier, London. Fig. 68.6 p 770.

- Reduce effort to do tasks (e.g. use a gadget)
- Change how you move: keep wrists up, fingers straighter and looser grip when working.

Joint protection principles are reviewed in Palmer and Simons (1991).

JOINT PROTECTION STRATEGIES

Joint protection is the application of ergonomics to everyday activities, work and leisure. Many people find ways of reducing pain and fatigue in daily activities through trial and error, but this takes time. Joint protection and energy conservation education should apply a systematic approach to changing habits, finding new solutions and speeding up change. Strategies include:

BOX 10.1   Joint protection and energy conservation principles

Joint protection

- Respect pain: use this as a signal to change activities
- Distribute load over several joints
- Reduce the force and effort required to perform activities by altering working methods, using assistive devices and reducing the weight of objects
- Use each joint in its most stable anatomic or functional plane
- Avoid positions of deformity and forces in their direction
- Use the strongest, largest joint available for the job
- Avoid staying in one position for too long
- Avoid gripping too tightly
- Avoid adopting poor body positioning, posture and using poor moving and handling techniques
- Maintain muscle strength and range of movement.

Energy conservation

- Pace activities by balancing rest and activity, alternating heavy and light tasks and performing activities more slowly
- Use work simplification methods, e.g. planning ahead, prioritising, using labour saving gadgets and delegating to others when necessary
- Avoid activities that cannot be stopped immediately if it proves beyond the person's ability
- Modify the environment to suit ergonomic/joint protection practices.
(College of Occupational Therapists 2003).

Respecting pain

Using aches and pains as a prompt to changing activities.

Altering working methods

E.g. altering movement patterns during tasks; more efficient positioning, e.g. sitting on a perch stool to iron; and reducing forces from lifting, pushing/pulling, stretching/reaching, carrying (Figs 10.2–10.5).

Restructuring activities

E.g. reordering task sequences within these, eliminating unnecessary steps to increase efficiency.

Using assistive technology

Reducing effort required performing activities, e.g. jar openers, dycem matting, key turners, easy-grip scissors, walking aids (see Ch. 9, Fig. 9.3).

Altering the environment

E.g. bringing objects within the person's reach envelope; reorganizing work areas to streamline activity processes; raising or lowering working heights.

Selecting appropriate product designs (universal designs)

E.g. equipment with non-slip handles (e.g. irons, screwdrivers, Good Grip kitchen equipment); electric alternatives (e.g. can openers, see Fig. 10.6); lightweight models (e.g. hand held vacuum cleaners for stairs); labour saving equipment (e.g. tumble drier, plug pulls, see Fig. 10.7); lever taps. Further details on assistive technology and environmental adaptation can be found in Chapter 9.

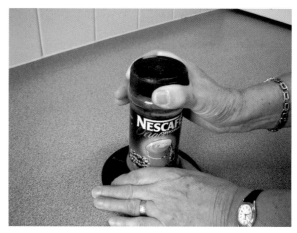

Figure 10.3 Opening a jar – alternate method avoiding ulnar deviation.

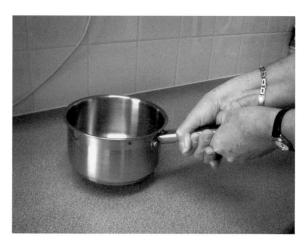

Figure 10.4 Carrying a pan with two hands.

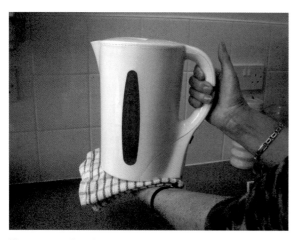

Figure 10.2 Carrying a kettle with two hands – distributing load, reducing metacarpophalangeal joint deviation.

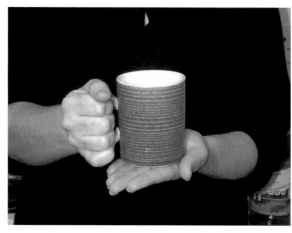

Figure 10.5 Holding a mug with two hands distributing load, avoiding metacarpophalangeal joint deviation.

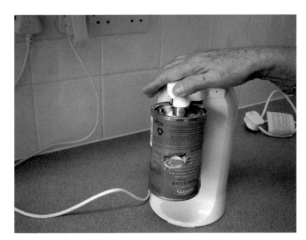

Figure 10.6 Electric can opener, avoiding ulnar deviation at the metacarpophalangeal joints.

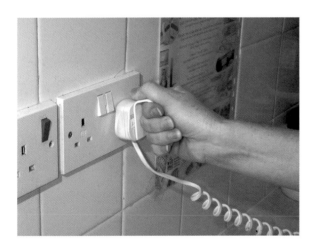

Figure 10.7 Electric plug pull, reducing forces on the wrist and metacarpophalangeal joints.

BOX 10.2   Examples of factors contributing to fatigue

Physical

- Pain
- The disease (e.g. inflammation, especially in a flare up).
- Physical demands due to biomechanical disruption of joints (e.g. lower limb OA, RA)
- Anaemia (due to the disease, medication or other heath/diet reasons)
- Poor sleep (e.g. due to pain, stress, the menopause)
- Deconditioning: insufficient physical activity causing muscle weakness
- Overdoing activities (boom-bust cycle)
- Other health problems (e.g. heart or lung disease)
- Poor nutrition: loss of appetite due to the disease; medication; difficulty cooking and shopping.

Psychosocial

- Depression, anxiety, helplessness, stress
- Poor self-efficacy
- Work pressures (e.g. difficulty fulfilling job demands)
- Problematic social support e.g. family and friends giving upsetting/unhelpful advice, lack of understanding.

Environmental

- Noise
- Poor lighting
- Temperature extremes
- Uncomfortable furniture (beds, chairs)
- Inefficient equipment positioning, work heights or room layout
- Transport issues, e.g. walking distance from car park, long commutes.

FATIGUE MANAGEMENT

Fatigue increases pain, cognitive disturbance (e.g. reduced concentration) and psychological effects (e.g. increased stress, low mood). There are many possible causes (see Box 10.2) and multiple solutions are needed. Helping people identify potential causes helps them prioritise changes. Practical strategies include:

ENERGY CONSERVATION

This aims to reduce fatigue, pain and increase activity tolerance to achieve overall greater productivity and quality of life without exacerbating pain. Energy conservation principles are included in Box 10.1 and Chapter 16 (Box 16.4). Usually taught alongside joint protection, practical strategies include:

Pacing

This significantly improves duration of physical activity (Furst et al 1987) and includes:

Taking rest breaks
Many find resting against their personal standards, feeling this is 'giving in' and preferring to remain

busy. Explain rest 'recharges the batteries' to keep going for longer. Recommend: regular short rest breaks, e.g. 3–5 minutes every 30–45 minutes sitting and relaxing joints; and/or 'microbreaks', i.e. 30 seconds every 5–10 minutes stretching and relaxing those joints and muscles being most used. Many express concerns that taking rests is seen as 'slacking' by managers at work, so microbreaks can be more achievable. Rest strategies are recommended to all workers by the Health and Safety Executive (2005) to reduce injury as they allow muscle recovery time. Developing habits is helped by e.g. setting a kitchen timer or mobile phone to ring/vibrate every 30 minutes; screen prompts every 5–10 minutes for microbreaks.

Balancing activities

Alternating heavy, medium and light activities during the day and week. Many do too much on 'good days' and suffer the consequences several days after (the boom and bust cycle). Breaking this habit requires attitudinal change. Many fear that, if they don't get things done, they won't meet work demands and family/home responsibilities. Activity diaries are useful in helping people identify and evaluate activity patterns (see Arthritis Research Campaign (2007) for an example).

Positioning

- Avoiding prolonged sitting and standing, change position regularly, taking a short stretch.
- Maintain efficient posture during activity, e.g. avoid sitting with the head 'poked forward' whilst reading or working at a desk. Book stands, writing slopes and document holders assist. Keep the back straighter using supportive seating, e.g. ergonomic office chairs. Poor posture and positioning use more energy, increasing fatigue and pain, than correct posture. Developing habits can be helped by the 'red dot' method, i.e. placing a red sticky dot at work/activity areas and associate seeing this with aligning posture and a microbreak.
- Analyse body positions during activities to identify more efficient movements and positions.

Planning

This includes using work simplification strategies. Can tasks be organised more efficiently? Can storage areas be more organised at home and work? Can certain tasks be avoided or eliminated, performed using different equipment, methods, or less often.

Or as a final solution, can someone else help? Offering to reciprocate doing another activity or function for that person helps reduce the feelings of obligation or dependency.

Problem solving

Teach task analysis; select an activity identified as problematic by the person; review each task in turn to identify if a change is beneficial or necessary; identify a range of possible solutions or alternative methods for each task; try these; determine which works best; then practice.

SLEEP HYGIENE

A sleep diary can be helpful (see Useful Websites). Solutions depend on the problems and can include: using more supportive mattresses and pillows; establishing a regular bedtime and evening routine, e.g. relaxation, soothing music, warm bath or shower, gentle exercise; avoiding stimulants 2–3 hours before bedtime (tea, coffee, caffeinated soft drinks, alcohol, smoking); reducing stimuli in the bedroom, e.g. avoiding television and computer use, turning clock faces away, black-out curtains, muted colour schemes.

COGNITIVE INTERVENTIONS

Evaluate potential common psychosocial causes of fatigue: loss of valued activities, poor self-efficacy, anxiety and problematic social support (Katz & Yelin 1995, Lorish et al 1991, Riemsma et al 1998, Wolfe et al 1996). Cognitive approaches used by OTs include: stress management (including managing automatic negative thinking, relaxation); mindfulness therapy; goal-setting to increase valued activity engagement (e.g. paid/unpaid work, leisure, social activities); assertiveness and communication training; liaising with family and carers. Stress and pain management can help improve self-efficacy, coping and perceptions of control (Rhee et al 2002) and referral for individually tailored cognitive-behavioural therapy is beneficial for those with more severe problems (Evers et al 2002).

PHYSICAL INTERVENTIONS

Regular physical activity and exercise reduce aches, pain and fatigue and improve sleep quality. Evaluate current level of physical activity and discuss benefits of and overcoming barriers to exercise (see Ch. 7). Recommend simple walking programmes (see Useful Websites) and referral to physiotherapy as necessary.

MEDICAL INTERVENTIONS

Good pain control can significantly reduce fatigue (Pollard et al 2006). Encourage taking analgaesia and prescribed medication effectively (see Ch. 15). Whilst providing specific medication advice is outside the professional competency of most therapists, explain the benefits of medication, mode of action and that timing or dosage may be improved. Recommend discussing medication with the rheumatology nurse (via the Rheumatology department's telephone advice line) or at their next Consultant, GP or rheumatology nurse appointment.

WHAT JOINT PROTECTION AND FATIGUE MANAGEMENT ARE NOT

Joint protection is often misperceived as meaning stopping activities, keeping joints immobile and excess rest. It can be seen as 'giving in'. Many find it confusing that the OT tells people to 'protect joints' (incorrectly perceived as limiting movement and activity) whilst the physiotherapist tells them to exercise as much as possible (incorrectly perceived as meaning all types of exercise causing pain and strain). These seem opposing messages. Rheumatology OTs and physiotherapists must give similar explanations to ensure patients are not confused. Emphasise 'looking after joints' means adapting activities and movements and reducing strain or force on joints. Exercise means being more physically active as well as stretching, strengthening and low-impact aerobic exercises. Exercise also applies joint protection principles, e.g. avoiding twisting (torque) forces or excess shock (e.g. high impact aerobics, wearing thin soled shoes whilst walking) and helps support joints so they are better able to tolerate forces that cannot be reduced. Fatigue management increases energy to be more physically active and do more enjoyable things in life. The combined benefits of all three help a more meaningful life to be lived (see Fig. 10.8).

HAND EXERCISES

Joint protection and fatigue management are normally provided alongside a) assessment for splints (see Ch. 12) and b) hand exercises, as joint

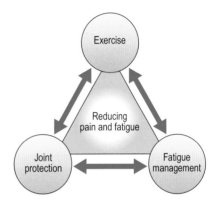

Figure 10.8 Joint protection, exercise and fatigue.

protection principles (Box 10.1) include maintaining muscle strength and range of movement. Maintenance hand exercise programmes should be easily integrated into normal daily routine, and help maintain all hand grips, combining strengthening and stretching (Hammond 2004, Hoenig et al 1993, O'Brien et al 2006). Strengthening hand muscles aids joint stability by compensating for ligamentous laxity. Keep the number of exercises to a minimum to ensure they can be achieved but ensure plenty of repetition. Lengthy, complex, hand exercise regimens are unlikely to be followed long-term. A simple home programme is described in Box 10.3.

HOW IS JOINT PROTECTION AND FATIGUE MANAGEMENT EDUCATION COMMONLY PROVIDED?

Education averages 1.5 hours over two appointments but is often less due to time constraints. Usual content is: education about the condition; how joints are affected by it; joint protection principles; demonstrations with short (e.g. 15–30 minutes) practice of common joint protection methods, e.g. making a cup of tea, rising from a chair; and discussing solutions to individuals' problems, supported by a self-help booklet (Hammond 1997). In general, behavioural approaches are not used. This is still usual practice but is it effective?

EVIDENCE FOR JOINT PROTECTION AND ENERGY CONSERVATION EFFECTIVENESS

USUAL JOINT PROTECTION EDUCATION

Barry et al (1994) evaluated in a randomized controlled trial (RCT) 1 hour of individual education,

---

BOX 10.3   A home hand exercise programme

Find a comfortable position: support the arm to avoid shoulder aching. Do one hand at a time for best movement. Warm-up for each exercise:

■ "Start with three slow repetitions: first about 70% as far as you can go, the second 90% and the third as far as you can comfortably go feeling a gentle pull, but not pain." Three days the first week, gradually increasing repetitions and number of days over 4–8 weeks, to 10 repetitions most/every day.

Range of movement

■ Wrist extension/flexion
■ Wrist pronation/supination:
■ Tendon gliding exercise
■ Radial finger walk.

Muscle strength and dexterity exercise

Use a pot of play-doh. (If difficult to open, keep wrapped firmly in a plastic bag). Do for five minutes on the first day, gradually increasing time or hands may ache later. Increase to 15–20 minutes (spread over several sessions if you need to).

■ Gently knead and squeeze
■ Roll into a sausage (two hands)
■ Pinch off dough with each finger/thumb in turn
■ Form a doughnut from the sausage. Put the fingers/thumbs in the hole; stretch out.

---

similar to the 'usual' content above, and identified improvement in joint protection knowledge. Two trials have evaluated usual joint protection education for 2.5 hours (as part of an 8 hour standard arthritis education programme). These also improved knowledge but not behaviour (Hammond & Freeman 2001, Hammond & Lincoln 1999a). Interviews identified only 25% of participants considered they had made changes (Hammond & Lincoln 1999a).

However, analysis of hand use patterns before and after education showed many cited changes were performed beforehand. Education raised awareness of changes already subconsciously made. For others, barriers to change were:

● considering joint protection not applicable as 'my hands are not that bad yet' or using techniques 'on bad days only', i.e. not perceiving joint protection is preventative and permanent change necessary (insufficient attitudinal change).

● difficulty recalling methods (insufficient knowledge change)
● difficulty getting used to different movements which felt 'clumsy and slow' (insufficient skill change)
● difficulty changing the habits and routines of a lifetime (insufficient behaviour change).

Interventions need to address these barriers to be effective.

BEHAVIOURAL JOINT PROTECTION EDUCATION

In contrast, structured group programmes, of 8–16 hours duration, emphasising active learning, problem solving, behavioural approaches, frequent practice and home programmes have been proven effective.

An RCT with people with early RA (n = 127) compared an 8 hour cognitive-behavioural approach joint protection programme with a standard arthritis education programme (including 2.5 hours of usual joint protection, not using behavioural approaches). At 1 year the behavioural group, compared to the standard group, significantly improved the use of joint protection, improved functional ability and reduced hand pain, general pain and early morning stiffness (Hammond & Freeman 2001). Benefits continued at 4 years and the behavioral group had fewer hand deformities (Hammond & Freeman 2004). Timing of education needs careful consideration as there is evidence it can be provided both too early and too late (Hammond 2004). Other studies in patients with established RA have also shown benefits:

● balance of rest and activity (Furst et al 1987);
● use of assistive devices (Nordenskiold 1994);
● functional ability (Nordenskiold et al 1998).

COMBINED JOINT PROTECTION, FATIGUE MANAGEMENT AND EXERCISE

RCTs in people with established RA have resulted in significant improvements in pain, functional and physical ability, self-efficacy and psychological status (Hammond et al 2008, Masiero et al 2007). An RCT in people with hand OA identified significant improvements at three months in grip strength and self-perceived hand function, in comparison to a control group receiving education about OA (Stamm et al 2002).

TEACHING JOINT PROTECTION AND FATIGUE MANAGEMENT

Facilitating behaviour change

Many attempts to change behaviour by making a change in knowledge (traditional handouts, demonstration, discussions) have been largely unsuccessful. Using cognitive, behavioural and learning theories to develop teaching programmes have been effective.

(Cordery & Rocchi 1998)

Groups provide a powerful modelling force for enabling joint protection behaviour change, enhancing self-efficacy (see Ch. 6) and increasing problem-solving activity with others facing similar difficulties. Group education can be more cost-effective. Treating six patients individually for 2 hours each (i.e. an ineffective level of education) takes 12 hours. Treating six patients in a group joint protection programme (e.g. Hammond & Freeman 2001, Hammond et al 2008) takes 12 hours and is proven effective. Therapists need to change services to deliver evidence-based practice.

Integrating behavioural approaches

The self-management cognitive-behaviour therapy approach is based on self-regulation and social cognitive theory (Kanfer & Gaelick 1989). This recommends four stages: creating a working relationship; creating and maintaining the motivation for change; developing and executing a behavioural change programme (including home programmes); and providing support to promote change and prevent relapse. (For further details see Hammond 2003).

Getting started – motivating for change and initial explanations

People must perceive joint protection and fatigue management are relevant now before they are likely to change, i.e. to be in contemplation (Prochaska & DiClemente 1992, Prochaska 2008, see Ch. 6). To help this attitudinal shift to contemplation, ask whether activities people have to do, need to do and enjoy doing are affected by arthritis and the causes (e.g. pain, fatigue, stiffness, frustration) and concerns for the future. This helps focus on the impact of arthritis and thus on contemplating the pros and cons of change (Prochaska 2008).

Do they want to reduce these causes? Explain joint protection and fatigue management are proven effective and discuss the benefits (pros) that can be gained (i.e. reduced pain and fatigue, staying independent, better function, less frustration, actively helping manage symptoms, better physical and psychological wellbeing). Allow time for the person to discuss their cons (e.g. concerns about negative self-image, embarrassment, not wanting to use assistive devices, wanting to remain as they are, not wanting to take the time to change, concerns joint protection is slower and more difficult) (Niedermann et al, 2009a, in review). If they have no pain or difficulties currently, joint protection is not relevant and they are unlikely to shift from precontemplation. Explain the education available, provide written information and discharge. Education too early is unlikely to be sufficiently recalled when applicable later so ensure mechanisms are in place for people to self-refer (Hammond 2004).

If they do have pain or difficulties and seem to be moving through the decisional balance stage into contemplation or preparation, then:

- explain how joints can be affected in arthritis, why forces on hands increase pain and hand deformities may develop
- examine their hands: Is there joint swelling? Can they move wrists, fingers and thumbs fully? Ask them to identify problems. Point out reduced wrist or finger extension/flexion, thumb web space or grip ability and likely functional consequences. Identify to them any deformities developing. This helps the person reflect if joint protection is personally relevant and provides motivation for change
- try common everyday activities. Ask them to explain the forces on their hands, e.g. lifting a full jug kettle. Discuss the ulnar forces on the MCPs and internal compression from the wrist extensors/flexors and thumb flexors/adductors. Trying two kettle designs (jug and traditional) helps people realise how object design influences forces
- try an alternate method (see Fig. 10.2) and ask them to explain the difference in forces felt. Several activities should be tried (Figs 10.3, 10.4)
- When people grasp the concept of altering forces through altering movement patterns, get them problem solving how different ways of holding objects or different object designs reduce forces

- Home programmes help increase commitment to change. The first 'home programme' should focus on further enabling the shift to contemplation and preparation. It can include watching using their hands during common activities (e.g. making a hot drink). Self-monitoring encourages awareness of movement patterns, aches and pains during activity and aids reflection on whether joint protection is personally relevant and the benefits are worth gaining. Supportive material is the booklet 'Looking after your joints when you have arthritis' (Arthritis Research Campaign 2007).

At the next session, discuss their attitudes to joint protection and ask if they are ready to commit to education. Have the pros now outweighed the cons for them? (Niedermann et al 2009a, in review). Learning facts is easy, but changing habits is harder. To shift from preparation to action, recommend attending a group joint protection programme (e.g. the Looking After your Joints Programme) (Hammond & Freeman 2001) or if, individual sessions, at least three further sessions as fewer are ineffective (Hammond & Freeman 2001).

Promoting change – practise, goal setting and home programmes

During practical training, apply the educational and skills training approaches described in Chapter 6. Everyday movement patterns are automatic movements using open-loop motor control, i.e. pre-programmed, often from childhood. Change requires shifting to closed-loop motor control whilst learning new movement patterns. Start with part-blocked practice, i.e. single tasks repetitively performed. This can be an early home programme activity. Each week practice with progressively more complex activities, e.g. a hot drink, then snack meal then a full meal. If performance errors are noted delay feedback initially (e.g. 3 seconds) to enable the person to identify and problem solve their own errors. Teach mental rehearsal to improve skills and practice opportunities. Further details on motor learning can be found in Ezekiel et al 2000, Lehto et al 2000, Marley et al 2000 and Wishart et al 2000.

BOX 10.4   Example of an action plan

Dates from:___Monday_____ to:_____Sunday_____

The Plan:

1. Practise the range of movement hand exercises three times *each* for 3 days.
2. Use the joint protection methods making a hot drink five times.
3. Imagine using the hot drink joint protection methods three times.
4. Listen to relaxing music tape before bedtime on three evenings.

I am sure I can complete this plan (circle):

0   1   2   3   4   5   6   ⑦   8   9   10
(not at all sure)   (totally sure)

When I complete the plan, my reward will be:

Put feet up with a cappuccino!

How well did I do with my plan?

Goal setting helps people commit to weekly home practice. Each session ask them to state and, preferably, write down an action plan (see Box 10.4). Goals should be determined by the person: and specify what, how often and how much (see Ch. 6). Encourage identifying rewards contingent on achieving their plan. Pushing people to practise too much is unlikely to be successful. Use a 10 point scale (see Box 10.4): how confident are they to complete each task on a scale of 0-10? Then the whole plan? If the answer is less than 7, ask them to revise their goal/plan to be more achievable.

At the start of the each session, always review goal progress. The home programme is an important, integral part of treatment. Failure should not be criticised. Rather, identify barriers and jointly problem-solve overcoming these (see also Ch. 6., Box 6.3). Finally, schedule a follow-up appointment 6–8 weeks after education finishes to review progress and promote continuing independently setting goals for longer term change.

OUTCOME MEASURES

In addition to measures described in Chapter 4, specific measures include:

KNOWLEDGE

The Joint Protection Knowledge Assessment (Hammond & Lincoln 1999b): 20 multiple choice items assessing ability to identify best methods. Some arthritis knowledge questionnaires also include joint protection and fatigue management items (see Ch.6).

SELF-EFFICACY

The Joint Protection Self-Efficacy Scale (Niedermann et al 2009b, in review): 10 items assessing confidence in caring for hand and finger joints, and applying joint protection methods. The RA Self-Efficacy Scale (Hewlett et al 2001) includes questions about confidence in using joint protection and fatigue management strategies.

ADHERENCE

Direct observation

The Joint Protection Behaviour Assessment (Hammond & Lincoln 1999c): analyses hand movements whilst making a hot drink and snack meal. Performance is recorded then analyzed, using an assessment manual, coding for correct, partially correct or incorrect movements in 20 tasks (e.g. lift a kettle). A 10-item version is equally reliable (Klompenhouwer et al 2000) and skilled assessors can do this without recording.

IMPACT ON FUNCTIONAL AND HEALTH STATUS

Relevant scales can be found in Chapters 4, 6 and 16 (Box 16.3). More specific questionnaires are:

The Evaluation of Daily Activities Questionnaire (Nordenskiold et al 1996, 1998) evaluating functional ability with and without assistive devices/altered working methods. This is used to evaluate joint protection and in clinical practice in Scandinavia. A UK version is in development.

Fatigue: the Multidimensional Assessment of Fatigue: 16 questions concerning the quantity, degree, distress, impact, and timing of fatigue (Tack 1991). The Vitality subscale of the SF-36 comprises four items (full of life, energy, worn out, tired) with six responses from 'all of the time' to 'none of the time' (Ware & Sherbourne 1992).

CONCLUSION

Joint protection and fatigue management are effective if taught effectively. How education is provided makes a significant difference to whether patients with rheumatological musculoskeletal conditions benefit. Educational, cognitive and behavioural approaches are significantly more effective than traditional techniques and should be provided (NICE 2009). The whole team needs to support people in committing to make the time to learn how to successfully apply these effective self-management strategies.

STUDY ACTIVITIES

1. Try the hand exercise programme (see Box 10.3). (You will need to buy a pot of Play-doh).
   - Write an action plan to do these everyday for a week. Keep an exercise diary.
   - What is the best way to do these and integrate them into your daily routine?
   - Identify what muscles are exercised in each.
2. Observe how you use your hands during activities at work/study and home (e.g. making a hot drink; using a computer; ironing).
   - Conduct a task analysis of two activities identifying the separate components and movements used for each task.
   - Apply joint protection and energy conservation principles to problem-solve alternate performance methods.
   - Write an action plan to practise alternate methods.
   - Reflect: how easy or difficult is it to change habitual, automatic behaviour patterns?
   - How much practice do you need to establish new habits?
3. Read the arc booklet: 'Looking after your joints when you have arthritis' (available from www.arc.org.uk).
   - Complete an activity diary for 2 days over the next week.
   - What is your balance of activity/rest?
   - Did you feel tired? Could you apply fatigue management strategies to increase efficiency? If so, set goals in your action plan to make changes.
   - Reflect: how easy or difficult was it to make changes?

USEFUL WEBSITES

Joint protection and fatigue

http:/www.arthritis.org/preventing-arthritis-pain.php/ (accessed March 2009).

www.arthritis.ca

Tips for Living Well section: joint protection and fatigue management ideas accessed March 2009

www.arc.org.uk

Arthritis information for patients: booklets on 'Looking after your joints when you have arthritis', 'Gardening with arthritis', 'Fatigue and arthritis' accessed March 2009.

http:/campus.dyc.edu/arthritis/homepage.htm/ (accessed March 2009).

http:/osteoarthritis.about.com/od/joint/protection/Joint_Protection.htm/ (accessed March 2009).

http:/www.mayoclinic.com/health/joint-protection/AR00027/ (accessed March 2009).

Hand exercises

http:/www.mayoclinic.com/health/arthritis/AR00030/ (accessed March 2009).

Walking plan

http:/www.arthritistoday.org/fitness/walking/tips-and-strategies/walking-plan.php/ (accessed March 2009).

Sleep information and diary

http:/www.patient.co.uk/leaflets/sleep_diary.htm/ (accessed March 2009).

http:/www.iboro.ac.uk/departments/hu/groups/csru/pdf/Daily%20Sleep%Diary+Hygiene.pdf/ (accessed March 2009).

References and further reading

Adams, J., Hammond, A., Burridge, J., et al., 2005. Static orthoses in the prevention of hand dysfunction in rheumatoid arthritis: a review of the literature. Musculoskeletal Care 3 (2), 85–101.

Arthritis Research Campaign, 2007. Looking After Your Joints when you have Arthritis. Arthritis Research Campaign, Chesterfield www.arc.org.uk.

Barry, M.A., Purser, J., Hazleman, R., et al., 1994. Effect of energy conservation and joint protection education in rheumatoid arthritis. Br. J. Rheumatol. 33, 1171–1174.

Brattstrom, M., 1987. Joint Protection and Rehabilitation in Chronic Rheumatic Diseases, third ed.. Wolfe Medical, London.

Chamberlain, M.A., Ellis, M., Hughes, D., 1984. Joint protection. Clin. Rheum. Dis 10 (3), 727–743.

College of Occupational Therapists, , 2003. Occupational Therapy Clinical Guidelines for Rheumatology: Joint Protection and Energy Conservation. College of Occupational Therapists, London.

Cordery, J.C., 1965. Joint protection; a responsibility of the occupational therapist. Am. J. Occup. Ther. 19, 285–294.

Cordery, J., Rocchi, M., 1998. Joint protection and fatigue management. In: Melvin, J., Jensen, G. (Eds.) Rheumatologic Rehabilitation vol 1: Assessment and Management. American Occupational Therapy Association, Bethesda, MD.

Eberhardt, K.B., Rydgren, L.C., Pettersson, H., et al., 1990. Early rheumatoid arthritis-onset, course and outcome over two years. Rheumatol. Int. 10, 135–142.

Evers, A.W., Kraaimaat, F.W., van Riel, P.L., et al., 2002. Tailored cognitive-behavioral therapy in early rheumatoid arthritis for patients at risk: a randomized controlled trial. Pain 100 (1–2), 141–153.

Ezekiel, H.J., Lehto, N.K., Marley, T.L., et al., 2000. Application of motor learning principles: the physiotherapy client as a problem-solver. III augmented feedback. Physiother. Can. 53 (1), 33–39.

Flatt, A., 1995. The Care of the Arthritis Hand, fifth ed.. Quality Medical Publishing, St Louis.

Furst, G.P., Gerber, L.H., Smith, C.C., et al., 1987. A program for improving energy conservation behaviours in adults with rheumatoid arthritis. Am. J. Occup. Ther. 41 (2), 102–111.

Hammond, A., 1997. Joint protection education: what are we doing?. Br. J. Occup. Ther. 60 (9), 401–406.

Hammond, A., 2003. Patient education in arthritis: helping people change. Musculoskeletal Care 1 (2), 84–97.

Hammond, A., 2004. What is the role of the occupational therapist? In: Sambrook, P., March, L. (Eds.), How to Manage Chronic Musculoskeletal Conditions. Best Pract. Res. Cl. Rheumatol. 18 (4), 491–505.

Hammond, A., Bryan, J., Hardy, A., 2008. Effects of a modular behavioural arthritis education programme: a pragmatic parallel group randomized controlled trial. Rheumatology 47 (11), 1712–1718.

Hammond, A., Freeman, K., 2001. One year outcomes of a randomised controlled trial of an educational-behavioural joint protection programme for people with rheumatoid arthritis. Rheumatology 40, 1044–1051.

Hammond, A., Freeman, K., 2004. The long term outcomes from a randomised controlled trial of an educational-behavioural joint protection programme for people with rheumatoid arthritis. Clin. Rehabil. 18, 520–528.

Hammond, A., Kidao, R., Young, A., 2000. Hand impairment and function in early rheumatoid arthritis. Arthritis Rheum. 43 (Suppl. 9), S285.

Hammond, A., Lincoln, N., 1999a. Effect of a joint protection programme for people with rheumatoid arthritis. Clin. Rehabil. 13, 392–400.

Hammond, A., Lincoln, N., 1999b. The joint protection knowledge assessment: reliability and validity. Br. J. Occup. Ther. 62 (3), 117–122.

Hammond, A., Lincoln, N., 1999c. Development of the joint protection behaviour assessment. Arthritis Care Res. 12 (3), 200–207.

Hammond, A., Lincoln, N., Sutcliffe, L., 1999. A crossover trial evaluating an educational-behavioural joint protection programme for people with rheumatoid arthritis. Patient Educ. Couns. 37, 19–32.

Health and Safety Executive, 2005. Aching arms (or RSI) in small businesses: is ill health due to upper limb disorders a problem in your workplace? http://www.hse.gov.uk/pubns/indg171.pdf/ (accessed 10.3.09.).

Heiburg, T., Kvien, T., 2002. Preferences for improved health examined in 1,024 patients with rheumatoid arthritis: Pain has highest priority. Arthritis Rheum. 47 (4), 391–397.

Hewlett, S., Cockshott, Z., Kirwan, J., et al., 2001. Development and validation of a self-efficacy scale for use in British patients with rheumatoid arthritis (RASE). Rheumatology 40, 1221–1230.

Hewlett, S., Cockshott, Z., Byron, M., et al., 2005. Patients' perceptions of fatigue in rheumatoid arthritis: overwhelming, uncontrollable, ignored. Arthritis Care Res. 53 (5), 697–702.

Hoenig, H., Groff, G., Pratt, K., et al., 1993. A randomized controlled trial of home exercise on the rheumatoid hand. J. Rheumatol. 20, 785–789.

Kanfer, FH., Gaelick, L., 1989. Self management methods. In: Kanfer, F.H., Goldstein, A.P. (Eds.) Helping People Change: A Textbook of Methods, third ed.. Pergamon Press, New York, pp. 283–345.

Katz, P.P., Yelin, E.H., 1995. The development of depressive symptoms among women with rheumatoid arthritis. Arthritis Rheum. 38, 49–56.

Klompenhouwer, P., Lysack, C., Dijkers, M., et al., 2000. The joint protection behaviour assessment: a reliability study. Am. J. Occup. Ther. 54 (5), 516–524.

Lehto, N.K., Marley, T.L., Ezekiel, H.J., et al., 2000. Application of motor learning principles: the physiotherapy client as a problem-solver. IV. Future directions. Physiother. Can. 53 (2), 109–114.

Lorish, C.D., Abraham, N., Austin, J., et al., 1991. Disease and psychosocial factors related to physical functioning in rheumatoid arthritis. J. Rheumatol. 18, 1150–1157.

Marley, T.L., Ezekiel, H.J., Lehto, N.K., et al., 2000. Application of motor learning principles: the physiotherapy client as a problem-solver. II. Scheduling practice. Physiother. Can. 52 (4), 315–320.

Masiero, S., Boniolo, A., Wassermann, L., et al., 2007. Effects of an educational-behavioural joint protection program on people with moderate to severe rheumatoid arthritis: a randomized controlled trial. Clin. Rheumatol. 26, 2043–2050.

Melvin, J.L., 1989. Rheumatic Disease in the Adult and Child: Occupational Therapy and Rehabilitation, third ed.. FA Davis, Philadelphia.

NICE (National Institute of Clinical Excellence), 2009. Ch. 6.3. Occupational Therapy. In: Rheumatoid arthritis: national clinical guideline for management and treatment in adults. Royal College of Physicians, London, pp. 87–94.

Niedermann, K., 2009a. Perceived Pros and Cons of joint protection among people with rheumatoid arthritis and occupational therapists (in review).

Niedermann, K., Forster, A., Ciurea, A., et al., 2009b Development and psychometric properties of a joint protection self-efficacy scale (JP-SES) for people with rheumatoid arthritis (in review).

Nordenskiold, U., 1994. Evaluation of assistive devices after a course of joint protection. Int. J. Technol. Assess. Health Care 10 (2), 293–304.

Nordenskiold, U., Grimby, G., Hedberg, M., et al., 1996. The structure of an instrument for assessing the effect of assistive devices and altered working methods in women with rheumatoid arthritis. Arthritis Care Res. 9, 21–30.

Nordenskiold, U., Grimby, G., Dahlin-Ivanoff, S., 1998. Questionnaire to evaluate effects of assistive devices and altered working methods in women with rheumatoid arthritis. Clin. Rheumatol. 17, 6–16.

O'Brien, A.V., Jones, P., Mullis, R., et al., 2006. Conservative hand therapy treatments in rheumatoid arthritis. A randomised controlled trial. Rheumatology 45 (5), 577–583.

Palmer, P., Simons, J., 1991. Joint protection: a critical review. Br. J. Occup. Ther. 54, 453–458.

Pollard, L.C., Choy, E.H., Gonzalez, J., et al., 2006. Fatigue in rheumatoid arthritis reflects pain, not disease activity. Rheumatology 45 (7), 885–889.

Prochaska, J.O., DiClemente, C.C., 1992. Stages of change in the modification of problem behaviours, In: Hersen, M., Eisler, R.M., Miller, P.M. (Eds.) Progress in Behaviour Modification. Sycamore Press, Champaign, IL.

Prochaska, J.O., 2008. Decision making in the transtheoretical model of behaviour change. Med. Decis. Making 28 (6), 845–849.

Rhee, S.H., Parker, J.C., Smarr, K.L., et al., 2002. Stress management in rheumatoid arthritis: what is the underlying mechanism? Arthritis Care Res. 13 (6), 435–442.

Riemsma, R.P., Rasker, J.J., Taal, E., et al., 1998. Fatigue in rheumatoid arthritis: the role of self-efficacy and problematic social support. Br. J. Rheumatol. 37, 1042–1047.

Stamm, T., Machold, K.P., Smolen, J.S., 2002. Joint protection and home hand exercises improve hand function in patients with hand osteoarthritis: a randomized controlled trial. Arthritis Care Res. 47, 44–49.

Tack, B.B., 1991. Dimensions and Correlates of Fatigue in Older Adults with Rheumatoid Arthritis [dissertation]. University of California, San Francisco Assessment available at http://www.son.washington.edu/research/maf/ (accessed 12.2.09.).

Ware Jr, J.E., Sherbourne, C.D., 1992. The MOS 36-Item short-form health survey (SF-36). I. Conceptual framework and item selection. Med. Care 30, 473–483.

Wishart, L.R., Lee, T.D., Ezekiel, H.J., et al., 2000. Application of motor learning principles: the physiotherapy client as a problem-solver. 1. Concepts. Physiother. Can. 52 (3), 229–232.

Wolfe, F., Hawley, D.J., Wilson, K., 1996. The prevalence and meaning of fatigue in rheumatic disease. J. Rheumatol. 23, 1407–1417.

Chapter 11

Applying psychological interventions in rheumatic disease

Elizabeth D. Hale BA(Hons) MSc Health Psychology C.Psychol. (Chartered Health Psychologist) Dudley Group of Hospitals NHS Foundation Trust, Russells Hall Hospital, Dudley and University of Birmingham, School of Sport and Exercise Sciences, Birmingham, UK

Gareth J. Treharne BSc (Hons) PhD University of Otago, Dunedin, Aotearoa/New Zealand Dudley, UK

CHAPTER CONTENTS

KEY POINTS

- The theories, research and professional practice approaches used by health psychologists provide a rich basis for the development of practical interventions for people with rheumatic disease that therapists can deliver
- There are many internet resources with information on health psychology, health and rheumatic disease (see Useful Websites)
- Experiencing a rheumatic disease is a chronic stressor with psychological as well as physical impact. Understanding an individual's illness perceptions might help the patient and their health professional make treatment decisions that are most acceptable for both parties
- Group based and individualised cognitive-behavioural programmes may enhance both psychological and physical outcomes of rheumatic disease.

INTRODUCTION

In this chapter we will consider how physiotherapists, occupational therapists, nurses and other allied health professionals benefit from understanding how psychological interventions can be applied to people with rheumatic disease. We will focus on cognitive-behavioural therapy (CBT) approaches you might consider applying and provide information about assessments of stress, illness perceptions and mood you can use in practice. The role of health psychologists in rheumatology was discussed in Chapter 1 and here we will also consider how they might add breadth to multidisciplinary teams (MDTs).

© 2010 Elsevier Ltd
DOI: 10.1016/B978-0-443-06934-5.00011-5

This volume is timely given the changing emphasis within the healthcare system, both in the UK and internationally. Health professionals are encouraged to promote self-care (or self-management) for patients with long-term conditions (Department of Health 2006). We will outline studies demonstrating the application of psychological theory and practice to facilitating self-management by enhancing concordance between patients and health professionals, building upon Chapter 5 (Biopsychosocial care) and Chapter 6 (Patient education and self-management). A recent meta-analytic review by Dixon et al (2007) identified that psychosocial interventions boost active coping efforts people with arthritis engage in. These interventions improve anxiety, joint swelling, as well as depression, functional ability and self-efficacy over pain. We will explain some of these concepts, like self-efficacy and coping in more detail (see also Chs 5 & 6). Finally, we provide some examples of practical tools to foster self-motivated behaviour change and improve outcomes of people with rheumatic diseases.

STRESS AND CHRONIC ILLNESS

The idea of effective 'coping' is related to how much 'stress' the person feels under. So we need to define these concepts and consider the theoretical background they arise from (Box 11.1).

Stress is normal. Most of us say we feel 'stressed' sometimes. You may find studying or elements of your job stressful, i.e. you perceive these stimuli or events as stressors. Lazarus & Folkman (1984) described how our reactions to such stressors include cognitions, emotions, behaviours and physiological changes. Cognitions are thoughts, such as the threat of how bad the outcome could be, how challenging it is and how much control you have over the situation (Lazarus & Folkman 1984). The emotional, behavioural and physical reactions might include feeling worried, thinking about the perceived problem a lot, working longer hours to complete work and experiencing physical symptoms of anxiety, such as 'butterflies' in the stomach (Lazarus & Folkman 1984).

Alternatively, you might view your courses or tasks at work as exciting, challenging and feel elated by the prospect. An individual's interpretation or perception of the stressful event and their response to it is the key element here. People experience different events, or different elements of events, as stressful or not based on their interpretation of the event. How you think about a given situation influences what you do. In reality, the experience of 'stress', and the ways in which we cope with it, is a process of interactions and adjustments in which we alter the impact of the stressful event or situation by making adjustments in our behaviours, cognitions and emotions (Lazarus & Folkman 1984, Fig. 11.1).

Chronic illnesses, like the rheumatic diseases, can be conceived as stressful events at both a physical and psychosocial level. They lead to coping

---

BOX 11.1   Frequently asked question: what is 'stress'?

In the language of the modern day we use the words 'stress' or 'stressed' to explain a feeling or emotion usually arising from a particular event or situation. We say we feel 'stressed' when we perceive that the demands of a situation outweigh the perceived resources that we have to meet it (Lazarus & Folkman 1984). The key word here is *perceived*.

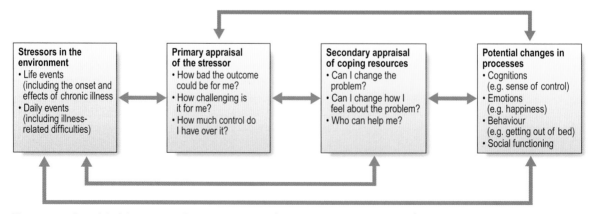

Figure 11.1 A model of the process of coping with stress (after Lazarus & Folkman 1984).

responses from early onset (Treharne et al 2004), which are revised and adjusted throughout the disease course. This is a specific application of the stress-appraisal-coping model. People constantly appraise their coping responses for their usefulness, make adjustments and re-appraise the situation as necessary (Lazarus & Folkman 1984).

The concept of coping was introduced in Chapter 5. Coping involves a process of managing the emotional and physical demands of the stressful situation. Although coping responses used may not actually solve the problem or alter the demands of the situation per se, they may enable the individual to alter their perception of the situation and reconstruct their thinking in more positive terms. Coping responses can act in two ways to reduce psychological stress (Lazarus & Folkman 1984):

PROBLEM-FOCUSED COPING

The individual acts to alter the problem causing the stress. This is employed when a person believes that the situation is changeable and they have, or can get, the resources to help them. These beliefs can easily be facilitated by a therapist offering practical interventions and psychological support enhancing active problem-focused coping strategies, such as making a plan of action and following it. Such coping strategies are associated with better psychological outcomes and less depression among people with rheumatic disease (Hampson et al 1996, Treharne et al 2007a, Zautra & Manne 1992).

EMOTION-FOCUSED COPING

The individual acts to cope with the emotional effects of a problem. Often people engage in this type of coping when they believe they cannot alter the stressor or have insufficient resources to cope with the problem (Lazarus & Folkman 1984). These strategies often involve avoidance, which can be active in nature, such as keeping busy with some other task, or passive in nature, such as social withdrawal. Emotion-focused coping does not always involve avoidant behaviour, for example trying to see the positive side of the situation is an active emotion-focused strategy (Treharne et al 2007a).

In the UK, facilitating coping strategies is becoming increasingly relevant as the government places further onus upon individuals to take responsibility for their own health and well-being, supported in full by multidisciplinary services within the NHS and

their selected partnerships (Department of Health 2006). 'Standards of care' have been published by the Arthritis and Musculoskeletal Alliance (ARMA) in the UK for a variety of rheumatic diseases, including back pain, connective tissue diseases, inflammatory arthritis and osteoarthritis (http://www.arma.net.uk). ARMA proposed self-management training should be available for individuals with rheumatic disease at any stage of their illness: via the Challenging Arthritis programme run by the charity Arthritis Care (see Barlow et al 1998): the generic Expert Patient Programmes, now available throughout the UK within NHS primary care trusts (see Expert Patients Programme 2009); and health professional led self management programmes. Many people will be happy to seek information and learn self-management strategies through group-based interventions, but not all are able to or comfortable with such courses (Hale et al 2006b). Ongoing individualised treatment plans by the multidisciplinary team are still required.

ASSESSING STRESS

Assessing causes of stress may form an important part of your baseline assessment, particularly if you provide relaxation therapy or other stress management interventions. Initially, psychologists assessed stress in terms of the impact of certain life events (Holmes & Rahe 1967). The death of a spouse or close family member was deemed more severe in impact than holidays, a notable stressor. The number of stressful life events, particularly recent ones, is linked to health status and onset of health problems (Holmes & Rahe 1967).

More recently, assessment has focused on impact of daily hassles, i.e. acute events having a direct daily impact (Kanner et al 1981), particularly for people with chronic illnesses like RA (Treharne et al 2002, Turner Cobb et al 1998). When these events become long-term (e.g. daily difficulties at work due to hand problems; frequent tense exchanges with a relative due to their limited understanding of the impact of rheumatic disease), the stressor becomes chronic. The impact of daily hassles can possibly be worse than some of the major life events mentioned (Pillow et al 1996).

Global assessments of stress levels can also be used without addressing the specific event causing the stress. For example, the Perceived Stress Scale (Cohen et al 1983) is a short measure of whether an individual is failing to cope with their perceived stress. This has been applied in several rheumatic disease studies. Scores predict worsening of anxiety over one year (measured using the Hospital Anxiety and Depression Scale; Zigmond & Snaith 1983) among people with rheumatoid arthritis (Treharne et al 2007a).

Assessing potentially stressful events in your patients' daily life can include the frequency, perceived impact and severity of the stressor for that individual. This can be measured with objective instruments, such as the Daily Stress Inventory (Brantley et al 1987). Alternatively, you can ask the patient to keep a simple daily diary of events and their responses (behaviours and moods) to help you design a tailored intervention to help them meet goals for improvement they set. Such diaries can be structured to cover various aspects of daily life (e.g. going shopping; when splints are used) in as much or as little detail as required. These do not have to meet psychometric standards necessary for research if being used as a clinical tool for information gathering, enabling the person to reflect on what they are experiencing on a day-to-day (or hour-by-hour) basis.

UNDERSTANDING STRESSORS

Common long-term daily stressors include frustration with daily activities, living with pain and fatigue and potentially limited understanding of family and friends. People with such long-term daily stressors may experience psychological and social changes that may be difficult to understand and accept (Katz & Neugebauer 2001). Health professionals need to respond to patient needs (which may not always be clearly articulated) and apply a range of approaches and models of self-care support. These approaches can be individual or group based. In order to target educational and therapeutic approaches appropriately we need to understand individual beliefs and capabilities, what knowledge patients have about their condition, the degree to which they have accepted their condition, their attitude, confidence and determination to achieve a progressive positive outcome (see Ch. 6).

COGNITIVE REPRESENTATIONS OF ILLNESS

As described earlier, cognitions are thought processes a person goes through to make sense of any situation or event. People form guides about what is expected in specific contexts, such as how to behave in a restaurant or lecture (e.g. not to throw food). These guides, called schemas, incorporate the norms and values appropriate to our society. However, people have individual beliefs and experiences that underpin the subtleties of their personal schemas (Greenberger & Padesky 1995).

Some well known illnesses have clear schemas, with labels attached to them, that people consider when searching for an explanation for a group of symptoms being experienced, for example 'influenza' (Bishop 1991). However, illnesses presenting with an array of rare, complex, variable and confusing symptoms are less easily interpreted. Individuals turn to other lay means of sense-making, for example, asking a relative or friend with a similar experience (Hale et al 2007). When it becomes necessary or apparent that formal medical assistance is required, diagnosis is not quick and the process may involve numerous tests and uncertainties. This can be common in rheumatic diseases, especially systemic lupus erythematosus (Hale et al 2006a), RA and fibromyalgia. This procedure contributes to the formation of patients' beliefs, attitudes and uncertainties and subsequently updates their illness schemas (see Ch. 5). Leventhal and colleagues laid much of the groundwork for our understanding of illness perceptions (Nerenz & Leventhal 1983, see Leventhal et al 2003).

Different types of information influence different responses to perceived threats to health and well-being. Leventhal and colleagues explored what adaptations and coping efforts need to be made and maintained in people experiencing chronic illness. They proposed an adaptive system model in which illness representations guide coping responses and performance of action plans followed by monitoring of the success or failure of coping efforts (Nerenz & Leventhal 1983). The model has similarities with other problem-solving behaviour theories, such as the transactional model of stress and coping described earlier (Fig. 11.1), wherein chronic illness is conceptualised as the stressful experience (Lazarus & Folkman 1984). Leventhal and colleagues described parallel thinking about the illness danger (e.g. 'What are these pains I keep getting, is there anything I can do about them?') and emotional control (e.g. "I am upset as my doctor said she can't cure it, what shall I do to make myself feel better about it?") (Nerenz & Leventhal 1983).

MEASURING ILLNESS PERCEPTIONS

Validated questionnaire measures of illness perceptions include the Revised Illness Perception Questionnaire (Moss-Morris et al 2002, see Box 11.2) and a shortened version, the Brief Illness Perception Questionnaire (Broadbent et al 2006). These can be applied in clinical practice to access patients' beliefs about their illness's impact and future health. These impacts include assessments about its consequences, its controllability (by the individual as a self-manager or via treatments they are prescribed), its emotional impact and its coherence (i.e. whether the symptoms and overall illness experience make sense to the patient). Moss-Morris et al (2002) describe how the patient's ongoing perceptions of the timeline of their illness relates to whether or not they think their illness will be permanent (i.e. chronic) and go through cycles (i.e. flare and remissions), as many rheumatic diseases can do (Hill & Ryan 2000).

REMODELLING ILLNESS PERCEPTIONS

By accessing patients' illness perceptions, health professionals can tailor patient education and

---

BOX 11.2 Illness cognitions (with example items from the Revised Illness Perception Questionnaire; Moss-Morris et al 2002)

1. Causes of the illness
   (e.g. 'A germ or virus'; 'smoking')
2. Consequences of the illness
   (e.g. 'My illness strongly affects the way others see me')
3. Controllability of the illness
   i. By the individual as a self-manager
   (e.g. 'I have the power to influence my illness')
   ii. Via treatments they are prescribed
   (e.g. 'My treatment can control my illness')
4. Emotional impact of the illness
   (e.g. 'My illness makes me feel angry')
5. Coherence of the illness
   (e.g. 'My illness doesn't make any sense to me')
6. Timeline of the illness
   i. Is it chronic?
   (e.g. 'I expect to have this illness for the rest of my life')
   ii. Does it go through cycles?
   (e.g. 'The symptoms of my illness change a great deal from day to day')

---

treatment plans to the individual emphasizing those elements causing most concern to the patient (Hale et al 2007). This helps people reassess any obviously erroneous illness beliefs they express. This can be achieved by sharing appropriate disease-related information, discussing treatment and working through any worries about potential side-effects. Patients' plans for the future can be constructed and revised as necessary using simple principles like carrying out activities that they enjoy (within their ability range) to distract them from worry and to facilitate a sense of achievement that is easily lost in a disease that can have severe psychosocial impact.

This approach to remodelling illness perceptions was formally tested in an intervention for people who had recently had a heart attack (Petrie et al 2002). After assessing participants' perceptions of their heart disease, an inpatient intervention provided general information about the need to avoid attributing all on-going symptoms to heart disease. A personalised approach then addressed the specific illness perceptions worrying participants (most of whom were men), as well as discussing their medications, discharge plan and importance of individual's lifestyle risks (e.g. poor diet, lack of exercise, smoking). This aimed to improve participants' sense of control by expanding their causal models beyond the common misconception that stress was the sole cause of their heart attack. Compared to a control group (given standard cardiac education), those receiving this personalised intervention showed improvements in perceptions of their ability to control symptoms, consequences of their heart disease and its timeline. After three months, they also felt more prepared for their discharge, had a faster rate of return to work and reported fewer symptoms of angina.

A similar approach was taken by Goodman et al (2005) among people with systemic lupus erythematosus. They used a group CBT intervention, including goal setting, writing action plans, carrying out 'behavioural experiments' to help challenge negative automatic thought patterns using cognitive restructuring, as well as relaxation, distraction and guided imagery. A limitation of Goodman et al (2005) study was that participants chose whether or not they were in the intervention group. This is not ideal for testing interventions because self-selection, rather than randomised allocation, means the two groups could be significantly different (for example, psychologically), even though reflective of how such interventions might be instigated in routine clinical practice (see Study activity 2). Patients reported increased perceptions that treatment could control their lupus but not in perceptions they could control their own illness. Despite this, there were decreases in perceived stress, feelings of helplessness and self-critical thinking after the intervention, demonstrating how the vicious circle of thoughts and behaviours can be broken (see Study activity 11.2).

Other group-based intervention studies have delivered patient education accessing patients' illness perceptions as part of the educative process. Brown et al (2004) described the benefits patients obtained from the groups 'Focus on Lupus' and 'Focus on Scleroderma' using qualitative analysis, providing depth to understanding the process. Patients reported feeling more in control, although people with lupus had a more positive collective response.

DEFINING MOOD DISORDERS AND ASSESSING MOOD

Psychological outcome measures are outlined in Chapter 4. It is important to identify whether mood states meet diagnostic criteria for psychiatric conditions before planning ways to help improve mood, as some may need mental health services. It is also important to monitor ongoing daily mood of the individual, and go beyond retrospective measures (e.g. the Hospital Anxiety and Depression Scale, Zigmond & Snaith 1983).

DEPRESSION AND ANXIETY

Like the word stress, the terms *depressed* and *anxious* have been assimilated into everyday language. These conditions are based on clear medical diagnoses (American Psychiatric Association 2000). Health professionals must listen to the mood symptoms their patients are describing and map these along the parallel continuum from happiness and calmness (the 'norm') through occasional bouts of dejectedness and worry (a transient problem) to enduring sadness or generalised anxiety (more chronic problems).

Depression

An 'episode' of major depression is classified by the American Psychiatric Association (2000) as at least two weeks of depressed mood or lack of interest in activities and anhedonia (the lack of pleasure from previously enjoyed activities). These problems are experienced most of the day and every day for this period. In addition to this, the individual should have four or more of the following associated problems:

- change in appetite or weight
- hypersomnia or insomnia (especially waking early)
- restlessness or feeling slowed down
- fatigue or loss of energy
- guilt and feelings of worthlessness
- inability to concentrate or indecisiveness
- suicidal ideation.

(American Psychiatric Association 2000)

There is some potential overlap with the effects of fatigue and disability from rheumatic disease, but the criterion of 'feeling slowed down' is meant as a cognitive rather than physical problem. Frank et al (1988) applied an earlier version of these criteria to a sample of people with rheumatoid arthritis using structured clinical interviewing finding the prevalence of major depression was 17%. A recent meta-analysis has confirmed depression is more common in RA than the general population (Dickens et al 2002).

A less intense but prolonged version of depression is called dysthymic disorder or minor depression. This is classified by the American Psychiatric Association (2000) as depressed mood most of the day, more days than not for at least two years, and is probably the most common type of depressed mood you will come across in your clinical practice (Frank et al 1988).

Anxiety

Generalised anxiety disorder is distinct from phobias and pure obsessive thought disorders. The American Psychiatric Association (2000) classifies this using criteria of excessive, uncontrollable worry about several events (which could include one's state of health) more days than not for a period of at least 6 months that has an impact on social functioning or work ability. In addition, the individual should have four or more of the following problems:

- feeling restless or 'edgy'
- easily fatigued
- difficulty concentrating
- irritability without reason
- muscle tension (particularly of the shoulders/neck)
- disturbed sleep (especially onset insomnia).

(American Psychiatric Association 2000)

ASSESSING DEPRESSION AND ANXIETY

Muscle tension may also be experienced in rheumatic disease (Treharne et al 2007b). It is also clear that (major) depression and (generalised) anxiety overlap in their listed symptoms and associated thought processes. The forthcoming revision to the American Psychiatric Association's criteria, due for publication in 2010, should clarify differences further (Kupfer et al 2002). Fortunately, both conditions are tackled by similar psychological therapies (Greenberger & Padesky 1995) and drug treatments (Joint Formulary Committee 2009).

Given the problems with accuracy of retrospective recall of psychological processes (Stone et al 1998), the criteria for depression and anxiety ideally require some form of daily mood assessment. Electronic completion of questionnaires is ideal given the ease of viewing questions and answer choices on-screen, saving on paper consumption and data entry time, whilst maintaining replicability of the meaning of questions (e.g. Wilson et al 2002, see Fig. 11.2).

Two classic measures of mood are the Positive and Negative Affect Schedule (Watson et al 1988, see also Crawford & Henry 2004, for normative data) and the bipolar Profile of Mood States (Lorr & McNair 1982, see also Treharne et al 2001, 2002, for applications of relevant subscales). Both these questionnaires assess depression (versus elation)

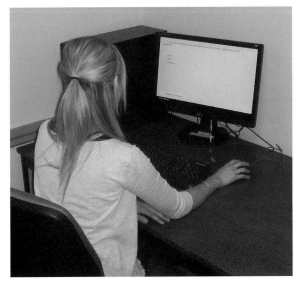

Figure 11.2 Electronic administration of questionnaires.

and anxiety (versus calmness) but, as with assessments of stress, a diary system for recording aspects of mood can be used. Alternatively, two screening questions can be used (Arroll et al 2003):

- During the past month have you often been bothered by feeling down, depressed, or hopeless?
- During the past month have you often been bothered by little interest or pleasure in doing things?

The responses help you direct your therapeutic skills to one or both of these issues (see below), or the basis for referral to local psychological services.

PRACTICAL COGNITIVE BEHAVIOURAL METHODS

So far we have examined how illness might be perceived as stressful, and how patients' symptoms, cognitions (i.e. thoughts), moods and behaviours combine to determine their coping responses. Appraisals of coping style and the effectiveness of that response guide further coping efforts. This applies to all of us in everyday life as well as to people with chronic illnesses. Many people find coping with the physical and the psychosocial effects of their disease difficult and may experience periods of depression and/or anxiety, which are troublesome even if they do not reach the formal criteria for a mood disorder (Lewinsohn et al 2000). This can occur at the initial stages of their disease journey (Treharne et al 2004), or any time particularly, during a flare or after a psychosocial loss like employment, a valued leisure activity or role within the home (Katz & Neugebauer 2001). It may also relate to any life event, such as a bereavement or moving house (Holmes & Rahe 1967). These kind of events (measured using inventories) relate to depression among people with RA (Turner Cobb et al 1998).

When coping becomes difficult, it is useful to understand what an individual believes about his or her disease and the likely impact of the disease. Understanding such thoughts and thought processes, the behavioural consequences of those thoughts and the physiological symptoms and reactions to those thoughts will give greater insight into those areas that might be hindering effective coping practices.

SELF-MANAGEMENT PROGRAMMES

The use of cognitive-behavioural approaches within rheumatology commenced on a large scale with the development of the Arthritis Self-Management Programme (ASMP; known as Challenging Arthritis in the UK), which facilitates effective coping within a group-based community programme led by people who have arthritis (Lorig & Holman 1989). Self-management, applying cognitive-behavioural techniques, builds upon the principle of self-efficacy (Bandura 1977) (see Chs 5 & 6). This approach aims to enhance the belief one can achieve a goal, even in the face of specific obstacles, for example, going for a walk even when feeling fatigued or when it is raining.

Participants in ASMP and Challenging Arthritis groups learn principles of self-help, i.e. taking responsibility for learning about and managing their condition. Within this, they are given disease-related information including: drug treatments; exercise; fatigue; pain management/relaxation techniques; nutrition; non-traditional treatments; problem-solving; communication skills; depression and contracting (learning to set achievable goals). Optimising the effectiveness of an intervention may require customising elements to individual difficulties and characteristics; for example, patients exhibiting heightened distress levels as opposed to those adjusting relatively well.

COGNITIVE-BEHAVIOURAL APPROACHES

Cognitive-behavioural approaches, on an individual basis or within small group settings (i.e. between 4 and 12 members), focus more specifically upon accessing those thoughts, moods and behaviours that lead to depression and anxiety (Dickens et al 2002). Classically, the type of thoughts indicative of depression focus upon loss, whereas thoughts about threat or challenge are typical in people with anxiety (Sanders & Wills 2005). Whilst there are formal measures of depression and anxiety (as outlined earlier and in Ch. 4), a flexibly structured clinical interview provides valuable information.

Cognitive approaches

People experiencing depression have a typically negative way of thinking about the self, the world and the future and may continue to appraise events in these terms, falling into a cycle of negative automatic thoughts, upon which they often ruminate, and find difficult to reconceptualise (Sanders & Wills 2005). An individual who has developed this negatively biased way of thinking will exhibit common cognitive biases, such as 'all-or-nothing' or 'black-and-white' thinking where the shades of 'grey' areas of life are overlooked, so that an individual might think, or even state out loud, that "I've completely failed, everyone else can do this". There may be 'catastrophic' thinking where the worst is always predicted "I'll never be able to do that again, I've lost everything." A particular challenge for the therapist might be working with those thoughts that involve 'gazing into a crystal ball' where the patient anticipates the future in a typically negative way so that their prediction will be "There's no point in trying this physiotherapy as it won't work." By structured questioning and listening to your patient carefully, you may be able to access the key areas of difficulty that you can work with.

Behavioural approaches

Setting acceptable staged goals that the individual can easily test that they can achieve (particularly if those goals are pleasurable) is a short-term behavioural experiment that will hopefully challenge the patient's hypotheses of overall failure and reduce anxieties. Like the well-known mantra of Alcoholics Anonymous (AA), they need to take things 'one day at a time'. Simple feedback, like plotting charts of achievement, exercise or activity diaries and suggesting personally-set rewards as an incentive, are useful maintenance tools the patient can use in the long-term. Such charts and diaries are best personally tailored to the needs of the individual rather than following a prescribed format. Suggestions you can use include structuring the records around various segments of the day (e.g. early morning, late morning, afternoon and evening, or before work, during work and after work) and the use of very small motivational rewards such as gold stars, which no one is too old for.

Cognitive therapy

Cognitive therapists will work to develop a 'conceptualisation' or 'formulation' that links schemas, salient or triggering events, mood, cognitions and behaviours to explain to the patient how vicious cycles arise that continue to feed negative repetitive thoughts and impact upon mood and, subsequently, behaviour. This may be beyond the scope of your practice, however, and it would be appropriate to work closely with the psychologist within your multidisciplinary team (if you work within such a team and have access to a psychologist). Occupational therapists can pursue post-graduate training in cognitive-behavioural therapy (as either short or long courses) and some essentials may be included in undergraduate courses. See Study activity 11.3 for details of an example case of a patient with systemic lupus erythematosus who experienced psychosocial difficulties.

Evidence for CBT approaches in rheumatology

CBT approaches can involve a number of broad methods focusing on breaking the cycle of thoughts and behaviours that may be perpetuating a psychological problem (Sanders & Wills 2005). Several studies have tested CBT approaches in rheumatic diseases. Sharpe et al (2001a, 2003) used the basis of the ASMP manual to deliver individually tailored one-to-one CBT sessions for people with rheumatoid arthritis. Reductions in depressed mood were found immediately after treatment and 6 and 18 months later for participants given the CBT intervention, whereas depressed mood worsened over the same period for those given just routine care (i.e. the control group). Swollen joint counts also reduced over time for the participants given CBT, more so than the control group. However, the individuals in the CBT group made significantly more coping efforts (over many strategies on an inventory where all efforts are summed) at the start of their study, therefore, the groups appeared unevenly matched for motivation to start with. It is also hard to convey a sense of what happened for individuals in the therapy sessions in a journal article. The additional report by Sharpe et al (2001b) on a series of these cases is more enlightening for select examples.

Another tailored CBT programme by Evers et al (2002) was developed for people with rheumatoid arthritis designated 'at risk' for psychological problems (i.e. characterised by higher levels of negative mood and anxiety, more passive coping with pain and stress, greater helplessness and less acceptance of disease and lower levels of social functioning, perceived support and network help). A selection of patient-preferred modules targeted, for example, negative mood or fatigue. People were selected in the 'early' stages of their disease. However, this was defined as within 8 years from diagnosis. This could be too wide a definition, providing a group with very varied experiences. Depression, helplessness and fatigue were significantly reduced post-treatment and 6 months later compared to the control group who received routine care. Furthermore, at the 6-month follow-up assessment perceived support, active coping with stress and adherence to prescribed medication had increased more in the CBT group than the control group. Of course it is not known at this stage how individualised treatments compare to more generalised CBT treatments for all people with rheumatoid arthritis or those not deemed 'at risk', nor how or what treatment effects might be seen in those with long-standing disease. However, although randomised controlled trials are hard to conduct, and inevitably still have limitations, the evidence currently suggests that CBT can show benefit for people with rheumatic disease, which are worth applying in practice.

CONCLUSION

Stress management, self-management programmes and using CBT approaches are all effective strategies in Rheumatology. These need to be an integral part of occupational and physiotherapists' daily practice. Further training in CBT approaches and liaison with health and clinical psychologists to develop services is recommended.

ACKNOWLEDGEMENTS

We thank Prof. George Kitas and Mrs Yvonne Norton MBE, Chair of Lupus West Midlands, for their support. We are also grateful to Miss S for consenting to share her experiences.

1. Think about a multidisciplinary team you have encountered or are part of. Did/does it have access to a psychologist or psychological services? If not, how does the team manage their patients' psychological issues? What suggestions would you make to improve this aspect of care?

2. Search for a recent article describing any type of psychological intervention for people with a rheumatic disease. (Use a database such as http://www.pubmed.com or http://scholar.google.com. Use search terms like 'cognitive behavioural therapy' or 'relaxation training.' Try adding other terms like 'knee' or 'hand' to find something more specific. Read how authors allocated patients to the control group (if they included one) and what this control group did (or did not do).

   ■ List some of the ethical considerations of group allocation and the practical problems that can arise.
   ■ How important is this for how useful the evidence is in practice?
   ■ Would you recommend practitioners apply the results as evidence on which to base practice?
   ■ What would you do differently if you did the study yourself?
   ■ How could you apply the intervention in everyday practice?

3. CASE STUDY: The impact of systemic lupus erythematosus.

   Miss S is a 35-year-old single woman with a confirmed diagnosis of systemic lupus erythematosus. She frequently experiences significant skin rashes and joint discomfort. She can no longer work as she experiences periods of severe fatigue and is often confined to the house which makes her feel isolated and depressed. Miss S had difficulty obtaining a diagnosis at the onset of her disease and was hospitalised for depression at this time. She used to be a dynamic out-going young woman, hard working and successful in her career. Since her diagnosis she has had significant psychosocial losses to adjust to: loss of satisfying work and income forcing a house move; loss of social life and friends and work colleagues; the prospect of losing a relationship due to her continuing ill-health and appearance concerns.

   Miss S would like to be more physically active, less dependent upon her family and work with animals at some point in the future. She continues to find it difficult to come to terms with her disease and experiences depression and anxiety about the future.

   Discuss with your colleagues or fellow students how you would approach the varied aspects of this case. If you work in a multidisciplinary team, how would your colleagues from other disciplines approach these issues? (For more details about this case, and other similar cases, see Hale et al 2006a.)

The Division of Health Psychology of the British Psychological Society
http://www.health-psychology.org.uk
Patient UK: A reference website aimed at the UK public. http://www.patient.co.uk
The Birmingham Arthritis Resource Centre: a community-based educational resource centre with information on several rheumatic diseases available in different languages.

http://www.barc.org.uk
The Arthritis and Musculoskeletal Alliance
http://www.arma.uk.net
The Oxford Cognitive Therapy Centre (Warneford Hospital, Oxford, UK): details of courses, booklets and textbooks on the cognitive approach to psychological therapy.
http://www.octc.co.uk

References and further reading

American Psychiatric Association, 2000. Diagnostic and Statistical Manual of Mental Disorders, fourth ed. text revision American Psychiatric Association, Washington, DC.

Arroll, B., Khin, N., Kerse, N., 2003. Screening for depression in primary care with two verbally asked questions: cross sectional study. Brit. Med. J. 327 (7424), 1144–1146.

Bandura, A., 1977. Self-efficacy: toward a unifying theory of behavioral change. Psychol. Rev. 84 (2), 191–215.

Barlow, J., Turner, A., Wright, C., 1998. Long-term outcomes of an arthritis self-management programme. Brit. J. Rheumatol. 37 (12), 1315–1319.

Bishop, G.D., 1991. Lay disease representations and responses to victims of disease. Basic Appl. Soc. Psych. 12 (1), 115–132.

Brantley, P.J., Waggoner, C.D., Jones, G.N., et al., 1987. A daily stress inventory: Development, reliability, and validity. J. Behav. Med. 10 (1), 61–74.

Broadbent, E., Petrie, K.J., Main, J., et al., 2006. The Brief Illness Perception Questionnaire. J. Psychosom. Res. 60 (6), 631–637.

Brown, S.J., Somerset, M.E., McCabe, C.S., et al., 2004. The impact of group education on participants' management of their disease in lupus and scleroderma. Musculoskeletal Care 2 (4), 207–217.

Cohen, S., Kamarck, T., Mermelstein, R., 1983. A global measure of perceived stress. J. Health Soc. Behav. 24 (4), 385–396.

Crawford, J.R., Henry, J.D., 2004. The Positive and Negative Affect Schedule (PANAS): construct validity, measurement properties and normative data in a large non-clinical sample. Brit. J. Clin. Psychol. 43 (3), 245–265.

Department of Health, 24 February, 2006. Supporting People with Long-Term Conditions to Self-Care: A Guide to Developing Local Strategies and Good Practice. Department of Health, London Online. Available: http://www.dh.gov.uk/en/Publicationsandstatistics/Publications/PublicationsPolicyAndGuidance/DH_4130725/Accessed 6.9.09.

Dickens, C., McGowan, L., Clark-Carter, D., Creed, F., 2002. Depression in rheumatoid arthritis: A systematic review of the literature with meta-analysis. Psychosom. Med. 64 (1), 52–60.

Dixon, K.E., Keefe, F.J., Scipio, C.D., et al., 2007. Psychological interventions for arthritis pain management in adults: a meta-analysis. Health Psychol. 26 (3), 241–250.

Evers, A.W.M., Kraaimaat, F.W., van Riel, P.L.C.M., et al., 2002. Tailored cognitive-behavioral therapy in early rheumatoid arthritis for patients at risk: a randomized controlled trial. Pain 100 (1-2), 141–153.

Expert Patients Programme. 2009. Find a course. Online. Available: http://www.expertpatients.co.uk/public/default.aspx?load=SearchCourses/ Accessed 6.9.09.

Frank, R.G., Beck, N.C., Parker, J.C., et al., 1988. Depression in rheumatoid arthritis. J. Rheumatol. 15 (6), 920–925.

Goodman, D., Morrissey, S., Graham, D., et al., 2005. The application of cognitive-behaviour therapy in altering illness representations of systemic lupus erythematosus. Behav. Change 22 (3), 156–171.

Greenberger, D., Padesky, C.A., 1995. Mind over Mood: Change How You Feel by Changing the Way You Think. Guilford, New York.

Hale, E.D., Treharne, G.J., Kitas, G.D., 2007. The common-sense model of self-regulation of health and illness: how can we use it to understand and respond to our patients' needs?. Rheumatology 46 (6), 904–906.

Hale, E.D., Treharne, G.J., Lyons, A.C., et al., 2006a. "Joining-the-dots" for systemic lupus erythematosus patients: personal perspectives of healthcare from a qualitative study. Ann. Rheum. Dis. 65 (5), 585–589.

Hale, E.D., Treharne, G.J., Macey, S.J., et al., 2006b. 'Big boys don't cry': a qualitative study of gender differences in self-management and coping with arthritis. Rheumatology 45 (Suppl. 1), i14. Abstract.

Hampson, S.E., Glasgow, R.E., Zeiss, A.M., 1996. Coping with osteoarthritis by older adults. Arthritis Care Res. 9 (2), 133–141.

Hill, J., Ryan, S., 2000. Rheumatology: A Handbook for Community Nurses. Whurr, London.

Holmes, T.H., Rahe, R.H., 1967. The social readjustment rating scale. J. Psychosom. Res. 11 (2), 213–218.

Joint Formulary Committee, March 2009. British National Formulary, 57th ed. British Medical Association and Royal Pharmaceutical Society of Great Britain, London Online. Available: http://bnf.org/bnf/ Accessed 6.9.09.

Kanner, A.D., Coyne, J.C., Schaefer, C., et al., 1981. Comparison of two modes of stress measurement: daily hassles and uplifts versus major life events. J. Behav. Med. 4 (1), 1–39.

Katz, P.P., Neugebauer, A., 2001. Does satisfaction with abilities mediate the relationship between the impact of rheumatoid arthritis on valued activities and depressive symptoms? Arthritis Care Res. 45 (3), 263–269.

Kupfer, D.J., First, M.B., Regier, D.A., 2002. A Research Agenda for DSM-V. American Psychiatric Association, Washington, DC.

Lazarus, R.S., Folkman, S., 1984. Stress, Appraisal, and Coping. Springer, New York.

Leventhal, H., Brissette, I., Leventhal, E.A., 2003. The common-sense model of self-regulation of health and illness. In: Cameron, L.D., Leventhal, H. (Eds.), The Self-Regulation of Health and Illness Behaviour. Routledge, London, pp. 42–65.

Lewinsohn, P.M., Solomon, A., Seeley, J.R., et al., 2000. Clinical implications of "subthreshold" depressive symptoms. J. Abnorm. Psychol. 109 (2), 345–351.

Lorig, K., Holman, H., 1989. Long-term outcomes of an arthritis self-management study: effects of reinforcement efforts. Soc. Sci. Med. 29 (2), 221–224.

Lorr, M., McNair, D., 1982. Profile of Mood States: Bi-Polar Form. Educational and Industrial Testing Service, San Diego.

Moss-Morris, R., Weinman, J., Petrie, K., et al., 2002. The revised illness perceptions questionnaire (IPQ-R). Psychol. Health 17 (1), 1–16.

Nerenz, D., Leventhal, H., 1983. Self-regulation in chronic illness. In: Burish, T.G., Bradley, L.A. (Eds.), Coping with Chronic Disease: Research and Applications. Academic Press, New York, pp. 13–37.

Petrie, K., Cameron, L., Ellis, C., et al., 2002. Changing illness perceptions after myocardial infarction: an early intervention randomized controlled trial. Psychosom. Med. 64 (4), 580–586.

Pillow, D.R., Zautra, A.J., Sandler, I., 1996. Major life events and minor stressors: identifying mediational links in the stress process. J. Pers. Soc. Psychol. 70 (2), 381–394.

Sanders, D., Wills, F., 2005. Cognitive Therapy: An Introduction, second ed.. Sage, London.

Sharpe, L., Sensky, T., Timberlake, N., et al., 2001a. A blind, randomized, controlled trial of cognitive-behavioural intervention for patients with recent onset rheumatoid arthritis: preventing psychological and physical morbidity. Pain 89 (2–3), 275–283.

Sharpe, L., Sensky, T., Timberlake, N., et al., 2001b. The role of cognitive behavioural therapy in facilitating adaptation to rheumatoid arthritis: a case series. Behav. Cogn. Psychoth. 29 (3), 303–309.

Sharpe, L., Sensky, T., Timberlake, N., et al., 2003. Long-term efficacy of a cognitive behavioural treatment from a randomized controlled trial for patients recently diagnosed with rheumatoid arthritis.. Rheumatology 42 (3), 435–441.

Stone, A.A., Schwartz, J.E., Neale, J.M., et al., 1998. A comparison of coping assessed by ecological momentary assessment and retrospective recall. J. Pers. Soc. Psychol. 74 (6), 1670–1680.

Treharne, G.J., Lyons, A.C., Tupling, R.E., 2001. The effects of optimism, pessimism, social support, and mood on the lagged relationship between daily stress and symptoms. Curr. Res. Soc. Psychol. 7 (5), 60–81 Online Available: http://www.uiowa.edu/~grpproc/crisp/crisp.7.5.htm/.

Treharne, G.J., Lyons, A.C., Booth, D.A., et al., 2002. Daily stress, coping, and helpful support in relation to symptoms and mood in rheumatoid arthritis (RA) patients. Rheumatology 41 (Suppl.), 73. Abstract.

Treharne, G.J., Lyons, A.C., Booth, D.A., et al., 2004. Reactions to disability in patients with early versus established rheumatoid arthritis. Scand. J. Rheumatol. 33 (1), 30–38.

Treharne, G.J., Lyons, A.C., Booth, D.A., et al., 2007a. Psychological well-being across 1 year with rheumatoid arthritis: coping resources as buffers of perceived stress. Brit. J. Health Psychol. 12 (3), 323–345.

Treharne, G.J., Lyons, A.C., Hale, E.D., et al., 2007b. Sleep disruption frequency in rheumatoid arthritis: predictors of change over 1 year and its impact on outcomes. Musculoskeletal Care 5 (1), 51–64.

Turner Cobb, J.M., Steptoe, A., Perry, L., Axford, J., 1998. Adjustment in patients with rheumatoid arthritis and their children.. J. Rheumatol. 25 (3), 565–571.

Watson, D., Clark, L.A., Tellegen, A., 1988. Development and validation of brief measures of positive and negative affect: the PANAS scales. J. Pers. Soc. Psychol. 54 (6), 1063–1070.

Wilson, A.S., Kitas, G.D., Carruthers, D.M., et al., 2002. Computerised information gathering in two specialist rheumatology clinics: an evaluation of an initial electronic version of the Short Form 36. Rheumatology 41 (3), 268–273.

Zautra, A.J., Manne, S.L., 1992. Coping with rheumatoid arthritis: a review of a decade of research. Ann. Behav. Med. 14 (1), 31–39.

Zigmond, A.S., Snaith, R.P., 1983. The hospital anxiety and depression scale. Acta Psychiat. Scand. 67 (6), 361–370.

Chapter 12

Orthotics of the hand

Jo Adams PhD MSc DipCOT School of Health Professions and Rehabilitation Sciences, University of Southampton, Southampton, UK

CHAPTER CONTENTS

KEY POINTS

- The most robust evidence to support the use of orthotics is for short-term pain relief.
- There is no evidence to indicate that static orthoses can prevent deformity from occurring nor correct established deformity
- Individuals prefer to wear orthotics made from soft rather than rigid material
- Orthotics that immobilise joints may contribute towards a reduction in range of motion. Teaching a hand exercise programme should be considered when providing these.
- Evidence is still required to support the most appropriate design of orthotics, the most appropriate time to prescribe orthotics and the optimal length of time to wear them.

INTRODUCTION

Static hand orthotics have been used in rheumatology for many years (Rotstein, 1965). They are recommended for helping individuals manage their arthritis (Scottish Intercollegiate Guidelines Network 2002) and are a popular, commonly used intervention (Henderson & McMillan 2002).

Hand orthotics are used in rheumatology:

- to rest/ immobilise weakened joint structures and decrease local inflammation (Janssen et al 1990)
- to decrease soft tissue and joint pain (Callinan & Mathiowetz 1996, Feinberg & Brandt 1981, Kjeken et al 1995, Pagnotta et al 2005).
- to correctly position joints (Nordenskiöld 1990, Ouellette 1991)
- to minimise joint contractures (McClure et al 1994)
- to increase joint stability (Kjeken et al 1995)
- to improve hand function (Janssen et al, 1990, Nordenskiöld 1990, Pagnotta et al 1998, 2005)
- to contribute towards self-management strategies in long-term disease management (Hammond 1998).

PRINCIPLES OF ACTION

RESTING THE JOINT AND PAIN REDUCTION

During periods of acute synovitis, resting affected joints in a biomechanically sound position may reduce joint friction and temperature. At a cellular level this may contribute to a reduction in the pro-inflammatory chemical environment within the joint (Hendiani et al 2003).

CORRECTLY POSITION JOINTS, MINIMISE CONTRACTURES AND DEFORMITIES AND INCREASE JOINT STABILITY

Static orthoses aim to support structures within the wrist and hand that are vulnerable. The radio-carpal, carpometacarpal joint (CMJ), metacarpophalangeal (MCPJ) and proximal interphalangeal (PIPJ) joints and the thumb web space are key anatomical areas for consideration when splinting. Where inflammation causes the potential for muscle imbalance, for example in swan neck and boutonnière deformities, orthotics apply a counterbalance force to prevent or correct extensor tendons slipping across normal joint fulcrums.

IMPROVE HAND FUNCTION

By adding support to proximal joints, applying counterbalanced force to deforming joints and improving biomechanical advantage splints have the potential to improve hand function (Prosser & Conolly 2003). In particular improving support to the wrist can improve grip strength and gross hand function (Nordenskiöld 1990).

Hand orthotics have some biological and biomechanical rationale for their use and action, however, evidence to support and clarify the clinical effectiveness of orthotics in rheumatology is still emerging (Adams et al 2005). This evidence is considered below in regard to five types of orthotics.

THE WRIST EXTENSION ORTHOSIS

Wrist extension orthoses may be custom-made using either thermoplastic or neoprene material or commercially manufactured from a soft or reinforced fabric with a possible addition of a volar metal support (Fig. 12.1). They may be prescribed to limit wrist circumduction and decrease torque during heavy tasks involving the wrist (Cordery & Rocchi 1998). They may also be used to increase the mobility of the arthritic hand. Wrist extension orthoses can stabilise the wrist in a functionally effective position (10-15 degrees of extension), and facilitate the action of the extrinsic finger flexors to improve handgrip strength (Stern et al 1996). Wrist orthoses provide support to the carpals and wrist joint and several designs of commercial wrist splints have been shown to significantly reduce the electrical activity of the wrist extensors during

lifting tasks in people without RA (Stegink- Jansen et al 1997). This may serve to reduce potentially deforming forces on the wrist and carpals.

When worn these orthosis can provide immediate pain relief and significantly reduce pain on functional use of the hand (Haskett et al 2004, Kjeken et al 1995, Nordenskiöld, 1990, Pagnotta et al 2005). Kjeken et al's (1995) randomised controlled trial analysed splint wear versus non-splint wear over 6 months (n = 69). There was no difference by group on pain, joint swelling, grip or hand motion. However, the control group (n = 33) without splints showed statistically significant improvement in wrist range of motion that was not evident in the splinted group. Both Kjeken et al (1995) and Sharma et al (1991) comment that these wrist orthoses can reduce wrist movement when worn over a number of months and the effects of this should be considered on provision.

In small-scale studies, elastic wrist orthoses have been shown to improve power grip strength for individuals with moderate to severe RA (Backman & Deitz 1988, Haskett et al 2004, Nordenskiöld 1990). However, they have been reported in a small sample (n = 36) to transiently reduce grip strength when first worn and to offer no improvement in grip strength (Stern et al 1996). Although both commercially available and custom made splints have contributed towards improvements in pain and grip strength after four weeks wear in the most able male patients elastic orthoses can hinder maximum grip strength (Sharma et al 1991).

Studies examining hand function have shown that these orthoses are particularly task specific, i.e.

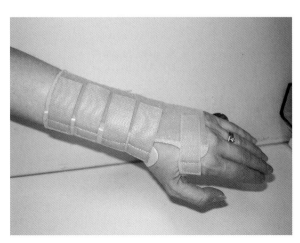

Figure 12.1 Wrist extension orthosis.

they may be able to assist one particular hand skill but reduce another (Pagnotta et al 1998, Stern et al 1996). Functional grip strength has been seen to increase significantly by up to 29% in a woman with RA when these orthoses were worn (Nordenskiöld 1990) yet dexterity, fine finger movement and speed of hand activity have not (Backman & Deitz 1988, Stern et al 1994, 1996).

In summary, wrist extension orthosis have been seen to increase handgrip strength, hand function and provided immediate hand pain relief in some patients. However, they may also contribute to a less dextrous and less mobile hand. There is little evidence to demonstrate the long-term effectiveness of these splints and the quality of evidence available to indicate the clinical effectiveness of these splints is weak (Egan et al 2003).

METACARPAL ULNAR DEVIATION ORTHOSES

These may be small palm-based orthoses or have the additional support of a wrist and forearm component. They may be used early in the rheumatoid disease process to limit the physical factors predisposing the MCPJs to ulnar deviation. By providing a medial force to the proximal phalanges, these orthotics can realign the metacarpals and phalanges during use to improve functional ability of the hand and to prevent further MCPJ ulnar drift and volar subluxation (Adams et al 2005). Therapeutic exercise MCP splints have also been designed to provide exercise options for extrinsic hand extensors and flexors and combat intrinsic plus deformities in the rheumatoid hand (Wijdenes et al 2003).

There is limited evidence for the clinical effectiveness of metacarpal ulnar deviation (MUD) orthoses. In a small repeated measures six months study patients (n = 26) rated them as highly acceptable and satisfactory (Rennie 1996). When worn they realigned the MCPJs and maintained that alignment during functional use of the hand and significantly improved ulnar drift in middle, ring and little finger. They also significantly improved three-point pinch grip strength but did not significantly improve scores on the Sollerman test of hand function (Sollerman 1984), reduce visual analogue pain levels nor improve gross power grip strength. There was no evidence to suggest that they had any long-term effect on correcting MCP joint alignment nor delayed the progression of ulnar deviation.

STATIC RESTING ORTHOSES

This orthosis aims to decrease localised pain and inflammation by resting the joint in a correct anatomical position, provide volar support for the carpus and proximal phalangeals to prevent subluxation realigning drifting MCP joints by providing an ulnar border to the orthosis and restricting carpal movement (Biese 2002). The rationale that correct joint positioning at rest can influence joint integrity has been challenged. Adams et al (2005) argue that the forces contributing towards joint deformity are present when the hand is used functionally thus correct positioning at rest is unlikely to address or correct these (Fig. 12.2).

It is the most commonly used orthosis for treating people with RA and the most frequently used to relieve wrist and hand pain (Henderson & McMillan 2002). These splints do not permit wrist or hand joint movement and are recommended to be worn whilst resting and/or during the night. There have been a few controlled studies examining clinical effectiveness.

Malcus Johnson et al's (1992) small, 18-month follow-up study of seven people with RA identified that the orthoses reduced nocturnal but not day time pain and MCPJ ulnar deviation continued unabated with splint use. Callinan and Mathiowetz's (1996) investigation (n = 39) demonstrated that for two types of resting orthosis (soft fabric and hard thermoplastic), there were significant reductions in overall pain levels when these orthoses were worn at night for a month. Hand function and morning stiffness were no different over time when wearing

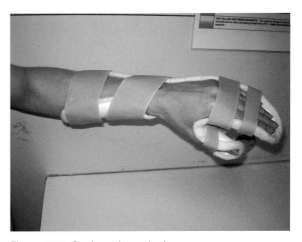

Figure 12.2 Static resting orthosis.

the splint. The majority of the study sample preferred the soft splints.

Janssen et al's (1990), 12-month, randomized, controlled trial of 29 patients reported a statistically significant reduction in hand joint swelling and a decrease in pain and tenderness scores when these splints were worn. There were improvements in grip strength but not hand function. These findings are difficult to interpret when changes in disease activity nor baseline values of outcomes were considered in the analysis.

Adams et al (2008) randomised controlled trial recruited (n = 116) controlled for baseline outcome value as well as disease activity at baseline in analysis. There were no significant differences in handgrip strength, self-report hand function using the Michigan Hand Outcomes questionnaire and MCPJ ulnar deviation by groups over 12 months follow-up. There was some evidence to indicate that early morning stiffness increased with splint wear (Adams et al 2006).

There is little evidence from longitudinal fully powered studies to indicate that these splints can impact on hand function and deformity, there is some evidence to suggest that hand pain may be improved.

FINGER SWAN NECK ORTHOSES

These small finger based splints apply a three-point force around the PIPJ to prevent PIPJ hyperextension and subsequent distal interphalangeal joint (DIPJ) flexion present in swan necking of the fingers. They are small functional orthoses that permit full PIP joint flexion but prevent hyperextension. They aim to decrease digital pain, correct or prevent swan necking in the digits and improve hand function (Zijlstra et al 2002).

These splints can be custom made using thermoplastic material or silver. Silver custom made options (Fig. 12.3) are more costly but have been reported as more durable than the thermoplastic alternatives, they are also more popular gaining higher adherence levels than thermoplastic alternatives (Macleod & Adams 2002, Macleod et al 2003).

There have only been three reported studies of clinical effectiveness. Ter Schegget and Knipping (2000) demonstrated in a crossover study of 18 individuals there was pain relief when worn but this did not reach statistically significant levels. There were significant improvements in digital stability

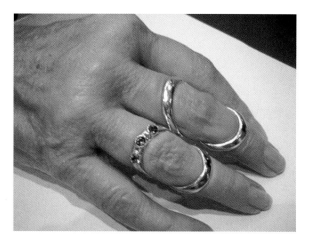

Figure 12.3 Silver ring swan neck orthoses.

and DIPJ extension. Zijlstra et al's (2002) small longitudinal study of 15 people with RA (using 48 ring orthoses) over a 12 month period demonstrated that these orthoses improved functional dexterity levels to statistically significant levels. These results were confirmed by their later study (Zijlstra et al 2004). Conversely, they were seen to have no effect on self-reported hand function, grip strength or hand pain (Zijlstra et al 2002, 2004).

THUMB SPLINTS

In CMCJ basal joint osteoarthrtis thumb splints are used for relief of thumb pain, weakness, contracture and improvement of function (Wajon & Ada 2005). Thumb splints may immobilise just the CMCJ: short opponens type (Fig. 12.4) or combine CMCJ with distal radio carpal joint immobilisation: long type (Fig. 12.5).

There have been no published studies that have compared splinting to no splint intervention. Studies that have examined both short and long type of splints in one study have reported no difference between the outcome of the splints. Weiss et al's, (2000) short, 2-week cross-over study, examined 26 hands using short and long splints. They reported that both types of splint appear to reduce subluxation of the first CMCJ. Pinch strength was not improved over 2 weeks of splinting, however patients reported anecdotally that they gained some pain relief on wear. Short splints were preferred to long. Soft neoprene splints are preferred to rigid

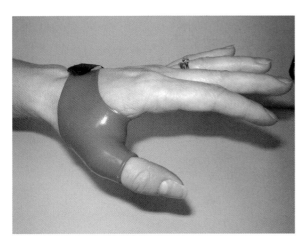

Figure 12.4 CMCJ short opponens type splint.

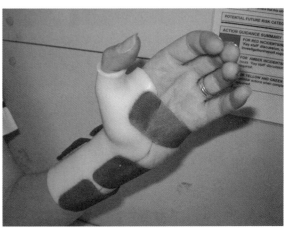

Figure 12.5 CMCJ and distal radio carpal immobilisation (long type) splint.

thermoplastic splints and patients prefer the soft splints for daily and long-term use. The beneficial effects have been seen to be amplified with the soft type of thumb splint (Weiss et al 2004).

Patients report preference for soft splints (Buurke et al 1999). In their cross-over study ten female patients were recruited and wore three types of manufactured splints (supple elastic, elastic and semi rigid material), over a period of 12 weeks. There was no difference in pain and pinch scores between the orthoses.

Wajon and Ada's (2005) randomised trial (n = 40) compared a short opponens type splint and a pinch exercise regime with a thumb strap splint and an abduction exercise regime over a 6 week period. Comparison of change scores over the 6 week follow-up assessments by a blinded assessor demonstrated no difference in outcome by groups for reported pain at rest, pinch grip strength and levels of hand function.

Swigart et al's retrospective study (1999) examined the effects of thumb splinting on 130 thumbs with varying stages of CMCJ osteoarthritis (OA). Some patients received surgical intervention but patients were excluded if they had been treated with exercise or steroid injections. Long thumb splints were reviewed after a maximum of 4 weeks wear. In milder forms of OA, 76% of patients benefited from some symptomatic improvement and in more severe cases of OA, 54% benefited. These benefits were maintained over 6 months.

Evidence that static thumb splinting may delay or prevent the need for surgical intervention has also been supported by Berggren et al's seven year follow-up study (Berggren et al 2001). The provision of occupational therapy including aids and equipment, joint protection advice and thumb splinting reduced the number of individuals requiring thumb joint surgery by 65% over a 7 year period (Berggren et al 2001).

Static thumb orthoses have been reported as being effective in long-term relief of OA symptoms when used alongside a single corticosteroid injection (Day et al 2004). A single corticosteroid injection combined with 3 weeks static splinting produced long-term relief from the symptoms of OA in stage I OA (n = 30 thumbs). Although individuals with later stage OA (stage IV) reported less benefit, 40% of participants received symptomatic improvement that was considered sufficient and sustained irrespective of their stage.

CONCLUSION

Static orthoses continue to be enthusiastically endorsed by therapists (Henderson & McMillan 2002). During an era when drug developments continue to assist with more effective control of disease activity and synovitis, continued research is needed into the most appropriate types of orthosis to recommend. The challenge is to provide objective evidence as to whether the continued use of orthoses is indicated for people with arthritis and if so which designs are the most effective and at which stage of the disease process.

1. Discuss and explore the typical progression of possible deformity in the arthritic hand.
2. Consider the research carried out examining the effectiveness of splints in preserving hand function in rheumatoid arthritis. Which prognostic and disease factors of those patients included in the studies would need to be evaluated when comparing the results from different studies?
3. Hand function is assessed and recorded using different methods. For example, one hand assessment may quantify time and speed as the indicator for hand function, whilst another quantifies pain level to define hand function. Compare and contrast the different indicators used in different standardized hand function assessments and discuss the benefits of each.

Scottish Intercollegiate Guidelines Network (SIGN): Management of early rheumatoid arthritis guidelines: http://www.sign.ac.uk/guidelines/fulltext/48/index.html/

Cochrane database: http://www.cochrane.org/index.htm/

National library for health: http://www.library.nhs.uk/Default.aspx/

British association of hand therapists: http://www.hand-therapy.co.uk/

College of Occupational Therapists Specialist Section: Rheumatology http://www.cot.org.uk/specialist/rheumatology/membership.php/

American Society of Hand Therapists http://www.asht.org/

References and further reading

Adams, J., Hammond, A., Burridge, J., Cooper, C., 2005. Static orthoses in the prevention of hand dysfunction in rheumatoid arthritis: A review of the literature. Musculoskeletal Care 3, 85–101.

Adams, J., Burridge, J., Hammond, A., et al., 2008. The clinical effectiveness of static resting splints in early rheumatoid arthritis: a randomised controlled trial. Rheumatology 45, 1548–1553.

Adams, J., Burridge, J., Hammond, A., et al., 2006. The potential side-effects of static resting splints in early rheumatoid arthritis. Ann. Rheum. Dis. 65, 657(abstract).

Backman, C., Deitz, J., 1988. Static wrist splint: its effect on hand function in three women with rheumatoid arthritis. Arthritis Care Res. 1, 151–160.

Berggren, M., Joost-Davidsson, A., Lindstrand, J., et al., 2001. Reduction in the need for operation after conservative treatment of osteoarthritis of the first carpometacarpal joint: a seven year prospective study. Scand. J. Plast. Reconstr. Surg. Hand Surgery 35, 415–417.

Biese, J., 2002. Therapist's evaluation and conservative management of rheumatoid arthritis in the hand and wrist. In: Mackin, E.J., Callahan, A.D., Skirven, T.M., Schneider, L.H., Osterman, A.L. (Eds.), Rehabilitation of the Hand and Upper Extremity. 5th ed., Mosby, St Louis pp 1569–1582.

Buurke, J., Grady, J., De Vires, J., Baten, C., 1999. Usability of thenar eminence orthoses: report of a comparative study. Clin. Rehabil. 13, 288–294.

Callinan, N.J., Mathiowetz, V., 1996. Soft versus hard resting splints in rheumatoid arthritis:pain relief, preference and compliance. Am. J. Occup. Ther. 50, 347–352.

Cordery, J., Rocchi, M., 1998. Joint protection and fatigue management. In: Melvin, J., Jensen, G. (Eds.) Rheumatologic Rehabilitation vol 1 Assessment and Management. American Occupational Therapy Association, Bethesda.

Day, C., Gelberman, R., Patel, A., et al., 2004. Basal joint osteoarthritis of the thumb: a prospective trial of steroid injection and splinting. J. Hand Surg. 29A, 247–251.

Egan, M., Brosseau, L., Farmer, M., et al., 2003. Splints/orthoses in the treatment of rheumatoid arthritis. Cochrane Dat. System. Rev. 1 CD004018.

Feinberg, J., Brandt, K.D., 1981. Use of resting splints by patients with rheumatoid arthritis. Am. J. Occup. Ther. 35, 173–178.

Hammond, A., 1998. The use of self-management strategies by people with rheumatoid arthritis. Clin. Rehabil. 12, 81–87.

Haskett, S., Backman, C., Porter, B., et al., 2004. A crossover trial of custom-made and commercially available wrist splints in adults with inflammatory arthritis. Arthritis Care Res. 51, 792–799.

Henderson, S., McMillan, I., 2002. Pain and function: occupational therapists use of orthotics in rheumatoid arthritis. Br. J. Occup. Ther. 65, 165–171.

Hendiani, J.A., Westlund, K.N., Lawand, N., et al., 2003. Mechanical sensation and pain thresholds in patients with chronic arthropathies. J. Pain 4, 203–211.

Janssen, M., Phiferons, J., Van de Velde, E., Dijkmans, B., 1990. The prevention of hand deformities with resting splints in rheumatoid arthritis patients. A randomised single blind one year follow-up study. Arthritis Rheum. 33, 123.

Kjeken, I., Moller, G., Kvien, T., 1995. Use of commercially produced elastic wrist orthoses in chronic arthritis. Arthritis Care Res. 8, 108–113.

Macleod, C., Adams, J., 2002. Improving patient adherence to swan neck ring splints. Rheumatology 41, 89.

Macleod, C., Adams, J., Cox, N., France, J., 2003. Ringing the change. Occup. Ther. News 11, 37.

Malcus Johnson, P., Sandkvist, G., Eberhardt, K., et al., 1992. The Usefulness of Nocturnal Resting splints in the Treatment of Ulnar deviation of the Rheumatoid Hand. Clin. Rheumatol. 11, 72–75.

McClure, P., Blackburn, L., Dusold, C., 1994. The use of splints in the treatment of joint stiffness. Biologic rationale and an algorithm for making clinical decisions. Phys. Ther. 74, 1101–1107.

Nordenskiöld, U., 1990. Reduction in pain and increase in grip force for women with rheumatoid arthritis. Arthritis Care Res. 3, 158–162.

Ouellette, E., 1991. The rheumatoid hand: orthotics as preventative. Semin. Arthritis Rheum. 21, 65–72.

Pagnotta, A., Baron, M., Korner-Bitensky, N., 1998. The effect of static wrist orthosis on hand function in individuals with rheumatoid arthritis. J. Rheumatol. 25, 879–885.

Pagnotta, A., Korner-Bitensky, N., Mazer, B., et al., 2005. Static wrist splint use in the performance of daily activities by individuals with rheumatoid arthritis. J. Rheumatol. 32, 2136–2143.

Prosser, R., Conolly, W.B., 2003. Rehabilitation of the Upper Limb. Butterworth Heinemann, Edinburgh.

Rennie, H.J., 1996. Evaluation of the effectiveness of a metacarpophalangeal ulnar deviation orthosis. J. Hand Ther. 9, 371–377.

Rotstein, J., 1965. Use of splints in conservative management of acutely inflamed joints in rheumatoid arthritis. Arch. Phys. Med. Rehab. 46, 198–199.

Scottish Intercollegiate Guidelines Network. 2002. Management of early arthritis Section 5 The role of the multidisciplinary team.

Sharma, S., Immonite, V., Schumacher, H.R., 1991. Relationship of wrist splint to wrist pain and grip strength in rheumatoid arthritis (RA) patients. Arthritis Care Res. 4(3), S25(c3).

Sollerman, C., 1984. Assessment of Grip Function: Evaluation of a New Test Method. Medical Innovation Technology (MITAB) Sjobo, Sweden.

Steglink-Jansen, C., Olson, S., Hasson, S., 1997. The effect of use of a wrist orthosis during functional activities on surface electromyography of the wrist extensors in normal subjects. J. Hand Ther. 10, 283–289.

Stern, E.B., Sines, B., Teague, T.R., 1994. Commercial wrist extensor orthoses. Hand function, comfort and interference across five styles. J. Hand Ther. 7, 237–244.

Stern, E.B., Ytterberg, S.R., Krug, H.E., et al., 1996. Immediate and short term effects of three commercial wrist extensor orthoses on grip strength and function in patients with rheumatoid arthritis. Arthritis Care Res. 9, 42–50.

Swigart, C., Eaton, R., Glickel, S., Johnson, C., 1999. Splinting in treatment of arthritis of the first carpometacarpal joint. J. Hand Surg. 24A, 86–91.

Ter Schegget, M., Knipping, A., 2000. A study comparing use and effects of custom-made versus prefabricated splints for swan neck deformity in patients with rheumatoid arthritis. Br. J. Occup. Ther. 59, 101–107.

Wajon, A., Ada, L., 2005. No difference between two splint and exercise regimens for people with osteoarthritis of the thumb: a randomised controlled trial. Aust. J. Physiother. 51, 245–249.

Weiss, S., La Stayo, P., Mills, A., Bramlet, D., 2000. Prospective analysis of splinting the first carpometacarpal joint: an objective, subjective, and radiographic assessment. J. Hand Ther. 13, 218–226.

Weiss, S., La Stayo, P., Mills, A., Bramlet, D., 2004. Splinting the degenerative basal joint:custom-made or prefabricated neoprene? J. Hand Ther. 17, 401–406.

Wijdenes, P., Formsma, S., Leysma, M., Van der Sluis, C., 2003. The MCP stabilisation splint: a new method to treat the intrinsic plus phenomenon in patients with rheumatoid arthritis. Ann. Rheum. Dis. 62, 547.

Zijlstra, T., Heijnsdijk-Rouwenhorst, L., Rasker, J., 2002. The effect of silver ring splints (SRS) on hand function in patients with rheumatoid arthritis (RA). Ann. Rheum. Dis. 61, 210.

Zijlstra, T., Heijnsdijk-Rouwenhorst, L., Rasker, J., 2004. Silver Ring Splints improve dexterity in patients with rheumatoid arthritis. Arthritis Care Res. 51, 947–951.

Chapter 13

Podiatry, biomechanics and the rheumatology foot

Jim Woodburn PhD MPhil BSc FCPodMed School of Health, Glasgow Caledonian University, Glasgow, UK

Deborah E. Turner PhD PGCert Medical Ultrasound, BSc (Hons), FCPodMed School of Health, Glasgow Caledonian University, Glasgow, UK

CHAPTER CONTENTS

KEY POINTS

- Foot involvement is common in rheumatic disease
- An understanding of foot and ankle biomechanics can help in assessing foot function and identifying treatment options
- Podiatrists are expertly placed to provide advice to patients and therapists on the management of foot health in rheumatic disease.

FOOT INVOLVEMENT IN THE RHEUMATIC DISEASES

This chapter describes the involvement of the foot in rheumatic diseases using examples of commonly presenting features. It outlines the biomechanics of the foot and how disruption of normal function can occur in rheumatic disease. The role of the podiatrist is described in relation to routine and extended scope practice in the management of foot health in patients with rheumatic conditions. Further information on specific rheumatic conditions can be seen in the chapters following.

INFLAMMATORY JOINT DISEASE

Rheumatoid arthritis

Small joint inflammation in the hands and feet is the hallmark of early rheumatoid arthritis (RA). Metatarsophalangeal (MTP) joint synovitis can be detected using magnetic resonance imaging (MRI) in 97% of patients (Boutry et al 2003). The MTP joints

DOI: 10.1016/B978-0-443-06934-5.00013-9

are involved early: MRI can detect bone oedema and synovitis even when the finger joints are normal (Ostendorf et al 2004). Erosive changes also occur early in these joints, and their grade of destruction is high (Belt et al 1998). Cardinal signs and symptoms are pain and stiffness which is worse in the early morning and after periods of standing and walking. Pain under the MTP joints is likened to 'walking on pebbles, glass or stones'. The feet can throb and burn and stiffness is a persistent background feature. The forefoot can rapidly widen with 'daylight sign' between the toes related to MTP synovitis, and joint capsule and periarticular ligament damage (Fig. 13.1). Patients report that normal footwear becomes tight, uncomfortable and difficult to wear. On examination the metatarsal squeeze test (gripping the MTP joints and compressing them together) may be positive and one or more MTP joints swollen and tender on palpation.

Early involvement in the peritalar region affects the tenosynovium of tibialis posterior in around 60% of patients (using MRI) and the midtarsal, subtalar and ankle joints in around 25% of patients

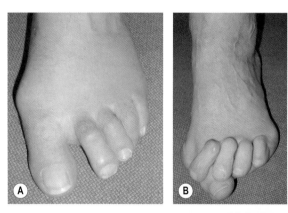

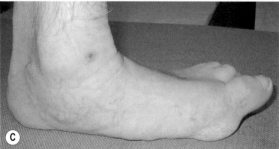

Figure 13.1 (A) Typical forefoot changes in the early stages of rheumatoid arthritis. (B) The forefoot of a patient with advanced, long-standing RA; and (C) pes planovalgus in RA.

(Bourty et al 2003, Fleming et al 1976). Pain and stiffness are common and subtle but clinically important changes in function can be detected within 2 years from onset (Turner et al 2006). Mild-to-moderate pes planovalgus (flat footedness) can be found. However, this tends to be passively correctable. In contrast to the MTP joints, ankle and subtalar joint erosions and destruction occur infrequently and in the later stages (>15 years). True bony ankylosis is rare (Belt et al 2001).

In established RA the prevalence of foot symptoms is over 90% (Michelson et al 1994). Synovial pannus and joint erosions weaken intra-articular and peri-articular structures, whilst joint effusion distorts the capsule. Therefore under normal weight-bearing loads progressive and severe deformities can develop. In the forefoot, fibular drift of the toes mimics ulnar deviation of the finger joints and if severe the subluxed or dislocated toes can over- or under-ride adjacent toes. Hallux valgus, tailors bunion and hammer, claw or mallet toe deformity can rapidly develop (Briggs 2003). Bursitis between or under the metatarsal heads is common and can be detected using MRI in around 60% of cases (Boutry et al 2003). Morton's interdigital neuroma may also be more prevalent in RA patients (Awerbuch et al 1982). Painful callosities can develop over the dorsum of prominent toe joints, medially on a hallux valgus joint or around the plantar metatarsal heads (Korda & Balint 2004).

Persistent disease in the peritalar region leads to the development of pes planovalgus and in severe cases the medial longitudinal arch may be completely collapsed (Turner et al 2008a). Pes planovalgus is associated with tendinopathy of tibialis posterior (Bouysset et al 2003, Jernberg et al 1999). Clinically the tendon may be swollen and inflamed medially at the ankle region (Woodburn et al 2002). MRI or ultrasound (US) imaging reveals tendon enlargement, tenosynovitis, tendinopathy, and intra-substance splits, however true rupture occurs in less than 5% of cases (Lehtinen et al 1996, Premkumar et al 2002). Pain and swelling in the posterior heel region may be associated with retrocalcaneal bursitis, Achilles enthesopathy and posterior calcaneal erosions (Falsetti et al 2003). Enthesopathy of the plantar fascia, or more rarely a plantar nodule, may lead to plantar heel pain.

Extra-articular manifestations such as peripheral arterial disease (nail fold infarcts, cutaneous vasculitis and digital gangrene), neuropathy, ulceration and subcutaneous nodules affect some patients with RA. Foot ulceration and infection are major clinical red flags, especially in patients treated with biologic therapies, glucocorticosteroids and some disease modifying antirheumatic drugs (DMARDs). Ulceration occurs most commonly over the dorsal aspect of hammer toes, over the metatarsal heads and the medial bunion with hallux valgus deformity. The overall prevalence of ulceration in people with RA is 9.7% (Firth et al 2008a) and common risk factors include deformity, elevated skin contact pressures, loss of protective sensation, peripheral vascular disease, active disease and steroid use (Firth et al 2008b). The risk of serious infection involving the skin is recognised in RA patients receiving anti-TNF therapy, and a number of case series have described infection associated with skin ulceration (Otter et al 2005) and spontaneous onychocryptosis (in-growing toenail) (Davys et al 2006a).

Seronegative spondlyoarthropathies

The seronegative spondyloarthropathies (SpAs) share a number of common clinical features, of which asymmetric oligoarthritis, peripheral small joint arthritis, enthesopathy, and dactylitis affect the feet. Peripheral enthesitis (characterised by inflammation at sites of tendon, ligament and joint capsule into bone) is regarded to be a hallmark feature of SpAs and may be associated with enthesophyte formation (bony proliferation). Inflammation may occur at any entheses, however, enthesitis at the heel is reported to be the most frequent and occurs at the attachment of the Achilles tendon (AT) and plantar fascia to the calcaneus (Olivieri et al 1992). In routine clinical practice enthesitis is diagnosed based on patient symptoms and clinical examination to determine tenderness on palpation. However, clinical examination underestimates the presence of enthesitis and detection is improved when imaging techniques such as MRI and high resolution US are used (Balint et al 2002, D'Agostino et al 2003, Galluzzo et al 2000).

Management of SpAs relies on DMARD and biologic drug therapy targeting the underlying disease mechanisms. However, ultrasonographic data suggest that despite intensive pharmacological management enthesitis in the foot is detectable in a high proportion of patients (approximately 60-80% of patients) and is poorly correlated with systemic parameters of disease activity (Borman et al 2006, D'Agostino et al 2003, Genc et al 2005). Biomechanical factors, including foot function, may contribute to the development of enthesopathies (Benjamin & McGonagle 2001) and

may help explain the discordance between disease activity parameters and enthesitis. It has been suggested poor alignment of the rearfoot and control of foot pronation, may make the enthesis at the heel more vulnerable to injury however, data are currently lacking to support this theory.

Forefoot deformity and nail pathologies are especially common in patients with PsA. A recent survey found 95% of patients had some deformity in the forefoot (Hyslop et al 2008). PsA will often present initially in the interphalangeal (IP) joints of the toes and then the MTP joints. Usually both IP joints in the toe are affected providing the characteristic clinical presentation dactylitis or 'sausage toe'. Inflammation at the IP and MTP joints can cause stretching and damage to the joint capsules and collateral ligaments leading to the typical toe joint deformities of RA. Inflammation can also lead to the formation of joint erosions, however, unlike in RA these tend to occur in the juxtaarticular region (adjacent to the articular surface). The course and progression of radiological damage can vary in patients with PsA, and a number of common features in the foot have been identified (Fig 13.2). These include the characteristic pencil in cup deformity (Gold et al 1988), the so called ivory shaft (increased bone density in the shaft of the phalanx), resorption of the distal phalanx, resulting in a characteristic pointed toe pulp (Moll 1987).

JUVENILE IDIOPATHIC ARTHRITIS

Foot problems such as synovitis, limited range of motion, malalignment and deformity have been reported in over 90% of children with juvenile idiopathic arthritis (JIA), generally increasing in severity with age, disease duration and in those with polyarticular disease (Spraul & Koenning 1994). Foot pain, deformity and impaired function are persistent problems even in those children optimally managed on DMARD and biologic therapy (Hendry et al 2008). Synovitis in the ankle and rearfoot joint occurs in approximately one-third of patients across all disease subtypes and is associated with limited ankle range of motion, pronated rearfoot and midfoot joints, and weakness of the ankle dorsiflexors/plantarflexors (Brostrom et al 2002, Spraul & Koenning 1994). Pes planovalgus is twice as common as varus heel alignment (pes cavus foot type) in these children (Mavidrou et al 1991).

Synovitis, effusion, erosive changes and deformity at affected MTP joints are observed in about

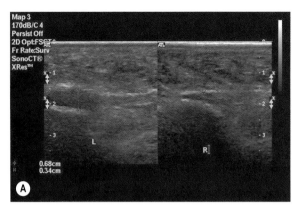 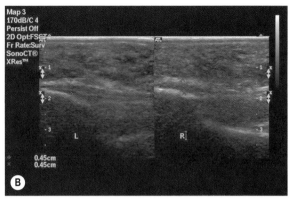

Figure 13.2 High resolution ultrasound image of the plantar fascia in a patient with PsA (A) Before, and (B) 6 weeks after a local corticosteroid injection.

one-fifth of JIA children and hallux valgus is common (Ferrari 1998). Deformities such as splaying of the forefoot; hammer, claw, and mallet toe deformity and MTP joint subluxation can rapidly develop. Leg length discrepancy, deformity and proximal joint malalignment resulting from growth disturbances can also impact on foot structure and function. Other problems such as Achilles tendinopathy, retrocalcaneal bursitis, tenosynovitis and plantar fasciitis occur in association with specific disease sub-types.

Disabling foot pain in JIA is associated with abnormalities in gait, either as a direct consequence of joint damage or as compensation to underlying impairments (Brostrom et al 2002, Hendry et al 2008, Witemeyer et al 1981). Typically these include reduced walking speed, increased double-limb support time, and step asymmetry. Gait can also be cautious and guarded with reduced heel-strike and push-off force (Brostrom et al 2002).

OSTEOARTHRITIS

The commonest sites for osteoarthritis in the foot are the 1st MTP joint (hallux rigidus), the ankle joint and the tarsometatarsal joints. Hallux rigidus is found in approximately 5% of adults above the age of 50 (Shereff & Baumhauer 1998) and is associated with trauma, metabolic and congenital disorders. The condition is often bilateral and affects more women than men. Patients may complain that the joint is stiff and painful and made worse by walking. Examination reveals a dorsal exostosis which is palpable and tender along the MTP joint line. Dorsiflexion motion is limited and painful.

Radiographs reveal loss of joint space, dorsal osteophytes, subchondral bone sclerosis and cysts.

Primary osteoarthritis of the ankle joint occurs in less than 10% of all cases and over 70% are post-traumatic (Saltzman et al 2005, Valderrabano et al 2008). The lower rate of primary disease in comparison to the hip and knee is attributed to anatomic, biomechanical, and cartilage properties which protect the joint from degenerative changes (Huch et al 1997). Trauma is usually associated with malleolar fractures and ankle ligament lesions. The ankle is stiff and painful with mild-moderate effusion. Pain can be elicited on specific movements such as dorsiflexion/inversion and crepitus can be felt. Range of motion will be limited, the joint unstable and gait adapted to achieve relief. Bony enlargement, malalignment and/or deformity, can progressively develop (Fig. 13.3). Malalignment is distributed in favour of varus across all etiologies (55% varus, 37% neutral, 8% valgus) (Valderrabano et al 2008). Joint space narrowing, osteophtye formation, subchondral bone sclerosis, and cyst formation are typical radiographic features as well as varus malalignment, anterior protrusion of the talus and flattening of the tibial plafond (articular surface of the distal end of the tibia).

CONNECTIVE TISSUE DISEASES

Foot involvement is prevalent but often overlooked in the two most common connective tissue diseases; scleroderma and systemic lupus erythematosus (SLE). The feet are involved less frequently and later than the hands in scleroderma but nevertheless 90% prevalence has been reported (La Montagna

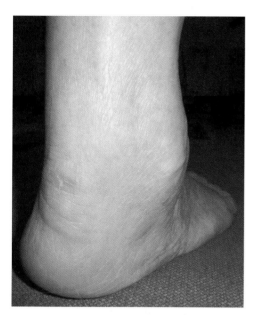

Figure 13.3 Malalignment and deformity of the ankle and subtalar joint in a patient with secondary, post-traumatic osteoarthritis.

et al 2002). Radiological changes in the joints in these patients include juxtaarticular demineralisation, distal phalange resorption, joint space narrowing, and extraarticular calcification. Radiological foot abnormalities have been reported in 26% of patients (Allali et al 2007). Approximately 90% of patients suffer from Raynaud's syndrome which can lead to pain in the feet and digital ulceration, scarring and in some cases gangrene and amputation (La Montagna et al 2002, Sari-Kouzel et al 2001).

Localised thickening and tightening of the skin of the toes (sclerodactyly) and flexion contractures have been reported in 6% of cases (La Montagna et al 2002) and are associated with atrophy of the underlying soft tissues. Subcutaneous calcinosis occurs infrequently (6%) but can be extremely painful and disabling if it occurs on a weight bearing area of the foot. Whilst problems in the feet occur less frequently than those in the hand they can be a major source of morbidity and disability in patients with scleroderma.

Non-erosive arthritic manifestations (Jaccoud's type arthropathy) involving the foot and ankle have been reported in patients with SLE. Common foot deformities found in these patients are hallux valgus, subluxation and fibular deviation of the MTP joints, and widening of the forefoot (Mizutani & Quismorio 1984, Reilly et al 1990). Erosive changes

are rare in this group; however, hook like erosions caused by pressure erosion beneath the distorted joint capsules in the deformed joints may appear and have been reported at the metatarsal heads. Accelerated atheroma is a well recognised complication of SLE and abnormal ankle brachial pressure indices have been reported in almost 40% of patients (Theodoridou et al 2003). However, it rarely leads to critical peripheral ischaemia and gangrene is a relatively uncommon finding (Jeffrey et al 2008). Raynaud's syndrome occurs in approximately 30% of cases (Bhatt et al 2007).

CRYSTAL JOINT DISEASE

Sudden onset of pain, swelling, erythema and limited movement in the foot or ankle is characteristic of acute gout. The 1st MTP joint is most commonly involved, although acute gouty arthritis can involve the dorsum of the foot or ankle. Diagnosis of gout is established when monosodium urate (MSU) crystals are found in joint aspirate. Tophi are chalky white deposits of MSU that are large enough to be seen on radiographs and may occur at virtually any site but commonly occur in the joints of the hand and foot (Harris et al 1999). The rate of tophi formation correlates with duration and severity of hyperuricaemia (Gutman 1973). Intra-articular tophi are associated with the formation of bone erosions. However in contrast to RA, these are ill defined with overhanging edges and are not associated with osteopenia (Dalbeth et al 2007). Compared with RA, joint space narrowing occurs late in the disease or joint space widening may also occur in advanced disease (Dalbeth et al 2007). Moreover there is a strong relationship between bone erosion and the presence of intraosseous tophus. This suggests that tophus infiltration into bone as the dominant mechanism for development of bone erosion and joint damage in gout (Dalbeth et al 2008).

Pseudogout is much less common than gout and usually presents with a less severe clinical picture. It is characterised by deposition of calcium pyrophosphate dehydrate (CPPD) crystals in the joint or periarticular tissues which produces an acute inflammatory synovitis. Whilst the disorder is more common in the knee, hip, shoulder and wrist, it can also affect the 1st MTP joint and ankle.

HYPERMOBILITY

Hypermobility (excessive mobility) can occur at a single joint or can be widespread throughout the body.

There are several conditions associated with hyper-mobility, including Ehlers-Danlos disease, Marfan syndrome, osteogenesis imperfecta and benign joint hypermobility syndrome (BJHMS) which is the most common and will be the focus of this section. BJHMS has been defined as generalised joint laxity and hyperextensibility of the skin in the absence of any systemic disease. The pattern and course of musculoskeletal problems can vary considerably in patients with BJHMS from intermittent problems in a single joint to persistent widespread involvement of joints and soft tissues. A high proportion of patients with BJHMS have intermittent joint and soft tissue pain, joint effusions, dislocations, and they also have a tendency to bruise and scar easily.

Patients with BJHMS have poorer proprioceptive feedback and muscle strength, although this can be improved with proprioceptive exercises (Hall et al 1995, Sahin et al 2008a, Sahin et al 2008b). The proprioceptive system plays a critical role in maintenance of joint stability, including body position and movement of joints. Therefore deficits in proprioceptive function can make joints and soft tissues more vulnerable to minor traumas and may allow acceleration of degenerative joint conditions (Hall et al 1995). Hypermobility at the ankle and foot has been reported in a high proportion of patients. In the foot it is common for patients with BJHMS to report ankle instability and recurrent ankle inversion sprains (Finsterbush et al 1982). Other common features include joint instability, pes planovalgus deformity, subluxation of the MTP joints and hallux valgus (Fig. 13.4). In a review of a 100 consecutive patients, the most frequent complaint (48% of cases) was pain in the feet and calf associated with pes planovalgus deformity. Both general and local hypermobility at the 1st MTP joint have been linked with hallux valgus deformity (Carl et al 1988, Myerson & Badekas 2000).

BIOMECHANICS OF THE FOOT AND ANKLE

FUNCTION OF THE FOOT AND ANKLE IN HEALTH

Normal foot function is required for efficient ambulation and is related to three events: shock absorption, weight-bearing stability and progression (Perry 1992). Subtalar joint eversion, with internal tibial rotation and midtarsal dorsiflexion are the shock

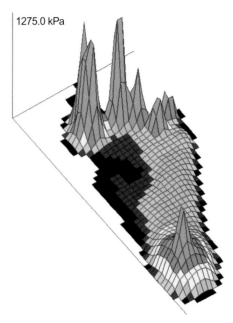

1275.0 kPa

Figure 13.4 Plantar pressure map showing high focal stresses at the MTP joints and weight bearing in the medial arch associated with pes planovalgus.

absorbing mechanisms that lessen the impact at initial foot-to-ground contact (~1.2-1.4 X body weight). This occurs during the first (heel) rocker when the body vector (centre-of-pressure) is located in the heel, behind the ankle to generate a plantarflexion moment. This causes rapid foot placement on the ground through ankle joint plantarflexion. Pretibial muscle activity (tibialis anterior and extensor hallucis and digitorum longus) controls the rate of plantarflexion until forefoot contact is made. Simultaneously, eversion at the subtalar joint, coupled with internal leg rotation serve to further absorb shock during this initial phase of gait. Tibialis anterior absorbs some of the shock during the heel rocker period as subtalar eversion is decelerated. Tibialis posterior initiates activity in the middle of this phase and serves as a reserve muscle force to control subtalar eversion. It also contributes to dynamic support of the midtarsal joint which dorsiflexes immediately following forefoot contact at the onset of midstance (Woodburn et al 2005). This movement also contributes to shock absorption and is further supported by the long flexor muscles of the leg and the intrinsic plantar foot muscles.

During the midstance period, the body moves forward across a plantargrade foot increasing the loading on the forefoot. The centre-of-pressure moves forward anterior to the ankle joint and a plantarflexion moment starts to develop. Weightbearing stability is established by synergistic ankle, subtalar and midtarsal joint motion aided by tightening of the plantar fascia (a ligament band extending from the calcaneus to the bases of the proximal phalanges). The tibia externally rotates and advances forward to dorsiflex the ankle joint and subtalar eversion reverses to inversion movement. This is the second ankle functional rocker. In combination these actions raise the talar head, dynamically lock the midtarsal joint and stabilise the medial and lateral columns of the foot. The third functional rocker is the forefoot rocker which characterises forward progression of the body. In the foot the centre-of-pressure reaches the metatarsal heads and terminates between the first and second metatarsal heads. The medial side of the foot is stabilised by plantarflexion of the first metatarsal by action of the peroneus longus. Dorsiflexion occurs through the MTP joints and the heel lifts from ground contact. The gastrocnemius and soleus calf muscles first act to control the rate of tibial advancement and then through concentric activity plantarflex the ankle joint. The foot pivots about the MTP joints and the body advances.

DISRUPTED FOOT AND ANKLE FUNCTION IN THE RHEUMATIC DISEASES

Across the rheumatic disorders pathological disease processes serve to disrupt the shock absorption, weight-bearing stability and progression functions of the foot and ankle. The clinical consequences are impairments such as pain, joint stiffness, and deformity which lead to degraded and adapted changes in gait. As a universal response to pain, independent of specific rheumatic diseases, patients adapt gait by slowing walking speed, reducing the step length, and increasing the period of double-limb support (Turner et al 2008a, 2008b, Woodburn et al 2004). In RA for example, in both early and established disease, the heel rocker can be absent as the foot is placed flat to the ground (Turner et al 2006, 2008a). The tibia is vertical with the centre-of-pressure located close to the ankle joint axis and the initial contact angle of the foot is parallel to the floor. This pattern occurs secondary to MTP disease and weak muscle action (e.g. gastrocnemius-soleus) and serves to reduce the rate of limb loading, and the joint and soft-tissue reaction forces. These actions lessen pain and protect joints vulnerable to progressive inflammatory damage (Turner et al 2008a).

In other diseases it may also be beneficial to reduce walking speed and shorten step length at initial heel contact to control symptoms. In the spondlyoarthropathies, these adapted changes may lessen the tensile and compressive forces on the Achilles tendon, plantar fascia and tibialis posterior; the classic and functional enthesis sites. Primary osteoarthritis of the ankle and or subtalar joints is rare but in post-traumatic secondary cases the large forces experienced during initial loading may serve to concentrate focal stresses on the articular surfaces when the geometry has changed as a result of instability or realignment. Malalignment and pain are associated so gait adaptation may beneficially improve symptoms and reduce stress on cartilage lesions.

Inflammatory joint disease most commonly disrupts the ankle rocker during the mid-stance period of gait when the weightbearing stability is required the most (Turner et al 2008a). Synovitis in the ankle, subtalar and midtarsal joints and tenosynovitis of tibialis posterior leads to stretching of the joint capsule and supporting ligaments, as well as attenuation (longitudinal tears or more rarely tendon rupture) (Woodburn et al 2005). Detailed gait studies have characterised the associated changes in joint motion and forces as well as plantar stresses and centre-of-pressure pathways (Turner et al 2008a, 2008b, Woodburn et al 2004). Excessive and prolonged subtalar eversion and ankle dorsiflexion occur, along with collapse of the medial weightbearing column. This is a highly unstable foot, which progresses to pes planovalgus. Reduced ankle plantarflexion moment and power both reflect the accompanying slow walking speed as well as gastrocnemius-soleus muscle weakness (Turner et al 2008a, 2008b). Keenan et al (1991) used electromyography to show that in patients with RA and pes planovalgus, tibialis posterior has elevated and prolonged activity in an attempt to stabilise the subtalar and midtarsal joints, even though the muscle is weak (Keenan et al 1991). The centre-of-pressure is directed more medially in the foot and focal stresses can appear on the medial mid-foot indicating column collapse (Turner et al 2008b).

Any of the rheumatic diseases associated with acute pain or swelling at the MTP joints (e.g. acute gout or synovitis) will normally disrupt the forefoot rocker during progression (Semple et al 2007). In RA for example, forward progression of the centre-of-pressure is delayed in the heel and mid-foot and rapidly advances through the forefoot as patients convert to a hip-pulling strategy. The adapted gait serves to minimise the time and magnitude of loading at painful joints (Semple et al 2007). In chronic disease, advanced deformity, joint stiffness, and pain are all associated with elevated areas of peak plantar pressure, irrespective of the underlying disease. Changes in joint motion and kinetics (forces) can also be detected during progression. In RA and PsA for example, motion analysis reveals reduced ankle plantarflexion in terminal stance, reduction in vertical and anterior/posterior ground reaction forces, and reduced peak ankle joint power (Turner et al 2008a, 2008b). Advancement of the tibia is slow and the foot is lifted from the ground further emphasising the loss of forefoot rocker. In severe forefoot disease, plantar callosities, bursa and ulceration are closely associated with localised sites of high pressure. Overall, the appearance is of a slow, shuffling style gait, with guarding and deliberate and cautious placement of the foot.

PODIATRY

OVERVIEW

Podiatry is a branch of the allied health professions dealing with the assessment, diagnosis and treatment of foot and ankle problems. Practitioners in specialist or extended scope roles are expertly placed to assess, advise and treat patients with the rheumatic diseases. Podiatry care is one of the most frequently requested service among RA patients (Martin & Griffith 2006) yet service provision throughout the UK is low (Redmond et al 2006). Encouragingly, the evidence base is growing for podiatry treatments (Brouwer et al 2005, Farrow et al 2005, Murley et al 2008).

BASIC FOOT HYGIENE, SELF-MANAGEMENT AND ADVICE

In patients with RA and foot problems, approximately half are unable to manage their own feet due to problems with reach and grip strength (Semple et al 2008). Podiatrists can assist patients and their family or carers to help them maintain good standards of personal foot hygiene. This can involve assistance with reaching the feet and using equipment such as nail-clippers and files. Self-management has benefits such as improved foot health outcomes, reduced demand on podiatry services, and develops self-monitoring for those with a history of problems such as ulceration and infection.

A small amount of well designed and validated patient information is available and focuses on causes and treatment of common problems as well as advice on self-management and footwear (e.g. 'Feet, footwear and arthritis', Arthritis Research Campaign patient information leaflet). Deformed toes, which cause pressure and thickening on the toenails may require periodic reduction using nail burrs to ease discomfort. Plantar or dorsal corns or callus require regular debridement and whilst effective, pain relief is short and the problem may rapidly recur within a few weeks (Davys et al 2005, Woodburn et al 2000). Surgical correction of underlying deformities is advised when callosities are persistent, or where skin tissue viability is poor and lesions have ulcerated. Given the high prevalence of dermatophytosis (superficial fungal infection or tinea) (Bicer et al 2003), advice on treatment for tinea pedis (athlete's foot) and onychomycosis (fungal infection of the nail) should be directed to the rheumatologist or GP.

FOOT ORTHOTICS

Foot orthotics are indicated in patients with rheumatic diseases to provide:

- joint stabilisation
- joint positioning to avoid excessive stress
- pain reduction
- prevention of deformity
- improvement of function
- joint rest
- reduction of inflammation
- improved range of motion and pressure distribution.

(after Kavlak et al 2003)

Across the rheumatic diseases complex foot problems are treated with customised orthoses to provide personalised fit and function (Fig. 13.5). Indeed, moderate-to-good levels of evidence suggest that in RA for instance, good outcome (pain reduction and increased function) can be achieved by customised functional orthoses, especially in early disease (Gossec, et al 2006, Woodburn et al 2002) and when combined with extra-depth shoes (Farrow et al 2005).

Customised orthoses comprise both cushioning, stability and correction elements. The basic orthotic shell will vary by stiffness according to the materials used and their thickness. For example, carbon graphite devices are thin and provide rigid functional control so are suitable for the early stages of inflammatory arthritis (Woodburn et al 2002). These devices are manufactured to plaster models, or digital scans which capture the optimal foot

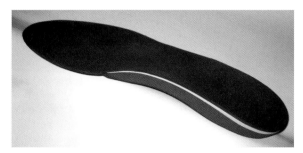

Figure 13.5 Customised foot orthotic for a patient with inflammatory joint disease. The orthosis has polypropylene middle shell to stabilise the subtalar and talonavicular joints and a cushioning top surface to protect painful MTP joints

pose in neutral alignments at the ankle, rearfoot and forefoot. Medial/lateral correction (for flexible eversion/inversion deformity) is created by heel and/or forefoot posts (or wedges), which are built externally or intrinsically into the shell. A top layer of cushioning material is added to reduce sheer and compressive stresses, which offload painful joints or plantar pressure lesions (Woodburn et al 2002). In pursuit of pain relief many patients with rheumatic foot conditions purchase off-the-shelf insoles and orthoses. Despite lacking robust data, many of these products do offer varying levels of symptom relief.

Total contact orthoses are custom-made to plaster or impression moulded casts of the feet and are indicated for moderate-to-severe deformity when joints are stiff and when secondary problems such as pressure lesions or ulceration exist. During manufacture, semi-rigid and cushioning materials are combined and shaped to closely fit the plantar foot geometry. This provides moderate stabilisation combined with maximum surface contact to cushion and support prominent and deformed joints. They are used in conjunction with extra-depth footwear. In ulcerated feet, devices such as the DH Off-Loading Walker™ (Ossur, Manchester, UK) and the Aircast SP Walker™ (DJO Incorporated, CA, USA) are used to off-load the ulcerated lesions. These lightweight walking braces permit near normal ambulation and provide total contact fit through mechanisms such as adjustable air cells. They also provide space to incorporate ulcer/wound dressings and/or insole systems to off-load the target ulcer site. Other walking braces such as the AirLift™ PTTD Brace (DJO Incorporated, CA, USA) can also be used for severe tendon and soft-tissue disease to mechanically off-load vulnerable tissues, and are also indicated

during episodes of acute inflammation, e.g. tibialis posterior tendinopathy in RA or Achilles tendinopathy in psoriatic arthritis.

Podiatrists are also involved in providing insoles and orthotics to treat osteoarthritis of the knee. Laterally wedged insoles reduce the knee adduction moment in medial compartment knee OA and offer short term pain relief (Hinman et al 2008, Kuroyanagi et al 2007). Longer term symptomatic effects are unclear, although nonsteroidal anti-inflammatory drug use may be reduced (Brouwer et al 2005, Gélis et al 2005, Pham et al 2004). Similarly, a medial-wedged insole, when combined with an ankle support, can achieve pain relief and provide functional improvement of valgus knee OA (Rodrigues et al 2008).

FOOTWEAR

Specialist footwear can be used to relieve pain, protect joints, and improve function in any of the rheumatic diseases (Chalmers et al 2000, Fransen & Edmonds 1997, Shakoor et al 2008). However, challenges exist to balance comfort and fit with style and design, especially for women. Indeed Williams concluded in a recent study of extra-depth shoe use in RA patients, 'Footwear replaces something that is normally worn and is part of an individual's body image. It has much more of a negative impact on the female patients' emotions and activities than previously acknowledged and this influences their behaviour with it' (Williams et al 2007a). This is often ignored as many clinicians do not have the time or necessary experience to properly advise patients. Ultimately this leads to poor treatment adherence and outcome (Williams & Meacher 2001).

Fully personalised orthopaedic shoes are the skilled domain of the orthotist and the appliance/footwear technician. They are indicated for patients with the severest and most complex foot deformities. Extra-depth footwear is used much more extensively these days as design, functionality and patient choice continue to improve. These shoes are either provided straight 'off-the-shelf' or assembled from modular sections which permit variation in width and depth of the toe box, and allow personalised modifications such as outer sole (e.g. rocker sole) and heel modifications (e.g. medial flare) to improve function, as well as adaptations such as Velcro fastenings, which are particularly helpful to those with hand disease (Helliwell et al 2007). These shoes are particularly useful in inflammatory joint disease when patients are unable to fit suitable retail shoes due to disabling foot pain and deformity. In RA there is evidence that extra-depth shoes are effective for pain relief and to improve function, particularly when combined with customised orthoses (Chalmers et al 2000, Fransen & Edmonds 1997, Williams et al 2007b). Overall satisfaction is raised when patients are involved in the design, supply and monitoring processes throughout treatment (Williams et al 2007b). Elsewhere, novel footwear concepts are being developed and tested to reduce knee joint loads (Shakoor et al 2008).

GAIT TRAINING, EXERCISE, AND MUSCLE STRENGTHENING

Muscle strengthening, proprioception training and gait re-education are undertaken in conjunction with orthotic, footwear and anti-inflammatory treatments. Since general aerobic condition might be poor and proximal limb involvement highly prevalent, rehabilitation (gait training, muscle and proprioception training and appliance/equipment supply) is routinely undertaken in a coordinated programme, working alongside other members of the multidisciplinary team.

TISSUE VIABILITY AND WOUND CARE

Foot ulceration can occur in patients with RA, connective tissue and crystal joint diseases (Firth et al 2008a, Jeffrey et al 2008, Kumar & Gow 2002). The management of foot wounds and prevention of infection, especially in those patients receiving biologic therapies, remains a key challenge (Davys et al 2006b). The podiatrist firstly has a key role to initiate preventative measures. This primarily involves joint protection to remove focal pressure from vulnerable sites using customised orthoses, braces or footwear. In those cases where ulcers develop, vascular assessment techniques and appropriate referral, wound care management/debridement, pain relief and orthoses and braces to facilitate off-loading are the cornerstones of practice.

Management of foot ulceration can be challenging for patients with rheumatic diseases. Systemic drug therapies may increase the risk of infection, delay wound healing, and may mask the classic signs of infection. Wounds may often extend down to the underlying bone and in the presence of joint erosions and deformities detection of osteomyelitis can be difficult. Severe foot deformity may make debridement and dressing of wounds challenging, furthermore, it may limit the choice of dressing

which can be applied (many may be too bulky and uncomfortable for patients). The newer biologic therapies are increasingly used to suppress inflammation in patients with rheumatic diseases; however, these drugs are powerful immunosuppressants and are associated with an increased risk of infection of skin/soft tissues (Otter et al 2005). Foot ulceration is a contraindication to treatment with any biologic agent as the risk of rapidly progressing infection is too great, therefore the treatment must be suspended. In these instances, ulcers need to be healed quickly so the patient can recommence drug therapy and strategies put in place to prevent recurrence.

EXTENDED SCOPE PRACTICE: INTRA-ARTICULAR AND LESIONAL INJECTIONS AND FOOT SURGERY

Podiatrists are trained in local anaesthesia at an undergraduate level and can perform regional anaesthesia of the foot or ankle to facilitate a number of treatments (usually surgery) and may use injections of local anaesthetics diagnostically. A number of AHPs including podiatrists can now access specialist training programs to undertake intra-articular (IA) or soft tissue (ST) injections as an adjunct to their practice and they can deliver injection therapy under a Patient Group Direction. Both IA and ST injections of corticosteroids can be an extremely effective method to reduce pain, inflammation, swelling and increase function at joints without exposing patients to the usual side effects associated with systemic drug therapy. However, a number of both local and systemic adverse effects have been identified including infection, bleeding, post injection flare, subcutaneous tissue atrophy/skin depigmentation, tendon rupture, nerve damage and delayed soft tissue healing (Saunders & Longworth 2006). Common sites for IA injection include the ankle, subtalar, talonavicular, MTP and IP joints. ST injections of the plantar fascia, retrocalcaneal bursa, interdigital neuroma/bursitis and the tendons of tibialis posterior and peroneal muscles also respond well. The effectiveness of IA or ST injection depends on the accuracy of placement.

The complex anatomy of the foot (particularly in the rearfoot) makes it hard to determine precisely which structures are involved from clinical examination alone and use of ultrasound (US) has been shown to influence sites selected for injection and positively influence short-term efficacy of injection (D'Agostino et al 2005). The use of US to guide injections is likely to occur more frequently as the

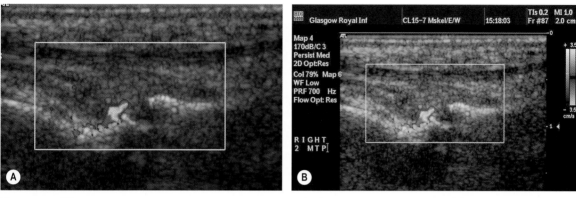

Figure 13.6 (A) Intra-articular corticosteroid injection into the 2nd MTP joint in an RA patient and (B) with high resolution ultrasound proven synovitis.

technology becomes cheaper and more accessible and more clinicians are appropriately trained in the technique (Fig. 13.6). It has been shown that with appropriate training and mentorship, podiatrists, can provide adequate sonographic images and reliably report features such as erosions, synovitis and bursitis with excellent levels of agreement when compared to expert radiologists (Bowen et al 2008). Therefore it is anticipated that US will become part of extended scope practice for podiatrists working in advanced/consultant practitioner roles. Podiatrists

routinely monitor response to rehabilitation therapies and when indicated (non-response, deteriorating foot health, and complications such as ulceration or infection) surgical opinion should be sought.

In 2008, there were approximately 150 surgically trained podiatrists and some may be undertaking forefoot reconstruction procedures in patients with rheumatic foot conditions. In more complex cases involving rearfoot and ankle conditions, techniques such as arthrodesis and joint replacement largely remain the remit of orthopaedics.

References and further reading

Allali, F., Tahiri, L., Senjari, A., et al., 2007. Erosive arthropathy in systemic sclerosis. BMC Public Health 7, 260.

Awerbuch, M.S., Shephard, E., Vernon-Roberts, B., 1982. Morton's metatarsalgia due to intermetatarsophalangeal bursitis

as an early manifestation of rheumatoid arthritis. Clin. Orthop. Relat. Res. 167, 214–221.

Balint, P.V., Kane, D., McInnes, I.B., et al., 2002. Ultrasonography of entheseal insertions in the lower limb in spondyloarthropathy. Ann. Rheum. Dis. 61, 905–910.

Belt, E.A., Kaarela, K., Lehto, M.U., 1998. Destruction and arthroplasties of the metatarsophalangeal joints in seropositive rheumatoid arthritis. A 20-year follow-up study. Scand. J. Rheumatol. 27, 194–196.

Belt, E.A., Kaarela, K., Mäenpää, H., et al., 2001. Relationship of ankle joint involvement with subtalar destruction in patients with rheumatoid arthritis. A 20-year follow-up study. Joint Bone Spine 68, 154–157.

Benjamin, M., McGonagle, D., 2001. The anatomical basis for disease localisation in seronegative spondylarthropathy at entheses and related sites. J. Anat. 199, 503–526.

Bhatt, S.P., Handa, R., Gulati, G.S., et al., 2007. Peripheral vascular disease in systemic lupus erythematosus. Lupus 16, 720–723.

Bicer, A., Tursen, U., Cimen, O. B., et al., 2003. Prevalence of dermatophytosis in patients with rheumatoid arthritis. Rheumatol. Int. 23, 37–40.

Borman, P., Koparal, S., Babaoglu, S., et al., 2006. Ultrasound detection of entheseal insertions in the foot of patients with spondyloarthropathy. Clin. Rheumatol. 25, 373–377.

Boutry, N., Lardé, A., Lapègue, F., et al., 2003. Magnetic resonance imaging appearance of the hands and feet in patients with early rheumatoid arthritis. J. Rheumatol. 30, 671–679.

Bouysset, M., Tebib, J., Tavernier, T., et al., 2003. Posterior tibial tendon and subtalar joint complex in rheumatoid arthritis: magnetic resonance imaging study. J. Rheumatol. 30, 1951–1954.

Bowen, C.J., Dewbury, K., Sampson, M., et al., 2008. Musculoskeletal ultrasound imaging of the plantar forefoot in patients with rheumatoid arthritis: inter-observer agreement between a podiatrist and a radiologist. J. Foot Ankle Res. 1, 5.

Briggs, P.J., 2003. Controversies and perils. Reconstruction of the rheumatoid forefoot. The Stainsby operation. Tech. Orthop. 18, 303–310.

Brostrom, E., Haglun-Akerlind, Y., Hagelbers, S., et al., 2002. Gait in children with juvenile chronic arthritis. J. Rheumatol. 31, 317–323.

Brouwer, R.W., Jakma, T.S., Verhagen, A.P., et al., 2005. Braces and orthoses for treating osteoarthritis of the knee. Cochrane Database Syst. Rev. 25 CD004020.

Carl, A., Ross, S., Evanski, P., et al., 1988. Hypermobility in hallux valgus. Foot Ankle 8, 264–270.

Chalmers, A.C., Busby, C., Goyert, J., et al., 2000. Metatarsalgia and rheumatoid arthritis: a randomised single-blind, sequential trial comparing 2 types of foot orthoses and supportive shoes. J. Rheumatol. 27, 1643–1647.

D'Agostino, M.A., Said-Nahal, R., Hacquard-Bouder, C., et al., 2003. Assessment of peripheral enthesitis in the spondylarthropathies by ultrasonography combined with power Doppler. Arthritis Rheum. 48, 523–533.

D'Agostino, M.A., Ayral, X., Baron, G., et al., 2005. Impact of Ultrasound Imaging on Local Corticosteroid Injections of Symptomatic Ankle, Hind-, and Mid-Foot in Chronic Inflammatory Diseases. Arthritis Rheum. 53, 284–292.

Dalbeth, N., Clarke, B., McQueen, F., et al., 2007. Validation of a radiographic damage index in chronic gout. Arthritis Rheum. 57, 1067–1073.

Dalbeth, N., Clark, B., Gregory, K., et al., August 15, 2008. Mechanisms of bone erosion in gout; a quantitative analysis using plain radiography and computed tomography. Ann. Rheum. Dis. Epub ahead of print.

Davys, H.J., Turner, D.E., Helliwell, P.S., et al., 2005. Debridement of plantar callosities in rheumatoid arthritis: a randomized controlled trial. Rheumatology 44, 207–210.

Davys, H.J., Woodburn, J., Bingham, S.J., et al., 2006a. Onychocryptosis (ingrowing toe nail) in patients with rheumatoid arthritis on biological therapies. Rheumatology 45 (Suppl. 1), i171.

Davys, H., Turner, D.E., Helliwell, P.S., et al., 2006b. Foot ulceration in patients with rheumatic diseases. Ann. Rheum. Dis. 65 (Suppl. II), 669.

Falsetti, P., Frediani, B., Fioravanti, A., et al., 2003. Sonographic study of calcaneal entheses in erosive osteoarthritis, nodal osteoarthritis, rheumatoid arthritis and psoriatic arthritis. Scand. J. Rheumatol. 32, 229–234.

Ferrari, J., 1998. A review of the foot deformities seen in juvenile chronic arthritis. The Foot 8, 193–196.

Farrow, S.J., Kingsley, G.H., Scott, D.L., 2005. Interventions for foot disease in rheumatoid arthritis: a systematic review. Arthritis Rheum. 53, 593–602.

Finsterbush, A., Pogrund, H., 1982. The hypermobility syndrome. Musculoskeletal complaints in 100 consecutive cases of generalized joint hypermobility. Clin. Orthop. Relat. Res. 168, 124–127.

Firth, J., Hale, C., Helliwell, P., et al., 2008a. The prevalence of foot ulceration in patients with rheumatoid arthritis. Arthritis Rheum. 59, 200–205.

Firth, J., Helliwell, P., Hale, C., et al., 2008b. The predictors of foot ulceration in patients with rheumatoid arthritis: a preliminary investigation. Clin. Rheumatol. 27, 1423–1428.

Fleming, A., Crown, J.M., Corbett, M., 1976. Incidence of joint involvement in early rheumatoid arthritis. Rheumatol. Rehabil. 15, 92–96.

Fransen, M., Edmonds, J., 1997. Off-the-shelf orthopedic footwear for people with rheumatoid arthritis. Arthrit. Care Res. 10, 250–256.

Galluzzo, E., Lischi, D.M., Taglione, E., et al., 2000. Sonographic analysis of the ankle in patients with psoriatic arthritis. Scand. J. Rheumatol. 29, 52–55.

Gélis, A., Coudeyre, E., Aboukrat, P., et al., 2005. Feet insoles and knee osteoarthritis: evaluation of biomechanical and clinical effects from a literature review. Annales de Réadaptation et de Médecine Physique 48, 682–689.

Genc, H., Cakit, B.D., Tuncbilek, I., et al., 2005. Ultrasonographic evaluation of tendons and enthesal sites in rheumatoid arthritis: comparison with ankylosing spondylitis and healthy subjects. Clin. Rheumatol. 24, 272–277.

Gold, R.H., Bassett, L.W., Seeger, L.L., 1988. The other arthritides. Roentgenologic features of osteoarthritis, ankylosing arthritis, psoriatic arthritis, Reiter's disease, multicentric reticulohistiocytosis, and progressive systemic sclerosis. Radiol. Clin. N. Am. 26, 1195–1212.

Gossec, L., Pavy, S., Pharm, T., et al., 2006. Non-pharmacological treatments in early rheumatoid arthritis: clinical practice guidelines based on published evidence and expert opinion. Joint Bone Spine 73, 396–402.

Gutman, A.B., 1973. The past four decades of progress in the knowledge with gout, with assessment of the present status. Arthritis Rheum. 16, 431–445.

Hall, M.G., Ferrell, W.R., Sturrock, R.D., et al., 1995. The effect of the hypermobility syndrome on knee joint proprioception. Brit. J. Rheumatol. 34, 121–125.

Harris, M.D., Seigel, L.B., Alloway, J.A., 1999. Gout hyperuricemia. Am. Fam. Physician 59, 925–934.

Helliwell, P.S., Woodburn, J., Redmond, A.C., et al., 2007. The Foot and Ankle in Rheumatoid Arthritis. A Comprehensive Guide. Elsevier Limited, London.

Hendry, G.J., Gardner-Medwin, J.G., Watt, G.F., et al., July 10, 2008. A survey of foot problems in Juvenile Idiopathic Arthritis. Musculoskeletal Care [Epub ahead of print].

Hinman, R.S., Payne, C., Metcalf, B.R., et al., 2008. Lateral wedges in knee osteoarthritis: what are their immediate clinical and biomechanical effects and can these predict a three-month clinical outcome?. Arthritis Rheum. 59, 408–415.

Huch, K., Kuettner, K.E., Dieppe, P., 1997. Osteoarthritis in ankle and knee joints. Semin. Arthritis Rheu. 26, 667–674.

Hyslop, E., Turner, D.E., McInnes, I.B., et al., 2008. An outpatient survey of foot problems in psoriatic arthritis. Ann. Rheum. Dis. 67 (Suppl. II), 527.

Jeffrey, R.C., Narshi, C.B., Isenberg, D.A., 2008. Prevalence, serological features, response to treatment and outcome of critical ischaemia in a cohort of lupus patients. Rheumatology 47, 1379–1383.

Jernberg, E.T., Simkin, P., Kravette, M., et al., 1999. The posterior tibial tendon and the tarsal sinus in rheumatoid flat foot: magnetic resonance imaging of 40 feet. J. Rheumatol. 26, 289–293.

Kavlak, Y., Uygur, F., Korkmaz, C., et al., 2003. Outcome of orthoses intervention in the rheumatoid foot. Foot Ankle Int. 24, 494–499.

Keenan, M.A., Peabody, T.D., Gronley, J.K., et al., 1991. Valgus deformities of the feet and characteristics of gait in patients who have rheumatoid arthritis. J. Bone Joint Surg. Am. 73, 237–247.

Korda, J., Balint, G.P., 2004. When to consult the podiatrist. Bailliéres Best Pract. Res. Clin. Rheumatol. 18, 587–611.

Kumar, S., Gow, P., 2002. A survey of indications, results and complications of surgery for tophaceous gout. N. Z. Med. J. 115, U109.

Kuroyanagi, Y., Nagura, T., Matsumoto, H., et al., 2007. The lateral wedged insole with subtalar strapping significantly reduces dynamic knee load in the medial compartment gait analysis on patients with medial knee osteoarthritis. Osteoarthritis and Cartilage 15, 932–936.

La Montagna, G., Baruffot, A., Tirri, R., et al., 2002. Foot involvement in Systemic Sclerosis: A longitudinal study of 100 patients. Semin. Arthritis Rheu. 31, 248–255.

Lehtinen, A., Paimela, L., Kreula, J., et al., 1996. Painful ankle region in rheumatoid arthritis. Analysis of soft-tissue changes with ultrasonography and MR imaging. Acta Radiologica 37, 572–577.

Martin, L.J., Griffith, S.M., 2006. High disease activity scores predict the need for additional health services in patients over 60 with rheumatoid arthritis. Musculoskeletal Care 4, 1–11.

Mavidrou, A., Klenerman, L., Swann, M., et al., 1991. Conservative management of the hindfoot in juvenile chronic arthritis. The Foot 1, 139–143.

Michelson, J., Easley, M., Wigley, F.M., et al., 1994. Foot and ankle problems in rheumatoid arthritis. Foot Ankle Int. 15, 608–613.

Mizutani, W., Quismorio, F.P., 1984. Lupus foot: deforming arthropathy of the feet in systemic lupus erythematosus. J. Rheumatol. 11, 80–82.

Moll, J.M.H., 1987. Seronegative arthropathies in the foot. Baillière's Clin. Rheumatol. 1, 289–314.

Murley, G.S., Landorf, K.B., Menz, H.B., et al., October 13, 2008. Effect of foot posture, foot orthoses and footwear on lower limb muscle activity during walking and running: A systematic review. Gait Posture [Epub ahead of print].

Myerson, M.S., Badekas, A., 2000. Hypermobility of the first ray. Foot Ankle Clin. 5, 469–484.

Olivieri, I., Foto, M., Ruju, G.P., et al., 1992. Low frequence of axial involvement in Caucasian pediatric patients with seronegative enthesopathy and arthropathy syndrome after 5 years of disease. J. Rheumatol. 19, 469–475.

Ostendorf, B., Scherer, A., Mödder, U., et al., 2004. Diagnostic value of magnetic resonance imaging of the forefeet in early rheumatoid arthritis when findings on imaging of the metacarpophalangeal joints of the hands remain normal. Arthritis Rheum. 50, 2094–2102.

Otter, S., Robinson, C., Berry, H., 2005. Rheumatoid arthritis, foot infection and tumour necrosis factor alpha inhibition-a case history. The Foot 15, 117–119.

Perry, J., 1992. Gait analysis. Normal and pathological function. Slack Incorporated, NJ. USA.

Pham, T., Maillefert, J.F., Hudry, C., et al., 2004. Laterally elevated wedged insoles in the treatment of medial knee osteoarthritis. A two-year prospective randomized controlled study. Osteoarth. Cartilage 12, 46–55.

Premkumar, A., Perry, M.B., Dwyer, A.J., et al., 2002. Sonography and MR imaging of posterior tibial tendinopathy. AJR Am. J. Roentgenol. 178, 223–232.

Redmond, A.C., Waxman, R., Helliwell, P.S., 2006. Provision of foot health services in rheumatology. Rheumatology 45, 571–576.

Reilly, P.A., Evison, G., McHugh, N.J., et al., 1990. Arthropathy of hands and feet in systemic lupus erythematosus. J. Rheumatol. 17, 777–784.

Rodrigues, P.T., Ferreira, A.F., Pereira, R.M., et al., 2008. Effectiveness of medial-wedge insole treatment for valgus knee osteoarthritis. Arthritis Rheum. 59, 603–608.

Sahin, N., Baskent, A., Cakmak, A., et al., 2008a. Evaluation of knee proprioception and effects on proprioception exercise in patients with benign joint hypermobility syndrome. Rheumatol. Int. 28, 995–1000.

Sahin, N., Baskent, A., Ugurlu, H., et al., 2008b. Isokinetic evaluation of knee extensor/flexor muscle strength in patients with hypermobility syndrome. Rheumatol. Int. 28, 643–648.

Saltzman, C.L., Salamon, M.L., Blanchard, G.M., et al., 2005. Epidemiology of ankle arthritis. Iowa Orthop. J. 25, 44–46.

Sari-Kouzel, H., Hutchinson, C.E., Middleton, A., et al., 2001. Foot problems in patients with systemic sclerosis. Rheumatology 40, 410–413.

Saunders, S., Longworth, S., 2006. Injection techniques in orthopaedics and sports medicine.

A practical manual for doctors and physiotherapists, third ed.. Elsevier, Edinburgh p7.

Semple, R., Turner, D.E., Helliwell, P.S., Woodburn, J., 2007. Regionalised centre of pressure analysis in patients with rheumatoid arthritis. Clin. Biomech. (Bristol, Avon) 22, 127–129.

Semple, R., Newcombe, L.W., Finlayson, G.L., et al., September 17 2008. The FOOTSTEP self-management foot care programme: Are rheumatoid arthritis patients physically able to participate? Musculoskeletal Care [Epub ahead of print].

Shakoor, N., Lidtke, R.H., Sengupta, M., et al., 2008. Effects of specialized footwear on joint loads in osteoarthritis of the knee. Arthritis Rheum. 59, 1214–1220.

Shereff, M.J., Baumhauer, J.F., 1998. Hallux rigidus and osteoarthrosis of the first metatarsophalangeal joint. J. Bone Joint Surg. Am. 80, 898–908.

Spraul, G., Koenning, G., 1994. A descriptive study of foot problems in children with juvenile rheumatoid arthritis (JRA). Arthrit. Care Res. 7, 144–150.

Theodoridou, A., Bento, L., D'Cruz, D.P., et al., 2003. Prevalence and associations of an abnormal ankle-brachial index in systemic lupus erythematosus: a pilot study. Ann. Rheum. Dis. 62, 1199–1203.

Turner, D.E., Helliwell, P.S., Emery, P., et al., 2006. The impact of rheumatoid arthritis on foot function in the early stages of disease: a clinical case series. BMC Musculoskelet. Disord. 7, 102.

Turner, D.E., Helliwell, P.S., Siegel, K.L., et al., 2008a. Biomechanics of the foot in rheumatoid arthritis: identifying abnormal function and the factors associated with localised disease 'impact'. Clin. Biomech. (Bristol, Avon) 23, 93–100.

Turner, D.E., Woodburn, J., 2008b. Characterising the clinical and

biomechanical features of severely deformed feet in rheumatoid arthritis. Gait Posture 28, 574–580.

Valderrabano, V., Horisberger, M., Russell, I., et al., October 2, 2008. Etiology of ankle osteoarthritis. Clin. Orthop. Relat. Res. [Epub ahead of print].

Williams, A., Meacher, K., 2001. Shoes in the cupboard: the fate of prescribed footwear? Prosthet. Orthot. Int. 25, 53–59.

Williams, A.E., Nester, C.J., Ravey, M.I., 2007a. Rheumatoid arthritis patients' experiences of wearing therapeutic footwear – a qualitative investigation. BMC Musculoskelet. Disord. 8, 104.

Williams, A.E., Rome, K., Nester, C.J., 2007b. A clinical trial of specialist footwear for patients with rheumatoid arthritis. Rheumatology 46, 302–307.

Witemeyer, S., Ansell, B.M., Ashburn, A., et al., 1981. Gait analysis: a pilot study- a possible mode of assessment of lower limb function in juvenile chronic arthritis. Rheumatol. Rehabil. 20, 31–37.

Woodburn, J., Barker, S., Helliwell, P.S., 2002. A randomized controlled trial of foot orthoses in rheumatoid arthritis. J. Rheumatol. 29, 1377–1383.

Woodburn, J., Stableford, Z., Helliwell, P.S., 2000. Preliminary investigation of debridement of plantar callosities in rheumatoid arthritis. Rheumatology 39, 652–654.

Woodburn, J., Nelson, K.M., Siegel, K.L., et al., 2004. Multisegment foot motion during gait: proof of concept in rheumatoid arthritis. J. Rheumatol. 31, 1918–1927.

Woodburn, J., Cornwall, M. W., Soames, R.W., et al., 2005. Selectively attenuating soft tissues close to sites of inflammation in the peritalar region of patients with rheumatoid arthritis leads to development of pes planovalgus. J. Rheumatol. 32, 268–274.

Chapter 14

Diet and complementary therapies

Dorothy Pattison PhD Bone & Joint Research Team, Knowledge Spa, Royal Cornwall Hospital (NHS) Trust, UK

Adrian White MA MD BM Bch General Practice and Primary Care, Peninsula Medical School, Plymouth, UK

CHAPTER CONTENTS

KEY POINTS

- A combination of weight loss/healthy eating and exercise is recommended in the management of osteoarthritis
- Weight loss and avoidance of alcohol can ameliorate the symptoms of gout and prevent future episodes
- Omega-3 fatty acids can give symptomatic benefits in rheumatoid arthritis
- Most other dietary supplements have no specific effect
- Evidence shows acupuncture can give lasting pain relief in osteoarthritis.

INTRODUCTION

Conventional medicine (pharmacological treatment) generally only offers symptom relief for chronic rheumatological conditions, and some patients are unwilling to take drugs for long periods, especially as they may have serious side-effects. Therefore, patients often seek out dietary or complementary approaches. These are discussed in turn in this chapter.

SECTION 1 DIET AND DIETARY THERAPIES

At some point, health professionals working in the area of musculoskeletal conditions will be asked by patients about the role that diet can play in managing their symptoms. Diet is one issue which is very important to many patients and may have a more important role than many health professionals acknowledge (Rayman & Pattison 2008). Dietitians are not yet widely viewed as core members of the rheumatology team and may not be easily accessed, thus it is important that some dietary issues can be safely addressed by other health professionals. This chapter will provide an overview of basic nutritional requirements for healthy eating in general and a more in depth examination of the available evidence for dietary advice in common musculoskeletal conditions. Dietary intervention

© 2010 Elsevier Ltd
DOI: 10.1016/B978-0-443-06934-5.00014-0

Table 14.1 Macronutrients, functions and dietary sources

NUTRIENT	PRINCIPLE ROLE	RECOMMENDED DAILY INTAKE AS % OF TOTAL ENERGY INTAKE	FOOD SOURCE
Protein (adults 19 years+)	Main nutrient required for muscle building and tissue repair	10–12%	Lean meat poultry, fish, eggs, dairy products, beans, pulses
Carbohydrate	Provides energy and vitamins, particularly 'B vitamins' which enable energy to be released from carbohydrate, protein and fat	50–60%	Wholegrain cereals, rye bread, wholegrain bread, wholegrain breakfast cereals, potatoes, cake, confectionary
Fat	Energy, fat soluble vitamins eg vitamin D, vitamin E	30% (total fat) 10% saturated fat (SFA) 6% polyunsaturated fat 12% monounsaturated 2% trans fatty acids 01–02 g/day n-3 PUFA (polyunsaturated fatty acid)	Butter, fatty meat, biscuits, cakes, pastry Sunflower oil/margarine Olive oil/margarine, nuts Processed foods Oily fish
Non-starch polysaccharide (NSP) or 'dietary fibre'	Bowel function – increases stool bulk. Cholesterol lowering, slows digestion	18 g/day	Wholegrain cereals and breads, legumes, fruits, vegetables

Source: Department of Health, 1991

usually involves adding a food, nutrient or substance to the diet for example a dietary supplement or removing food from the diet or making a total change to dietary intake. In general, diets are perceived to be harmless but, uninformed and unnecessary dietary restrictions will disturb normal diet and lifestyle patterns, increase the risk of nutritional deficiencies and even adversely affect medical treatment. Therefore, it is important to recognise when expert advice is necessary. To deal with this, two scenarios are discussed in the case studies at the end of this chapter.

HEALTHY EATING

A healthful diet is based on a varied intake of wholegrain cereals, low fat dairy products, fish and lean meats, olive oil based oils and margarines, fruit and vegetables, beans and pulses, is therefore low in fat, especially saturated fat, salt and sugar but adequate in energy, protein and fibre (Tables 14.1, 14.2).

NUTRITION IN MUSCULOSKELETAL CONDITIONS

There is an enormous amount of dietary advice aimed at people with arthritis, particularly rheumatoid arthritis (RA). Unfortunately, the vast majority of

Table 14.2 Food groups and targets for intake

FOOD GROUP	TARGETS FOR DIETARY INTAKES
Bread, potato, cereals, rice, flour, pasta	Average 6–11 portions/day (eg 1 portion = 1 slice bread) Use wholegrain and white
Sugars, sweets, biscuits, cakes	Eat 'in moderation'
Fats: butter, margarine, oil	Use olive oil & olive oil-based products Grill, poach, bake, steam instead of frying
Dairy products	½–1 pint milk/day (any type) 4–5 yogurts a week 4–6 portions cheese a week (1 portion = 25 g) Use low fat products
Lean meat (beef, pork, lamb)	2–3 portions a week
Poultry	>2–3 portions a week
Fish (all types)	≥2 portions a week
Eggs	2–3 a week
Fruit & vegetables	5 portions daily: 1 portion = 1 apple, 3 dried apricots, 1 cereal bowl of mixed salad, 2 broccoli florets
Alcohol	Women ≤ 14 units/week Men ≤ 21 units/week (1 unit = ½ pint lager/beer (3–4% ABV); 125 ml glass wine (~12% ABV); 1 pub measure of spirits)

Source: http://wwweatwellgovuk/healthydiet/

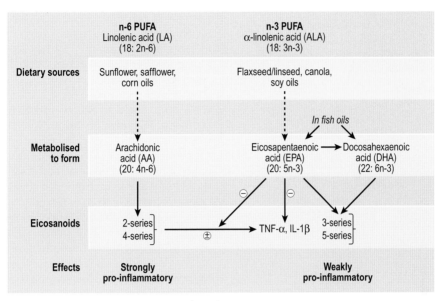

Figure 14.1 Metabolism of polyunsaturated fatty acids (PUFA).

claims made by self-styled diets for arthritis such as The Dong diet, Sister Hill's diet, Norman F. Childer's diet, and many more, are unsubstantiated, based on individual experience and cannot be generalised to everyone with the condition. Undertaking high-quality dietary intervention studies is complex and extremely difficult to do, thus 'high-level' evidence of efficacy of a dietary intervention is often lacking. Also, studies measure diverse outcomes making interpretation of the results more difficult. For example, global measures of well being and assessment of pain are more susceptible to placebo effect and convey a different message than measurements of objective, clinical outcomes. In addition, dietary advice recommended for other clinical conditions may be contradictory, thus adding confusion. The following section summarises dietary advice for which there is some evidence of efficacy in the rheumatic diseases.

FISH OILS AND OMEGA–3 FATTY ACIDS

The majority of evidence for the beneficial effects of fish oils in the management of arthritis comes from studies in RA. Long chain omega-6 (n-6) and omega-3 (n-3) polyunsaturated fatty acids (PUFAs) are precursors of inflammatory mediators such as eicosanoids (Fig. 14.1) Metabolism of n-6 PUFA, yields arachidonic acid, a precursor of strongly inflammatory leukotrienes, prostaglandins and thromboxanes (two and four series) (Fig. 14.1), whereas

n-3 PUFA are converted to eicosapentaenoic acid (EPA) and further to docosahexaenoic acid (DHA) which yield less inflammatory eicosanoids (three and five series). EPA and DHA are obtained from dietary sources found mainly in oily fish such as mackerel, sardines, halibut, herring, salmon, trout and fresh tuna (not tinned), whereas n-6 PUFAs are much more abundant in the diet for example in seeds, vegetable oils and margarines. The conversion pathways of n-3 and n-6 PUFA are shared, consequently they are in competition for the same enzyme necessary for adaptation (Fig. 14.1). So, in addition to advising patients to increase their intake of n-3 PUFA from fish or supplements, a reduction in the intake of n-6 PUFA may increase the effectiveness of n-3 PUFA supplements. This could be achieved by replacing sunflower oils/margarines with olive or rapeseed oils and olive oil based margarines.

There is good evidence for a therapeutic benefit of n-3 PUFA (EPA + DHA) in patients with RA if taken as fish oil supplements (Fortin et al 1995). A more recent systematic review of the same intervention studies, but specifically exploring pain control in people with RA, concluded that the amount of n-3 PUFA necessary to achieve a reduction in pain is 2.7–3 g/day (total EPA + DHA) for 3–4 months, that is, the maximum duration of these studies (Goldberg & Katz 2007).

The proportion of EPA and DHA in fish oil supplements varies greatly between products but it is

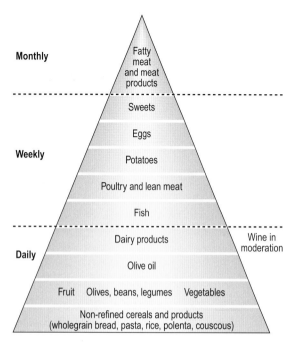

Figure 14.2 Typical Mediterranean-type diet.

possible to achieve an intake of 2 g n-3 PUFA from four or five fish oil capsules, containing 500 mg or more n-3 PUFA. The number of capsules required will also vary depending on oily fish consumption. Liquid fish oil preparations are more concentrated sources of n-3 PUFA and are often flavoured to improve tolerance.

Many 'one-a-day' type cod liver oil capsules contain high amounts of the fat soluble vitamins A and D. It is considered unsafe to take high doses of vitamin D long-term because of the risk of hypercalcaemia and hypercalciuria and also unsafe to take high doses of vitamin A because of toxicity or a possible increase in hip fracture. Pregnant women should avoid cod liver oil supplements because of the unknown tetratogenic effects of vitamin A at high doses (Rayman & Callaghan 2006a). Therefore, all patients should be advised to use fish body oil supplements.

N-3 PUFA rich fish oils have also been shown to be effective in secondary cardiovascular disease prevention (Mead et al 2006). Given that people with RA are at an increased risk of cardiovascular disease (Goodson & Solomon 2006), eating oily fish more than twice a week can be recommended. There has been concern over high levels of toxic substances such as dioxins, polychlorinated biphenyls (PCBs), and mercury levels in oily fish and fish oil supplements. The Food Standards Agency (FSA) recommends two portions of fish a week one of which should be oily for the general population. For people who want to eat more oily fish, the FSA has set a maximum of four portions of oily fish per week (Food Standards Agency 2002). Women of reproductive age and girls should limit their intake of oily fish to one portion a week and should avoid swordfish, marlin or shark because of high mercury levels. There is also a Europe wide dioxin limit which manufacturers of fish oil supplements adhere to so toxicity from these should not be a problem. People on anti-coagulation therapy should seek guidance from their medical practitioner before taking high doses of fish oil.

In summary, the evidence currently available suggests that there is a beneficial effect for people with RA from high dose long-chain n-3 PUFA, for 3 to 6 months duration. However, longer term safety of high dose fish oil supplementation has not been adequately monitored. The effect of n-3 PUFA from food sources on joint symptoms has not been investigated.

PLANT SOURCES OF N-3

EPA and DHA can be synthesised from α-linolenic acid (ALA) found most commonly in green leafy vegetables, flaxseeds, rapeseeds and canola oils, although the conversion of ALA to EPA and DHA is relatively inefficient. There is little evidence to support the efficacy of these oils in the management of rheumatic diseases (Rennie et al 2003). On the other hand, there is some supporting evidence for gamma-linolenic acid (GLA) supplementation. GLA is produced from n-6 linoleic acid and is found in plant oils such as evening primrose oil, blackcurrant seed and borage seed oils (Leventhal et al 1993, Little & Parsons 2001a, 2001b, Watson et al 1993). However, results are inconsistent and more research is required in this area before recommendations can be made.

NUTRITION IN OTHER CONDITIONS

There is some evidence 'in vitro' that long chain n-3 PUFAs, can affect the metabolism of osteoarthritic cartilage (Curtis et al 2002), but this is not sufficient to recommend high dose fish oil therapy in this group of patients. Patients with gout may be required to follow a diet low in dietary purines. Oily fish are rich in purines and may need to be avoided if gouty symptoms are exacerbated by the consumption of oily fish.

FRUIT, VEGETABLES AND ANTIOXIDANTS

Dietary antioxidants are of particular interest in the management of arthritis. These 'phytochemicals' are found extensively in fruits and vegetables particularly brightly coloured varieties such as oranges, apricots, mangos, carrots, peppers/capsicum, and tomatoes and in green leafy vegetables. The most common antioxidants are vitamins C, E and A, but there are many more, such as the carotenoids β-carotene and β-cryptoxanthin. Antioxidants play a crucial role in our internal defence system protecting against harmful metabolites and other substances. There is some evidence that higher dietary intakes of some antioxidants may lower the risk of developing inflammatory arthritis (Pattison et al 2004, 2005) and possibly dampen down the inflammatory response in established disease (Pattison et al 2007). However, this theory is based on epidemiological evidence of dietary intake in inflammatory arthritis. A recent systematic review did not support the use of individual antioxidant supplementation (vitamins A, C, E and selenium) in the treatment of any type of arthritis (Canter et al 2007).

In OA, a higher dietary intake and higher serum levels of vitamin D were associated with a lower risk of knee OA progression (McAlindon et al 1996) but more recent data from two large epidemiological studies of OA have not confirmed this association (Felson et al 2007). Results from a UK intervention study of vitamin D supplementation in established OA knee are awaited.

Anaemia is common in people with RA, usually as a manifestation of the anaemia of chronic disease associated with RA. Mild iron deficiency may actually be beneficial and suppress joint inflammation (Rayman & Callaghan 2006b). Therefore iron supplementation may be detrimental and is not recommended unless under medical supervision.

Overall, the practice of mega-dosing with nutritional supplements should be strongly discouraged. Not only is there no scientific evidence to support this treatment in rheumatic diseases, high doses of individual nutrients can be harmful. For example, long term, excessive vitamin C intake (>1000 mg/day) can result in gastrointestinal disturbances. A high intake of selenium can lead to selenosis (loss of hair, skin and nails) and for many other nutrients the effect of high doses may yet be unknown.

VEGETARIAN AND VEGAN DIETS

The effects of vegetarian and vegan diets have been investigated in people with RA but not OA (Hafström et al 2001). The pooled results of the only four controlled studies found long-term clinical benefit for patients with RA after fasting followed by a vegetarian diet for three months or more (Müller et al 2001). If followed appropriately, vegetarian diets should not cause nutritional problems. However, vegan diets are much more nutritionally restrictive and may result in excessive weight loss. Patients should be encouraged to seek dietetic support. 'Living food' diets (uncooked, vegan diet) (Hänninen et al 2000) and gluten-free diets have also been evaluated in patients with RA but there is as yet little consistent evidence of their efficacy.

MEDITERRANEAN–TYPE DIET

This way of eating is based on daily intakes of fresh fruits and vegetables, nuts, beans and pulses, olive oil, wholegrain cereals and regular oily fish and poultry consumption (Fig. 14.2). Thus, the diet contains n-3 PUFAs, olive oil, antioxidants, dairy products and unrefined carbohydrates. In a recent study, Swedish patients with RA who followed a modified Mediterranean diet for 3 months reported reduced inflammatory activity, increased physical functioning and improved vitality compared with those who followed the control diet (Sköldstam et al 2003). No such studies have been undertaken in people with OA.

BODY WEIGHT

'Rheumatoid cachexia' is a common occurrence, which in some can cause weight loss. Increased catabolism, muscle wasting and anorexia develop as a result of excess cytokine production (Morley et al 2006). Thus, nutritional support may not be effective unless given in combination with adequate pharmacological control of the inflammatory response. Elderly patients with hip fracture are often frail and of low body weight. Nutrition support is paramount in this group of patients to encourage healing and recovery. Efficacy has been demonstrated in randomized controlled trials (Avenell & Handoll 2003, Hedström et al 2006).

Epidemiological studies have shown that obesity precedes OA knee and people who are overweight in their 30s are at an increased risk of developing OA knee in their 70s (Felson 1988). There is limited but increasing evidence supporting the efficacy of weight loss as an intervention in overweight and obese patients with OA knee (Woolf 2007). The most successful intervention is a combination of exercise with a weight reduction plan (Messier et al 2004, NICE 2006).

Current dietary guidelines for the management of gout recommend weight loss in those who are overweight and a reduction or avoidance of alcohol (especially beer). Low animal purine diets are still prescribed for patients with gouty symptoms not adequately controlled by drugs (e.g. Allopurinol) (Zhang et al 2006). For further information on gout see Chapter 23.

FOOD AVOIDANCE

True food allergy is no more prevalent in people with RA than in the general population. Food intolerance is more common and dietary exclusion is a popular intervention with patients. A dietary exclusion programme is used to detect food intolerances in a minority of patients under strict dietetic supervision. Specific food stuffs identified by patients as causing flare-ups of symptoms are very individual and cannot be generalised to all people with RA. The risk of nutrient deficiencies must be emphasised if groups of foods are avoided and dietary assessment is recommended. The common belief that tomatoes and citrus fruits are 'acidic' and that consumption will exacerbate joint inflammation is not supported by human science. Stomach acids are far stronger than naturally occurring plant acids, plus the body is very efficient at maintaining an optimal pH. In fact these foods are rich in antioxidants such as vitamin C, lycopene and β-cryptoxanthin and should be included in a healthy diet.

A low starch diet has been investigated in the treatment of ankylosing spondylitis (Ebringer & Wilson 1996) but there is no evidence supporting use of this dietary regime in routine practice (Zochling et al 2006) (Table 14.3).

DIETARY SUPPLEMENTS

There is little convincing evidence that dietary supplements influence the course of RA (Table 14.3). However, dietetic consultation may be warranted if dietary intake is obviously insufficient to meet an individual's nutritional requirements.

Table 14.3 Evidence for commonly used dietary supplements for management of arthritic symptoms

SUPPLEMENT	OSTEOARTHRITIS	RHEUMATOID ARTHRITIS
Avocado/Soybean Unsaponifiables (ASU)	Good - hip and knee*	None
New Zealand green-lipped mussel (Perna canaliculus)	Inconclusive**	Inconclusive**
Shark cartilage	None – risk of toxic side effects	
Methylsulfonylmethane (MSM)	Limited – knee***	None
Cider vinegar	None	None
Green Tea extract	None	None
Ginger	No effect***	No effect
Curcumin	None	None
Rosehip extract	Limited for knee	None

*Cobb & Ernst 2006
**Ernst E 2003
***Ameye & Chee 2006

Glucosamine and chondroitin supplements have been extensively studied for the relief of symptoms in knee osteoarthritis. A review by Towheed et al (2005) concluded that glucosamine (sulphate or hydrochloride) was not superior to placebo for pain, stiffness and function as measured by the Western Ontario and McMaster University Osteoarthritis Index (WOMAC). There is some evidence that for patients with joint pain, who want to control symptoms with dietary supplements, taking 1500 mg with glucosamine sulphate may have beneficial symptomatic effects (Clegg et al 2006). However, there is no consensus regarding the use of glucosamine sulphate between international OA management guidelines. For example in the UK, NICE guidelines do not support the use of glucosamine sulphate in the management of OA (NICE 2008), whereas EULAR guidelines state that glucosamine sulphate and chondroitin sulphate have symptomatic effects in OA knee (Jordan et al 2003). Concerns have been raised about whether glucosamine causes abnormal glucose metabolism, asthma, hypersensitivity, or arteriosclerosis but there is little evidence to support these concerns.

DAIRY PRODUCTS, CALCIUM AND VITAMIN D

Of particular dietary importance to people with RA is calcium and vitamin D intake, necessary for maintaining strong and healthy bones and reducing the risk of osteoporosis (Department of Health 1998). Lower fat dairy products i.e. semi-skimmed or skimmed milk, reduced fat cheeses have the same calcium, if not more than the full fat products. Calcium enriched soya milks or other alternatives must be recommended to people who do not or cannot use dairy products as soya milk per se does not contain calcium. Vitamin D is generated by the action of UVB rays on the skin and is the most efficient source of vitamin D. There are some good dietary sources of vitamin D including fish oils, egg yolk, margarine and meat.

SECTION 2 COMPLEMENTARY THERAPIES

Patients and therapists often seek out complementary treatment to manage their rheumatic condition. Alternative therapies are used as a substitute for conventional approaches. Complementary therapies are used in addition to conventional treatment. These are described below. Many are used by appropriately trained therapists as adjuncts to conventional modalities (see Chs 8 & 11).

ACUPUNCTURE/ACUPRESSURE

Acupuncture involves the stimulation of points in the body with needles. Often, electrical stimulation is applied to the needles – electroacupuncture. In acupressure, the stimulation is by pressure from the fingers or sometimes special devices, such as the wrist-bands for treating nausea in pregnancy. Acupuncture was first discovered by the Chinese, and many modern practitioners still use ancient concepts, for example, that the needles influence the flow of energy in meridians. However, there is plenty of evidence that the needles stimulate several areas of the nervous system, releasing opioid peptides (popularly known as 'endorphins'). Therefore, many western practitioners are discarding the traditional concepts and regard acupuncture as a particular form of nerve stimulation. However, it is important to distinguish acupuncture from transcutaneous electrical nerve stimulation (TENS): TENS usually only has a temporary effect, whereas acupuncture's effect accumulates as the treatment is repeated. Usually a course of six or eight treatments is needed.

Although traditional Chinese theory seems to suggest that acupuncture can in some way treat the fundamental cause of the disease, in practice there is no evidence that acupuncture can modify the course of systemic diseases such as rheumatoid arthritis or ankylosing spondylitis. Its main contribution is in pain control. For example, reviews of nearly a dozen randomized controlled trials (RCTs) in osteoarthritis of the knee have shown acupuncture to be at least as effective as, and probably more effective than, non-steroidal anti-inflammatory drugs (NSAIDs) – for both controlling pain and improving function (White et al 2007). What was also impressive was that the effect of a course of treatment was still measurable after 6 months. These studies showed that true acupuncture alone was statistically significantly superior to placebo or 'sham' acupuncture alone.

For fibromyalgia, individual RCTs have reached different conclusions as to whether acupuncture, given as an adjunct to other treatments, reduces patients' symptoms. A recent review found that the overall evidence was not high quality, but that all the studies that used electroacupuncture were positive (Mayhew & Ernst 2006).

OSTEOPATHY AND CHIROPRACTIC

These complementary therapies, though differing slightly in training and approach, both use the techniques of massage, mobilisation and manipulation. They are most often used for spinal problems (neck pain, back pain), which are beyond the scope of this chapter. These treatments seem to have a good reputation for safety, though manipulation of the spine has been known to cause injuries to the nervous system, and to interfere with its blood supply causing stroke. Treatment should be given only by registered practitioners.

Some techniques, particularly mobilization, are used for arthritis in peripheral joints, such as OA of the hip or knee. This approach is similar to conventional manual therapy which is discussed in the Physical Therapies chapter (Ch. 8). Overall, mobilisation in rheumatic diseases seems best used as part of a comprehensive treatment programme (Fiechtner & Brodeur 2002). One small study suggested that manipulative therapy could provide additional pain relief to other treatments for fibromyalgia (Gamber et al 2002).

HOMEOPATHY

In homeopathy, natural substances are given in highly diluted preparations – so dilute that often none of the original substance may be present. Although this appears to be contrary to the laws of physics, and homeopaths have not yet demonstrated how it could work, nevertheless many patients have reported significant benefits from homeopathy. It seems likely that the very detailed history that is needed in finding the exact remedy can itself act as a powerful therapy. Homeopathy would appear to be very safe.

One RCT found no effect of homeopathy compared with placebo in rheumatoid arthritis (Fisher & Scott 2001), but a systematic review of homeopathy for people with OA found four RCTs which provided some supportive evidence, and recommended more research (Long & Ernst 2001). In fibromyalgia, two small studies found homeopathy significantly better than placebo in lessening tender point pain (Fisher et al 1989) and improving the quality of life and global health (Bell et al 2004).

HERBAL MEDICINE

This section refers to medicines made from plants or plant extracts, and not to the food supplements or individual phytochemicals discussed in the previous section or listed in Table 14.3. Several herbs, such as Devil's claw (*Harpagophytum procumbens*), willow bark extract, and nettle (*Urtica dioica*) are traditional folk treatments for painful conditions in many cultures. Recent research has increased the level of awareness of their side-effects as well as their interactions with many drugs.

Two reviews found no good evidence that any herb is beneficial for rheumatoid arthritis (Little & Parsons 2001a) or for osteoarthritis (Little & Parsons 2001b), other than those mentioned in the previous section. Many herbs are available for patients to purchase, but it seems sensible for health practitioners not to make recommendations unless they are qualified to do so. The situation also applies to Chinese herbs: prescribing them is a highly specialised skill that has to take into account individual dosage, particular combinations of herbs, significant variations in quality of the products, and toxicity.

BALNEOTHERAPY

This is treatment by bathing in warm water, usually with natural or added minerals or mud packs. Also known as 'spa therapy', it is often used on the European mainland and in Israel for inflammatory arthritis. Trials in patients with rheumatoid arthritis have generally shown that patients feel better after a course of balneotherapy, but the evidence is not good enough to draw conclusions (Verhagen et al 2003). In ankylosing spondylitis, one trial showed a short-lived effect compared with exercise alone (Altan et al 2006), but another study showed no effect of mud packs compared with fresh water (Codish et al 2005). There is some evidence that balneotherapy may be effective in fibromyalgia (Evcik et al 2002).

MAGNET THERAPY

There has been a considerable amount of laboratory research on the effects of magnetic fields in reducing the severity of pain, but rather few clinical trials. Magnets may be applied over the joint itself, or in wrist-bands in the hope of producing a systemic effect. Although there are some positive RCTs that seem to show magnets reduce pain from arthritis in the hip or knee (Harlow et al 2004, Wolsko et al 2004), because of problems with blinding the trials do not provide evidence strong enough to make recommendations.

TAI CHI

This eastern approach to physical exercise is suitable for older people, and includes a meditative element. It shows no overall effects in RA, but does improve the range of movement in ankle joints. It is also popular with patients, and it is one form of exercise that patients tend to continue to use (Han et al 2004). In elderly people with hip or knee OA, a recent study showed a trend to less benefit from tai chi than from hydrotherapy (Fransen et al 2007).

YOGA

A literature review found a small number of studies in patients with musculoskeletal conditions show some benefits, when compared with patients who did not practise yoga (Raub 2002).

SUMMARY

Diet is a popular intervention for people with musculoskeletal conditions. This might involve the exclusion of certain foodstuffs thought to aggravate symptoms, the addition of a supplement believed to ameliorate symptoms or a change of eating habits towards healthy eating for weight loss or weight maintenance and heart health. Although there is only limited scientific evidence to support either exclusion diets or dietary supplementation in the management of musculoskeletal conditions, dietary advice relevant to cardiovascular and bone health would benefit the majority and should be more widely available.

Alternative and complementary therapies are often used for chronic conditions. Acupuncture can produce pain relief in rheumatological conditions but there is no evidence that it can alter the course of the disease. Mobilisation of joints by osteopaths and chiropractors may be used as part of a multi-therapy approach. Homeopathy is safe and can be effective, though how much of the effect is due to the actual remedies is not known. Currently, there is insufficient evidence to recommend herbal remedies or other therapies.

STUDY ACTIVITIES

1. Further details of specific vitamins and minerals can be found in nutrition textbooks. Compile a 'pocket reference table' for your own use of vitamins and minerals. Headings might include: 'sources'; 'main role'; 'deficiency state'; and 'musculoskeletal relevance'.
2. Record exactly what you eat and drink over 4 days including at least one weekend day. Does your diet meet current dietary guidelines? Think of your vitamin and mineral requirements as well as protein, fat, carbohydrate and alcohol. How could you 'improve' your diet – what do you need to eat more of and what could you cut down on? How difficult would it be to make a major dietary change?
3. Undertake a dietary survey of patients you see over a week. How many of them have questions about diet and arthritis? How many of them have taken herbal medicines? What questions do they ask? Could you answer them? Where could you find the answers if you don't know? Where can you access patient advice regarding diet and arthritis?

CASE STUDY 14.1

Miss Hall has rheumatoid arthritis and is postmenopausal. In the past treatment has included intermittent oral steroids. Miss Hall's physical activity levels are reduced due to her disease state. Miss Hall has been trying a 'special diet' for six months during which time she has avoided all dairy products and red meat. She is suffering from tiredness and fatigue, more so than usual and has lost weight, which she puts down to her RA. When challenged, Miss Hall admits she doesn't really think that the 'diet' makes her feel any better and she admits that she finds it difficult and frustrating sticking to the diet. She feels hungry a lot of the time and her friends have commented on how thin she has become. Despite these effects, Miss Hall has continued with the diet hoping it will improve her arthritis.

Advice: Provide Miss Hall with an information leaflet on healthy eating. Discuss the nutritional requirements for a healthy diet and a healthy weight. Point out the risks of being underweight to bone health. Highlight the need for calcium and vitamin D for healthy bones and the benefits of fruit and vegetables for bone health and general health. As Miss Hall wishes to re-introduce the foods that she has excluded, suggest she keeps a record of everything she eats and drinks and note how she feels afterwards for example, if any symptoms of arthritis are provoked after eating dairy foods or meat. This action may help her assess for herself if the diet is appropriate and if not, how she can re-introduce the excluded foods.

CASE STUDY 14.2

Patient Gary Sowden
Male, aged 65 years   Height: 170 m Weight: 102 kg
Medical history
Hypertension 5 years

Myocardial Infarction (MI) 3 years ago
Dyslipidaemia
Clinical diagnosis of knee osteoarthritis
    6 months ago

(Continued)

CASE STUDY 14.2 (CONTINUED)

DXA (bone density scan) osteopaenia at lumbar spine and femoral neck

Medication

Paracetamol, NSAIDs, Antacid

Statins

Self-prescribed glucosamine sulphate

Social history

- Lives with wife (and dog)
- Non-smoker
- Alcohol: ~7–10 units per week

Lifestyle

- Exercise limited because of weight
- Diet: low fat, avoids dairy products because of raised cholesterol level, and uses Soya milk
- Avoids 'acidic' foods because of painful joints and 'heartburn'
- Patient feels that bowels are easily upset and medication causes constipation and nausea
- Mr Sowden is fed up with taking so many pills and is bored with his diet

Advice:

- Work out his body mass index (BMI = weight in kg/height in metres^2) and explain, sensitively, where this figure appears on a BMI chart – in the 'obese' category. Allow him to respond – how does this make him feel? Begin to explore his feelings and his attitude towards his weight. How does he feel his weight impacts on his life, for example, on his health, his hobbies, activities, marriage etc? Does he want to and feel able to address this? Is he at the stage where he is ready for change?
- In the first instance, suggest he keeps a food diary for a week or two to reveal his dietary intake. This may have some immediate impact on Mr Sowden himself. A completed food diary is a very useful tool for dietitians to use with patients at their initial appointments.
- Another suggestion might be that he could attend a slimming group – men do go and often do very well with peer support.
- Given his other dietary issues (raised cholesterol, osteopaenia and food avoidance), this is a more complex case and Mr Sowden should be referred to a registered dietitian in the hospital or community but your advice will have started Mr Sowden thinking about his eating habits and weight which will be very helpful when he attends his dietetic appointment.
- Discuss possible ways that Mr Sowden could safely increase his activity levels.
- What advice would you give if he asked you if he should see an osteopath or an acupuncturist?

USEFUL WEBSITES AND PATIENT INFORMATION

Arthritis Research Campaign (arc) website (www.arc.org.uk) accessed January 2009 – Diet and Arthritis.

Arthritis Care (www.arthritiscare.org.uk) accessed January 2009 Healthy Eating and Arthritis.

CAMEOL (Complementary and Alternative Medicine Evidence On line) at (www.rccm.org.uk/cameol) accessed January 2009.

Complementary and Alternative Medicine Specialist Library (/www.library.nhs.uk/CAM/) accessed January 2009.

National Osteoporosis Society (www.nos.org.uk) accessed January 2009 – Healthy Eating for Strong Bones.

British Dietetic Association 'Food facts' (www.bda.uk.com) accessed January 2009 – Diet and rheumatoid arthritis, Diet and osteoarthritis, Osteoporosis plus various information sheets for weight management and healthy eating.

Food Standards Agency (FSA) (www.eatwell.gov.uk) accessed January 2009.

Arthritis: Improve your health, ease pain, and live life to the full Dorling Kindersley, London, 2006.

Arthritis: Your questions answered Dorling Kindersley, London, 2007.

Ernst, E., Pittler, M., Wider, B., 2006. The Desktop Guide to Complementary and Alternative Medicine. Mosby: Edinburgh.

References and further reading

Altan, L., Bingol, U., Aslan, M., et al., 2006. The effect of balneotherapy on patients with ankylosing spondylitis. Scand. J. Rheumatol. 35 (4), 283–289.

Ameye, L.G., Chee, S.S., 2006. Osteoarthritis and nutrition. From nutraceuticals to functional foods: a systematic review of the scientific evidence. Arthritis Res. Ther. 8, R127.

Avenell, A., Handoll, H.H., 2003. A systematic review of protein and energy supplementation for hip fracture aftercare in older people. Eur. J. Clin. Nutr. 57 (8), 895–903.

Bell, I.R., Lewis, D.A., Brooks, A.J., et al., 2004. Improved clinical status in fibromyalgia patients treated with individualized homeopathic remedies versus placebo. Rheumatology (Oxford) 43 (5), 577–582.

Canter, P.H., Wider, B., Ernst, E., 2007. The antioxidant vitamins A, C, E and selenium in the treatment of arthritis: a systematic review of randomized controlled trials. Rheumatology Advance Access published May, 23.

Clegg, D.O., Reda, D.J., Harris, C.L., et al., 2006. Glucosamine, chondroitin sulfate, and the two in combination for painful knee osteoarthritis. N. Eng. J. Med. 354 (8), 795–808.

Cobb, C.S., Ernst, E., 2006. Systematic review of a marine nutriceutical supplement in clinical trials for arthritis: the effectiveness of the New Zealand green-lipped mussel Perna canaliculus. Clin. Rheumatol. 25 (3), 275–284.

Codish, S., Dobrovinsky, S., Abu, S.M., et al., 2005. Spa therapy for ankylosing spondylitis at the Dead Sea. Isr. Med. Assoc. J. 7 (7), 443–446.

Curtis, C.L., Rees, S.G., Little, C.B., et al., 2002. Pathologic indicators of degradation and inflammation in human osteoarthritis cartilage are abrogated by exposure to n-3 fatty acids. Arthritis Rheum. 46 (6), 1544–1553.

Department of Health. 1991. Dietary Reference Values for Food Energy and Nutrients for the United Kingdom: Report of the Panel on Dietary References Values of the Committee on Medical Aspects of Food Policy. The Stationary Office, London.

Department of Health. 1998. Nutrition and Bone Health: with particular reference to calcium and vitamin D., Report of the Subgroup on Bone Health, Working Group on the Nutritional Status of the Population of the Committee on Medical Aspects of Food and Nutrition Policy. The Stationary Office, London.

Ebringer, A., Wilson, C., 1996. The use of a low starch diet in the treatment of patients suffering from ankylosing spondylitis. Clin. Rheumatol. 15 (Suppl. 1), 62–66.

Ernst, E., 2003. Avocado-soybean unsaponifiables (ASU) for osteoarthritis - a systematic review. Clin. Rheumatol. 22 (4-5), 285–288.

Evcik, D., Kizilay, B., Gokcen, E., 2002. The effects of balneotherapy on fibromyalgia patients. Rheumatol. Int. 22 (2), 56–59.

Felson, D.T., 1988. Epidemiology of hip and knee osteoarthritis. Epidemiol. Rev. 10, 1–28.

Felson, D.T., Niu, J., Clancy, M., et al., 2007. Low levels of vitamin D and worsening of knee osteoarthritis: results of two longitudinal studies. Arthritis Rheum. 56, 129–136.

Fiechtner, J.J., Brodeur, R.R., 2002. Manual and manipulation techniques for rheumatic disease. Med. Clin. N. Am. 86 (1), 91–103.

Fisher, P., Scott, D.L., 2001. A randomized controlled trial of homeopathy in rheumatoid arthritis. Rheumatology (Oxford) 40 (9), 1052–1055.

Fisher, P., Greenwood, A., Huskisson, E.C., et al., 1989. Effect of homeopathic treatment on fibrositis (primary fibromyalgia). Brit. Med. J. 299 (6695), 365–366.

Food Standards Agency. 2002. Survey of Dioxins and Dioxin-like PCBs in Fish Oil Supplements (Number 26/02) www.food.gov.uk/multimedia/pdfs/26diox.pdf.

Fortin, P.R., Lew, R.A., Liang, M. H., et al., 1995. Validation of a meta-analysis: the effects of fish oil in rheumatoid arthritis. J. Clin. Epidemiol. 48, 1379–1390.

Fransen, M., Nairn, L., Winstanley, J., et al., 2007. Physical activity for osteoarthritis management: a randomized controlled clinical trial evaluating hydrotherapy or Tai Chi classes. Arthritis Rheum. 57 (3), 407–414.

Gamber, R.G., Shores, J.H., Russo, D.P., et al., 2002. Osteopathic manipulative treatment in conjunction with medication relieves pain associated with fibromyalgia syndrome: results of a randomized clinical pilot project. J. Am. Osteopath. Assoc. 102 (6), 321–325.

Goldberg, R.J., Katz, J., 2007. A meta-analysis of the analgesic effects of omega-3 polyunsaturated fatty acid supplementation for inflammatory joint pain. Pain 129, 210–223.

Goodson, N.J., Solomon, D.H., 2006. The cardiovascular manifestations of rheumatic diseases. Curr. Opin. Rheumatol. 18, 135–140.

Hafström, I., Ringertz, B., Spångberg, A., et al., 2001. A vegan diet free of gluten improves the signs and symptoms of rheumatoid arthritis: the effects on arthritis correlate with a reduction in antibodies to food antigens. Rheumatology 40 (10), 1175–1179.

Han, A., Robinson, V., Judd, M., et al., 2004. Tai chi for treating rheumatoid arthritis, Cochrane. Database Syst. Rev. (3) CD004849.

Hänninen, O., Kaartinen, K., Rauma, A.L., et al., 2000. Antioxidants in vegan diet and rheumatic disorders. Toxicology 155 (1-3), 45–53.

Harlow, T., Greaves, C., White, A., et al., 2004. Randomised controlled trial of magnetic bracelets for relieving pain in osteoarthritis of the hip and knee. Brit. Med. J. 329 (7480), 1450–1454.

Hedström, M., Ljungqvist, O., Cederholm, T., 2006. Metabolism and Catabolism in hip fracture patients. Nutritional and anabolic intervention-a review. Acta Orthop. 77 (5), 741–747.

Jordan, K.M., Arden, N.K., Doherty, M., et al., 2003. EULAR Recommendations: an evidence based approach to the management of knee osteoarthritis: Report of a task force of the standing committee for international clinical studies including therapeutic trials (ESCISIT). Ann. Rheum. Dis. 62, 1145–1155.

Leventhal, L.J., Boyce, E.G., Zurier, R.B., 1993. Treatment of rheumatoid arthritis with gamma-linolenic acid. Ann. Int. Med. 119, 867–873.

Little, C., Parsons, T., 2001a. Herbal therapy for treating rheumatoid arthritis. Cochrane Database Syst. Rev. CD002948.

Little, C.V., Parsons, T., 2001b. Herbal therapy for treating osteoarthritis. Cochrane Database Syst. Rev. CD002947.

Long, L., Ernst, E., 2001. Homeopathic remedies for the treatment of osteoarthritis: a systematic review. Brit. Homeopathic J. 90 (1), 37–43.

Mayhew, E., Ernst, E., 2006. Acupuncture for fibromyalgia–a systematic review of randomized clinical trials. Rheumatology (Oxford) 46 (5), 801–804.

McAlindon, T.E., Felson, D.T., Zhang, Y., et al., 1996. Relation of dietary intake and serum levels of vitamin D to progression of osteoarthritis of the knee among participants in the Framingham Study. Ann. Int. Med. 125, 353–359.

Mead, A., Atkinson, G., Albin, D., et al., 2006. Dietetic Guidelines on food and nutrition in the secondary prevention of cardiovascular disease – evidence from systematic reviews of randomized controlled trials. J. Hum. Nutr. Diet. 19 (6), 401–419 second update, January 2006.

Messier, S.P., Loeser, R.F., Miller, G.D., et al., 2004. Exercise and dietary weight loss in overweight and obese older adults with knee osteoarthritis: the Arthritis, diet and activity promotion trial. Arthritis Rheum. 50, 1501–1510.

Morley, J.E., Thomas, D.R., Wilson, M.G., 2006. Cachexia: pathophysiology and clinical relevance. Am. J. Clin. Nutr. 83, 735–743.

Müller, H., de Toledo, F.W., Resch, K.L., 2001. Fasting followed by vegetarian diet in patients with rheumatoid arthritis: a systematic review. Scand. J. Rheumatol. 30 (1), 1–10.

NICE, 2006. Clinical Guideline 43. Obesity: Guidance on the Prevention, Identification, Assessment and Management of Overweight and Obesity in Adults and Children. National Collaborating Centre for Chronic Conditions. Royal College of Physicians, London.

NICE, 2008. Clinical guideline 59. Osteoarthritis: the care and management of osteoarthritis. National Collaborating Centre for Chronic Conditions. Royal College of Physicians, London.

Pattison, D.J., Lunt, M., Welch, A., et al., 2007. Diet and Disability in Early Inflammatory Polyarthritis. Rheumatology 46 (Suppl. 1), i122.

Pattison, D.J., Silman, A.J., Goodson, N.J., et al., 2004. Vitamin C and the risk of developing inflammatory polyarthritis: prospective nested case-control study. Ann. Rheum. Dis. 63, 843–847.

Pattison, D.J., Symmons, D.P.M., Lunt, M., et al., 2005. Dietary β–cryptoxanthin and inflammatory polyarthritis: results from a population-based prospective study. Am. J. Clin. Nutr. 82, 451–455.

Raub, J.A., 2002. Psychophysiologic effects of Hatha Yoga on musculoskeletal and cardiopulmonary function: a literature review. J. Altern. Complem. Med. 8 (6), 797–812.

Rayman, M., Callaghan, A., 2006a. Polyunsaturated fatty acids in the treatment of arthritis. In: Nutrition and Arthritis. Blackwell Publishing, Oxford, pp. 146–183.

Rayman, M., Callaghan, A., 2006b. Role of micronutrients in the amelioration of rheumatoid arthritis and osteoarthritis. In: Nutrition and Arthritis. Blackwell Publishing, Oxford, pp. 112–145.

Rayman, M., Pattison, D.J., 2008. Dietary manipulation in musculoskeletal conditions. Best Pract. Res. Clin. Rheumatol. 22, 535–561.

Rennie, K.L., Hughes, J., Lang, R., et al., 2003. Nutritional Management of rheumatoid arthritis: a review of the evidence. J. Hum. Nutr. Diet. 16, 97–109.

Sköldstam, L., Hagfors, L., Johansson, G., 2003. An experimental study of a Mediterranean diet intervention for patients with rheumatoid arthritis. Ann. Rheum. Dis. 62, 208–214.

Towheed, T.E., Maxwell, L., Anastassiades, T.P., et al., 2005. Glucosamine therapy for treating osteoarthritis (Review). Cochrane Database Syst. Rev. (2) CD002946pub2.

Verhagen, A.P., Bierma-Zeinstra, S.M., Cardoso, J.R., et al., 2003. Balneotherapy for rheumatoid arthritis. Cochrane Database Syst. Rev. CD000518.

Watson, L., Byars, M.L., McGill, P., et al., 1993. Cytokine and prostaglandin production by monocytes of volunteers and rheumatoid arthritis patients treated with dietary supplements of blackcurrant seed oils. Brit. J. Rheumatol. 32, 1055–1058.

White, A., Foster, N.E., Cummings, M., et al., 2007. Acupuncture treatment for chronic knee pain: a systematic review. Rheumatology (Oxford) 46 (3), 384–390.

Wolsko, P.M., Eisenberg, D.M., Simon, L.S., et al., 2004. Double-blind placebo-controlled trial of static magnets for the treatment of osteoarthritis of the knee: results of a pilot study. Altern. Ther. Health Med. 10 (2), 36–43.

Woolf, A.D., 2007. What healthcare services do people with musculoskeletal conditions need? The role of rheumatology. Ann. Rheum. Dis. 66, 293–301.

Zhang, W., Doherty, M., Bardin, T., et al., 2006. EULAR evidence based recommendations for gout Part II: Management Report of a task force of the EULAR Standing Committee For International Clinical Studies Including Therapeutics (ESCISIT). Ann. Rheum. Dis. 65 (10), 1312–1324.

Zochling, J., van der Heijde, D., Dougados, M., et al., 2006. Current evidence for the management of ankylosing spondylitis: a systematic literature review for the ASAS/EULAR management recommendations in ankylosing spondylitis. Ann. Rheum. Dis. 65, 423–432.

Chapter 15

Pharmacological treatments in rheumatic diseases

Benazir Saleem MBChB MRCP Leeds Teaching Hospitals NHS Trust, Leeds, UK

Philip G. Conaghan MBBS PhD FRACP FRCP Leeds Institute of Molecular Medicine, University of Leeds and Leeds Teaching Hospitals NHS Trust, Leeds, UK

CHAPTER CONTENTS

KEY POINTS

- The pathogenesis of rheumatic diseases is diverse and often involves a complex mix of immunological and biomechanical mechanisms.
- Prior to prescribing pharmacological therapy, the needs of the patients, alternative non-pharmacological remedies and drug interactions (the pharmaco-dynamics and pharmaco-kinetics) need to be considered.
- Symptomatic management of pain involves analgesics (e.g. paracetamol, NSAIDs, opioids) and therapy is titrated according to severity of pain with such therapies tailored to individual needs and co-morbidities.
- For people with osteoarthritis, current therapies are aimed at symptom control. However for people with inflammatory arthritis, treatment of the underlying inflammatory process is required. This will involve anti-inflammatory drugs, glucocorticosteroids, and disease modifying anti-rheumatic drugs (DMARDs). There is evidence that DMARDs are able to modulate the disease process in inflammatory arthritis and especially with the newer biologic drugs, prevent progression of joint damage and even induce remission.

> ■ While increased understanding and knowledge of the pathogenesis of rheumatic diseases has resulted in increased therapeutic options, all pharmacological therapies are associated with adverse events. For optimal outcomes consumer and clinician education are essential, together with a multi-disciplinary approach for complex problems.

INTRODUCTION

In rheumatic diseases, pharmacotherapies are largely used for control of inflammatory processes or for pain control; such therapies are usually used in conjunction with non-pharmacological therapies such as muscle strengthening. Over the past decade, a greater understanding of the underlying mechanism involved in inflammatory arthritides has facilitated the development of new drugs and raised therapeutic goals. The aims of modern therapy are early diagnosis and prompt initiation of therapy to control inflammation, thereby preventing pain and subsequent joint damage with associated impaired function.

The decision regarding initiation and selection of drug therapy is not only based on the diagnosis, but on a person's age, past medical history (e.g. previous peptic ulcer), the presence of co-morbidities (e.g. renal impairment) and the presence of concomitant medications. Compliance with medication and patient expectations are other important concepts to be taken into consideration when prescribing. It is worth briefly reviewing the underlying processes for which pharmacotherapies are employed.

PAIN

The word pain comes from Latin 'poena' meaning fine or penalty. Pain is a complex phenomenon involving biopsychosocial interactions, and detailed mechanisms are beyond the scope of this chapter. In brief, pain perception peripherally is mediated by the terminal endings of finely myelinated A delta and of non-myelinated C fibres. Chemicals produced locally as a result of injury produce pain by direct stimulation or by sensitizing the nerve endings. A-delta fibres are responsible for the acute pain sensation, which may be followed by a slower onset, more diffuse pain mediated by the slower conducting C fibres. Most sensory input enters the spinal cord via the dorsal spinal roots. When the signal reaches the spinal cord, a signal is immediately sent back along motor nerves to the original site of the pain, triggering the muscles to contract (Kidd et al 2007). The pain signal is also sent to the brain. Only when the brain processes the signal and interprets it as pain do people become conscious of the sensation. Pain receptors and their nerve pathways differ in different parts of the body and the type of pain felt depends on the stimuli. These stimuli may be mechanical, thermal or chemical.

It is worth noting that the anatomical source of pain in many arthritic conditions is not always clear, and may often be multifactorial in nature. In early rheumatoid arthritis (RA) where synovitis is the primary pathology, the pain is presumably derived from inflammatory mediators in the synovium. In osteoarthritis (OA), the sources of pain are more controversial and may arise from the synovium or subchondral bone. The source of pain in lateral epicondylitis may be different again and relate to specific entheseal pathology. Musculoskeletal pain may be present without the classical signs of inflammation.

INFLAMMATION

Inflammation results in heat, redness, swelling, pain and loss of function. Acute inflammation involves: increased blood supply in the region of injury; an increase in local capillary permeability; exudation of vascular fluid; migration of inflammatory cells out of the blood vessels and into the surrounding tissue; and the release of mediators of inflammation. Acute inflammation may resolve or can lead to chronic inflammation, tissue death (necrosis), scarring or fibrosis.

However, the triggering event for inflammation in many inflammatory arthritides is unclear and both environmental and genetic triggers have been considered i.e. exposure to an environmental antigen in a genetically predisposed individual. It is known that a foreign antigen activates T-cells resulting in an inflammatory response. This process is paramount in the body's normal defence against infection, when the process is controlled and subject to inhibitory mechanisms. Uncontrolled and autonomous, this process can result in diseases such as rheumatoid arthritis (RA). In RA, activated T-cells secrete inflammatory cytokines that lead to chronic activation of B cells and immunoglobulin synthesis

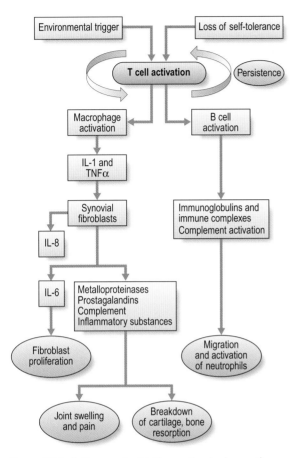

Figure 15.1 Pathogenesis of inflammation in rheumatic disease.

(see Fig. 15.1). The pro-inflammatory cytokines include interleukin (IL)-1 and tumour necrosis factor α (TNF) that in turn stimulate the production of more cytokines such as IL-6 and IL-8 (Jovanovic et al 1998). The result is pain, chronic synovitis and eventually local tissue and bone destruction.

PRINCIPLES OF CLINICAL PHARMACOLOGY

Before prescribing a therapeutic agent, two main questions must be answered:

- What does this drug do to the person? (pharmaco-dynamics)

Pharmadynamics is the study of the biochemical and physiological effects of drugs and the mechanism of drug action, and the relationship between drug concentration and effect.

- What does the person do to this drug? (pharmaco-kinetics).

Pharmacokinetics is a branch of pharmacology dedicated to the determination of the fate of substances administered externally to a living organism. In practice, this discipline is applied mainly to drug substances, though in principle it concerns itself with all manner of compounds ingested or otherwise delivered externally to an organism, such as nutrients, metabolites, hormones, toxins, etc. Pharmacokinetics is often divided into several areas including, but not limited to, the extent and rate of absorption, distribution, metabolism and excretion.

Absorption is the process of a substance entering the body. Distribution is the dispersion or dissemination of substances throughout the fluids and tissues of the body. Metabolism is the transformation of the substance and its daughter metabolites. Excretion is the elimination of the substances from the body. In rare cases, some drugs irreversibly accumulate in a tissue in the body.

When calculating dosage, it is important to know the half-life of the drug. This refers to the time required for the amount in the body to fall to 50% and is influenced by drug clearance and the volume of distribution. Drug clearance is defined as the volume of plasma that would contain the amount of drug excreted per minute. Drug clearance is a measure of the ability of the body to eliminate a drug from the circulation. It determines daily dosage. Drugs may be cleared by the renal system (mostly excreted, e.g. penicillin) or by the hepatic system (mostly metabolised e.g. paracetomol). Some drugs undergo substantial removal from the portal circulation by the liver after oral administration (e.g. Buprenorphine). This 'first-pass' effect can significantly reduce the amount of active drug that reaches the systemic circulation. The volume of distribution for a drug is determined by its degree of water or lipid solubility, the extent of plasma- and tissue-protein binding, and the perfusion of tissues. It gives an indication of initial or loading dose e.g. hydroxychloroquine (see later).

DRUGS USED IN RHEUMATIC DISEASES

ANALGESICS

Paracetamol

Paracetamol, also known as acetaminophen in the USA, is one of the most commonly used non-narcotic analgesics; it is also an anti-pyretic agent (lowers temperature). It is recommended as the first line analgesic in OA by the American College of Rheumatology (ACR) and European League against Rheumatism (EULAR). It is usually taken orally but may be used per rectum. Orally it is well absorbed and peak plasma concentrations are reached in 30–60 minutes. A proportion is bound to plasma proteins and the drug is inactivated in the liver. The plasma half-life of paracetamol is 2–4 hours. It is a weak inhibitor of cyclo-oxygenase (COX-1) (Warner et al 1999) at therapeutic doses.

The usual dose of paracetamol in adults is in the range of 1 gram three or four times daily. The incidence of side effects at therapeutic levels is low so routine monitoring is not required. Toxic doses (two to three times the maximum therapeutic dose) can cause fatal renal and liver failure. This effect is exacerbated by concomitant alcohol ingestion and in patients with active liver disease (Clissold 1986).

OPIOIDS

This group of drugs are used to relieve moderate to severe pain. The term opioid applies to substance that produces morphine-like effects. Opium is an extract of the juice of the poppy 'papaver somniferum' which has been used for social and medicinal purposes for thousands of years to induce euphoria, analgesia and sleep, and prevent diarrhoea. These effects are reflected in the potential toxicity of opioids in clinical use: nausea, constipation and confusion. Repeated administration can result in mild tolerance and (much more uncommonly) cause dependence. The most severe and serious adverse reaction associated with opioid use is respiratory depression, the mechanism behind fatal overdose.

Opioids are available in a variety of forms, and are usually used parenterally for acute pain, while oral and transdermal preparations have been developed for chronic ambulatory use. Some oral agents are also available in slow release preparations. A number of common drugs are now highlighted.

Morphine

Morphine can be administered parenterally (intramuscularly, subcutaneously, intravenously) and orally. The former route is preferred as the drug undergoes substantial first pass effect after oral dosing. Morphine has a half-life of 2–3 hours. Morphine commonly causes nausea and vomiting (and therefore is often given with an anti-emetic), constipation and drowsiness. It may also lead to respiratory depression and hypotension.

Pethidine

Unlike morphine, pethidine is a synthetic opioid, but has the same mechanism of action. It produces prompt but short lasting analgesia and is not recommended for chronic use because of a high risk of tolerance and dependency. Like morphine, it is absorbed well orally but undergoes extensive first pass metabolism and so is only used parenterally. The side-effect profile is similar to morphine but pethidine can also cause convulsions and other central nervous system disorders.

Codeine and codeine/paracetomol preparations

Codeine is an opium derivative pro-drug; once metabolised about 5–10% of codeine will be converted to morphine. It is usually prescribed orally as it is not as extensively metabolised on first pass through the liver. Codeine is effective for mild to moderate pain but may be too constipating for long-term use. The combination of codeine with paracetomol (generic name, co-codomol) is also effective for patients with mild to moderate pain, though evidence for superior efficacy of the combination is minimal.

Tramadol

Tramadol is a centrally acting analgesic, which possesses opioid agonist properties and activates monoaminergic spinal inhibition of pain. It is metabolised in the liver and excreted via the kidneys. It may be administered orally, rectally, intravenously or intramuscularly for patients with moderate to severe pain. Tramadol is about 10% as potent as morphine and consequently may have fewer of the typical opioid side effects. Tramadol is well tolerated in short term use with dizziness, nausea, sedation, dry mouth and sweating being the principal adverse effects.

Buprenorphine

Buprenorphine is a thebaine derivative, and its analgesic effect is due to partial agonist activity at μ-opioid receptors, i.e. when the molecule binds to a receptor, it is only partially activated in contrast to a full agonist such as morphine. Buprenorphine also has very high binding affinity for the μ receptor such that opioid receptor antagonists (e.g. naloxone) only partially reverse its effects. Buprenorphine is administered via a transdermal route in 35, 52.5 and 70 mcg/hour patches that deliver the dose over 96 hours. It is not administered orally, due to very high first-pass metabolism. Buprenorphine is metabolised by the liver and the metabolites are eliminated mainly through excretion into bile. The elimination half-life of buprenorphine is 20–73 hours (mean 37). Common adverse drug reactions associated with the use of buprenorphine are similar to those of other opioids and include: nausea and vomiting, drowsiness, dizziness, headache, itch, dry mouth, miosis, orthostatic hypotension, male ejaculatory difficulty, decreased libido and urinary retention. Constipation and central nervous system (CNS) effects are seen less frequently than with morphine. Hepatic necrosis and hepatitis with jaundice have been reported with the use of buprenorphine, especially after intravenous injection of crushed tablets.

Fentanyl

Fentanyl transdermal patches work by releasing fentanyl into body fats, which then slowly release the drug into the bloodstream over 72 hours, allowing for long lasting relief from pain. Fentanyl patches are manufactured in five patch sizes: 12.5 micrograms/h, 25 μg/h, 50 μg/h, 75 μg/h, and 100 μg/h. Rate of absorption is dependent on a number of factors and body temperature, skin type and placement of the patch can have major effects. Fentanyl is metabolised by the liver and excreted renally. The side effect profile is similar to buprenorphine.

ANTI-INFLAMMATORY DRUGS

Anti-inflammatory drugs are used extremely commonly across the world for acute and chronic musculoskeletal pain. The drugs may be classified into three categories:

1. Non-steroidal anti-inflammatory drugs (NSAIDs)
2. Glucocorticosteroids
3. Disease modifying anti-rheumatic drugs (DMARDs).

NSAIDs

This very commonly used group of drugs is effective in reducing the immediate signs and symptoms of

Table 15.1 Common non-steroidal anti-inflammatory drugs (NSAIDs) with usual oral daily dosage

NSAID	DAILY DOSE (MG)
Meloxicam	7.5–15
Ibuprofen	1200–2400
Diclofenac	75–150
Naproxen	500–1000
Indometacin	50–150
Celecoxib	100–400
Etoricoxib	60–120

inflammation, although much of their use is as analgesics in conditions where the underlying inflammatory nature of the condition is not always clear (e.g. commonly used over-the-counter for headaches and lower back pain). NSAIDs are commonly used in patients suffering from all types of inflammatory arthritis and are also recommended for patients with OA if paracetamol is ineffective.

There are many different NSAIDs currently available and a list of common NSAIDs with their usual daily doses are shown in Table 15.1. The dose used in inflammatory arthritis is often higher than that used in osteoarthritis or soft tissue problems. The usual rule in dosing is to use the lowest effective dose for the shortest possible period of time.

In general the NSAID mechanism of action is by inhibition of cyclooxygenase and thus inhibition of the production of prostaglandins and thromboxanes. There are two cyclooxygenase enzymes, COX-1 and COX-2. COX-1 is important in producing prostaglandins with physiological functions such as protection of the gastrointestinal mucosa and vascular homeostasis; its levels are reasonably constant. On the other hand, COX-2 is up-regulated at sites of inflammation and it is responsible for the production of inflammatory mediators. All NSAIDs vary in their degree of COX-1 and COX-2 selectivity.

NSAIDs can be given orally, topically, intramuscularly or per rectum. The drugs tend to be well absorbed in the gastrointestinal tract and are highly plasma bound. They only have a small first pass effect. There is no consistent evidence that one NSAID is superior to another in terms of analgesic or anti-inflammatory efficacy. However they do have different pharmacokinetic properties according to half life. Drugs such as indometacin, diclofenac and ibuprofen have short half lives (<6 hours), whilst naproxen and meloxicam have long

Table 15.2 Common side-effects of NSAIDs

Gastrointestinal	Nausea, diarrhoea Dyspepsia, bleeding, ulceration
Hypersensitivity	Rashes, angio-oedema, bronchospasm
Cardiovascular	Potential increased risk of ischaemic heart disease and stroke, hypertension
Renal	Fluid retention, renal impairment
Central nervous system	Headache, dizziness, depression

half lives (>10 hours). In addition, many of these agents come in slow-release or modified release preparations to extend their half-life. This difference in half life is important for daily dosing regimens, and it is worth considering what time of day the person's symptoms are greatest.

Topical NSAIDs may be useful for knee and hand OA (Moore et al 1998). They generally require multiple daily applications. Their advantages are fewer serious side effects because they do not achieve high plasma levels. The most common problems are rash and pruritis (itching) at the application site.

As a class, oral NSAIDs are associated with a large number of side effects, as presented in Table 15.2. The gastrointestinal side effects are the most frequent, and risk factors for gastrointestinal side effects include: age over 65 years, history of peptic ulcer disease, use of oral corticosteroids or anticoagulants. Given the large numbers of people who use NSAIDs, they are associated with a significant mortality and morbidity. There are also important clinical pharmacodynamic interactions associated with NSAID use: they can antagonise antihypertensive medication leading to high potassium levels.

NSAIDs and cardiovascular risk

In order to overcome the considerable gastrointestinal (GI) toxicity (see Table 15.2) and mortality associated with NSAIDs, selective COX-2 inhibitors were developed (e.g. celecoxib, etoricoxib), and initial studies suggested some benefit from these agents in reducing serious gastrointestinal complications. However the withdrawal from the market of one of these agents, rofecoxib, due to an increased risk of thrombotic vascular complications, led to a re-evaluation and understanding that both COX-2 and traditional NSAIDs have a pro-thrombotic

tendency. All COX-2 agents and NSAIDs should be used with caution (lowest dose for shortest period of time) or where possible avoided completely in people with cardiovascular risk factors or who are taking aspirin (as aspirin is used in people with increased cardiovascular risk, but also because of concerns about an interaction between NSAIDs and aspirin that may reduce the benefits of aspirin) (Graham 2006). Another strategy for reducing GI side effects is co-prescription of gastroprotective agents such as proton-pump inhibitors (PPI eg omeprazole); in the UK, the National Institute for Health and Clinical Excellence (NICE) have recommended that all people with osteoarthritis requiring NSAIDs for moderate to long term use should have a PPI co-prescribed, based on a cost-effectiveness analysis (Conaghan et al 2008).

CORTICOSTEROIDS

Oral corticosteroids (also known as glucocorticosteroids) have been used in patients with RA and other inflammatory joint conditions for many years. Corticosteroids are effective in rapidly reducing inflammation. Some patients require low dose maintenance doses of corticosteroid (<10 mg/day) but long-term usage and higher doses are associated with increased side effects. Patients with severe RA, vasculitis or active systemic lupus erythematosus (SLE) may require intravenous, high-dose corticosteroids.

Corticosteroids are powerful immunosuppressants. The corticosteroid receptor is a transcription factor, and after binding the receptor –steroid complex enters the cell nucleus and binds to specific DNA sequences modifying DNA transcriptions. The result is inhibition of various leucocytes, especially lymphocytes and macrophages. Corticosteroids can reduce prostaglandin and leukotriene production and antagonise the effect of some pro-inflammatory cytokines.

The pharmacokinetics of corticosteroids depends on the preparation. The most widely used, prednisolone, has a half-life of 2–3 hours. Other preparations include methylprednisolone, hydrocortisone and triamcinolone. Corticosteroid therapy may be associated with adverse effects (see Table 15.3), which are generally related to the cumulative dose of drug. Of particular concern is the ability of corticosteroids to induce bone loss and osteoporosis. All patients requiring long-term steroid therapy (e.g. prednisolone >7.5 mg/day for 3 months) require bone protection therapy with a calcium supplement and probably a bisphosphonate (e.g. alendronate).

Table 15.3 The adverse effects of corticosteroid therapy

Musculoskeletal	Osteoporosis
	Myopathy
	Avascular necrosis of the femoral head
Immunological	Increased susceptibility to infection
Endocrine	Truncal obesity, moon-like face
	Hyperglycaemia or frank diabetes
	Acne
	Hirsuitism
	Salt and water retention
Dermatological	Thinning of skin
	Increased fragility of skin
Cardiovascular	Hypertension
	Exacerbation of congestive heart failure
Gastrointestinal	Peptic ulceration
	Reduced rate of ulcer healing
	Pancreatitis
Neurological	Cataracts
	Psychosis
	Change in mood (especially high doses)

Long-term oral corticosteroid therapy leads to suppression of the body's own hypothalamic pituitary – adrenal axis. Abrupt cessation of the drug may induce a withdrawal syndrome involving fatigue, myalgia, anorexia, weight loss and sometimes collapse with hypotension and electrolyte imbalance. To prevent this all patients should be educated, wear medi-alert bracelets and undergo gradual reduction of steroid dose prior to cessation.

Intra–articular corticosteroid

Intra-articular corticosteroids are important in the management of mono-articular inflammatory arthritis and therapy-resistant joints in polyarthritis. They are also used for their short-term (up to approximately 4 weeks) analgesic efficacy in common musculoskeletal disorders such as OA knee, subacromial impingement syndrome, tennis elbow and carpal tunnel syndrome. Corticosteroids are also used in caudal epidurals for patients suffering from radicular-pattern leg pain.

Most commonly used corticosteroid preparations for intra articular joint injections are hydrocortisone, methylprednisolone and triamcinolone. The dose used depends largely on the joint to be injected, although there is little consensus across clinicians on the type or dose of steroid recommended. For example, a knee may require 80 mg of methylprednisolone and an elbow may require 40 mg. 4 mg of

methylprednisolone or triamcinolone and 20 mg of hydrocortisone are equivalent to 5 mg prednisolone.

The long-term side-effects of intra-articular corticosteroids are unclear with no good human studies and animal model evidence for both beneficial (related to effects on synovitis) and detrimental effects on cartilage. However, the detrimental consequences of persistent synovitis versus the side effects of the steroid need to be considered. As a general rule, an individual joint should not be injected more than 3–4 times a year. Following an intra-articular corticosteroid patients are advised to rest the relevant joint for 24 hours and monitor for signs and symptoms of infection. Serious side-effects are highly unlikely, with the most important being septic arthritis. Occasionally patients notice a flare in their joint pain within the first 24 hours after an injection. This usually settles on its own within a couple of days. Occasionally with intra-articular and peri-articular injections some thinning (loss of subcutaneous fat) or change in the colour of the skin may occur at the injection site, so care needs to be taken in areas where appearance may be important. The risk of side-effects, particularly thinning of the skin, is greatest with the stronger corticosteroid preparations.

DISEASE MODIFYING ANTI–RHEUMATIC DRUGS

These drugs modify the inflammatory process in patients with RA and other inflammatory arthritides. In modern management of RA, disease modifying anti-rheumatic drugs (DMARDs) are initiated at time of diagnosis to control inflammation, prevent joint damage and preserve function and quality of life. These drugs are slow to work and it often takes weeks before any clinical effect is noticeable. There is no consensus on the order of usage if a drug is stopped due to lack of efficacy or toxicity, and there is increasing use of combination therapies with evidence-based therapeutic synergy. The more commonly prescribed DMARDs are now briefly reviewed.

Methotrexate

Methotrexate (MTX) is an established treatment for inflammatory joint conditions and is commonly the first DMARD used for RA. The use of MTX has escalated since the 1980s with good evidence now available for its long term effectiveness as a single agent and part of combination therapy with other DMARDs and biologic agents. The safety profile has been carefully studied and documented with guidelines for its use and monitoring (Pincus et al 2003).

Methotrexate acts as a folate antagonist by inhibiting the enzyme dihydrofolate reductase, which reduces intracellular folate. This folate is required for the synthesis of purines, important in cell replication. Methotrexate is commonly prescribed orally with a bioavailability of about 65%. It can also be given subcutaneously if the oral route is not tolerated. The half-life is 5–6 hours and about 50% is excreted via the renal route.

Most patients require a dose of methotrexate of about 15–20 mg given once per week (maximum dose 25 mg per week). Patients are prescribed folic acid supplements to reduce the common, mild adverse effects of MTX such as nausea or mouth ulcers. Other serious side-effects include bone marrow suppression and abnormal liver function tests. The incidence of serious adverse events is reduced by regular monitoring of full blood count (FBC) and liver function tests (LFT). It must be used with caution in patients with renal impairment as the risk of adverse events is increased. Methotrexate is potentially teratogenic (causing birth defects) so pregnancy is contraindicated whilst the patient is taking the drug and for 3 months after stopping. The consumption of alcohol is also contraindicated in patients on MTX.

Sulphasalazine

Sulphasalazine (SAS) is a combination of sulphapyridine, an antibacterial agent, and 5 aminosalicylic acid, which has anti-inflammatory properties. It is commonly used for the treatment of RA, peripheral joint disease in ankylosing spondylitis (AS) and psoriatic arthritis (PsA) and inflammatory bowel conditions such as ulcerative colitis (UC).

SAS is administered orally at doses of 1–1.5 grams twice a day. The dose is gradually increased as this improves tolerability. Side effects include nausea, upper abdominal pain and rash. Rarely a leucopenia (low white blood cells) is observed. Regular blood monitoring (FBC) will allow early detection of haematological abnormalities. There have been no accounts of teratogenicity (abnormalities to the developing foetus) but it can induce a reversible reduction in sperm count.

Antimalarials, e.g. hydroxychloroquine (HCQ)

Hydroxychloroquine is probably the weakest acting of the DMARDs. It tends to be used in combination with other drugs in patients with RA and in the arthritis of SLE. The exact mechanism of action is unknown but it is thought to have an effect on the signal transduction pathway, inhibiting pro-inflammatory gene expression. The bioavailability is variable and ranges from 20–100% but is constant within an individual. It has a long half-life of 40 days and hence may take 3 months to achieve its full effect. As a consequence, a loading dose of 200 mg twice a day is given for 1 month before reducing to a standard dose of 200 mg once a day.

The anti-malarials are the least toxic of all DMARDs. Rarely, they can cause myopathy, abnormal skin pigmentation and peripheral neuropathy. Of most concern, although rare, is irreversible retinopathy resulting in permanent visual loss. It is recommended that baseline ophthalmology screening (visual acuity and assessment for blurred vision) is performed if patients have pre-existing ocular pathology or visual disturbance, impaired renal function or are over the age of 60.

Leflunomide

Leflunomide is a competitive inhibitor of pyrimidine synthesis. It is primarily used in RA and prevents the multiplication of pro-inflammatory lymphocytes. After oral administration it undergoes rapid chemical conversion to its active metabolite. This metabolite has a long half-life of 15 to 18 days. Therefore, like HCQ, leflunomide requires a loading dose to achieve steady state concentrations. The loading dose of 100 mg once a day for 3 days is however often omitted in clinical practise because of poor tolerability. The usual maintenance dose is 10–20 mg per day. The most important adverse reactions to leflunomide are hepatic. Other side effects include diarrhoea, nausea, weight loss, rashes, hair loss, teratogenicity and hypertension. Regular monitoring of blood pressure, full blood count (FBC), urea and electrolytes (U&E's) and lung function tests (LFTs) are required.

TUMOUR NECROSIS FACTOR ANTAGONIST AGENTS

Tumour necrosis factor (TNF α) is a pivotal pro inflammatory cytokine that is released by activated monocytes, macrophages and T lymphocytes (see Fig. 15.1). It promotes inflammatory responses that are important in the pathogenesis of RA (Bazzoni & Beutler 1996, Taylor et al 2000) TNF binds to

2 receptors, the type 1 receptor (p55) and the type 2 receptor (p75). The advent of TNF antagonist therapies (etanercept, adalimubab, infliximab) has markedly improved control of inflammation in RA and reduced radiographic damage progression (Klareskog et al 2004, Maini et al 1999, Weinblatt et al 2006). They have also successfully been used in AS (Baraliakos et al 2005, Marzo-Ortega et al 2005), PsA (Antoni et al 2005, Mease et al 2006) and inflammatory bowel disease. Superior efficacy is observed when TNF antagonists are used in combination with MTX. Currently in the UK, the use of these therapies is limited to patients that have failed traditional DMARDs and have high levels of disease activity.

Etanercept is a soluble fusion protein composed of two dimers, each with an extra cellular, ligand-binding portion of the higher affinity type 2 TNF receptor (p75) linked to the Fc portion of human IgG1, thereby preventing each from binding to its respective receptors (Olsen & Stein 2004). It is administered subcutaneously (50mg once a week or 25mg twice a week) and takes 50 hours to reach peak concentrations. The half-life is around 4 days. It can be prescribed as mono-therapy but data from clinical trials show superior efficacy when taken with methotrexate (Klareskog et al 2004).

Adalimubab is a recombinant human IgG1 monoclonal antibody that binds to human TNF α with high affinity. Therefore it impairs both cytokine binding to its receptors and lysing cells that express TNF α on their surface. It is administered subcutaneously reaching peak concentrations after 130 hours. Adalimubab may be prescribed as mono-therapy but like etanercept superior efficacy is seen when combined with methotrexate.

Infliximab is a chimeric IgG1 anti-TNF α antibody containing the antigen binding region of a mouse antibody and the constant region of a human antibody. It binds to soluble and membrane bound TNF α with high affinity, impairing the biding of TNF α to its receptor. In pharmacokinetic terms, there appears to be marked variations among patients, with trough levels varying by a factor of 100 following the standard dose of 3mg per kilogram every 8 weeks given intravenously. However when used as mono-therapy patients often experienced a loss of response over time due to the development of anti-infliximab antibodies (human anti-chimeric antibodies). Combination therapy with methotrexate reduces the tendency to form antibodies.

Table 15.4 The adverse events of TNF antagonist agents

Infection	Serious bacterial and opportunistic infections (e.g. aspergillosis) have been reported Increased risk of tuberculosis (TB)
Malignant disease	TNF antagonists do not confer an increased risk of malignancy above that of RA with the possible exception of skin malignancy
Heart disease	May exacerbate heart failure
Injection site/ infusion reactions	Redness and itching at injection site Infusion reactions include mild headache or nausea or in 2% hypersensitivity reaction
Autoimmune response	Induction of anti-nuclear antibody (ANA), double stranded DNA and anti-nuclear cytoplasmic antibody. However, clinical manifestations of drug induced lupus or vasculitis are surprisingly rare
Lung disease	Exacerbation of existing lung fibrosis

Adverse effects of TNF antagonist therapy

Similar adverse events have been documented in all 3 TNF antagonist agents (see Table 15.4). They form the basis of the screening (including TB screening) and monitoring procedures for all patients prior to starting and whilst receiving TNF antagonist therapy.

OTHER BIOLOGIC AGENTS

Rituximab

Rituximab is a chimeric anti-CD20 monoclonal antibody that causes a selective depletion of CD20+ B cells. B cells can produce autoantibodies that, in some diseases, are directly pathogenic (Dass et al 2006). This drug was originally developed for the treatment of refractory CD20+ B cell non Hodgkin's lymphoma. In 2006, Rituximab in conjunction with methotrexate was licensed in the US and the EU for use in patients with active, moderate to severe RA that is refractory to treatment with TNF antagonist agents. The results from two major trials (Cohen et al 2006, Emery et al 2006) highlight successful clinical outcomes in terms of laboratory, patient-reported and radiographic measures.

Rituximab is given as two infusions of 1g on days 1 and 15 with infusions of methylprednisolone. The mean half-life is 20 days. The main adverse events are minor infections and there have been no reported cases of TB. Most adverse infusion reactions occur during or immediately after the infusion. Up to 30% of patients experience pruritis, urticaria (allergic reaction in which red round wheals develop on the skin), pyrexia, throat irritation and hypo- and hypertension. The incidence of infusion reactions is reduced by concomitant intravenous corticosteroid. Small studies have also shown rituximab to be beneficial in connective tissue disease such as SLE (Eisenberg 2006).

Abatacept

The pathogenesis of RA is dependent on T cell activation. This requires two signals: firstly presentation of the antigen to the T cell receptor and secondly various co-stimulatory molecules. Abatacept is a soluble fusion protein that targets co-stimulation. It has demonstrated good results in patients with RA that are non responsive to MTX or failed previous TNF antagonist therapy (Genovese et al 2005, Kremer 2005). Abatacept (10 mg per kg) is given as an infusion every month and has a favourable safety profile, with no increase in malignancy or TB.

CONCLUSION

The therapeutic options for rheumatic diseases continue to expand and modern biologic therapies

mean that at least RA patients are reaching levels of disease control previously thought impossible; these drugs are expensive and place a huge burden on health systems. For the vast majority of musculoskeletal patients with OA or mechanical joint pain, our use of pharmacological analgesia remains largely empiric with few good trials of how to optimally use individual drugs or combination therapies. Despite increasing therapeutic options, a multi disciplinary approach remains key to the management of patients with rheumatic diseases.

STUDY ACTIVITIES

1. Access the NICE web site (http://guidance.nice.org.uk/) and identify the published guidelines for the management of 1) OA and 2) RA. Prepare a list of all pharmacological approaches.
2. Access the Arthritis Research Campaign (http://www.arc.org.uk), the Arthritis Foundation (http://www.arthritis.org) and Arthritis Care (http://www.arthritiscare.org.uk/home) websites.
   - Identify all patient information leaflets that would be applicable to a patient presenting to a therapist with difficulties with pain control. Consider five main messages on pharmacological approaches that you can identify from the information in these leaflets. List these and keep them for future reference.

References and further reading

Antoni, C.E., Kavanaugh, A., Kirkham, B., et al., 2005. Sustained benefits of infliximab therapy for dermatologic and articular manifestations of psoriatic arthritis: results from the infliximab multinational psoriatic arthritis controlled trial (IMPACT). Arthrit. Rheum. 52 (4), 1227–1236.

Baraliakos, X., Brandt, J., Listing, J., et al., 2005. Outcome of patients with active ankylosing spondylitis after two years of therapy with etanercept: clinical and magnetic resonance imaging data. Arthrit. Rheum. 53 (6), 856–863.

Bazzoni, F., Beutler, B., 1996. The tumor necrosis factor ligand and receptor families. N. Engl. J. Med. 334 (26), 1717–1725.

Clissold, S.P., 1986. Paracetamol and phenacetin. Drugs 32 (Suppl. 4), 46–59.

Cohen, S.B., Emery, P., Greenwald, M.W., et al., 2006. Rituximab for rheumatoid arthritis refractory to anti-tumor necrosis factor therapy: Results of a multicenter, randomized, double-blind, placebo-controlled, phase III trial evaluating primary efficacy and safety at twenty-four weeks. Arthrit. Rheum. 54 (9), 2793–2806.

Conaghan, P.G., Dickson, J., Grant, R.L., 2008. Care and management of osteoarthritis in adults: summary of NICE guidance. Br. Med. J. 336, 502–503.

Dass, S., Vital, E.M., Emery, P., et al., 2006. Rituximab: novel B-cell depletion therapy for the treatment of rheumatoid arthritis. Expert Opin. Pharmaco. 7 (18), 2559–2570.

Eisenberg, R., 2006. Targeting B cells in SLE: the experience with rituximab treatment (anti-CD20). Endocr. Metab. Immune Disord. Drug Targets 6 (4), 345–350.

Emery, P., Fleischmann, R., Filipowicz-Sosnowska, A., et al., 2006. The efficacy and safety of rituximab in patients with active rheumatoid arthritis despite methotrexate treatment: results of a phase IIB randomized, double-blind, placebo-controlled, dose-ranging trial. Arthrit. Rheum. 54 (5), 1390–1400.

Genovese, M.C., Becker, J.C., Schiff, M., et al., 2005. Abatacept for rheumatoid arthritis refractory to tumor necrosis factor alpha inhibition. N. Engl. J. Med. 353 (11), 1114–1123.

Graham, D.J., 2006. COX-2 Inhibitors, other NSAIDs and cardiovascular risk; the seduction of common sense. J. Am. Med. Assoc. 296 (13), 1653–1656.

Jovanovic, D.V., Di Battista, J.A., Martel-Pelletier, J., et al., 1998. Il-7 stimulates the production and expression of pro-inflammatory cytokines, IL-beta and TNF-alpha by human macropgages. J. Immunol. 160, 3513–3521.

Kidd, B.L., Langford, R.M., Wodehouse, T., 2007. Arthritis and pain. Current approaches in the treatment of arthritic pain. Arth. Res. Ther. 9 (3), 214.

Klareskog, L., van der Heijde, D., de Jager, J.P., et al., 2004. Therapeutic effect of the combination of etanercept and methotrexate compared with each treatment alone in patients with rheumatoid arthritis: double-blind randomised controlled trial. The Lancet 363 (9410), 675–681.

Kremer, J.M., 2005. Selective costimulation modulators: a novel approach for the treatment of rheumatoid arthritis. J. Clin. Rheumatol. 11 (Suppl. 3), S55–S862.

Maini, R., St Clair, E.W., Breedveld, F., et al., 1999. Infliximab (chimeric anti-tumour necrosis factor alpha monoclonal antibody) versus placebo in rheumatoid arthritis patients receiving concomitant methotrexate: a randomised phase III trial. ATTRACT study group. The Lancet 354 (9194), 1932–1939.

Marzo-Ortega, H., McGonagle, D., Jarrett, S., et al., 2005. Infliximab in combination with methotrexate in active ankylosing spondylitis: a clinical and imaging study. Ann. Rheum. Dis. 64 (11), 1568–1575.

Mease, P.J., Kivitz, A.J., Burch, F.X., et al., 2006. Continued inhibition of radiographic progression in patients with psoriatic arthritis following 2 years of treatment with etanercept. J. Rheumatol. 33 (4), 712–721.

Moore, R.A., Tramèr, M.R., Carroll, D., et al., 1998. Quantitative systematic review of topically applied non-steroidal anti-inflammatory drugs. Br. Med. J. 316 (7128), 333–338.

Olsen, N.J., Stein, C.M., 2004. New drugs for rheumatoid arthritis. N. Engl. J. Med. 350 (21), 2167–2179.

Pincus, T., Yazici, Y., Sokka, T., et al., 2003. Methotrexate as the "anchor drug" for the treatment of early rheumatoid arthritis. Clin. Exp. Rheumatol. 21 (5 Suppl. 31), S179–S185.

Taylor, P.C., Peters, A.M., Paleolog, E., et al., 2000. Reduction of chemokine levels and leukocyte traffic to joints by tumor necrosis factor alpha blockade in patients with rheumatoid arthritis. Arthrit. Rheum. 43 (1), 38–47.

Warner, T.D., Giuliano, F., Vojnovic, I., et al., 1999. Nonsteroid drug selectivities for cyclo-oxygenase-1 rather than cyclo-oxygenase-2 are associated with human gastrointestinal toxicity: a full in vitro analysis. Proc. Natl. Acad. Sci. USA 96 (13), 7563–7568.

Weinblatt, M.E., Keystone, E.C., Furst, D.E., et al., 2006. Long-term efficacy and safety of adalimu-mab plus methotrexate in patients with rheumatoid arthritis: ARMADA 4 year extended study. Ann. Rheum. Dis. 65 (6), 753–759.

Chapter 16

Inflammatory arthritis

Anne O'Brien MPhil Grad Dip Phys MCSP School of Health and Rehabilitation, MacKay Building, University of Keele, Keele, UK

Catherine Backman PhD OT(C) FCAOT Department of Occupational Science & Occupational Therapy, The University of British Columbia, Vancouver, BC, Canada

CHAPTER CONTENTS

KEY POINTS

- Initial detailed assessment is important in identifying where therapies can be most efficacious – opportunities for subsequent review allow timely response, especially in flares.
- Early therapy interventions minimise inflammation, pain, joint damage, deconditioning, and functional limitation.
- Self-management programmes that emphasize self efficacy and behaviour change improve health outcomes in RA.
- Physical activity is vital to maintaining activities of daily living and quality of life.
- Work disability can be delayed or prevented.
- Relate any exercise to improving performance of individually relevant functional tasks; individualise range, resistance, eccentric, concentric muscle work, length of hold of contraction

© 2010 Elsevier Ltd
DOI: 10.1016/B978-0-443-06934-5.00016-4

- Wherever possible, minimise pain first
- Avoid uncontrolled end of range movements
- Aim to improve exercise tolerance as well as increasing range of movement/muscle strength and joint stability
- Reassure new exercisers that joint/muscle aches may last up to 30–60 minutes after exercise – this is normal!
- Dosage should be individualised – most benefit from some daily exercise (ARC, Keep Moving leaflet 2005)
- Modify exercise during a flare; focus on maintaining range but without resistance
- Minimise use of equipment so exercise can easily be performed at home
- Written information should support exercise instructions and include 'SOS' contact details.

INTRODUCTION

Inflammatory arthritis is a category of rheumatic conditions involving inflammation of the synovial joints and includes specific forms such as rheumatoid arthritis, psoriatic arthritis, systemic lupus erythematosus, ankylosing spondylitis, reactive arthritis and juvenile idiopathic arthritis, among others. This chapter will focus on rheumatoid arthritis (RA), as a common presentation of inflammatory arthritis.

RA is a systemic, autoimmune disease characterized by symmetrical involvement of the peripheral joints, especially the small joints of the hands and feet, wrists, elbows, shoulders, knees and cervical spine. Symptoms include joint pain, stiffness and generalized fatigue, with exacerbations and remissions. Its aetiology is unknown and there is no cure. Despite significant recent improvements in medical management, RA remains a chronic condition resulting in mild to severe limitations in mobility and participation in everyday activities. RA has an impact across the spectrum of International Classification of Functioning, Disability and Health (ICF: World Health Organization, 2002) (see Ch. 4). In terms of body structure and function, joint mobility, muscle function, hand strength and dexterity are frequently impaired. Activity limitations, such as difficulty walking or handling objects, may subsequently restrict participation in self care, household work, employment, social relationships and leisure. The available resources and way a person responds to their illness and the challenges it presents

(personal characteristics) influences perceived health, as will the environment, such as accessibility of the physical or built environment or support provided by institutional policies. For example, work disability begins early in RA, affecting over one-third, depending on disease severity, age of onset and job demands (Burton et al 2006). RA has a substantive physical, psychosocial, and economic impact. Rehabilitation services are important in maintaining, restoring and improving patient function as well as enhancing quality of life.

CHARACTERISTICS OF RHEUMATOID ARTHRITIS

PREVALENCE AND INCIDENCE

The prevalence of RA is remarkably consistent at 0.5–1% of the population in Western nations and women are affected twice as much as men (Kremers & Gabriel 2004, Symmons et al 2002). There is a genetic susceptibility, supported by a higher prevalence in North American aboriginal populations (up to 7%) and lower rates in China, Japan and rural Africa (Ferucci et al 2004). Incidence varies but is typically close to 40 per 100,000 (Symmons 2002), although declining over the past few decades, possibly due to increased oral contraceptive use, dietary influences and cohort effects (Symmons 2002). However, a recent cohort study suggested rising incidence of RA in women after four decades of decline (Gabriel et al 2008). Mortality studies show RA decreases life expectancy, possibly due to its associated co-morbidities, including cardiovascular, respiratory and gastrointestinal problems (Kremers & Gabriel 2004). Co-morbidities may be due to chronic illness effects (e.g. de-conditioning leading to cardiovascular problems) or treatments (e.g. non-steroidal anti-inflammatory drugs leading to gastrointestinal problems). The increased mortality associated with RA has been relatively stable over the past few decades. Recent changes in medical management will take several years to effect mortality rates (Kremers & Gabriel 2004).

PATHOLOGY AND IMMUNOLOGY

RA is an autoimmune disease with abnormal antibody and T-cell responses to an auto-antigen (Haynes 2004). The result is a wide-spread inflammatory process in the synovial cells lining joint capsules and other body tissues, manifesting as a range of extra-articular features. The normal joint has a thin synovium lining the joint capsule. These cells produce synovial fluid which lubricates and provides nutrition to the articular cartilage. In early RA, lymphocytes infiltrate the joint capsule, proliferation of the synovial lining occurs, resulting in increased synovial fluid production. This presents as swollen, warm, red and painful joints. Prolonged periods of inflammation stress the surrounding ligaments and tendons causing laxity and subsequent joint instability. Therefore, intervention focuses on reducing the inflammatory response. In more advanced stages pannus forms: the synovium proliferates with fibroblasts, macrophages, T cells, and blood vessels. The pannus invades and erodes articular cartilage, eventually exposing the bone. Bone resorption and remodelling may occur in end-stage disease when cartilage destruction may be unavoidable. Intervention for end-stage disease is typically joint replacement.

Synovitis (inflammation of synovium) is not limited to joint capsules. The long tendons of the hand pass through synovial sheaths and this *tenosynovitis* may restrict tendon gliding, causing stiffness and limited finger mobility. Other tendon sheaths may be similarly affected. RA is said to be 'active' or 'exacerbated' when joints are inflamed and laboratory indicators of disease activity, such as erythrocyte sedimentation rate (ESR) are elevated. RA is said to be 'in remission' or 'controlled' when inflammation is minimal.

Extra-articular features of RA include a range of inflammatory processes: cutaneous changes such as vasculitis (inflammation of the small blood vessels) and rheumatoid nodules (fibrosis nodes in subcutaneous tissue, commonly near the elbow); inflammation of tissues in the eye (scleritis, uveitis); cardiac disease (myocarditis, pericarditis and effusions); lung and pleural disease; kidney disease and peripheral neuropathies (Haynes 2004). Generally speaking, extra-articular manifestations suggest more severe disease. Therapeutic recommendations and interventions need to accommodate systemic symptoms and impairments as well as joint disease.

DIAGNOSIS, DIFFERENTIAL DIAGNOSIS AND SPECIAL TESTS

Diagnosis results from a careful history together with physical examination, radiological and serological tests. The American College of Rheumatology (ACR)

Table16.1 Revised criteria for classification of RA (Arnett et al 1988)

CRITERION	DEFINITION
1. Morning stiffness	Morning stiffness in and around the joints, lasting at least 1 hour before maximal improvement
2. Arthritis of 3 or more joint areas	At least 3 joint areas simultaneously have had soft tissue swelling or fluid (not bony overgrowth alone) observed by a physician. The 14 possible areas are right or left PIP, MCP, wrist, elbow, knee, ankle and MTP joints.
3. Arthritis of the hand joints	At least 1 area swollen (as defined above) in a wrist, MCP or PIP joint
4. Symmetrical arthritis	Simultaneous involvement of the same joint areas (as defined in 2) on both sides of the body (bilateral involvement of PIPs, MCPs or MTPs is acceptable without absolute symmetry)
5. Rheumatoid nodules	Subcutaneous nodules, over bony prominences or extensor surfaces or in juxta-articular regions, observed by a physician
6. Serum rheumatoid factor	Demonstration of abnormal amounts of serum rheumatoid factor by any method for which the results have been positive in <5% of normal control subjects
7. Radiographic changes	Radiographic changes typical of rheumatoid arthritis on postero-anterior hand and wrist radiographs, which must include erosions or unequivocal bony decalcification localized in or most marked adjacent to the involved joints (osteoarthritis changes alone do not qualify)

Key: MCP, metacarpophalangeal; MTP, metatarsophalangeal; PIP, proximal interphalangeal

established criteria for the diagnosis of RA (Arnett et al 1988), listed in Table 16.1. Diagnosis is confirmed if a patient has at least four of the seven criteria. The first four must have been present for at least 6 weeks. Rheumatoid factor (RF) is important for both diagnosis and prognosis of RA (Shin et al 2005).

Other tests aid monitoring disease activity. Most commonly ESR and C-reactive protein (CRP) blood tests assess levels of inflammation and are known as 'inflammatory markers'. CRP is a better indicator of the acute phase response in the first 24 hours, but a more expensive test. (See Chapter 3 for details). Raised markers often indicate a 'flare' of RA, but the possibility of infection causing this elevation should always be considered.

Therapists should be aware of a patient's haemoglobin (Hb) because, not only may RA patients present with 'anaemia of chronic disease', but as inflammatory markers rise, Hb may fall and vice versa. Consequently, a patient with low Hb, may not be as able to actively participate with therapy; appearing pale and possibly reporting overwhelming fatigue.

MONITORING DISEASE ACTIVITY, PROGRESSION AND PROGNOSIS

Predicting prognosis is challenging, but outlook is now more positive with recent significant pharmacological advances and the advent of anti-TNF therapies (see Ch. 15). A sero-positive rheumatoid factor (RF), at, or soon after diagnosis, indicates a worse prognosis in terms of long term erosive joint disease (Shin et al 2005). Auto-antibodies against cyclic citrullinated peptide (CCP) may be more specific than RF, not only for predicting prognosis (Kastbom et al 2004), but also diagnosing RA (Nishimura et al 2007). El Miedany et al (2008) suggest longer duration of early morning stiffness (EMS), greater percentage change in health assessment questionnaires (HAQ) and anti-CCP positivity are all predictors of persistent arthritis. Ongoing disease activity, both clinically and serologically, has been linked to increasing morbidity, loss of function and mortality. Therapists should be aware of anticipated prognosis and pro-actively target therapies accordingly.

Felson et al (1993) published a core set of disease activity measures for use in RA clinical trials. These include articular indices (joint counts), the patient's assessment of their pain and physical function and both the patient and clinician's global assessment of disease activity, as well as results of one acute inflammatory marker. Therapists should be aware of these valid and reliable measures, but may use them in isolation and/or combination with other functional measures of therapy progress. Twenty percent, 50% and 70% response criteria (known as ACR 20, 50 and 70) have been defined to identify improvement in RA (Felson et al 1995), which therapists should understand. The Disease Activity Score, calculated on 28 specific joints (DAS-28), is a standard approach to monitoring RA progress and drug response (Prevoo et al 1995).

RADIOGRAPHIC FEATURES

Conventional plain film x-rays remain the most frequently used method of evaluating disease

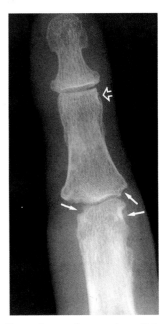

Figure 16.1 Illustrating erosions on the radial and ulnar aspects of the proximal interphalangeal joint as seen on radiology. With permission from: Theodorou DJ et al 2003 Ch. 71 Imaging of rheumatoid arthritis. In: Hochberg MC et al (eds) Rheumatology 3rd edn, Elsevier, London. Fig. 71.1 p801.

progression in RA and assisting in diagnosis (Cimmino et al 2004). Bony erosions caused by RA may be visible from a few months following symptom onset. They are found at lateral joint margins, typically first seen in the small joints of the hands and feet (Fig. 16.1). Joint spaces may also be narrowed as the thickness of hyaline cartilage of synovial joints is reduced. Osteopaenia and peri-articular osteoporosis may be seen around these small joints on x-ray, but are more accurately quantified on DEXA scans, used to quantify the osteoporosis presenting in many RA patients (Tourinho et al 2005) particularly in early inflammatory arthritis (Murphy et al 2008).

Synovial joint subluxation may also be seen on x-ray. On examination, the hands can present with deformities associated with RA: the swan-neck, boutonnière and ulnar-deviation affecting the interphalangeal (IP) and metacarpo-phalangeal (MCP) joints and Z deformity affecting the thumbs. Any level of the cervical spine can also be affected. The consequences of subluxation of the atlanto-axial and atlanto-occipital joints are the most serious (compression of the spinal cord, nerve roots or cervical artery). Lateral views with the cervical spine in flexion or extension help assess this as well as views of the odontoid peg from an anterior to posterior view through the mouth.

Magnetic resonance imaging (MRI) aids evaluating synovitis, tenosynovitis and bursitis in the hands and feet of newly diagnosed patients (Boutry et al 2003). MRI may be used more in future for monitoring purposes (Cimmino et al 2004) as it is more sensitive, detecting both soft tissue and bony changes (Uetani 2007).

More recent research has focussed on using ultrasound scanning (USS) imaging in RA (Filippucci et al 2007), particularly to detect sub-clinical synovitis or bony erosions not evident with conventional radiology.

CLINICAL EVALUATION

Initial assessment and ongoing evaluation will be undertaken by many multidisciplinary team members. Although overlap is inevitable, therapists have a unique line of inquiry to establish a baseline level of function, particularly related to activities of daily living, as well as identifying current clinical problems. Ay et al (2008) reported that RA patients experience most functional challenges with gripping, hygiene and grooming, running errands and shopping. For those in acute flare up, only a subjective history may be possible, perhaps with part of an objective examination. Therapists work collaboratively with patients to establish functional goals and devise plans to achieve them.

SUBJECTIVE ASSESSMENT

History of presenting condition

The patient's main problems must be identified from the outset. Some information may be provided on referral documentation. Therapists may have access to in-patient or on-line records, but a careful and logical history will elicit:

● Current symptoms, e.g. joint pain or EMS (which may signal a flare up of arthritis).
● Any difficulty with family, work or leisure life.
● Recent changes triggering referral to therapies.

Past medical history

A relevant past medical history is needed, as certain treatments may be contraindicated or alter a patient's capacity for therapy. Key questions include:

● Previous surgery?
● Previous hospital admissions with outcomes?
● Co-morbidities: cardio-vascular, respiratory, neurological or other conditions?
● Diabetes or epilepsy?
● Fractures of unknown cause, indicating possible osteoporosis?
● Ongoing/outstanding medical investigations?

Ask the patient if there is anything they believe to be important to assess that has not yet been discussed.

Drug history

This provides clues to disease severity and helps determine optimal timing for therapy. Relevant aspects to note are:

● Current prescribed and recently discontinued medication.
● Current or recently prescribed corticosteroids (orally, inhaled, intra-articular, intramuscular or intravenous) or anticoagulant therapy.
● Non-prescribed alternative or complimentary medicines – patients may need prompting to discuss these.

The timing of medication may also be relevant, especially for patients who have recently started or stopped disease-modifying anti-rheumatic drugs (DMARD's), biologics or received intra-articular injections. Knowing the timescale for drugs to reach full efficacy is important when planning therapy. See Chapter 15 for further details.

It will be important for therapists to be aware of allergic reactions, including latex (for Theraband™ purposes or if gloves are required).

Social and functional history

This provides an understanding of the patient's roles and responsibilities, typical daily activities and any difficulties encountered in these as a result of symptoms or joint impairment. Understanding the activities the patient needs and wants to do helps establish functional goals. Occupational performance areas should be assessed (Law et al 2005):

● Self care: eating, bathing, grooming, toileting, dressing, taking medication
● Productivity: household work, caring for children/family members, employment, going to school

● Leisure: engaging in recreational pursuits and socializing with others, both within the home and community.

The context in which these are performed is also important to query, such as where the patient lives and works, household members, sociocultural expectations, community resources and transportation. This helps establish priorities for intervention relevant to the patient.

When problems are noted in self-care, productivity or leisure, probe for contributing factors, including pain, physical factors (strength, endurance, mobility), or environmental factors (physical barriers, lack of proper equipment for a particular task). This determines which observational assessments are necessary. Discussing social roles provides an opportunity to inquire about psychological status, such as depression resulting from withdrawal from valued activities or roles (Katz & Yelin 1994), cultural beliefs and expectations, intimate relationships or coping issues. Although not feasible to assess every area in an initial evaluation, one should be alert to those most relevant to the individual, their circumstances and stage of illness. Some may be ready to act while others may still be adjusting to the diagnosis or a change in functional status and wondering how to cope. People with more established disease may come to therapy for specific and well-delineated purposes, as they are already experienced in managing their illness.

Asking the patient to describe their usual levels of mobility (including mobility aids and if mobility level has recently changed) helps the therapist plan objective assessment safely. Ask about estimated walking distance, what limits this, e.g. pain or shortness of breath, whether steps or stairs have to be negotiated (with or without banisters/stair lifts, etc.) and corroborate ability in objective examination. Subjective evaluation may include self-report measures of health and functional status (discussed later, and in Chs 4 & 5).

These two case examples illustrate how subjective findings will guide organizing the objective examination. The presenting issues and functional priorities differ for each patient. When time or patient tolerance is limited, focus on a few key issues for the objective examination and begin priority interventions to establish the therapeutic relationship. When necessary, evaluation and intervention planning can evolve over subsequent visits. See the clinical pathway in Fig. 16.2 for a comparison of functional goals, assessment and intervention plan for Ms Jones and Mrs Edwards.

CASE STUDY 16.1 NEWLY DIAGNOSED PATIENT-SUBJECTIVE HISTORY

Ms Sarah Jones, aged 38, a part-time computer programmer and mother of two young children, consults her general practitioner. She complains of a 6 month history of wrist and hand pain, increasing weakness in her grip and general fatigue. Initially, she thought her symptoms related to a house move, but on questioning, she admits things have not improved over time. She reports general body stiffness experienced in the mornings, recently lasting over an hour, and episodes of swelling in the small joints of her fingers. This has made it difficult for her to work and she is concerned as she has had to take some time off. She describes how she has 'trouble dressing my two-year-old' and 'peeling vegetables'. She has had some relief taking Ibuprofen medication.

CASE STUDY 16.2 PATIENT WITH MORE ESTABLISHED DISEASE-SUBJECTIVE HISTORY

Mrs Edwards, aged 62, has had RA for 22 years. She is referred to out-patient therapy following a right total knee arthroplasty 10 days previously. Medically, her RA is managed with combination therapy (methotrexate and sulfasalazine). Over the years, she has learned to 'listen to her body' and recognizes how to pace activities to manage fatigue. As a result of increasing knee pain and decreasing mobility prior to surgery, she was unable to maintain her exercise routine, and reports declining general strength and stamina. She is a little concerned about the stress placed on her hand and wrist while using a walking stick/cane as she recovers from surgery, because several joints are subluxed. Mrs Edwards is a retired office manager and lives in a small, one-level house with her husband. Both are avid gardeners.

OBJECTIVE EXAMINATION

If possible objective examination should follow the subjective history, but if a patient is acutely unwell, this may not be feasible. A logical approach ensures nothing of great importance should be missed if performed over several sessions. Whilst the focus will usually be the musculoskeletal system, a full respiratory or neurological assessment may be required with some patients (see Table 16.2).

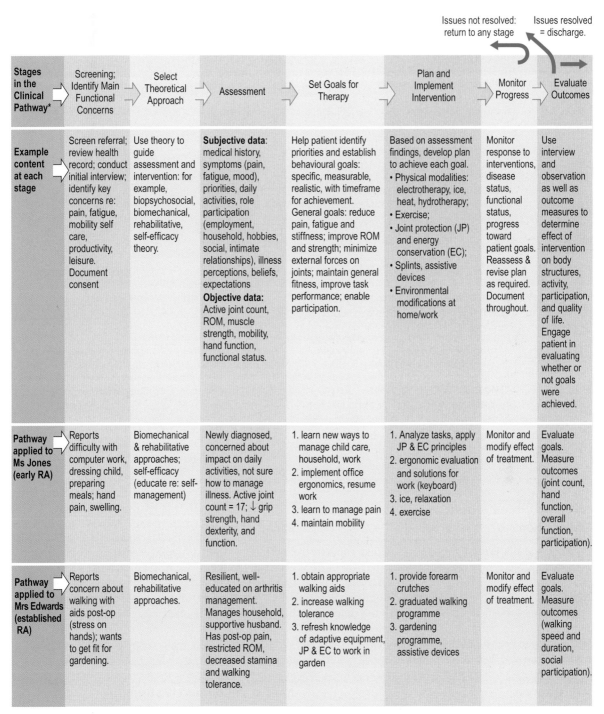

Stages in the Clinical Pathway*	Screening; Identify Main Functional Concerns	Select Theoretical Approach	Assessment	Set Goals for Therapy	Plan and Implement Intervention	Monitor Progress	Evaluate Outcomes
					Issues not resolved: return to any stage	Issues resolved = discharge.	
Example content at each stage	Screen referral; review health record; conduct initial interview; identify key concerns re: pain, fatigue, mobility self care, productivity, leisure. Document consent	Use theory to guide assessment and intervention: for example, biopsychosocial, biomechanical, rehabilitative, self-efficacy theory.	**Subjective data**: medical history, symptoms (pain, fatigue, mood), priorities, daily activities, role participation (employment, household, hobbies, social, intimate relationships), illness perceptions, beliefs, expectations **Objective data**: Active joint count, ROM, muscle strength, mobility, hand function, functional status.	Help patient identify priorities and establish behavioural goals: specific, measurable, realistic, with timeframe for achievement. General goals: reduce pain, fatigue and stiffness; improve ROM and strength; minimize external forces on joints; maintain general fitness, improve task performance; enable participation.	Based on assessment findings, develop plan to achieve each goal. • Physical modalities: electrotherapy, ice, heat, hydrotherapy; • Exercise; • Joint protection (JP) and energy conservation (EC); • Splints, assistive devices • Environmental modifications at home/work	Monitor response to interventions, disease status, functional status, progress toward patient goals. Reassess & revise plan as required. Document throughout.	Use interview and observation as well as outcome measures to determine effect of intervention on body structures, activity, participation, and quality of life. Engage patient in evaluating whether or not goals were achieved.
Pathway applied to Ms Jones (early RA)	Reports difficulty with computer work, dressing child, preparing meals; hand pain, swelling.	Biomechanical & rehabilitative approaches; self-efficacy (educate re: self-management)	Newly diagnosed, concerned about impact on daily activities, not sure how to manage illness. Active joint count = 17; ↓ grip strength, hand dexterity, and function.	1. learn new ways to manage child care, household, work 2. implement office ergonomics, resume work 3. learn to manage pain 4. maintain mobility	1. Analyze tasks, apply JP & EC principles 2. ergonomic evaluation and solutions for work (keyboard) 3. ice, relaxation 4. exercise	Monitor and modify effect of treatment.	Evaluate goals. Measure outcomes (joint count, hand function, overall function, participation).
Pathway applied to Mrs Edwards (established RA)	Reports concern about walking with aids post-op (stress on hands); wants to get fit for gardening.	Biomechanical, rehabilitative approaches.	Resilient, well-educated on arthritis management. Manages household, supportive husband. Has post-op pain, restricted ROM, decreased stamina and walking tolerance.	1. obtain appropriate walking aids 2. increase walking tolerance 3. refresh knowledge of adaptive equipment, JP & EC to work in garden	1. provide forearm crutches 2. graduated walking programme 3. gardening programme, assistive devices	Monitor and modify effect of treatment.	Evaluate goals. Measure outcomes (walking speed and duration, social participation).

*stages in this pathway based upon the Occupational Performance Process Model (Fearing & Clark 2000)

Figure 16.2 Clinical pathway for physiotherapy and occupational therapy for individuals with rheumatoid arthritis.

Table 16.2 Components of the objective examination

COMPONENT	DESCRIPTION	ADDITIONAL NOTE
General observation	Transfers, amount of assistance required, quality of movement, sitting/standing postures, eye contact	Observe patient's response to proposed therapy, willingness to actively participate
UL joint observations	Swelling and/or erythema – especially MCP, IP and wrist joints	Severity of hand signs and symptoms may not correlate with poorer hand function
LL joint observations	Foot posture whilst weight-bearing; medial arch flattening, tendo-achilles angle, subluxation of MTP joints, tread on footwear	Document regularly used assistive, orthotic devices
Palpation	Small joints of hands especially but any symptomatic joints; active or inactive synovitis, tenderness	DAS-28 joint scoring adopted internationally (Prevoo et al 1995)
Range of movement	For UL, LL and spinal joints – measure actively and passively. Note reason for limitation of range, muscle length and neurodynamics as appropriate. Measure with manual or electronic goniometry or "eye-ball" technique	Should be linked with a functional goal. Reliability of goniometry disputed: standard errors between 15 and 30°
Muscle strength	Note hand dominance – power grip and key grip most functional. Individual and key muscle groups should be assessed depending on functional challenges. UL – wrist extensors and rotator cuff muscles. LL – quadricep and gluteal muscle groups	Jamar dynamometry and pinch/key grip dynamometry (Mathiowetz et al 1984). Oxford scale method (Medical Research Council, 1976)
Joint stability	Some agonist muscles may be a lot stronger than antagonist exacerbating instability at a joint	Key joints: wrists, MCP and IP joints in hands, knees, MTP joints and cervical spine
Mobility	Gait patterns +/− mobility aids and support required. Steps/stairs. Note ability and safety	Note "quality of gait" including stride length, cadence, heel strike, and distance the patient can (or cannot) walk
Transfers	Sit to stand, lie to sit +/− assistive devices. Note ability and safety	Make as functional and replicate home circumstances as much as possible
Exercise tolerance	Borg scale (Borg 1985) is a speedy and pragmatic method where patients state their "rate of perceived exertion" (RPE)	Most patients have reduced exercise tolerance

Key: UL, upper limbs; LL, lower limbs; MTP, metatarsophalangeal, MCP, metacarpophalangeal; IP, interphalangeal

Observation

Welsing et al (2001) identified that functional capacity is most reduced with higher disease activity in early RA and with joint damage in late RA. Very often initial impressions can be deceptive; someone with apparently established and significant hand deformities may have accommodated and adapted over time and have good residual hand function. However, the opposite can also be true (see Fig. 16.3A-D).

Palpation

The DAS-28 joint scoring method identifies pain and swelling on joint palpation and is part of a disease activity score (DAS), including patient and clinician opinion, questionnaires and ESR levels as part of disease and drug monitoring (Prevoo et al 1995). Knowing which joints are most affected helps therapists to plan relevant and targeted treatment.

Range of movement

Caution is needed when assessing passive range, especially in the cervical spine. In most instances this is not advisable and could elicit symptoms of cervical artery insufficiency. Assessing joint range can be very time consuming if all spinal, UL and LL joints are included. The therapist may direct range of movement (ROM) assessment to specific joints impacting on previously identified key functional difficulties.

Joint stability/muscle strength

RA often affects joints bilaterally, but a symmetrical distribution of either joint range or muscle power should not be presumed. Power grip can be reliably measured using a Jamar dynamometer (Mathiowetz et al 1984) but may not always be comfortable for patients with RA (see Fig. 16.4). Key grip however, is rarely uncomfortable to assess (e.g. using B&L

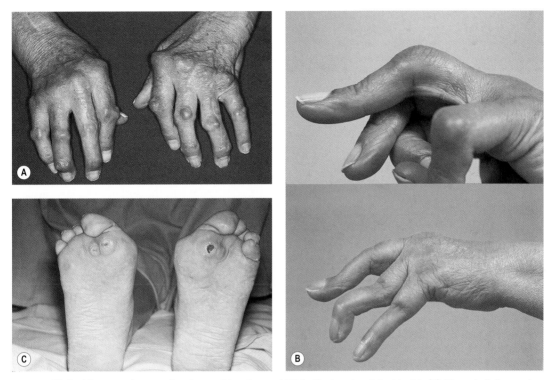

Figure 16.3 Clinical features that may be observed in advanced RA in the hand and foot in RA. (A) Ulnar deviation and rheumatoid nodules, (B) Swan-neck and Boutonniere deformities, (C) RA- forefoot deformity with callosity under MT head. With permission from: (A) Matteson EL Ch.69 Extra-articular features of rheumatoid arthritis and systemic involvement, Fig 69.4 p782, (B) Gordon DA and Hastings DE 2003 Ch. 68 Clinical features of rheumatoid arthritis Fig 68.7 p771, (C) Gordon DA and Hastings DE 2003 Ch. 68 Clinical features of rheumatoid arthritis Fig 68.15 p776. In: Hochberg MC et al (eds) Rheumatology 3rd edn, Elsevier, London.

Engineering Pinch Gauge) and other dynamometers are valid and reliable tools to use (e.g. MIE digital grip measures (MIE Medical Research, Leeds UK); Grippit digital measure, AB Detektor, Sweden).

Some units may have more sophisticated electronic methods of measuring muscle strength (e.g. isokinetic machines), both isometrically as well as isotonically within a stated range of motion. Whilst affording more accuracy for research, it is not essential for patients in standard clinical settings. Using isokinetic machines may, however, be contraindicated in patients with active inflammatory joint disease.

Functional mobility and transfers

The 'get up and go' test quantifies mobility, especially in more elderly patients (Wall et al 1998, Podsiadlo & Richardson 1991). Alternatively, a quick timed '10 metre walk test' needs only a measured walk way and stop watch for equipment. Slippers and soft-soled slip-on shoes with minimal

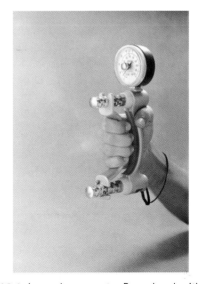

Figure 16.4 Jamar dynamometer. Reproduced, with permission, from the 'Benefits Now' website-http://www.benefitsnowshop.co.uk/

support should be discouraged and 'trainer' type footwear, possibly with velcro fastening, promoted for both safety and joint protection reasons.

ASSESSMENT OF OCCUPATIONAL PERFORMANCE (FUNCTIONAL ASSESSMENT)

The initial interview identifies priority occupational performance issues and guides selecting additional evaluations to determine underlying performance components or environmental conditions contributing to the problem (Backman & Medcalf 2000). In addition to ROM, strength, and mobility, evaluation may include:

- Hands-on evaluation of soft-tissue integrity
- Hand dexterity (e.g. pegboard tests)
- Hand function
- Symptoms affecting occupational performance, e.g. pain and fatigue
- Specific activities of daily living (ADL), instrumental ADL (IADL), work, or leisure assessments, as indicated by the client's problems and priorities.

Useful measures are summarized in Table 16.3 and outcome measures for baseline and follow up assessments are discussed in Chapters 4 and 5. During formal evaluation, particular attention is given to assessing hand function because RA typically affects these joints and the hands are involved in almost all daily activities. Early hand involvement is one of the strongest predictors of poor outcomes in RA (Schumacher et al 2004). Early detection and intervention through hand therapy may be one way to improve outcomes. Questionnaires measuring overall function may not be sensitive enough to capture specific problems with hand use in every-day activity (O'Connor et al 1999). Detailed observations of joint effusions, synovial proliferation, ligamentous integrity and deformity also contribute to a comprehensive hand assessment. Combining subjective and objective measures gives an overall picture of functional status.

The ICF (World Health Organization, 2002) distinguishes between activity limitations and participation restrictions. To capture these changes, specific measures of activity and participation are being developed or refined, potentially as part of a core set of outcome measures (Uhlig et al 2007). Staying abreast of emerging tools will improve comprehensive and valid functional assessment.

IMPORTANT FIRST TREATMENTS – EARLY RECOGNITION OF SIGNS AND SYMPTOMS

Because RA is episodic, recognising when a patient is entering a 'flare up' phase is very important. Patients should be aware of a sudden increase in joint swelling with associated pain, increasing EMS as well as over-whelming fatigue. Experienced patients will recognise signs and symptoms and appropriately self-manage, but the newly diagnosed may need guidance. Therapists are ideally positioned to help the patient to identify tell-tale signs, and manage the situation to best advantage. For example, for acute joint effusions (red, warm, swollen and painful joints), local treatments like ice and resting splints are indicated. To alleviate more systemic pain and fatigue, balancing rest and activity will help significantly. Some gentle daily activity (pottering in the home, gentle stretching) is important to prevent soft tissue shortening, but during the acute few days of a flare many patients will benefit from additional chair or bed rest. The balance is specific to each individual and dependant upon which joints are involved. Ensuring family members and significant others understand this principle is essential and therapists can often play an important role acting as an advocate for the individual.

Flare ups can be induced by stress and significant life events (Curtis et al 2005, Straub et al 2005) but the aetiology may also be unexplained. Early recognition and prompt management can minimise effects. Appropriate medication, as well as using ice (with hot joints, unless Raynaud's phenomenon is an issue) or heat in the form of hot packs, warm showers or baths when muscular spasms are painful, can all ease symptoms.

IDENTIFICATION OF RED FLAGS

- Joint instability of the cervical spine occurs as a consequence of repeated flare ups and over-stretching of the surrounding ligaments (Dreyer & Boden, 1999). Patients may report sensory or motor changes, e.g. paraesthesia/anaesthesia, a history of dropping items or recent falls without obvious cause. A detailed neurological examination should follow to include dermatomes, myotomes and reflexes for both upper and lower limbs. Symptoms should be promptly reported to the Rheumatology Consultant. Follow-up may include onward referral to either orthotists for assessment for

Table 16.3 Selected functional tests/measures of activity and participation

TEST	DESCRIPTION	REFERENCE
	Performance-based Tests of hand function	
Arthritis Hand Function Test (AHFT)	11-item test of hand strength, dexterity, and functional tasks for adults with RA, osteoarthritis, and scleroderma	Backman et al 1991; Poole et al 2000
Sequential Occupational Dexterity Assessment (SODA)	Measures ability to do 12 functional tasks, with difficulty scored by both occupational therapist and client	van Lankveld et al 1996
	Self-report assessments of hand and upper limb function	
Cochin Rheumatoid Hand Disability Scale	Evaluates level of difficulty performing 18 functional tasks	Duruoz et al 1996
Disabilities of the Arm, Shoulder and Hand (DASH) Questionnaire	30-items evaluate level of pain and difficulty with functional tasks; optional modules for sports, work, and musicians; for any diagnosis	Beaton et al 2001 (includes entire questionnaire)
Michigan Hand Outcomes Questionnaire (MHQ)	Scores symptoms, function, and aesthetics for pre- and postoperative evaluations	Chung et al 1998 (includes entire questionnaire)
	Overall health and functional status	
Arthritis Impact Measurement Scales 2 (AIMS-2)	Self-report of mobility, physical, household and social activities, ADL, pain, depression & anxiety	Meenan et al 1992
Canadian Occupational Performance Measure (COPM)	Semi-structured interview, rating performance and satisfaction with performance in self care, productivity, leisure on 1–10 scale	Law et al 2005
Evaluation of Daily Activities Questionnaire (EDAQ)	Self-report or interview rating performance of 102 ADL with and without assistive devices/ adapted methods	Nordenskiold et al 1998 (UK version in development)
Health Assessment Questionnaire Disability Index (HAQ) and HAQ-II	HAQ: Self-report of difficulties performing 20 ADL tasks (in 8 categories). HAQ-II: 10 item version.	Fries et al 1980 Wolfe 2005
Medical Outcomes Study Short Form-36 (SF-36)	Health survey with 8 subscales: physical function, social function, mental health, pain, physical role limitations, emotional role limitations, energy/fatigue, and general health	Ware & Kosinski, 2001
	Impact of fatigue on function	
Multi-dimensional Assessment of Fatigue (MAF)	16-item questionnaire addressing fatigue severity, frequency, distress and impact on ability to perform 11 activities	Belza 1995
	Parenting disability	
Parenting Disability Index	Self-report of difficulty caring for children ≤5 yrs, 6–12 yrs, and/ or >12 yrs	Katz et al 2003
	Participation	
Keele assessment of participation	Self-report, 11-item questionnaire; measures whether or not one is engaging in activities when and as they would like	Wilkie et al 2005
Social role participation questionnaire	Self-report questionnaire rating salience and satisfaction with 10 domains of social participation	Gignac et al 2008
	Work disability	
Ergonomic Assessment Tool for Arthritis	Customized self-assessment and semi-structured interview re: work organization, job demands and environment	Backman et al 2008
Work Limitations Questionnaire	Self-report questionnaire rating difficulty performing 25 specific job demands	Lerner et al 2001
Work Instability Scale	Self-report, 23-item questionnaire to identify risk for problems believed to lead to work disability	Gilworth et al 2003

cervical collar/brace or to spinal surgeons. For approximately 50% of patients, neurological deficit can subside following surgery to improve cervical instability, but mortality rates can be significant (Ronkainen et al 2006). Neurosurgeons may be the preferred first option, but many orthopaedic surgeons also manage RA patients with spinal instability. Ignoring signs of spinal instability could lead to tetraplegia, so vigilance by the therapist is required.

● RA patients receiving steroid therapy may notice excessive bruising often due to low platelet counts. Consequently, it is important therapists handle patients carefully to avoid skin damage. Healing in general may be slow in RA (Boardman et al 2001) and ulceration from skin abrasions can take months to heal. Precautions include keeping nails short, removing jewellery (e.g. wrist watches or rings) that may 'catch' on the skin and ensuring that foot plates are correctly positioned to avoid calf contact during wheelchair transfers. Patients receiving anti-TNF therapies may also have slower healing rates and more infection complications, especially post surgery, although some dispute this (Bibbo & Goldberg 2004).

REHABILITATION INTERVENTIONS FOR RA

Guidelines for pharmacological and non-pharmacological management of RA have been documented in both the United States (American College of Rheumatology 2002) and Britain (Luqmani et al 2006, NICE 2009). Special attention has been given to early RA management to minimize disability (Hennell & Luqmani 2008), and to rehabilitation interventions (Hammond 2004). There is some evidence to show RA symptoms are relieved by thermotherapy, laser therapy, acupuncture, splints and assistive devices; and that pain and function can improve with patient education, joint protection behaviours, exercise therapy, hand exercises, and cognitive-behavioural therapy. However since Hammond's review in 2004 few treatment studies have been published and well-designed rehabilitation trials are still required to identify which treatments work best for patients at different disease stages.

Figure 16.2 introduced a clinical pathway from assessment to outcome evaluation, providing an overview of occupational therapy and physical therapy management. Specific interventions are summarized in turn below.

PHYSIOTHERAPY EVIDENCE–BASED TREATMENT PROGRAMMES

The Association of Rheumatology Health Professionals has published standards of care documenting physical therapy competencies in rheumatology (2006), based on work by Moncur (1988). Treatment programmes must be individualised and devised in agreement and collaboration with the patient

(Heller & Shadick 2007). The purpose and intended outcome for each stage of therapy should be discussed to clarify realistic expectations. As a rule the earlier a referral is made to therapists, the more successful interventions will be, especially if joint protection principles are adopted early on in joint disease. However for some individuals the shock of diagnosis may mean time is required to contemplate, before any actions can be positively adopted. Therapists should include promotion of long term health in their treatment strategies (see Ch. 6) and facilitate the patient to remain in work or education. In the context of inter-professional practice, physiotherapy and occupational therapy colleagues work collaboratively with patients to achieve shared therapy objectives. Increasingly, therapy will be delivered in community settings and the emphasis will continue to be on empowering the individual to manage their own symptoms.

Exercise therapy

Exercise therapy, in its many possible settings, is the mainstay of physiotherapy treatment (Hurley et al 2002, Lineker et al 2006). Exercise is prescribed to: improve joint range and muscle power, maximise joint stability, increase exercise tolerance, reduce morning stiffness/muscle spasm and thereby associated pain. The overall aim is to optimise function in ADL. Physiological benefits are well known, but Hurley et al (2003) also documented many psychosocial benefits of exercising in osteoarthritis, much of which is applicable in RA. Lee et al (2006) evaluated exercising three times a week for at least 20 minutes for more than 6 months and found that exercisers with RA experienced significantly less fatigue and disability compared with non-exercisers. Patients report that pain remains a significant barrier to their exercising (Bajwa & Rogers 2007) so unless this is addressed and an end purpose understood, exercise may seem irrelevant at best, painful at worst and therefore rarely undertaken independently.

Key features of exercising with RA:

- Relate any exercise to improving performance of individually relevant functional tasks; individualise range, resistance, eccentric, concentric muscle work, length of hold of contraction
- Wherever possible, minimise pain first
- Avoid uncontrolled end of range movements

- Aim to improve exercise tolerance as well as increasing range of movement/muscle strength and joint stability
- Reassure new exercisers that join/muscle aches may last up to 30-60 minutes after exercise – this is normal!
- Dosage should be individualised – most benefit from some daily exercise (ARC, Keep Moving leaflet, 2005)
- Modify exercise during a flare; focus on maintaining range but without resistance
- Minimise use of equipment so exercise can easily be performed at home
- Written information should support exercise instructions and include "SOS" contact details.

Within the United Kingdom, 'Arthritis Care' and 'Young Arthritis Care' organisations encourage individuals to exercise in groups. This is popular and helps individuals remain motivated. Similarly, 'People with Arthritis Can Exercise' (PACE) programmes operate in the USA and "JointWorks" and "Waterworks" are offered by the Arthritis Society in Canada. These group initiatives are cost effective and for many peer support is invaluable. For others, exercising 1:1 with a therapist or alone is preferred (Bajwa & Rogers 2007) and therapists should select or produce audio-visual material to support this.

Tai Chi has become increasingly popular among people with arthritis. Whilst evidence is limited, Han et al (2004) report no detrimental affects in RA patients. A higher level of participation and generally greater enjoyment was also documented, compared with a traditional range of movement exercise class.

Previously, concern has been raised about exercise potentially increasing joint pain and exacerbating inflammatory disease, especially during a flare up. However, many studies reassure therapists and patients alike that appropriately prescribed exercises are significantly beneficial (Bearne et al 2002, Kennedy 2006, American Physical Therapy Association Ottawa Panel 2004a, Panel 2004, Van den Ende et al 2000, 2006).

The frequency of exercise required remains generally poorly documented and evaluated. Many recommend daily practice of simple stretching exercises to maintain or improve joint range for all large joints e.g. shoulder, hip and knee, and strength exercises most days (ARC 2005).

For all, early exercise therapy should be encouraged. Prophylactic exercises to prevent contractures, muscle atrophy and general deconditioning help the individual to maximise quality of life long term. Patients should be reassured it is never too late to start and regular exercise can be beneficial for everyone.

Research has demonstrated that hand exercises improve hand function over a six month period (O'Brien et al 2006). A combination of daily stretching and strengthening exercises improved hand function as measured by the Arthritis Impact Measurement Scales upper limb function subscale. Further research into this is ongoing.

Hydrotherapy

Hydrotherapy uses the properties of water, buoyancy, turbulence and drag during exercise to achieve an end functional goal. Hydrotherapy remains popular, despite efficacy having been challenged in some studies (Verhagen et al 1997, 2004). However, benefit has been demonstrated (Hall et al 1996) with patients reporting continued pain relief and reduced morning stiffness by diminishing muscle spasm. Some consider this an expensive resource (Epps et al 2005) not available to all. Consequently, therapists should be clear about their rationale for prescribing hydrotherapy as opposed to land-based exercise. However, it may be cost-effective if sufficient numbers utilise the resource throughout the day.

Cryotherapy

For many patients cryotherapy can be a useful adjunct to treatment of hot swollen joints (Robinson et al 2006) before or after exercise. For most patients a simple ice pack can be replicated at home by using 'frozen peas' or equivalent to ease symptoms temporarily (Hirvonen et al 2006). Information relating to optimal dosage and frequency remains illusive. Contraindications should be checked prior to treatment, e.g. a significant number of RA patients have Raynaud's phenomenon.

Thermotherapy

Some patients experiencing muscle spasm or morning stiffness report benefits from applying heat and many report a morning shower minimises morning stiffness. Simple hot packs can be used, heated up in microwaves at home. Evidence for thermotherapy remains limited, but no detrimental effects have been reported (Welch et al 2002). Wax therapy, previously popular especially for hands, is less favoured today as being too passive a treatment. Benefit is only maintained if followed by hand exercises (Dellhag et al 1992). Therapists should be cautious of applying heat to joints with active synovitis. Some evidence indicates that metalloproteinases are activated with increasing temperature which could accelerate degeneration of hyaline cartilage (Yasura et al 2006). However, the clinical relevance of this is yet to be established in RA patients.

Electrotherapy

Many electrotherapy modalities have historically been used, but studies have been criticised for lack of methodological rigour as well as low sample sizes. The American Physical Therapy Association Ottawa Panel has published practice guidelines (2004b) for electrotherapy in RA. This panel recommends the use of therapeutic ultrasound, low level laser, transcutaneous electrical nerve stimulation (TENS), electrical stimulation and thermotherapy.

Berliner & Piegsa (1997) studied the physiological effects of continuous therapeutic ultrasound in a water bath on skin microcirculation and temperature in RA patients. Comparing healthy participants with patients with high and low disease activity, they concluded (based on a single treatment intervention) that microcirculation increased significantly in healthy participants, but least in those with high inflammatory activity.

A meta-analysis of low level (non-thermal) laser therapy concluded this has small short term effects on pain relief, range of movement and reduction in morning stiffness (Brosseau et al 2005). This systematic review highlights that future research must investigate dosage, wavelength, site of application and treatment duration.

Transcutaneous electrical nerve stimulation (TENS) is used for pain relief. It can be independently applied by the patient and used with many peripheral and spinal joints at home. Brosseau et al (2003) systematically reviewed effects of TENS in the rheumatoid hand. TENS significantly reduced resting pain and joint tenderness, and improved grip strength. However there were conflicting results between the differing modalities of TENS ('conventional' and 'acupuncture-like' TENS). Further research is needed, with increased power, to draw more meaningful conclusions.

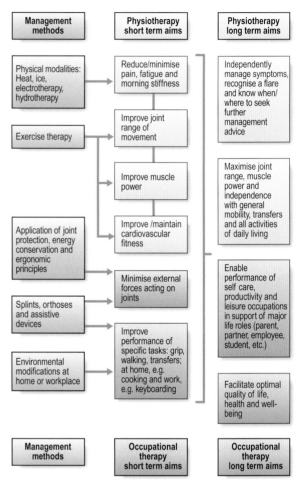

Figure 16.5 Management of RA by occupational and physiotherapists.

Acupuncture

Acupuncture has been reported to have anti-inflammatory properties (Zijlstra et al 2003) and is increasingly used for symptomatic treatment of RA. As with many other modalities, data are not compelling and there are often methodological limitations in trials, but its popularity with patients suggests an anecdotal analgesic benefit. Casimiro et al (2005) report benefit from electro-acupuncture in knee pain in RA, but conclusions are limited due to few trials and small sample sizes. Results to date suggest no effect on inflammatory markers, swollen or tender joint counts or analgesic intake. Figure 16.5 summarises the management of a patient with RA from a physiotherapy and occupational therapy perspective.

OCCUPATIONAL THERAPY INTERVENTIONS

Occupational therapy interventions are directed at resolving functional limitations identified by the patient while managing symptoms like pain and fatigue. It is important to stay involved and connected with family, friends, and community, because withdrawal from everyday activities, including housework, leisure and social activities, is more closely linked to poor psychological outcomes than difficulty with ADL (Katz & Alfieri 1997). Patients may grieve the loss of participation in valued roles or experience mood changes, such as depression or anxiety, as they negotiate living with chronic illness. Engaging in meaningful activities is critically important to maintaining a sense of identity and positive self-worth. To have the greatest impact on health and well-being, it is highly recommended that occupational therapists take time to evaluate the occupations of greatest value to the client and focus on improving participation in these.

Comprehensive occupational therapy programmes have demonstrated sustained improvements in function (Helewa et al 1991, Steultjens et al 2002). Typical programmes involve: patient education (including joint protection, energy conservation, psychosocial support and cognitive-behavioural approaches to improve coping); splinting; assistive devices and environmental modifications; and activity adaptation.

PATIENT EDUCATION: SUPPORTING SELF-MANAGEMENT

Arthritis self-management programmes improve health outcomes for people with RA (Lorig & Holman 2006, Riemsma et al 2003). Successful programmes are based on enhancing self efficacy, i.e. the patient's confidence that they can adopt behaviours to control disease symptoms and enhance function. Facilitating new habits through counselling on joint protection, energy conservation and cognitive-behavioural approaches are the cornerstone of occupational therapy patient education, which focuses on practical strategies to engage in life despite pain, fatigue, depression, and physical challenges.

Joint protection principles are based upon biomechanical and ergonomic guidelines and aim to reduce pain and local inflammation during task performance, preserve the integrity of vulnerable joint structures and improve function (Backman et al 2004). Energy conservation principles involve planning and pacing activities, to balance energy and fatigue in support of valued activities (Backman et al 2004). To be effective, general principles of joint protection and energy conservation need to be demonstrated and applied to the patient's specific roles and activities (see Table 16.4). Compared to standard care, comprehensive joint protection education has been shown to reduce pain and morning stiffness, and improve ADL performance (Hammond et al 1999; Hammond & Freeman 2001). See Chapters 1 and 6 for further descriptions of techniques and evidence.

The psychosocial impact of RA cannot be underestimated: symptoms may significantly impact daily routines, and depression often accompanies RA. For example, morning stiffness can delay self care routines and present a challenge getting to work on time, or frustrate a mother needing to care for a young child waking early or during the night. Fatigue may limit participation in family events or recreational activities if all one's energy is expended in obligatory paid and unpaid work activities. Ongoing disruption to daily routines creates distress and coping difficulties for many patients. There may be added worries regarding employment, financial issues, or family obligations.

One-to-one and group educational programmes (including joint protection and energy conservation mentioned above) help patients develop self-management skills and identify reasonable ways to plan ahead and adjust routines where possible to minimize pain and fatigue while doing daily activities. Cognitive-behavioural approaches and counselling assist patients to recognize ineffective thought processes, feelings and behaviours, then set goals and implement practical strategies to cope with the emotional consequences of RA (Backman 2006). For example, stress management and relaxation techniques might focus on changing attitudes and responses to challenging situations, rhythmic breathing and guided imagery. Because of differing priorities among patients and the episodic nature of RA, it is wise to offer a range of strategies and encourage patients to select those most applicable to their unique situation.

Involving family members in education and counselling sessions may be welcomed, as social support is important to living with RA. In many ways, RA affects the entire family, and spouses, parents or children may have questions of their own. Sometimes, problem-solving involves coordinating the efforts of several members of the health care team, for example, coordinating medications, ROM exercises, and joint protection techniques to optimize performance, or engaging the services of a

Table 16.4 Joint-protection and energy-conservation principles and sample techniques

PRINCIPLE	SAMPLE TECHNIQUES OR APPLICATION
Respect your pain	Reduce time and/or effort spent on an activity if pain occurs and lasts for more than 2 hours after the activity has been discontinued. Avoid nonessential activities that aggravate your pain
Balance rest and work	Take short breaks during your work. For example, take a 5-minute rest at the end of an hour of work. Intersperse more active tasks with more passive or quiet work
Reduce the amount of effort needed to do the job	Use assistive devices such as a jar opener or lever taps. Slide pots across the counter instead of lifting. Use a trolley to transport heavy items. Use a raised toilet seat and seat cushion to reduce stress on hips, knees, and hands. Use frozen vegetables to minimize peeling and chopping
Avoid staying in one position for prolonged periods of time	Change position frequently to avoid joint stiffness and muscle fatigue. For example, take a 30-second range of motion break after 10–20 minutes of typing or holding a tool; after standing for 20 minutes perch on a stool for the next 20 minutes; walk to the mailroom after 20–30 minutes sitting at your desk
Avoid activities that cannot be stopped immediately if you experience pain or discomfort	Plan ahead. Be realistic about your abilities so you don't walk or drive too far, or leave all your shopping and errands to a single trip
Reduce unnecessary stress on your joints while sleeping	Use a firm mattress for support. Sleep on your back with a pillow to support the curve in your neck. If you prefer to lay on your side, place a pillow between your knees and lay on the least painful side
Maintain muscle strength and joint range of motion	Do your prescribed exercises regularly. Strong muscles will help support your joints. Regular exercise will reduce fatigue
Use a well-planned work space	Organize your work space so that work surfaces and materials are at a convenient height for you, to ensure good posture. Place frequently used items within close reach. Reduce clutter by getting rid of unnecessary items, or storing less frequently used items away from the immediate work space

Note. From the Mary Pack Arthritis Program, Vancouver Coastal Health, Vancouver, BC Canada. Used with permission.

vocational counsellor, social worker or psychologist to resolve complex employment, family, or emotional issues.

Splinting

Splints support and protect joints, minimize pain, and enhance function. They may provide localized rest to reduce pain and inflammation (e.g. a hand resting splint, see Fig. 16.6a); enhance joint stability to improve function (e.g. a wrist splint to improve ability to grasp, lift and carry items, see Fig. 16.6b); align joints in a stable anatomical plane to minimize deformity and stretching of the joint capsule and ligaments (e.g. a silver ring splint to position a swan-neck deformity of the finger into a slightly flexed posture, see Fig. 16.6c); or facilitate recovery from surgery (e.g. dynamic flexion or extension splints following arthroplasty or tendon repairs to encourage early finger motion in a controlled range (Backman et al 2004).

A more comprehensive discussion of splinting is presented in Chapter 12. With respect to RA, evidence suggests that wrist splints improve hand strength (Haskett et al 2004, Pagnotta et al 1998) and reduce pain (Haskett et al 2004, Veehof et al 2008), and after a break-in period, do not compromise

dexterity (Haskett et al 2004). During flares, resting splints may be recommended for the wrists and hands, knees, or elbow, at night use or during daytime rests. A systematic review concluded there is little evidence that resting splints improve function, yet patients prefer using them rather than going without, suggesting they alleviate pain (Egan et al 2001).

For prolonged MCP joint effusion, MCP protection splints may be indicated. These restrict flexion and ulnar deviation at the MCP joints with the intent to prevent or minimize subluxation. One study, using x-rays to evaluate 27 hands with RA, showed that while worn the splints corrected the alignment of all MCP joints except the index finger (Rennie 1996), although long-term benefits have not been evaluated.

Foot orthoses in combination with supportive shoes (Fig. 16.6d) support the transverse and longitudinal arches of the foot, alleviate metatarsalgia, and enable people with RA to walk comfortably (Chalmers et al 2000, Hawke et al 2008) (see also Ch. 13).

Assistive devices and environmental modifications

Dozens of assistive devices are available to accommodate physical limitations or promote adherence to

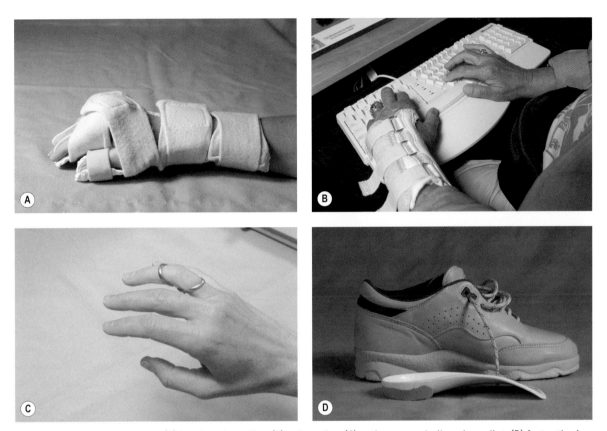

Figure 16.6 Splints used in RA. (A) hand resting splint; (B) wrist splint; (C) anti-swan neck silver ring splint; (D) foot orthosis and supportive shoe.

joint protection principles. Common devices include jar openers (to accommodate for weak grasp), long-handle shoe horns, sock aids, or dressing sticks (to accommodate limited motion), and raised toilet seats (to reduce stress on hips, knees, and hands, because the higher seat means less need to push up). Once only available through therapy departments and medical supply catalogues, the move toward universal accessibility means many helpful devices can be found in department, hardware, office supply and other shops. For example, cook shops have an array of utensils with large grips, making grasp easier for all, not just people with RA. They also have lightweight dishes and small appliances for easy use at counter height. Ergonomic office equipment, appropriately selected, facilitates improved posture to minimize pain and fatigue.

Not all assistive devices will 'fit' all patients, and careful assessment and patient education may be necessary to prevent inappropriate suggestions. The long-handled reacher that accommodates decreased range of motion may present a mechanical disadvantage in some situations, putting greater stress on the hands and wrists, counteracting the intended benefit. Devices that fail to resolve the functional problem are not used. However, in one follow-up study, as many as 91% of kitchen devices reduced pain and were still in use by women with RA 6 to 12 months after they were first provided (Nordenskiold 1994). Not all patients are ready to consider multiple assistive devices and environmental modifications at once, and some devices reinforce beliefs about 'being disabled'. Limit recommendations to the most important problems first, and build on successes as they occur.

Home modifications may enhance independence and functional capacity. Physical environment modifications can be divided into three categories (Mann et al 1999): re-arranging the living environment, such as moving dishes to lower shelves; adding to the environment, such as the placement of hooks and storage bins to keep frequently used supplies within easy reach; and structurally modifying the environment, such as installing a walk-in shower or ramps in place of stairs. Such modifications help people compensate for physical limitations arising from RA. In a small qualitative study, women described physical modifications, such as stair lifts and grab bars, accessing services such as home delivery of groceries, and involving friends and family to assist with tasks like home maintenance to successfully adapt to living with RA (Moss 1997). Similar accommodations, individualized to the patient's chosen activities, delay or prevent disability at home and work.

Activity adaptation at home and work

For many patients, what matters most is actively engaging in parenting, household work, employment, socializing and similar roles. Mothers with arthritis describe learning to adjust expectations and set priorities, and recommend strategies such as omitting non-essential tasks, delegating to others, and 'figuring out' how to adapt tasks to match their physical ability and energy (Backman et al 2007). Work place transitions are also common (Gignac et al 2008), with patients identifying fluctuations in productivity, job changes, and job loss. Assessing workplace ergonomics (Backman et al 2008a, Backman 2008b) and adapting the workplace to accommodate arthritis symptoms may support productivity. Specific education on job accommodation legislation, vocational rehabilitation resources, and problem-solving in the workplace may reduce work disability (Lacaille et al 2007, 2008).

REFERRAL TO SPECIALIST SERVICES

Ideally patients with RA should have access to a diverse multi-disciplinary team (Hennell & Luqmani 2008). Within a secondary care environment this may include specialist nurses, podiatrists, social welfare staff, dieticians, orthotists and others. In the primary care setting staff involved include general practitioners with a 'specialist interest' in rheumatology and specialist community nurses. Employers may need to be advised of their employee's health challenges, if the patient is willing to disclose their arthritis. Therapists are often the key staff who undertake workplace assessments with their patients and may involve a Disability Employment Advisor. Within a school or college environment, therapists may assess young people and liaise closely with parents and dedicated 'special needs' staff.

CONCLUSION

Proactive therapists will enjoy working with patients who have diverse and challenging problems arising from inflammatory arthritis. Therapists have an integral role within multi-disciplinary teams and their early targeted intervention maximises functional outcome. Evidence is increasing to support therapy interventions and further studies are essential to advance the practice of physical and occupational therapy and improve the health and well-being of people living with arthritis.

STUDY ACTIVITIES

1. Log on to Jointzone-www.jointzone.org.uk
   - Identify the inflammatory disorders section then the RA extra-articular manifestations section
   - Read how the systems of the body may potentially be affected by RA
   - Make notes relevant to your clinical practice.
2. Ms Sarah Jones (introduced earlier) continues to experience inflammation in her MCP joints, and upon examination you notice joint subluxation, ulnar deviation and ligamentous laxity.
   - What evidence is there for the effectiveness of splinting the MCP joints in terms of preventing deformity, reducing pain, or improving hand function?
   - List three principles of joint protection and advise Sarah on how to specifically apply them to household work and family leisure activities.
   - Subsequently, Sarah is referred to a hand surgeon and receives MCP joint replacements (index, middle, ring and little fingers in her right hand). Investigate the typical post-operative protocol.
3. Consider your own clinical practice working with patients with inflammatory arthritis –
   - Select three new outcome measures you are not familiar with but think you could usefully employ.
   - With a few colleagues obtain and critically appraise the original papers and subsequent papers reporting on their validity and reliability
   - Establish if you need to obtain a licence to use them
   - Pilot their use in your own clinical environment over a 3-month period

USEFUL WEBSITES

Arthritis and Musculoskeletal Alliance (ARMA). Standards of Care for people with inflammatory arthritis. http://www.arma.uk.net.

Association of Rheumatology Health Professionals (ARHP), 2006. Standards of practice: Physical therapy competencies in rheumatology http://www.rheumatology.org/arhp/practice/standards.

Musculoskeletal Services Framework Document – Department of Health UK. http://www.dh.gov.uk/en/Publicationsandstatistics/Publications/PublicationsPolicyAndGuidance/DH_4138413

Arthritis Research Campaign (UK). http://www.arc.org.uk. To obtain the exercise leaflet - "Keep moving". http://ww.arc.org.uk/arthinfo/patpubs/6282/6282.asp.

Hydrotherapy Association of Chartered Physiotherapists – UK guidelines. http://www.csp.org.uk/director/groupandnetworks/ciogs/skillsgroups/hydrotherapy.cfm.

Joint zone – a study of rheumatology – UK. http://www.jointzone.org.uk/.

National Rheumatoid Arthritis Society (NRAS) –UK. http://www.rheumatoid.org.uk.

NHS Evidence (UK): Musculoskeletal Specialist Library. http://www.library.nhs.uk/musculoskeletal.

British Health Professionals in Rheumatology (BHPR). http://www.rheumatology.org.uk/bhpr.

The Health Talk Online Website personal experiences of health and illness – Rheumatoid Arthritis. http://www.healthtalkonline.org.

The Wright Stuff Arthritis Supplies. www.arthritissupplies.com.

Able Data, hundreds of assistive devices and technologies. www.abledata.com.

Arthritis Foundation (US), includes community-based self-management, exercise programs and resources for living well. http://ww.arthritis.org/resources.php.

Arthritis Society (Canada), includes Arthritis Self-Management

Program information and a storefront for patients to purchase educational materials and assistive devices. http://www.arthritis.ca.

Psychometric Laboratory for Health Sciences – references to useful scales & outcome measures. http://home2.btconnect.com/Psylab_at_Leeds/scales.htm.

The DAS-28 for disease activity monitoring. http://www.dasscore.nl.

References and further reading

American College of Rheumatology, 2002 Guidelines for the management of rheumatoid arthritis 2002 update. Arthritis Rheum. 46 (2), 328–346.

American Physical Therapy Association Ottawa Panel 2004a Evidence-based clinical practice guidelines for therapeutic exercises in the management of rheumatoid arthritis in adults. Phys. Ther. 84, 934–972.

American Physical Therapy Association, Ottawa Panel 2004b Evidence-based clinical practice guidelines for electrotherapy and thermotherapy interventions in the management of rheumatoid arthritis in adults 2004. Phys. Ther. 84 (11), 1016–1143.

ARC, 2005. Keep Moving Education Leaflet. Chesterfield, UK. Online. Available: http://www.arc.org.uk (accessed 9.2.09.).

Arnett, F.C., Edworthy, S.M., Bloch, D.A., et al., 1988. The American Rheumatism association 1987 revised criteria for the classification of rheumatoid arthritis. Arthritis Rheum. 31 (3), 315–324.

Association of Rheumatology Health Professionals, 2006. Standards of practice: Physical therapy competencies in rheumatology. Online. Available: http://www.rheumatology.org/arhp/practice/standards 17 July 2007. (accessed 9.2.09.).

Ay, S., Tur, B.S., Kucukdeveci, A., 2008. Evaluation of disability

in patients with degenerative and inflammatory arthritis. Int. J. Rehabil. Res. 31 (2), 159–163.

Backman, C.L., 2006. Psychosocial aspects in the management of arthritis pain. Arthritis Res. Ther. 28, 221. (doi:10.1186/ar2083).

Backman, C., Mackie, H., Harris, J., 1991. Arthritis Hand Function Test: Development of a standardized assessment tool. Occup. Ther. J. Res. 11, 245–256.

Backman, C., Medcalf, N., 2000. Identifying components and environmental conditions contributing to occupational performance issues. In: Fearing, V.J., Clark, J. (Eds.) Individuals in Context: A Practical Guide to

Client Centred Practice. Slack Inc, Thorofare, NJ, pp. 55–67.

Backman, C.L., Fairleigh, A., Kuchta, G., 2004. Occupational therapy. In: St Clair, E.W., Pisetsky, D.S., Haynes, B.F. (Eds.) Rheumatoid Arthritis. Lippincott Williams & Wilkins, Philadelphia, pp. 431–439.

Backman, C.L., Del Fabro Smith, L., Smith, S., et al., 2007. The experiences of mothers living with inflammatory arthritis. Arthritis Rheum. 57 (1), 381–388.

Backman, C.L., Village, J., Lacaille, D., 2008a. The ergonomic assessment tool for arthritis (EATA): development and pilot testing. Arthritis Rheum. 59 (10), 1495–1503.

Backman, C., 2008b. The Ergonomic Assessment Tool for Arthritis (Ergotool). http://ergotool.arthritisresearch.ca (accessed 14.1.09.).

Bajwa, H.A., Rogers, L.Q., 2007. Physical activity barriers and program preferences among indigent internal medicine patients with arthritis. Rehabil. Nurs. 32 (1), 31–34 40.

Bearne, L.M., Scott, D.L., Hurley, M.V., 2002. Exercise can reverse quadriceps sensorimotor dysfunction that is associated with rheumatoid arthritis without exacerbating disease activity. Rheumatology 41 (2), 157–166.

Beaton, D.E., Katz, J.N., Fossel, A.H., et al., 2001. Measuring the whole or the parts? Validity, reliability, and responsiveness of the disabilities of the arm, shoulder and hand outcome measure in different regions of the upper extremity. J. Hand Ther. 14 (2), 128–146.

Belza, B., 1995. Comparison of self-reported fatigue in rheumatoid arthritis and controls. J. Rheumatol. 22 (4), 639–643.

Berliner, M., Piegsa, M., 1997. Effects of therapeutic ultrasound in a water bath on skin microcirculation and skin temperature in rheumatoid arthritis. Eur. J. Phys. Med. Rehabil. 7 (2), 46–49.

Bibbo, C., Goldberg, J.W., 2004. Infectious and healing complications after elective orthopaedic foot and ankle surgery during tumor necrosis factor-alpha inhibition therapy. Foot Ankle Int. 25 (5), 331–335.

Boardman 3rd, N.D., Cofield, R.H., Bengtson, K.A., et al., 2001. Rehabilitation after total shoulder arthroplasty. J. Arthroplas. 16 (4), 483–486.

Borg, G.E., 1985. An Introduction to Borg's RPE scale. Ithaca, New York.

Boutry, N., Lardé, A., Lapègue, F., et al., 2003. Magnetic resonance imaging appearance of the hands and feet in patients with early rheumatoid arthritis. J. Rheumatol. 30 (4), 671–679.

Brosseau, L., Welch, V. & Wells, G.A., et al., 2005. Low level laser therapy (Classes I, II and III) for treating rheumatoid arthritis. *Cochrane Database of Systematic Reviews* (4) Art. No.: CD002049. DOI: 10.1002/14651858.CD002049.pub2.

Brosseau, L., Yonge, K.A. & Welch, V., et al., 2003. Transcutaneous electrical nerve stimulation (TENS) for the treatment of rheumatoid arthritis in the hand. *Cochrane Database of Systematic Reviews* (2) Art No. CD004377. DOI: 10.1002/14651858.CD004377.

Burton, W., Morrison, A., Maclean, R., et al., 2006. Systematic review of studies of productivity loss due to rheumatoid arthritis. Occup. Med. 56 (1), 18–27.

Casimiro, L., Barnsley, L. & Brosseau, L., et al., 2005. Acupuncture and electroacupuncture for the treatment of rheumatoid arthritis. *Cochrane Database of Systematic Reviews* (4) Art No. CD003788. DOI: 10.1002/14651858.CD003788.pub2.

Chalmers, A.C., Busby, C., Goyert, J., et al., 2000. Metatarsalgia and rheumatoid arthritis: A randomized, single blind, sequential trial comparing 2 types of foot orthoses and

supportive shoes. J. Rheumatol. 27, 1643–1647.

Chung, K.C., Pillsbury, M.S., Walters, M.R., et al., 1998. Reliability and validity testing of the Michigan Hand Outcomes Questionnaire. J. Hand Surg. [Am] 23, 575–587.

Cimmino, M.A., Parodi, M., Silvestri, E., et al., 2004. Correlation between radiographic, echographic and MRI changes and rheumatoid arthritis progression. Reumatismo 56 (1), 28–40.

Curtis, R., Groarke, A., Coughlan, R., et al., 2005. Psychological stress as a predictor of psychological adjustment and health status in patients with rheumatoid arthritis. Patient Edu. Counsel. 59 (2), 192–198.

Dellhag, B., Wollersjo, I., Bjelle, A., 1992. Effect of active hand exercise and wax bath treatment in rheumatoid arthritis patients. Arthritis Care Res. 5, 87–92.

Dreyer, S.J., Boden, S.D., 1999. Natural history of rheumatoid arthritis of the cervical spine. Clin. Orthop. Relat. Res. 366, 98–106.

Duruoz, M.T., Poiraudeau, S., Fermanian, J., et al., 1996. Development and validation of a rheumatoid hand functional disability scale that assesses functional handicap. J. Rheumatol. 23 (7), 1167–1172.

Egan, M., Brosseau, L. & Farmer, M., et al., 2001. Splints and Orthosis for treating rheumatoid arthritis. *Cochrane Database of Systematic Reviews* (4) Art No. CD004018. DOI: 10.1002/14651858.CD004018.

El Miedany, Y., Youssef, S., Mehanna, A.N., et al., 2008. Development of a scoring system for assessment of outcome of early undifferentiated inflammatory synovitis. Joint, Bone, Spine 75 (2), 155–162.

Epps, H., Ginnelly, L., Utley, M., et al., 2005. Is hydrotherapy cost-effective? A randomised controlled trial of combined hydrotherapy programmes compared with physiotherapy land techniques in children with juvenile idiopathic arthritis. Health Technol. Ass. 9 (39), 1–59 iii-iv, ix-x.

Fearing, V.G., Clark, J., 2000. Individuals in context: A practical guide to client centred practice. Slack Inc, Thorofare, NJ.

Felson, D.T., Anderson, J.J., Boers, M., et al., 1993. The American College of Rheumatology preliminary core set of disease activity mea-sures for rheumatoid arthritis clinical trials. Arthritis Rheum. 36, 729–740.

Felson, D.T., Anderson, J.J., Boers, M., et al., 1995. The American College of Rheumatology preliminary definition of improvement in rheumatoid arthritis. Arthritis Rheum. 38, 727–735.

Ferucci, E.D., Templin, D.W., Lanier, A.P., 2004. Rheumatoid arthritis in American Indians and native Alaskans: A review of the literature. Semin. Arthritis Rheum. 34, 662–667.

Filippucci, E., Iagnocco, A., Meenagh, G., et al., 2007. Ultrasound imaging for the rheumatologist VII. Clin. Exp. Rheumatol. 25 (1), 5–10.

Fries, J.F., Spitz, P.W., Kraines, R.G., et al., 1980. Measurement of patient outcome in arthritis. Arthritis Rheum. 23, 137–145.

Gabriel, S., Crowson, C.S., Kremers, H.M., et al., 2008. The rising incidence of rheumatoid arthritis. Arthritis Rheum. 58 (conference supplement), 773. [abstract].

Gignac, M.A.M., Cao, X., Lacaille, D., et al., 2008. Arthritis-related work transitions: A prospective analysis of reported productivity losses, work changes and leaving the labor force. Arthritis Rheum. 59 (12), 1805–1813.

Gilworth, G., Chamberlain, A., Harvey, A., et al., 2003. Development of a work instability scale for rheumatoid arthritis. Arthritis Rheum. 49 (3), 349–354.

Hall, J., Skevington, S.M., Maddison, P.J., et al., 1996. A randomised and controlled trial of hydrotherapy in rheumatoid arthritis. Arthritis Care Res. 9, 206–215.

Hammond, A., Lincoln, N., Sutcliffe, L., 1999. A crossover trial evaluating an educational-behavioural joint protection programme for people with rheumatoid arthritis. Patient Edu. Counsel. 37, 19–32.

Hammond, A., Freeman, K., 2001. One-year outcomes of a randomized controlled trial of an educational-behavioural joint protection programme for people with rheumatoid arthritis. Rheumatology 40, 1044–1051.

Hammond, A., 2004. Rehabilitation in rheumatoid arthritis: a critical review. Musculoskeletal Care 2 (3), 135–151.

Han, A., Judd, M. & Welch, V., et al., 2004. Tai chi for treating rheumatoid arthritis. *Cochrane Database of Systematic Reviews* (3) Art No. CD004849. DOI: 10.1002/14651858.CD004849.

Haskett, S., Backman, C., Porter, B., et al., 2004. A crossover trial of commercial versus custom-made wrist splints in the management of inflammatory polyarthritis. Arthritis Rheum. 51, 792–799.

Hawke, F., Burns, J. & Radford, J.A., et al., 2008. Custom-made foot orthoses for the treatment of foot pain. *Cochrane Database of Systematic Reviews* (3) Art No. CD006801. DOI: 10.1002/14651858.CD006801. pub2.

Haynes, B.F., 2004. Pathology. In: St Clair, E.W., Pisetsky, D.S., Haynes, B.F. (Eds.) Rheumatoid Arthritis. Lippincott Williams & Wilkins, Philadelphia, pp. 118–139.

Helewa, A., Goldsmith, C.H., Lee, P., et al., 1991. Effects of occupational therapy home service on patients with rheumatoid arthritis. Lancet 337, 1453–1456.

Heller, J.E., Shadick, N.A., 2007. Outcomes in rheumatoid arthritis: incorporating the patient perspective. Curr. Opin. Rheumatol. 19 (2), 101–105.

Hennell, S., Luqmani, R., 2008. Developing multidisciplinary guidelines for the management of early rheumatoid arthritis.

Musculoskeletal Care 6 (2), 97–107.

Hirvonen, H.E., Mikkelsson, M.K., Kautiainen, H., et al., 2006. Effectiveness of different cryotherapies on pain and disease activity in active rheumatoid arthritis. A randomised single blinded controlled trial. Clin. Exp. Rheumatol. 24 (3), 295–301.

Hurley, M.V., Mitchell, H.L., Walsh, N., 2003. In osteoarthritis, the psychosocial benefits of exercise are as important as physiological improvements. Exerc. Sport Sci. Rev. 31 (3), 138–143.

Hurley, M.V., Dziedzic, K., Bearne, L., et al., 2002. The clinical and cost-effectiveness of physiotherapy management of elderly people with common rheumatological conditions. The Chartered Society of Physiotherapy, London.

Kastbom, A., Strandberg, G., Lindroos, A., et al., 2004. Anti-CCP antibody predicts the disease course during 3 years in early rheumatoid arthritis. Ann. Rheum. Dis. 63, 1085–1089.

Katz, P.P., Alfieri, W.S., 1997. Satisfaction with abilities and well-being: Development and validation of a questionnaire for use among persons with rheumatoid arthritis. Arthritis Care Res. 10 (1), 89–98.

Katz, P.P., Pasch, L.A., Wong, B., 2003. Development of an instrument to measure disability in parenting activity among women with rheumatoid arthritis. Arthritis Rheum. 48, 935–943.

Katz, P.P., Yelin, E.H., 1994. Life activities of persons with rheumatoid arthritis with and without depressive symptoms. Arthritis Care Res. 7 (2), 69–77.

Kennedy, N., 2006. Exercise therapy for patients with rheumatoid arthritis: safety of intensive programmes and effects upon bone mineral density and disease activity: a literature review. Phys. Ther. Rev. 11 (4), 263–268.

Kremers, H.M., Gabriel, S.E., 2004. Epidemiology. In: St Clair, E.W.,

Pisetsky, D.S., Haynes, B.F. (Eds.) Rheumatoid Arthritis. Lippincott Williams & Wilkins, Philadelphia, pp. 1–10.

Lacaille, D., White, M.A., Backman, C.L., et al., 2007. Problems faced at work due to inflammatory arthritis: new insights gained from understanding patients' perspective. Arthritis Rheum. 57 (7), 1269–1279.

Lacaille, D., White, M.A., Rogers, P.A., et al., 2008. Employment and arthritis: making it work – A proof of concept study. Arthritis Rheum. 59 (11), 1647–1655.

Law, M., Baptiste, S., Carswell, A., et al., 2005. Canadian Occupational Performance Measure, fourth ed. CAOT Publications, Ottawa, ON.

Lerner, D., Amick, B.C., Rogers, W.H., et al., 2001. The work limitations questionnaire. Med. Care 39, 72–85.

Lee, E.O., Kim, J.I., Davis, A.H., et al., 2006. Effects of regular exercise on pain, fatigue and disability in patients with rheumatoid arthritis. Fam. Commun. Health 29 (4), 320–327.

Lineker, S.C., Hurley, L., Wilkins, A., et al., 2006. Investigating care provided by physical therapists treating people with rheumatoid arthritis: pilot study. Physiother. Can. 58 (1), 53–60.

Lorig, K.R., Holman, H., 2006. Self-management education: history, definition, outcomes, and mechanisms. Ann. Behav. Med. 26, 1–7.

Luqmani, R., Hennell, S., Estrach, C., et al., 2006. British Society for Rheumatology and British Health Professionals in Rheumatology guideline for the management of rheumatoid arthritis (the first 2 years). Rheumatology 45, 1167–1169.

Mann, W.C., Tomita, M., Hurren, D., et al., 1999. Changes in health, functional and psychosocial status and coping strategies of home-based older persons with arthritis

over three years. Occup. Ther. J. Res. 19, 126–146.

Mathiowetz, V., Weber, K., Volland, G., et al., 1984. Reliability and validity of grip and pinch strength evaluations. J. Hand Surg. (Am) 9, 222–226.

Medical Research Council, 1976. Aids to the Investigation of Peripheral Nerve Injuries. HMSO, London, UK.

Meenan, R.F., Mason, J.H., Anderson, J.J., et al., 1992. AIMS2: the content and properties of a revised and expanded Arthritis Impact Measurement Scales Health Status Questionnaire. Arthritis Rheum. 35 (1), 1–10.

Moncur, C., 1988. Discipline-specific standards of care: Physical therapy competencies in Physical Therapy Management of Arthritis. Churchill Livingstone, New York p 29-41.

Moss, P., 1997. Negotiating spaces in home environments: older women living with arthritis. Soc. Sci. Med. 45, 23–33.

Murphy, E., Bresnihan, B., Fitzgerald, O., 2008. Measurement of periarticular bone mineral density in the hands of patients with early inflammatory arthritis using dual energy x-ray absorpitometry. Clin. Rheumatol. 27 (6), 763–766.

NICE. (2009). Rheumatoid Arthritis: National clinical guideline for management and treatment in adults http://www.nice. org.uk/nicemedia/pdf/ CG79FullGuideline.pdf(accessed 13.9.09)

Nishimura, K., Sugiyama, D., Kogata, Y., et al., 2007. Meta-analysis: diagnostic accuracy of anti-cyclic citrullinated peptide antibody and rheumatoid factor for rheumatoid arthritis. Ann. Intern. Med. 146 (11), 797–808.

Nordenskiold, U., 1994. Evaluation of assistive devices after a course in joint protection. Int. J. Technol. Assess. Health Care 10, 293–304.

Nordenskiold, U., Grimby, G., Dahlin-Ivanoff, S., 1998. Questionnaire

to evaluate the effects of assistive devices and altered working methods in women with rheumatoid arthritis. Clin. Rheumatol. 17, 6–16.

O'Brien, A.V., Jones, P., Mullis, R., et al., 2006. Conservative hand therapy treatments in rheumatoid arthritis. Rheumatology 45, 577–583.

O'Connor, D., Kortman, B., Smith, A., et al., 1999. Correlation between objective and subjective measures of hand function in patients with rheumatoid arthritis. J. Hand Ther. 12, 323–329.

Pagnotta, A., Baron, M., Korner-Bitensky, N., 1998. The effect of a static wrist orthosis on hand function in individuals with rheumatoid arthritis. J. Rheumatol. 25, 879–885.

Podsiadlo, D., Richardson, S., 1991. The timed "Up & Go": a test of basic functional mobility for frail elderly persons. J. Am. Geriat. Soc. 39 (2), 142–148.

Poole, J.L., Gallegos, M., O'Linc, S., 2000. Reliability and validity of the Arthritis Hand Function Test in adults with systemic sclerosis (scleroderma). Arthritis Care Res. 13 (1), 69–73.

Prevoo, M.L., van't Hof, M.A., Kuper, H.H., et al., 1995. Modified disease activity scores that include twenty-eight joint counts. Development and validation in a prospective longitudinal study of patients with rheumatoid arthritis. Arthritis Rheum. 38 (1), 44–48.

Rennie, R.J., 1996. Evaluation of the effectiveness of a metacarpophalangeal ulnar deviation orthosis. J. Hand Ther. 9, 371–377.

Riemsma, R.P., Kirwan, J.R. & Taal, E., et al., 2003. Patient education for adults with rheumatoid arthritis. *Cochrane Database of Systematic Reviews* (2) Art No. CD003688. DOI: 10.1002/14651858.CD003688.

Ronkainen, A., Niskanen, M., Auvinen, A., 2006. Cervical

spine surgery in patients with rheumatoid arthritis: longterm mortality determinants. J. Rheumatol. 33 (3), 517–522.

Shin, Y., Choi, J., Nahm, D., et al., 2005. Rheumatoid factor is a marker of disease activity in Korean rheumatoid arthritis. Yonsei Med. J. 46 (4), 464–470.

Straub, R.H., Dhabhar, F.S., Bijlsma, J.W.J., et al., 2005. How psychological stress via hormones and nerve fibers may exacerbate rheumatoid arthritis. Arthritis Rheum. 52 (1), 16–26.

Schumacher, HR., Habre, W., Meador, R., Hsia, E.C., 2004. Predictive factors in early arthritis: long-term follow-up. Semin. Arthritis Rheum. 33 (4), 264–272.

Steultjens, E.M.J., Dekker, J., Bouter, L.M., et al., 2002. Occupational therapy for rheumatoid arthritis: a systematic review. Arthritis Rheum. 47, 672–685.

Symmons, D., Turner, G., Webb, R., et al., 2002. The prevalence of rheumatoid arthritis in the United Kingdom: New estimates for a new century. Rheumatology 41, 793–800.

Symmons, D.P.M., 2002. Epidemiology of rheumatoid arthritis: Determinants of onset, persistence and outcome. Best Prac. Res. Clin. Rheumatol. 16 (5), 707–722.

Tourinho, T.F., Stein, A., Castro, J. A., et al., 2005. Rheumatoid arthritis: evidence for bone loss in premenopausal women. J. Rheumatol. 32 (6), 1020–1025.

Uetani, M., 2007. Imaging approach for the evaluation of the bone and joint destruction in rheumatoid arthritis. Clin. Calcium 17 (4), 453–462.

Uhlig, T., Lillemo, S., Moe, R.H., et al., 2007. Reliability of the ICF Core Set for rheumatoid arthritis. Ann. Rheum. Dis. 66, 1078–1084.

Van den Ende, C.H., Breedveld, F.C., le Cessie, S., et al., 2000. Effect of intensive exercise on patients with active rheumatoid arthritis: a randomised clinical trial. Ann. Rheum. Dis. 59, 615–621.

Van den Ende, C.H., Vliet Vlieland, T.P.M., Munneke, M., et al., 2006. Dynamic exercise therapy for treating rheumatoid arthritis: a systematic review. Coch. Lib. (4).

van Lankveld, W., van't Pad Bosch, P., Bakker, J., et al., 1996. Sequential occupational dexterity assessment (SODA): a new test to measure hand disability. J. Hand Ther. 9 (1), 27–32.

Veehof, M.M., Taal, E., Heijnsdijk-Rouwenhorst, L.M., et al., 2008. Efficacy of wrist working splints in patients with rheumatoid arthritis: A randomized controlled study. Arthritis Rheum. 59 (12), 1698–1704.

Verhagen, A.P., de Vet, H.C.W., de Bie, R.A., et al., 1997. Taking baths: the efficacy of balneotherapy in patients with arthritis. A systematic review. J. Rheumatol. 24, 1964–1971.

Verhagen, A.P., Bierma-Zeinstra, S. M.A. & Boers, M., et al., 2004. Balneotherapy for rheumatoid arthritis. *Cochrane Database of Systematic Reviews* (1) Art No. CD000518. DOI: 10.1002/14651858. CD000518.

Wall, J.C., Bell, C., Campbell, S., et al., 1998. The expanded timed get up and go test. Gait Post. 7, 187.

Ware, J.E., Kosinski, M., 2001. The SF-36® Physical and Mental Health Summary Scales: A Manual for users of Version 1, second ed. Quality Metric, Lincoln, RI.

Welch, V., Brosseau, L. & Casimiro, L., et al., 2002. *Thermotherapy* for treating rheumatoid arthritis. *Cochrane Database of Systematic Reviews* (2) Art No. CD002826. DOI: 10.1002/14651858.CD002826.

Welsing, P.M., van Gestel, A.M., Swinkels, H.L., et al., 2001. The relationship between disease activity, joint destruction and functional capacity over the course of rheumatoid arthritis. Arthritis Rheum. 44, 2009–2017.

Wilkie, R., Peat, G., Thomas, E., et al., 2005. The Keele assessment of participation: A new instrument to measure participation restriction in population studies. Combined qualitative and quantitative examination of its psychometric properties. Qual. Life Res. 14, 1889–1899.

Wolfe, F., 2005. Why the HAQ-II can be an effective substitute for the HAQ. Clin. Exp. Rheumatol. 23 (Suppl 39), S29–S30.

World Health Organization, 2002. International Classification of Functioning, Disability and Health. World Health Organization, Geneva.

Yasura, K., Nakagawa, Y., Kobayashi, M., et al., 2006. Mechanical and biochemical effect of monopolar radiofrequency energy on human articular cartilage: an in vitro study. Am. J. Sports Med. 34 (8), 1322–1327.

Zijlstra, F.J., van den Berg-de-Lange, I., Huygen, F.J., et al., 2003. Anti-inflammatory actions of acupuncture. Mediators Inflam. 12 (2), 59–69.

Chapter 17

Osteoarthritis

Krysia Dziedzic PhD MCSP Arthritis Research Campaign National Primary Care Centre, Primary Care Sciences, Keele University, Keele, UK

Susan L. Murphy ScD, OTR/L Department of Physical Medicine and Rehabilitation, University of Michigan and Veterans Affairs Ann Arbor Health Care System, Ann Arbor, MI, USA

Helen Myers PhD MSc BSc Arthritis Research Campaign National Primary Care Centre, Primary Care Sciences, Keele University, Keele, UK

CHAPTER CONTENTS

KEY POINTS

- Osteoarthritis (OA) is a common condition, particularly in older adults affecting the joints such as the knee, hip, hand and foot.

DOI: 10.1016/B978-0-443-06934-5.00017-6

- As the population ages in the western world the proportion of people with OA in the population is increasing. The impact of OA is significant and will be the fourth largest cause of disability by 2020.
- Core treatments such as exercise, physical activity and information about OA are recognised as important for all patients considered to have the diagnosis, and therapists have an active role to play in the management of people with OA.
- Positive messages that something can be done for people with OA should be conveyed to patients.
- OA is a chronic long-term condition and should therefore be managed as such with appropriate review and reassessment throughout the course of the condition.

INTRODUCTION

The following chapter provides an overview of osteoarthritis (OA), its impact on functioning and the effectiveness of current treatments, including prevention efforts. OA is a complex disorder. The most commonly affected sites are the knees, hips and hands, followed by other areas such as the low back, neck and feet (Dieppe & Lohmander 2005). OA causes pain, stiffness and disability. Structures in and around the joint are considered to be the primary cause of signs and symptoms (Felson et al 2000). It is now recognised that OA should not be considered a wear and tear disease but a dynamic process of changes within a joint followed by repair and remodelling (Doherty & Dougados 2001). OA develops when excessive mechanical loads are placed on normal joints, when normal loads are placed on an abnormal joint (Brandt et al 2006), or where there is an inherent susceptibility for acquiring OA.

RISK FACTORS

Whilst there is no one single identifiable cause of OA, a number of risk factors for the onset of OA have been identified. These include increasing age, female gender, genetics, obesity, trauma, occupational activities, and local mechanical factors (Doherty 2001, Hunter & Felson 2006).

GENETICS

There is evidence of a strong hereditary component to OA in the hand, from studies of twins, and of an increased risk of hand OA in first-degree relatives (siblings, parents, offspring) of people with hand OA (Doherty 2000). Sisters of women with Heberden's nodes are more likely than expected to have Heberden's nodes themselves in their fifties (Stecher 1941). Early changes in the knee joint such as loss of medial cartilage volume and muscle strength have been found to have a high hereditary component (Zhai et al 2005).

OBESITY

Being overweight has been found to precede the development of knee OA (Felson et al 1997). Obesity increases the mechanical load on the knee joint and being overweight also increases the risk of disease progression (Dougados et al 1992, Schouten et al 1992).

TRAUMA

A previous injury to knee, hip or hand joints has been associated with development of OA (Dieppe & Lohmander 2005).

OCCUPATIONAL FACTORS

Specific jobs are associated with development of OA. Jobs which require repetitive pincer motions have been associated with OA of the distal interphalangeal (DIP) joints (Hadler et al 1978). Other jobs, such as farming, that require squatting and kneeling along with heavy lifting have been associated with knee and hip OA (Croft et al 1992).

LOCAL MECHANICAL FACTORS

In knee OA, the malalignment of the hip, knee, and ankle (an angle measured by full-limb radiography) has been shown to be a predictor of OA progression (Issa & Sharma 2006). Malalignment can be either varus (bow-legged) or valgus (knock-kneed) (Issa & Sharma 2006) and depending upon the type of malalignment, knee OA progression is higher in specific compartments of the knee joint (Sharma et al 2001).

PREVALENCE AND INCIDENCE

Arthritis affects approximately 43 million adults in the USA and is a leading cause of disability (Center for Disease Control 2001, Hootman et al 2005). A report by Arthritis Care (2004) identified 8.5 million adults in the UK with pain and disability that could be attributed to arthritis, with OA the most common form of all the arthritis conditions.

OA generally affects more females than males, (Felson et al 1987, Lawrence et al 1998, van Saase et al 1989) however, a recent meta-analysis showed that these gender differences may be dependent on the joint site. Specifically, females tended to show a higher prevalence of knee and hand OA compared to men but no differences were found in prevalence of hip OA (Srikanth et al 2005).

The prevalence of OA increases with age as OA is irreversible. Approximately 10% of the world's population over 60 years will have symptoms that can be attributed to OA (Symmons et al 2003). Based on estimates from US population data, nearly everyone over the age of 65 years will have at least minimal radiographic signs of osteoarthritis at one joint site (Lawrence et al 1998). There have been very few studies of the incidence of OA despite this being the commonest form of arthritis. Oliveria et al (1999) report the incidence of OA to be 671 in women and 399 in men per 100,000 adults.

OA is often asymptomatic in individuals, but by far the most common symptom that leads an individual to seek a diagnosis and treatment is pain. Figure 17.1 describes a 'staircase' of the prevalence of OA of the knee presenting in primary care (Peat et al 2001). It shows how the association between joint signs on x-ray and joint pain experienced strengthens as people progress up the 'staircase'.

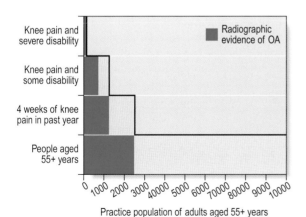

Figure 17.1 The prevalence staircase. Shading represents the proportion in each category with radiographic evidence of knee osteoarthritis. The proportion with radiographic evidence in the knee pain and severe disability category is not known, although expected to be high. (Source: Peat et al. Ann Rheum Dis 2001:60:91–97 with permission)

MORBIDITY AND MORTALITY

OA is common in older adults and as the western population increases in age the proportion of people with OA in the community will increase. It has been estimated that OA will be the fourth leading cause of disability by 2020 and the 6th leading cause of years lived with disability (Woolf & Pfleger 2003).

GLOBAL IMPACT

In the UK in 1999–2000, 36 million working days were lost due to OA, at a cost of £3.2 billion in lost productivity (Department for Work and Pensions cited in: Arthritis Research Campaign 2002). At this time, £43 million was also spent on community services and £215 million was spent on social services tackling OA-related problems (ARMA 2004). The total cost of OA in the UK has been estimated to be equivalent of 1% of Gross National Productivity per year (ARMA 2004, Doherty et al 2003, Levy et al 1993).

Arthritis treatment is associated with a large economic burden on the US healthcare system (estimated at $86 billion in 1997) (Murphy et al 2004). This burden is likely to become even greater with the projected increase of arthritis to 20% of the US population by 2030 (Center for Disease Control 2003).

AETIOLOGY, PATHOLOGY, IMMUNOLOGY

The pathophysiological changes in OA are considered to be dynamic. In OA, there is focal loss of cartilage covering the bone ends of the synovial joint with associated changes underneath the cartilage (subchondral) and formation of bone growths called osteophytes (Dieppe & Lohmander 2005). As the disease progresses, fluid filled cysts form in the bone, and fragments of bone or cartilage may float loosely in the joint space. The synovium also can become inflamed in advanced stages of the disease, which can further irritate the cartilage.

It has been suggested that OA may be classified based on potential cause; primary and secondary (Mitchell & Cruess 1977). Primary OA is more of a 'generalised' disease arising from systemic or genetic predisposition (Fig. 17.2). Secondary OA is a 'local' disease in which there is a definite history of injury or trauma to a particular joint (Felson et al 2000). Local OA, such as OA of the knee, is often seen in

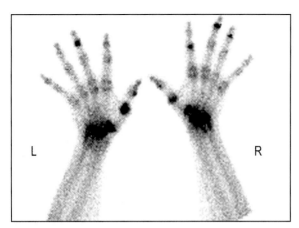

Figure 17.2 ^{99m}Tc-MDP bone scan delayed planar image of the hands demonstrates increased tracer uptake within bilateral first CMC joints and bilateral radiocarpal joints, as well as within the left third DIP joint, right third and fourth DIP and second PIP joints. Patient had history of prior trauma to the bilateral wrists and had a distribution of findings on radiographs consistent with osteoarthritis. From Hochberg MPH (2008) Figure 31.14 Nuclear medicine with permission from Elsevier Ltd, London.

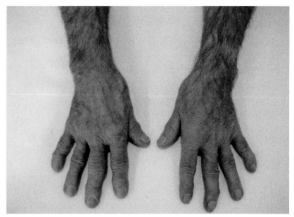

Figure 17.3 Osteoarthritis in the hands with Heberden's nodes seen on the distal interphalangeal joints and enlargement at the proximal interphalangeal joints. Copyright, Smooth study.

athletes and people at younger ages while primary OA, in which one or more joints are affected, is most prevalent among older adults.

DISEASE ACTIVITY, PROGRESSION, PROGNOSIS, INFLAMMATION

OA is commonly known as a non-inflammatory condition, however, it is increasingly recognised that variable degrees of local inflammation can occur (Symmons et al 2003) and that treatment approaches targeted at inflammation may be appropriate at certain stages of the disease (NICE 2008, Zhang et al 2007a, 2007b).

DIAGNOSIS, DIFFERENTIAL DIAGNOSIS, SPECIAL TESTS

Whilst it is recognised that asymptomatic radiographic OA exists, in clinical practice patients frequently present with symptomatic joints with or without accompanying changes on X-ray. OA pain may be accompanied by morning stiffness, which occurs on first wakening in the morning and lasts less than 30 minutes. The sensation of joint stiffness

can also be present when mobilising after resting for a prolonged period of time. The hip, knee (tibiofemoral, tibia and patellofemoral joints) and hand (carpometacarpal joint, distal interphalangeal and proximal interphalangeal joints) are the most frequently affected sites. In the hands, nodes, which were first described by William Heberden (1710–1801) can be present. If nodes are present in the distal interphalangeal joints they are classed as Heberden's nodes (Fig. 17.3) and in the proximal interphalangeal joints, Bouchard's nodes.

OA is diagnosed either by X-ray, clinical examination, or a combination of the two. Radiographic confirmation of OA involves examination of the presence of joint changes and severity of the disease and is often measured on the Kellgren and Lawrence scale (Box 17.1) (Kellgren & Lawrence 1957).

Some studies have found that radiographic severity of OA is not highly correlated with joint pain, (Birrell et al 2005, Hannan et al 2000) therefore a clinical examination is recommended (ARMA 2004). The American College of Rheumatology (ACR) has established clinical criteria used to classify knee, hip and hand OA for research studies which includes symptoms as well as joint changes. To establish knee OA according to the ACR clinical criteria, patients need to report knee pain and have 3 of the 6 following criteria:

- age >50 years
- morning stiffness of the knee ≤30 minutes duration

- crepitus on active motion
- tenderness of the bony margins of the knee joint (tested by palpating)
- bony enlargement noted on examination
- or no palpable synovial warmth.

(Altman et al 1986)

To establish hip OA, patients need to report hip pain and have either:

- limited range of motion in internal rotation and hip flexion (<15 degrees and ≤115 degrees respectively) or
- range of motion in hip internal rotation ≥15 degrees plus pain present, morning stiffness of the hip for ≤60 minutes duration, and age >50 years (Altman et al 1991).

To establish hand OA, patients need to meet the following criteria:

- hand pain, aching or stiffness lasting most days or all days in the past month, plus three out of four of the following:
- fewer than three swollen MCPJs (metacarpophalangeal joints);
- enlargement ≥2 of 10 selected joints;
- deformity ≥1 of 10 selected joints;
- enlargement in ≥2 DIPJs (distal interphalangeal joints)

(Altman et al 1990)

The 10 selected joints are the CMCJ, index and middle finger – DIPJs and PIPJs – on each hand.

In primary care the use of X-rays to establish a diagnosis of OA is limited (NICE 2008) as this does not direct future management in this setting. Whilst initial studies provided support for the use of clinical criteria to classify OA without radiographs, a recent study found that in the knee the criteria may only be sensitive in detecting later stages of OA (Peat et al 2006). X-ray is often still considered the gold standard in OA diagnosis (Altman et al 1986 & 1991).

A differential diagnosis is helpful to exclude patients who have inflammatory arthritis. No special laboratory tests are indicated to confirm OA but patients who have suspected inflammatory arthritis may need blood tests to rule out these conditions (Zhang et al 2009). As OA affects a high proportion of older adults, it is essential to recognise that such individuals may also have a number of co-existing conditions e.g. cardiovascular problems, diabetes (Kadam et al 2004).

CLINICAL PRESENTATION, CLINICAL FEATURES, CLINICAL SUBSETS

Joint pain in older people can be attributed to the joint itself and/or structures supporting the surrounding joint. The cartilage and underlying bone are degraded by the process of OA and whilst cartilage does not contain nerve endings that may generate pain the underlying bone does. Figure 17.4 illustrates the common sites that may be affected in isolation, bilaterally or in combination.

Different sub-sets of OA have been identified in the literature. Often a number of joints are affected. For instance, it is projected that up to 50% of people with knee or hip OA also have back pain (Wolfe et al 1996a). Generalised OA describes multi-site involvement. Nodal OA involves nodes at the IP joints of the hands in combination with OA at other sites. Erosive hand OA has been defined radiographically, where severe destruction of a joint and erosions can be identified. This form of OA is considered aggressive and disabling (Punzi et al 2004, Verbruggen & Veys 2000). Thumb base involvement is considered to have more severe functional consequences in hand OA (Zhang et al 2009).

SYMPTOMS AND SIGNS

The following section covers the predominant symptoms and signs of OA.

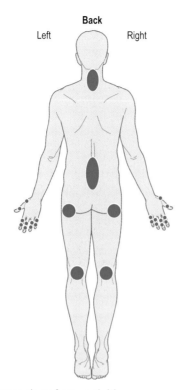
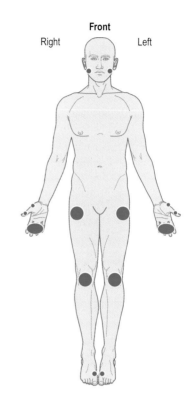

Figure 17.4 Common sites of osteoarthritis.

PAIN

The most common and important symptom of OA is pain. Pain may be localised and mild or can refer to other areas e.g. the hip joint may refer pain to the knee. Tenderness around the joint can be localised on palpation of soft tissues structures. Pain is often described as episodic with 'flaring' of symptoms. Pain may be very severe affecting an individual's ability to sleep.

> "I mean, if I sit too long, that doesn't help either. But the worst part is if I'm asleep and my legs are bent and I haven't woke up, the pain, I can't tell you what it is like. I cannot move it…and what I do is I grip both hands round the knee and try to force my leg straight and I break out in a hot sweat. All I can say is that it is a bony pain. I could shout out with the pain."
>
> (Susan, in Jinks et al 2007).

In the knee or hip, pain may also be felt during activities such as bending or stair climbing. Another source of OA pain may result from altering movement patterns to favour the less affected knee or hip. In this case, controlateral muscle pain may be felt. The unpredictability of intermittent pain in the lower limb often has a greater impact on the individual than constant pain (Hawker et al 2008).

STIFFNESS

Stiffness is a symptom of OA occurring particularly in the morning or after long stretches of inactivity. Stiffness usually dissipates as people begin to move or perform gentle stretching exercises. The symptoms of joint stiffness are felt in and around the joints commonly affected by OA and are often described by patients as being short-lived. Stiffness lasting more than 30 minutes may be an indicator of inflammatory joint disease, e.g. RA.

> "Had some pain and stiffness in my knees later in the day when squatting/stooping down for a short while looking in a low cupboard….This faded away when I stood up and flexed the joint – getting erect was a struggle. I find this frustrating at times, but accept it as one of the disadvantages of growing old."
>
> (Peter, in Jinks et al 2007).

FATIGUE

Fatigue is an understudied but prevalent symptom in OA. It is associated with decreased physical function and disability in mobility activities (Avlund et al 2003, Wolfe 1999). Fatigue is also highly associated with pain (Wolfe et al 1996b, Zautra et al 2007). The mechanisms of fatigue, however, in people with OA remain unclear. In knee OA, it is hypothesized that quadriceps fatigue during prolonged walking in older, obese people may contribute to OA development and progression (Syed & Davis 2000). The experience of fatigue is likely to be multi-faceted for people with OA. For instance, people who have higher daily fatigue are found to have less positive emotions within the day (Zautra et al 2007) and decreased physical activity (Murphy et al 2008). Whereas OA pain has been well studied, future work will need to examine the symptom of fatigue in OA in order to best refine treatment strategies.

JOINT ENLARGEMENT AND NODES

Joint enlargement is one of the hallmarks of OA, however the reliability of clinical assessment of joint enlargement is variable. The clinical classification of hand OA using the ACR clinical criteria (Altman et al 1990) uses joint enlargement as a feature to distinguish OA from RA. Heberden's nodes are found at the DIP joints and are seen as pea-like structures on the dorsolateral aspect of the joint (Fig. 17.3). Bouchards' nodes are seen at the PIP joints. Finger nodes and joint deformities do not always cause significant pain or disability however they might cause dissatisfaction with hand appearance.

JOINT DEFORMITIES

Structural changes within the OA joint can lead to joint deformity. Figures 17.5 and 17.6 illustrate common joint deformities of the lower limb and hands. Malalignment can be either varus (bow-legged) or valgus (knock-kneed) (Issa & Sharma 2006). A quadriceps lag and fixed flexion deformity are features seen at the knee joint and flexion contractures may occur at the hip. Lateral deviation and flexion of the finger joints and subluxation and adduction at the thumb base are common hand deformities.

EFFUSION

Mild joint effusions in the knee are not uncommon and the prepatella and anserine bursae may show

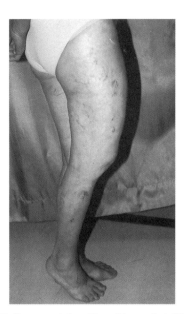

Figure 17.5 Common deformities of lower limb OA. Bowing of the right femur. A forward and lateral deformity provoking excruciating pain, due to varus osteoarthritis of the knee and shortening of the right lower limb. From Hochberg MC et al (2008) Figure 195.4 with permission from Elsevier, London.

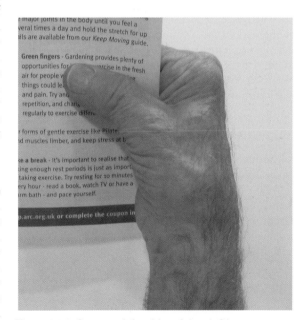

Figure 17.6 Common deformities of thumb OA.

signs of inflammation (bursitis). In the hand, if more than two metacarpophalangeal joints are swollen then inflammatory arthritis should be considered (Altman et al 1990). A hot, swollen joint is a red flag for OA and warrants immediate investigation.

CREPITUS

The patellofemoral joint commonly presents with crepitus which can be heard as cracking sounds and can be identified through palpation of the patella whilst a patient raises from a chair to stand and then slowly sits with equal weight through both feet (Peat et al 2004). The presence of crepitus may not, however, be associated with the severity of knee OA.

MUSCLE WASTING

Whether muscle is involved prior to joint change or whether joint changes, pain and stiffness lead to muscle weakness is uncertain. However, reduced strength in key muscle groups around OA joints is a feature of OA (e.g. weak quadriceps muscles, weakness of grip and pinch strength, Trendelenburg gait – an abnormal gait caused by weakness of the hip abductors allowing the pelvis to drop down on the opposite side in the weight-bearing phase).

LOSS OF RANGE OF MOVEMENT

Loss of range of movement and pain and the end of movement are common clinical features of OA (Dieppe & Lohmander 2005). Restriction in range of movement has been found to be predictive of the presence of OA in people newly presenting to primary care with hip pain (Birrell et al 2001).

BALANCE AND PROPRIOCEPTION

Individuals with joint signs and symptoms may have difficulty in sustaining normal balance e.g. standing on one leg for a timed period. Reasons for this can be multi-factorial but this may be an indicator of severity of OA (Pai et al 1997). Impaired balance and proprioception can lead to difficulties with mobility.

LOSS OF FUNCTIONING

There is a well-established link between pain and reduced physical function. Chronic pain is common among people with OA and is associated with problems in performing daily activities, decreased physical activity, and diminished quality of life. People with OA have reported that pain affects many areas of their lives such as functional and social activities, interpersonal relationships, emotional well-being, and body image (Carr 1999). An individual with OA may be referred for physical or occupational therapy because of pain or problems with function or mobility, e.g. walking up or down stairs, or difficulty in performing daily activities (e.g. washing, dressing).

PSYCHOSOCIAL FACTORS

Psychosocial factors may explain some of the discordance between reported knee pain and OA changes on x-ray (Creamer at al 1999). In the community, women reporting knee pain in the absence of radiographic OA had higher anxiety scores than women without pain (Creamer at al 1999), however depression was not significantly related to knee pain in this population.

Frustration with activities of daily living is a commonly reported problem (Hill 2005). Asking patients about the specific tasks they get frustrated with may help them to identify strategies for managing frustration.

CLINICAL EVALUATION, ASSESSMENT, SUBJECTIVE AND OBJECTIVE EXAMINATION

A clinical diagnosis of OA will depend on a number of presenting features, including symptoms and signs. The European League against Rheumatism (EULAR) for example has produced recommendations for the diagnosis of hand OA (Zhang et al 2009).

OA can be assessed through a variety of methods including self-complete questionnaires (see Ch. 4). Lower limb function is frequently measured with instruments such as the Western Ontario and McMaster Universities Arthritis Index (WOMAC) (Bellamy et al 1988) and Lequesne Index (Lequesne et al 1987). The WOMAC is a validated questionnaire for adults with knee or hip OA. Patients rate their currently experienced pain and difficulty performing physical activities.

For self-reported hand assessment a number of instruments can be used (Dziedzic et al 2005), including the AUSCAN, the Australian Canadian index for the hand (Bellamy et al 2002). The WOMAC and the AUSCAN follow the same principles, a three-section tool that covers pain on activity, stiffness and functional difficulty because of arthritis.

Objective assessments can be performed to establish the severity of presentation and to evaluate improvement or maintenance of abilities over time.

Choice of functional test or measurement tool will be dependent on a variety of factors, such as the clinical setting, time available and purpose of assessment. Hand function can be measured using a variety of performance based standardized tests, such as the Grip Ability Test (Dellhag & Bjelle 1995) and physiological tests such as grip and pinch strength (measured using the Jamar dynamometer and B & L pinch gauge respectively) (Mathiowetz et al 1985). Quadriceps strength testing (Sharma et al 2003) and timed physical function (Guralnik et al 1994) have been shown to be valid and reliable for the knee.

The International Classification of Functioning (ICF see Ch. 4) provides a useful model for the mapping of specific assessment tools. It may be more appropriate to identify a measure of participation (Wilkie et al 2004) or social networking for some patients with OA than identifying the severity and location of joint pain. Understanding a patient's workplace requirements is also important for those continuing in work (see Ch. 9).

IMAGING

Whilst x-ray is considered the gold standard, Magnetic Resonance Imaging (MRI) has been shown to identify not only OA features in the joint but those elsewhere, e.g. synovitis (Conaghan et al 2005a, Tan et al 2003). It is currently recognised that there is a very poor correlation between x-ray changes and patients' signs and symptoms, except in those who are in the severe stages of their condition, where severe pain and disability correlate with severe x-ray change (Peat et al 2001) (Fig. 17.1).

Ultrasound is another method of imaging joint structures and again, work in this field is looking to identify the association of pain and disability with joint damage (Conaghan et al 2005b, D'Agostino et al 2005). Future research may give a greater indication as to the relationship between joint damage and patients' signs and symptoms.

TREATMENT APPROACHES

Guidelines provide a synthesis of approaches to the management of OA. The National Institute of Health and Clinical Excellence (http://guidance. nice.org.uk/) has published guidelines for the management of OA in the NHS in England and Wales, OMERACT/OARSI have published international

recommendations for the management of OA (Zhang et al 2007b) and the European League Against Rheumatism (http://www.eular.org/) has published EULAR recommendations for hip, knee and hand OA.

In all guidelines there is emphasis on evidence-based programmes, condition specific recommendations and systematic reviews. Whilst many of the treatments are not evidence based they are considered a best care approach and have been agreed by consensus (e.g. Zhang et al 2007a, b).

All guidelines recognise that there are common core treatments that should be available to all people with OA. Core treatments include access to information, advice on activity and exercise therapy, weight loss if overweight and the optimal use of paracetamol and topical NSAIDs for pain relief.

AIMS AND PRINCIPLES OF MANAGEMENT

The optimal management of OA requires a combination of non-pharmacological and pharmacological interventions. Treatments should be individualised and should acknowledge the patient's expectations and health beliefs (Zhang et al 2007a). One of the fundamental mistakes that a health professional can make is to assume that a person with OA will have a benign condition. It has been reported that disability associated with OA can be as severe as that with RA, and someone with OA may have significant needs in terms of treatment (Zhang et al 2009).

The following quotes highlight what it means to an individual to be given a diagnosis of OA:

> "I've been …I've seen him…but all he said to me, you see (is), it's wear and tear. When he describes wear and tear if it's …it's just age and it's just a 'whatsit'…as if nothing can be done for you […] . With him telling me it was wear and tear that meant they couldn't do anything, but I don't know whether they can or not."
>
> (Geoff, in Jinks et al 2007)

> "I went to the GP (he) gave me a form…with OA or something, whatever they call it. I thought that wasn't very helpful. 'Nothing we can do about it' he said and at the time I'd got really bad pain, which was why I went…. down the thumb. I honestly wouldn't ever go back and tell them my hands are playing up 'cause he said there was nothing they could do"
>
> (Hill 2005)

If a patient has been given a diagnosis of OA then the therapist should provide support and positive messages about treatments that can be offered (ARMA 2004, NICE 2008).

The aims of treatment are to control symptoms, limit deterioration and maintain functional status. Therapists need a comprehensive understanding of the impact of OA on the person's physical, psychological and social well-being, quality of life, daily activities, occupation, mood, relationships and hobbies.

Occupational performance can be affected by arthritis, leading to absenteeism and job disruptions, reduced hours, changing jobs, and leaving employment (Gignac et al 2008). Even when individuals are able to remain in employment, productivity losses are common, e.g. being unable to take on extra work. The impact that OA has on work leads to diverse employment changes that may occur in the lives of many individuals and difficulties with remaining employed (Gignac et al 2008).

The management plan should include review (e.g. annual) and reassessment of health status and needs (ARMA 2004), as OA is a chronic, long-term condition that requires monitoring over time. Information should be made available to people on how to relieve symptoms and when to consult a health professional for further help, for example if symptoms and functional capacity are worsening despite treatment (ARMA 2004).

Treatment should be patient-centred and plans should be developed in partnership. Figure 17.7 illustrates an example of a clinical pathway for an individual presenting with generalised OA.

Individuals with symptoms from OA are frequently managed in primary care. In this setting OA is defined as a clinical syndrome, where adults 45 years and over presenting with joint pain and

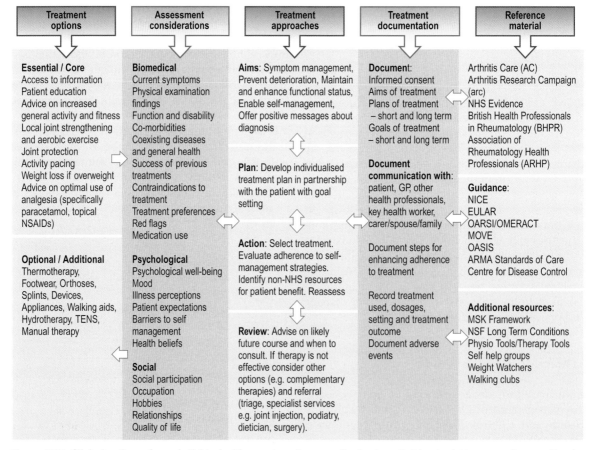

Figure 17.7 Clinical pathway for an individual with symptomatic generalised osteoarthritis: physiotherapy and occupational therapy treatment options.

problems, in the absence of red flags, e.g. inflammatory arthritis, injury or hot swollen joint, are considered to have OA and can be managed as such without the requirement for an x-ray (NICE 2008).

NON-PHARMACOLOGICAL TREATMENT APPROACHES

PATIENT EDUCATION

Education on the likely course of their OA and possible treatments available needs to be provided. Qualitative studies in OA have demonstrated that patients frequently report that they are told by health professionals that nothing can be done (Jinks et al 2007, Sanders et al 2002 & 2004). Positive messages about what can be done need to be conveyed (ARMA 2004).

Different patients have different information needs and it is therefore desirable to provide many forms of information support e.g. written, verbal, web sites. The Arthritis Research Campaign (http://www.arc.org.uk), Arthritis Care (http://www.arthritiscare.org.uk), the Arthritis Foundation (http://www.arthritis.org) and the ARMA Standards of Care (http://www.arma.uk.net/pdfs/oa06.pdf) are useful Internet locations for health care practitioners and patients with OA.

Information should cover pharmacological and non-pharmacological options and should be evidence-based where possible. This should address the specific needs of the individual, e.g. work, role as carer.

CORE THERAPY INTERVENTIONS: EXERCISE, SELF-MANAGEMENT AND JOINT PROTECTION

PHYSICAL ACTIVITY INTERVENTIONS

These interventions are most commonly structured exercise programmes that attempt to alter the mechanics of arthritic joints by maintaining joint flexibility, increasing muscle strength, and reducing pain. Two recent syntheses of exercise guidelines for people with hip and knee OA (OASIS: Osteoarthritis of the knee and hip and activity: a systematic international review and synthesis (Vignon et al 2006); and the MOVE consensus (Roddy et al 2005)) recommend regular physical activity as a core disease management strategy. Of the different types of exercise, such as strengthening versus aerobic or group versus home exercise, no one type is recommended over another. The OASIS group found that physical activity in daily life may be a risk factor for developing OA, but maintains that activities should be engaged in, even at a high intensity, if the activity performed is not painful and does not predispose to further trauma (Vignon et al 2006).

Different types of programmes designed for people with OA include:

● The PACE programme from the Arthritis Foundation (USA). This programme combines flexibility and low-impact aerobic exercise. (http://www.cdc.gov/arthritis/intervention/ accessed March 2009).

● Aquatics and hydrotherapy. Aquatic programmes are popular among people with OA because the water may relieve joint pain and stiffness as well as provide an environment that protects joints while exercising.

● Land-based exercise programmes.

● Strengthening programmes. These are usually done in a progressive fashion in which strength is built up gradually over time. Weights or theraband are often used with the goal of strengthening muscles around affected joints (e.g. Fig. 17.8A,B, Fig. 17.9)

● Aerobic programmes such as walking or other endurance-based programs are important to impact overall fitness and have effects on strength and balance. (e.g. http://www.arthritistoday.org/fitness/walking/tips-and-strategies/walking-plan.php accessed March 2009).

There is a misconception that exercise is only suitable for those who are fit and well and who experience no joint pain during exercise. It is important to remember that exercise should be a component of all therapy for OA, no matter the age of the patient and irrespective of co-morbid problems, severity of pain and disability. Exercise programmes should be adapted according to the ability of the patient, and strategies to manage pain before, during, and after exercise should be discussed.

Structured exercise programmes have been shown to reduce difficulty in performing activities of daily living among people with knee OA (Ettinger et al 1997, Penninx et al 2001). Several studies have supported the effectiveness of exercise on pain and physical function among older adults who have hip or knee OA (Baker & McAlindon 2000, Borjesson et al 1996, Hay et al 2006, Hurley et al 2007, McCarthy

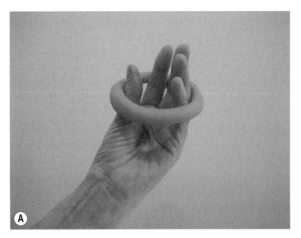 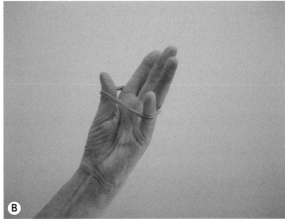

Figure 17.8 (A) (B) Putty, elasticated bands or theraband are often used with the goal of strengthening muscles around affected joints in OA. Examples for the hand are illustrated.

et al 2004, Roddy et al 2005, van Baar et al 1998, van Baar et al 1999). Much of the evidence for the use of exercise has been conducted in the knee and there is limited evidence for the benefit of exercise in the hip and hand. However, the consensus of experts is that exercise should be considered in other joints and aerobic exercise will benefit the individual with OA in any joint (NICE 2008, Zhang et al 2007a, 2007b). As no one programme is considered more effective than another, patients should be encouraged to participate in at least one type of programme based on their personal preference. This is particularly critical given that many people do not adhere to these programmes over time and adherence is necessary to best limit OA progression.

Adherence to exercise programmes is related to better outcomes (Hurley et al 2007) and strategies to promote adherence need to be employed (see Ch. 7), for example some patients can prefer group activities. Health eating and healthy weight are important in reducing the impact of pain and functional limitation with OA. Weight loss programmes seem to be most effective when combined with exercise (Christensen et al 2007).

BEHAVIOURAL SELF-MANAGEMENT INTERVENTIONS

Interventions such as self-management programmes employ a psychological approach to increase coping skills and problem-solving abilities related to the disease (Hawley 1995). Behavioural programmes do not forestall the progression of disability in OA, but have been shown to have positive effects on other health outcomes (Calfas et al 1992, Hawley 1995, Lorig et al 1993, Lorig et al 2001) and are thought to be a very important adjunct to physical activity interventions (Vignon et al 1996). The Arthritis Self-Management Program (Lorig et al 1985) is an established behavioural intervention for older adults with osteoarthritis. The programme is given by lay people who often have the disease and the content includes the management of symptoms, medications, and emotions, problem-solving and decision-making abilities, use of community resources, adoption of exercise programmes and joint protection (Lorig et al 2001). This intervention and other behavioural interventions have been shown to have positive effects on pain, depression, and health care utilisation over time (Hawley 1995, Keefe et al 1990, Lorig et al 1993, Superio-Cabuslay et al 1996). Guidelines suggest that self-management strategies are most effective when based on specific approaches e.g. enhancing exercise adherence (see Ch. 7).

JOINT PROTECTION

Joint protection and fatigue management should be an essential component of therapy. Effective approaches should be used including educational, cognitive and behavioural approaches (see Ch. 10). Access to devices and assistive equipment that would improve the ability to undertake activities of everyday life is important and referral for specialist assessment is important for those with severe disease. Joint protection in combination with hand exercises is thought to be beneficial for people with hand OA (Stamm et al 2002).

Personal Exercise Program

Your Organisation Name
your address/your telephone/fax/email/website
you can have more than one header

General Exercises

Provided for: Patient's name _____

Provided by: Your name _____

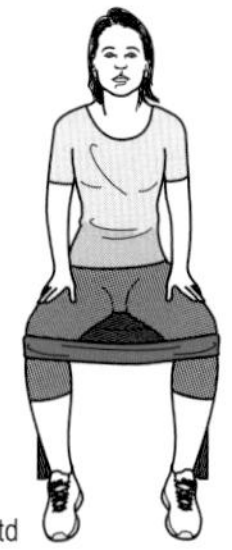

© PhysioTools Ltd

Sit on a chair. Put a rubber exercise band around your knees.
Spread knees apart. Slowly bring knees back together

Repeat _____ times

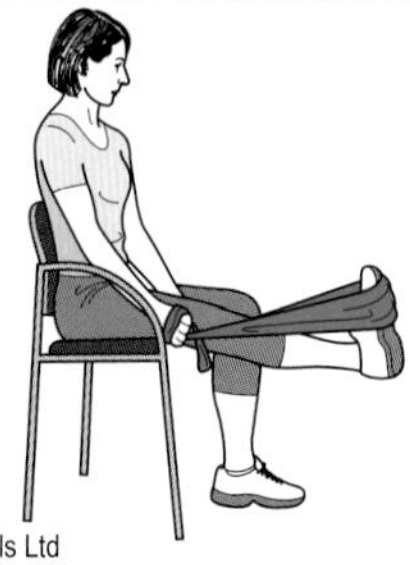

© PhysioTools Ltd

Put a rubber exercise band under your foot and hold on to the ends.
Straighten and bend your leg keeping your hands still

Repeat _____ min

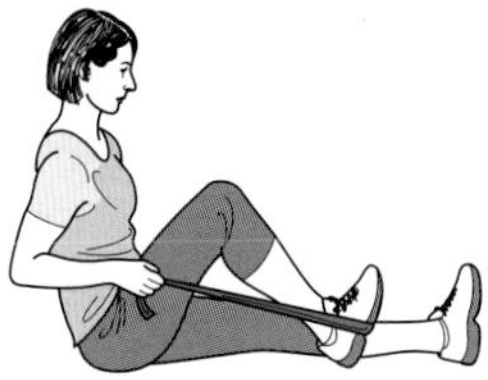

© PhysioTools Ltd

Long sitting. Put a band around your foot.
Bend your knees as far as possible. Gently pull the band to bend
your knee a little more. Hold _____ secs.

Repeat _____ times

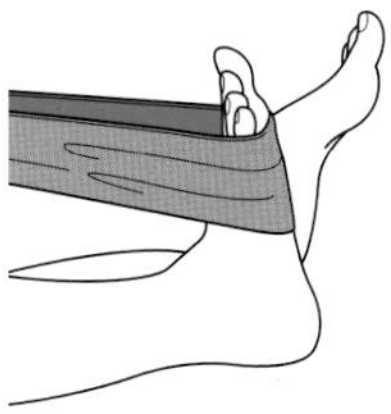

© PhysioTools Ltd

Sit with one leg straight out in front of you. Put a band around your foot.
Gently pull the band and feel the stretch in your calf. Hold approx _____ secs.

Repeat _____ times

Figure 17.9 PhysioTools offers a wide range of exercises (www.physiotools.com).

OTHER THERAPEUTIC MODALITIES

Alongside these core treatments, other modalities may be required if symptoms and disability persist. These include weight loss advice for those overweight (see Ch. 14), transcutaneous electrical nerve stimulation (TENS) (Ch. 8), thermotherapy (Ch. 8), manual therapy (Ch.8), orthoses and footwear (Ch. 13), assistive equipment and devices (Ch. 9) and splinting (Ch. 12). Walking aids, such as canes, are considered beneficial for lower limb OA. These modalities are all discussed in previous chapters.

PHARMACOLOGICAL APPROACHES

Common pharmacological approaches include paracetamol, topical NSAIDs, oral NSAIDs, COX-2s and joint injection (see Ch. 15). Other less common approaches include injectable glucocorticoids, which are injected directly into the joint for fast pain relief. Viscosupplementation (for knee OA only) involves a series of injections into the joint. The injected material is hyaluronic acid, a naturally occurring substance found in the synovium. Capsaicin and glucosamine sulphate (NICE 2008) are other alternative and complementary treatments options. These are all discussed in Chapters 14 and 15.

INDICATIONS FOR SURGERY

People with OA may require joint replacement surgery. Patients should have at least received the core treatment approaches for OA prior to consideration of surgery (NICE 2008). A pre-surgical assessment is needed to determine treatment options including surgery and the balance of benefits and risks of these treatments.

In 2005, patients with osteoarthritis accounted for at least 55,495 primary knee joint arthroplasties in England and Wales (NJR 2005). Exercise after discharge results in short term benefit after elective primary total knee arthroplasty although effects are small to moderate, and only in the short term (Minns Lowe et al 2007).

SELF-MANAGEMENT EDUCATION AND PREVENTION EFFORTS

In the US where arthritis is a rapidly growing public health problem, the Center for Disease Control (CDC) has created a national arthritis action plan to try to hinder and prevent OA (Meenan et al 1999). The goals of the programme include education for better self-management of arthritis as well as guidance on engaging in physical activity. Currently none of the health care systems recently evaluated in 25 US states met targeted objectives for including these areas in arthritis treatment (Hootman et al 2005). A clear and optimal method for disseminating and providing interventions to a large number of people does not currently exist.

Physiotherapists and occupational therapists now have a unique opportunity given their skills and background to become more active in OA prevention. Given the growing public health problem in the western world, there need to be better-funded healthcare initiatives to combat this problem. Current guidelines for physical activity for all adults are, as given by Healthy People 2010, engaging in:

- at least 30 minutes of moderate intensity activity (such as brisk walking, vacuuming, or gardening) on at least 5 days a week
- up to 20 minutes of vigorous activity (running, aerobics, heavy yard work) on at least 3 days a week (Center for Disease Control, http://www.cdc.gov/nccdphp/dnpa/physical/stats/definitions.htm).

CONCLUSION

Osteoarthritis (OA) is a common condition, affecting the joints such as the knee, hip, hand and foot. As the population ages in the western world the proportion of people with OA in the population will increase and OA will be the fourth largest cause of disability by 2020. Core treatments such as exercise, physical activity and information about OA are recognised as important for all patients, and therapists have an active role to play in the management of people with OA. Positive messages that something can be done for people with OA should be conveyed to patients. As OA is a chronic long-term condition it should therefore be managed as such with appropriate review and reassessment throughout the course of the condition.

STUDY ACTIVITIES

1. Access the NICE web site (http://guidance.nice.
   org.uk/) and identify the published guidelines for
   the management of OA. Prepare a list of all non-
   pharmacological approaches for the management of OA.
2. Access the Arthritis Research Campaign (http://www.
   arc.org.uk), the Arthritis Foundation (http://www.
   arthritis.org) and Arthritis Care (http://www.
   arthritiscare.org.uk/home) websites. Identify all
   patient information leaflets that would be applicable
   to an older adult presenting to a therapist with joint
   pain, and difficulties with activities of daily living.
   Consider five main messages that you would convey
   to a patient based on the information in these
   leaflets. List these and keep them for future
   reference.

3. The NHS Evidence – Musculoskeletal (www.
   library.nhs.uk/musculoskeletal) holds a National
   Knowledge Week on Osteoarthritis (OA) with an
   annual update of articles published each year (see
   http://www.library.nhs.uk/MUSCULOSKELETAL/Page.
   aspx?pagename=NKWAEU).
   Conduct a literature search and prepare a
   reference list, for the past year, of articles related to
   the management of OA, with a brief summary of the
   findings of each.
4. Identify and read a published high quality qualitative
   study investigating the personal experiences of
   living with OA. Consider the impact of OA on the
   individual in the context of social, environmental and
   occupational factors.

CASE STUDY 17.1

Denry is a 54-year-old plumber who enjoys fishing and
golf. He went to his doctor complaining of pain in his
thumbs, which first started when he was working, but
now trouble him at other times. He finds gripping small
items painful and his hands feel generally clumsier
than before. He hasn't been able to go fishing and play
golf because of the pain. He occasionally has to ask
his son to undo things, especially opening new jars. He
reports increased frustration with his thumb pain and, at
times, wanting to throw his tools across the room. He's
currently self-employed and is worried that he will be
unable to work. His knees sometimes ache after being
in one position for too long and he finds them very stiff
when getting up from kneeling.

He has been given paracetamol by the doctor but
doesn't think he should take tablets for his pain. In all
other respects he is fit and well. He believes that nothing
can be done because he works his hands and knees hard
at his job and these problems are part of getting older.
On examination, he has signs of OA in the bases of both
thumbs, the left is worse than the right but he is right
handed. He has subluxation and adduction deformities
of his thumb bases and there is evidence of wasting in
the hypothenar eminences. He has no finger nodes but
several finger joints look more enlarged than normal.

There is pain on palpation of the thumb bases of both
hands. Grip and pinch strength are reduced mainly on
the left hand. Other joints in the upper limb are normal.
On examination of the knees there is evidence of mild

quadriceps wasting and slight loss of full range of knee
extension on the right knee. Gait is normal but balancing
on one leg is more difficult than Denry expects.

The aims of treatment are to optimise pain relief,
improve range of movement and muscle strength,
offer positive messages about what can be done for
OA and inform Denry about joint protection, assistive
devices and appliances that can be helpful for everyday
tasks. Denry is encouraged to use paracetamol in the
way the GP prescribed it and to attend a group session
on joint protection and exercise for people with arthritis.
Here he is taught exercises, ways of performing tasks
by modifying his grip and how to use heat and ice
to relieve pain. Exercises include how to use putty to
perform hand strengthening and stretching exercises.
The possibility of using a topical NSAID is raised if
the paracetamol, thermotherapy and exercise are not
adequate for pain relief. To reinforce education, an
exercise list from Physiotools (http://www.physiotools.
com/(S(mmjricmOnovaqOy40wmsiwz3))/Home.
aspx?PageId=Home) is printed out for Denry for the
hands and knees and Internet resources are provided
for continuing self-care. The OT also provides
individualised assessment, advice, and modifications
for work (including ergonomic tool design), and for his
valued activities of fishing and golf to help make this
easier.

Following the classes Denry has met another man in a
similar position and they have joined a local swimming

(Continued)

CASE STUDY 17.1 (CONTINUED)

group and a walking group to maintain overall levels of fitness. The swimming has been beneficial to the hand pain and hand strength. Denry has declined the option of a thumb splint for work and doesn't feel he needs further physiotherapy for pain relief. Denry feels more confident that he can cope with his symptoms and modify his work practices so that he may continue his job. He hopes to start playing golf and go fishing again shortly.

CASE STUDY 17.2

Mrs Machin is an 84-year-old widow who enjoys knitting and visiting her grandchildren. She went to her doctor complaining of pain and loss of function in her hands and hips, which she has had on and off for years, but these problems now make it difficult to walk down stairs and dress. Increasingly Mrs Machin uses two hands to do everything. She reports that her pain and fatigue increase throughout the day and become so severe that she needs to rest for long periods later in the afternoon. She is not able to accomplish her usual daily tasks and is worried that if things get any worse she won't be able to drive or live in her own home.

Mrs Machin has been given paracetamol by the doctor and has had her right thumb base injected. Her general health is declining as her levels of fitness have reduced. She believes it's all an inevitable consequence of ageing. She has had physiotherapy before but can't remember what this was. On examination, she has signs of severe OA in the hips and hands. There are deformities and enlargements of most joints and there is evidence of muscle wasting. Mrs Machin has finger nodes in all distal interphalangeal joints. There is minimal pain on palpation of the affected joints. Grip and pinch strength are reduced but other joints in the upper limb are normal. On examination of the hips there is evidence of marked quadriceps wasting and loss of full range of hip movement. Gait is normal on flat surfaces but slow and cautious. Balancing on one leg would be impossible.

The aims of treatment are to optimise pain relief and functional ability, improve range of movement and muscle strength, offer positive messages about what can be done for OA and inform Mrs Machin and her daughter about assistive devices and appliances that can be helpful for everyday tasks. Mrs Machin attends group sessions on joint protection and exercise for people with arthritis as well as instruction on activity pacing. Here she is taught exercises, joint protection strategies, how to use heat and ice to relieve pain, and how to plan activities in accordance with her symptom severity. She asks about the best way of continuing her hobby of knitting without aggravating her hands. To reinforce education, an exercise list from PhysioTools (http://www.physiotools.com/(S(mmjricm0novaq0y40wmsiwz3))/Home.aspx?PageId=Home) is printed out for hands and hips and patient information leaflets are provided for continuing self-care. Her daughter has put a handrail in at home for the stairs.

The OT also conducts an individual assessment of personal and domestic ADL. Recommendations for easier clothing designs, height of chair and bed and bath aids are made – with referral to Social Services for the latter. Mrs Machin's fitness to drive is tactfully discussed with her and she is recommended to inform her insurance company and Vehicle Licensing Authority about her health. Information about Community Transport schemes is also provided.

Following the classes Mrs Machin has joined a local group who meet regularly for gentle exercises. Mrs Machin is surprised at how she has regained some of her independence and notices she is more active throughout her day. She reports that she feels less pain and fatigue by breaking up some of the challenging activities she used to pack into her mornings when she felt the best, like shopping and housecleaning, and no longer requires the long rest periods in the afternoon. She feels more knowledgeable about services in the community that could help her. She has discussed the option of referral for hip surgery. She has been instructed to contact the practice nurse for a review of her general health in 6 months.

References and further reading

Altman, R., Asch, E., Bloch, G., et al., 1986. Development of criteria for the classification and reporting of osteoarthritis: classification of osteoarthritis of the knee. Arthritis. Rheum. 29, 1039–1049.

Altman, R., Alarcón, G., Appelrouth, D., et al., 1990. The American college of rheumatology criteria for the classification and reporting of osteoarthritis of the hand. Arthritis. Rheum. 33, 1601–1610.

Altman, R., Alarcón, G., Appelrouth, D., et al., 1991. The American College of rheumatology criteria for the classification of osteoarthritis of the hip. Arthritis. Rheum. 34, 505–514.

ARMA, 2004. Standards of Care for people with osteoarthritis. http://www.arma.uk.net/pdfs/oa06.pdf/ (accessed March 2009).

Arthritis Care, 2004. OA Nation. www.arthritiscare.org.uk/OANation/ (accessed March 2009).

Arthritis Research Campaign, 2002. Arthritis: the Big Picture. http://www.arc.org.uk/ (accessed March 2009).

Avlund, K., Vass, M., Hendriksen, C., 2003. Onset of mobility difficulty among community-dwelling old men and women. The role of tiredness in activities. Age Aging 32, 579–584.

Baker, K., McAlindon, T., 2000. Exercise for knee osteoarthritis. Curr. Opin. Rheumatol. 12, 456–463.

Bellamy, N., Buchanan, W.W., Goldsmith, C.H., et al., 1988. Validation study of WOMAC: a health status instrument for measuring clinically important patient relevant outcomes to antirheumatic drug therapy in patients with osteoarthritis of the hip or knee. J. Rheumatol. 15, 1833–1840.

Bellamy, N., Campbell, J., Haraoui, B., et al., 2002. Clinimetric properties of the AUSCAN Osteoarthritis Hand Index: an evaluation of reliability, validity and responsiveness. Osteoarthrit. Cartil. 10 (11), 863–869.

Birrell, F., Croft, P., Cooper, C., et al., 2001. Predicting radiographic hip osteoarthritis from range of movement. Rheumatology 40, 506–512.

Birrell, F., Lunt, M., MacFarlane, G., et al., 2005. Association between pain in the hip region and radiographic changes of osteoarthritis: results from a population-based study. Rheumatology 44, 337–341.

Borjesson, M., Robertson, E., Weidenhielm, L., et al., 1996. Physiotherapy in knee osteoarthrosis: effect on pain and walking. Physiother. Res. Int. 1 (2), 89–97.

Brandt, K.D., Radin, E.L., Dieppe, P.A., et al., 2006. Yet more evidence that osteoarthritis is not a cartilage disease. Ann. Rheum. Dis. 65, 1261–1264.

Calfas, K.J., Kaplan, R.M., Ingram, R.E., 1992. One-year evaluation of cognitive behavioural intervention in osteoarthritis. Arthritis. Care Res. 5, 202–209.

Carr, A.J., 1999. Beyond disability: measuring the social and personal consequences of osteoarthritis. Osteoarthr. Cartil. 7 (2), 230–238.

Center for Disease Control, 2001. Prevalence of disabilities and associated health conditions among adults-United States, 1999. Morb. Mortal. Wkly. Rep. 50, 120–125.

Center for Disease Control, 2003. Projected prevalence of self-reported arthritis or chronic joint symptoms among persons ages ≥65 years: United States, 2005–2030. Morb. Mortal. Wkly. Rep. 52, 489–491.

Christensen, R., Bartels, E.M., Astrup, A., et al., 2007. Effect of weight reduction in obese patients diagnosed with knee osteoarthritis: a systematic review and meta-analysis. Ann. Rheum. Dis. 66, 433–439.

Conaghan, P., Felson, D., Gold, G., et al., 2005a. MRI and non-cartilaginous structures in knee osteoarthritis. Osteoarthr. Cartil. 14, 87–94.

Conaghan, P., D'Agostino, M.A., Ravaud, P., et al., 2005b. EULAR report on the use of ultrasonography in painful knee osteoarthritis. Part 2: Exploring decision rules for clinical utility. Ann. Rheum. Dis. 64 (12), 1710–1714.

Creamer, P., Lethbridge-Cejku, M., Costa, P., et al., 1999. The relationship of anxiety and depression with self-reported knee pain in the community: data from the Baltimore Longitudinal Study of Aging. Arthritis. Care Res. 12, 3–7.

Croft, P., Coggon, D., Cruddas, M., et al., 1992. Osteoarthritis of the hip: an occupational disease in farmers. Br. Med. J. 304, 1269–1272.

D'Agostino, M.A., Conaghan, P., Le Bars, M., et al., 2005. EULAR report on the use of ultrasonography in painful knee osteoarthritis. Part 1: prevalence of inflammation in osteoarthritis. Ann. Rheum. Dis. 64, 1703–1709.

Dellhag, B., Bjelle, A., 1995. A grip ability test for use in rheumatology practice. J. Rheumatol. 41, 138–163.

Department for Work and Pensions. Analytical Services Division cited in: Arthritis Research Campaign, Arthritis the Big Picture 2002. http://www.ipsos-mori.com/_assets/polls/2002/pdf/arthritis.pdf/ (accessed March 2009).

Dieppe, P.A., Lohmander, L.S., 2005. Pathogenesis and management of pain in osteoarthritis. Lancet 365, 965–973.

Doherty, M., 1994. Colour Atlas and Text of Osteoarthritis. Wolfe, London, UK.

Doherty, M., 2000. Genetics of hand osteoarthritis. Osteoarthr. Cartil. 8 (Suppl.), 8–10.

Doherty, M., 2001. Risk factors for progression of knee osteoarthritis. Lancet 358 (9284), 775–776.

Doherty, M., Dougados, M., 2001. Evidence-based management of osteoarthritis: practical issues relating to the data. Best Pract. Res. Clin. Rheumatol. 15, 517–525.

Doherty, M., Mazieres, B., Le Bars, M., 2003. Eular recommendations for the treatment of osteoarthritis of the knee in general practice. CD ROM Bristol-Myers Squibb, UPSA.

Dougados, M., Gueguen, A., Nguyen, M., et al., 1992. Longitudinal radiologic evaluation of osteoarthritis of the knee. J. Rheumatol. 19, 378–383.

Dziedzic, K.S., Thomas, E., Hay, E.M., 2005. A systematic search and critical review of measures of disability for use in a population survey of hand osteoarthritis. Osteoarthr. Cartil. 13, 1–12.

Ettinger, W.H., Burns, R., Messier, S.P., et al., 1997. A randomized trial comparing aerobic exercise and resistance exercise with a health education program in older adults with knee osteoarthritis: the fitness arthritis seniors trial. J. Am. Med. Assoc. 277 (1), 25–31.

Felson, D.T., Lawrence, R.C., Dieppe, P.A., et al., 2000. Osteoarthritis: new insights: Part 1: the disease and its risk factors. Ann. Intern. Med. 133, 635–646.

Felson, D.T., Naimark, A., Anderson, J., et al., 1987. The prevalence of knee osteoarthritis in the elderly. The Framingham Osteoarthritis Study. Arthritis. Rheum. 30, 914–918.

Felson, D.T., Zhang, Y., Hannan, M.T., et al., 1997. Risk factors for incident radiographic knee osteoarthritis in the elderly: the Framingham Study. Arthritis. Rheum. 40, 728–733.

Gignac, M.A., Cao, X., Lacaille, D., et al., 2008. Arthritis-related work transitions: a prospective analysis of reported productivity losses, work changes, and leaving the labor force. Arthritis. Rheum. 59 (12), 1805–1813.

Guralnik, J.M., Simonsick, E.M., Ferrucci, L., et al., 1994. A short physical performance battery assessing lower extremity function: association with self-reported disability and prediction of mortality and nursing home admission. J. Gerontol. 49, M85–M94.

Hadler, N.M., Gillings, D.B., Imbus, H. R., et al., 1978. Hand structure and function in an industrial setting. Arthritis. Rheum. 21, 210–220.

Hannan, M.T., Felson, D.T., Pincus, T., 2000. Analysis of the discordance between radiographic changes and knee pain in osteoarthritis of the knee. J. Rheumatol. 27, 1513–1517.

Hawker, G.A., Stewart, L., French, M.R., et al., 2008. Understanding the pain experience in hip and knee osteoarthritis – an OARSI/OMERACT initiative. Osteoarthr. Cartil. 16, 415–422.

Hawley, D.J., 1995. Psycho-educational interventions in the treatment of arthritis. In: Baillières Clin. Rheumatol. 9 (4), 803–823.

Hay, E.M., Foster, N.E., Thomas, E., et al., 2006. Effectiveness of community physiotherapy and enhanced pharmacy review for knee pain in people aged over 55 presenting to primary care: pragmatic randomised trial. Br. Med. J. 333, 995–999.

Hill, S., 2005. Illness perceptions of people with hand problems: a population survey and focus group enquiry. Keele University, London (published thesis).

Hochberg, M.C., Silman, A.J., Smolen, J.S., et al., 2008. Rheumatology edition, (fourth ed.) Text with Continually Updated Online Reference, 2-Volume Set Elsevier. http://www.elsevier.com/wps/find/bookdescription.cws_home/712501/description#description/ (accessed March 2009).

Hootman, J.M., Langmaid, G., Helmick, C.G., et al., 2005. Monitoring progress in arthritis management – United states and 25 states, 2003. Morb. Mortal. Wkly. Rep. 54, 19. http://ww.cdc.gov/nccdphp/dnpa/physical/stats/definitions.htm.

Hunter, D.J., Felson, D.T., 2006. Osteoarthritis. Br. Med. J. 332 (7542), 639–642.

Hurley, M.V., Walsh, N.E., Mitchell, H.L., et al., 2007. Clinical effectiveness of a rehabilitation program integrating exercise, self-management, and active coping strategies for chronic knee pain: a cluster-randomized trial. Arthritis. Rheum. 57 (7), 1211–1219.

Issa, S.N., Sharma, L., 2006. Epidemiology of osteoarthritis: an update. Curr. Rheumatol. Rep. 8, 7–15.

Jinks, C., Ong, B.N., Richardson, J., 2007. A mixed methods study to investigate needs assessment for knee pain and disability:

population and individual perspectives. BMC Musculoskelet. Disord. 8, 59.

Kadam, U.T., Jordan, K., Croft, P.R., 2004. Clinical comorbidity in patients with osteoarthritis: a case-control study of general practice consulters in England and Wales. Ann. Rheum. Dis. 63 (4), 408–414.

Keefe, F.J., Caldwell, D.S., Williams, D.A., et al., 1990. Pain coping skills training in the measurement of knee pain. II. Follow-up results. Behav. Ther. 21, 435–447.

Kellgren, J., Lawrence, J., 1957. Radiologic assessment of osteoarthritis. Ann. Rheum. Dis. 16, 494–501.

Lawrence, R.C., Helmick, C., Arnett, F.C., et al., 1998. Estimates of the prevalence of arthritis and selected musculoskeletal disorders in the United States. Arthritis. Rheum. 41, 778–799.

Lequesne, M.G., Mery, C., Samson, M., et al., 1987. Indexes of severity for osteoarthritis of the hip and knee: validation: value in comparison with other assessment tests. Scand. J. Rheumatol. 65 (Suppl.), 85–89.

Levy, E., Perme, A., Perodeau, D., et al., 1993. Les coûts Socio-économiques de l'arthrose en France [Socio-economic costs of osteoarthritis in France]. Rev. Rhum. Ed. Fr. 60, 635–675.

Lorig, K., Lubeck, D., Kraines, R.G., et al., 1985. Outcomes of self-help education for people with arthritis. Arthritis. Rheum. 28, 680–685.

Lorig, K.R., Mazonson, P.D., Holman, H.R., 1993. Evidence suggesting that health education for self-management in patients with chronic arthritis has sustained health benefits while reducing health care costs. Arthritis. Rheum. 36, 439–446.

Lorig, K.R., Ritter, P., Stewart, A.L., et al., 2001. Chronic disease self-management program: 2-year health status and health care utilization outcomes. Med. Care 39, 1217–1223.

McCarthy, C.J., Mills, P.M., Pullen, R., et al., 2004. Supplementing a home exercise programme with a class-based exercise programme is more effective than home exercise alone in the treatment of knee osteoarthritis. Rheumatology (Oxford) 43, 880–886.

Mathiowetz, V., Kashman, N., Volland, G., et al., 1985. Grip and pinch strength: normative data for adults. Arch. Phys. Med. Rehabil. 66, 69–74.

Meenan, R.F., Callahan, L.F., Helmich, C.G., 1999. The national arthritis action plan: a public health strategy for a looming epidemic. Arthritis. Care Res. 12, 79–81.

Minns Lowe, C.J., Barker, K.L., Dewey, M., et al., 2007. Effectiveness of physiotherapy exercise after knee arthroplasty for osteoarthritis: systematic review and meta-analysis of randomised controlled trials. Br. Med. J. 335 (7624), 812.

Mitchell, N.S., Cruess, R.L., 1977. Classification of degenerative arthritis. Can. Med. Assoc. J. 117, 763–765.

Murphy, L., Cisternas, M., Yelin, E., et al., 2004. Update: direct and indirect costs of arthritis and other rheumatic conditions-United States, 1997. Morb. Mortal. Wkly. Rep. 53, 388–389.

Murphy, S.L., Smith, D.M., Clauw, D.J., et al., 2008. The impact of momentary pain and fatigue on physical activity in women with osteoarthritis. Arthritis. Rheum. 59 (6), 849–856.

NICE, 2008. Osteoarthritis: the care and management of adults with osteoarthritis. National Institute of Health and Clinical Excellence. http://www.nice.org.uk/Guidance/CG59/ (accessed March 2009).

NJR, 2005. National Joint Registry for England and Wales. 3rd Annual clinical report: 8–9. www.njrcentre.org.uk/documents/reports/annual/3rd/NJR_AR2_LR.pdf/. (accessed March 2009).

Oliveria, S.A., Felson, D.T., Cirillo, P.A., et al., 1999. Body weight, body mass index, and incident symptomatic osteoarthritis of the hand, hip, and knee. Epidemiology 10, 161–166.

Pai, Y.-C., Rymer, W.Z., Chang, R.W., et al., 1997. Effect of age and osteoarthritis on knee proprioception. Arthritis. Rheum. 40, 2260–2265.

Peat, G., McCarney, R., Croft, P., 2001. Knee pain and osteoarthritis in older adults: a review of community burden and current use of primary health care. Ann. Rheum. Dis. 60, 91–97.

Peat, G., Thomas, E., Handy, J., et al., 2004. The Knee Clinical Assessment Study – CAS(K). A prospective study of knee pain and knee osteoarthritis in the general population. BMC Musculoskelet. Disord. 5, 4.

Peat, G., Thomas, E., Duncan, R., et al., 2006. Clinical classification criteria for knee osteoarthritis: performance in the general population and primary care. Ann. Rheum. Dis. 65, 1363–1367.

Penninx, B.W., Messier, S.P., Rejeski, J., et al., 2001. Physical exercise and the prevention of disability in activities of daily living in older persons with osteoarthritis. Arch. Intern. Med. 161, 2309–2316.

Punzi, L., Ramonda, R., Sfriso, P., 2004. Erosive osteoarthritis. Best Pract. Res. Clin. Rheumatol. 18 (5), 739–758.

Roddy, E., Zhang, W., Doherty, M., et al., 2005. Evidence-based recommendations for the role of exercise in the management of osteoarthritis of the hip or knee – the MOVE consensus. Rheumatology 44, 67–73.

Sanders, C., Donovan, J., Dieppe, P., 2002. The significance and consequences of having painful and disabled joints in older age: co-existing accounts of normal and disrupted biographies. Sociol. Health Illness 24, 227–253.

Sanders, C., Donovan, J.L., Dieppe, P., 2004. Unmet need for joint replacement: a qualitative investigation of barriers to treatment among individuals with severe pain and disability of the hip and knee. Rheumatology 43, 353–357.

Schouten, J.S., van den Ouweland, F., Valkenburg, H.A., 1992. A 12 year follow up study in the general population on prognostic factors of cartilage loss in osteoarthritis of the knee. Ann. Rheum. Dis. 51, 932–937.

Sharma, L., Dunlop, D.D., Cahue, S., et al., 2003. Quadriceps strength and osteoarthritis progression in malaligned and lax knees. Ann. Intern. Med. 138 (8), 613–619.

Sharma, L., Song, J., Felson, D.T., et al., 2001. The role of knee alignment in disease progression and functional decline in knee osteoarthritis. J. Am. Med. Assoc. 286, 188–195.

Srikanth, V.K., Fryer, J.L., Zhai, G., et al., 2005. A meta-analysis of sex differences prevalence, incidence, and severity of osteoarthritis. Osteoarthr. Cartil. 13, 769–781.

Stamm, T.A., Machold, K.P., Smolen, J.S., et al., 2002. Joint protection and home hand exercises improve hand function in patients with hand osteoarthritis: a randomized controlled trial. Arthritis. Rheum. 47 (1), 44–49.

Stecher, R.M., 1941. Heberden's nodes: heredity in hypertrophic arthritis of the finger joints. Am. J. Med. Sci. 201, 801–809.

Superio-Cabuslay, E., Ward, M.M., Lorig, K.R., 1996. Patient education interventions in osteoarthritis and rheumatoid arthritis: a meta-analytic comparison with nonsteroidal antiinflammatory drug treatment. Arthritis. Care Res. 9, 292–301.

Syed, I.Y., Davis, B.L., 2000. Obesity and osteoarthritis of the knee: hypotheses concerning the relationship between ground reaction forces and quadriceps fatigue in long-duration walking. Med. Hypoth. 54, 182–185.

Symmons, D., Mathers, C., Pfleger, B., 2003. Global Burden of Osteoarthritis in the Year 2000. World Health Organization, Geneva Available from: URL: http://www3.who.int/whosis/menu.cfm?path=evidence,burden, burden_gbd2000docs&language=english accessed March 2009.

Tan, A.L., Wakefield, R.G., Conaghan, P.G., 2003. Imaging of the musculoskeletal system: magnetic resonance imaging, ultrasonography and computed tomography. Best Pract. Res. Clin. Rheumatol. 17, 513–528.

The Atlas of Standard Radiographs of Arthritis, 2005. Rheumatology 44, iv43–iv72.

van Baar, M.E., Dekker, J., Oostendorp, R.A.B., et al., 1998. The effectiveness of exercise therapy in patients with osteoarthritis of hip or knee: a randomised clinical trial. J. Rheumatol. 25, 2432–2439.

van Baar, M.E., Assendelft, W.J.J., Dekker, J., et al., 1999. Effectiveness of exercise therapy in patients with osteoarthritis of the hip or knee: a systematic review of randomized clinical trials. Arthritis. Rheum. 43, 1361–1369.

van Saase, J.L., van Romunde, L.K., Cats, A., et al., 1989. Epidemiology of osteoarthritis: Zoetermeer survey. Comparison of radiological osteoarthritis in a Dutch population with that in 10 other populations. Ann. Rheum. Dis. 48, 271–280.

Verbruggen, G., Veys, E.M., 2000. Erosive and non-erosive hand osteoarthritis. Use and limitations of two scoring systems. Osteoarthr. Cartil. 8 (Suppl.), S45–S54.

Vignon, E., Valat, J.-P., Rossingnol, M., et al., 2006. Osteoarthritis of the knee and hip and activity: a systematic international review and synthesis (OASIS). Joint Bone Spine 73, 442–455.

Wilkie, R., Peat, G., Thomas, E., et al., 2004. Measuring the consequences of osteoarthritis and joint pain in population-based studies. Can existing health measurement instruments capture levels of participation? Arthritis. Rheum. 51, 755–762.

Wolfe, F., 1999. Determinants of WOMAC function, pain, and stiffness scores: evidence for the role of back pain, symptom counts, fatigue and depression in osteoarthritis, rheumatoid arthritis, and fibromyalgia. Rheumatology 38, 355–361.

Wolfe, F., Hawley, D.J., Peloso, P.M., et al., 1996a. Back pain in osteoarthritis of the knee. Arthritis. Care Res. 9 (5), 376–383.

Wolfe, F., Hawley, D.J., Wilson, K., 1996b. The prevalence and meaning of fatigue in rheumatic disease. J. Rheumatol. 23, 1407–1417.

Woolf, A.D., Pfleger, B., 2003. Burden of major musculoskeletal conditions. Bull. World Health Organ. 81 (9), 646–656.

Zautra, A.J., Fasman, R., Parish, B.P., et al., 2007. Daily fatigue in women with osteoarthritis, rheumatoid arthritis, and fibromyalgia. Pain 128, 128–135.

Zhai, G., Ding, C., Stankovich, J., et al., 2005. The genetic contribution to longitudinal changes in knee structure and muscle strength: a sibpair study. Arthritis. Rheum. 52, 2830–2834.

Zhang, W., Doherty, M., Leeb, B.F., et al., 2007a. EULAR evidence based recommendations for the management of hand osteoarthritis: report of a Task Force of the EULAR Standing Committee for International Clinical Studies Including Therapeutics (ESCISIT). Ann. Rheum. Dis. 66 (3), 377–388.

Zhang, W., Moskowitz, R.W., Nuki, G., et al., 2007b. OARSI recommendations for the management of hip and knee osteoarthritis, Part I: critical appraisal of existing treatment guidelines and systematic review of current research evidence. Osteoarthr. Cartil. 15 (9), 981–1000.

Zhang, W., Doherty, M., Leeb, B.F., et al., 2009. EULAR evidence based recommendations for the diagnosis of hand osteoarthritis – report of a task force of the EULAR standing committee for international clinical studies including therapeutics (ESCISIT). Ann. Rheum. Dis. 68 (1), 8–17.

Chapter 18

Fibromyalgia syndrome and chronic widespread pain

Joseph G. McVeigh PhD DipOrthMed BSc(Hons) Physiotherapy, School of Health Sciences, University of Ulster, Jordanstown, Northern Ireland, UK

Rachel O'Brien PhD, MSc DipCOT Faculty of Health & Well Being, Sheffield Hallam University, Broomhall Road, Sheffield, UK

KEY POINTS

- FMS has a significant impact on the quality of life of those with the condition
- Management of FMS must be multidisciplinary
- Treatment programmes should be multimodal, addressing the physical and psychological aspects of the condition
- Exercise, tailored to the individual, is an important component of any treatment programme
- Improving self efficacy is crucial in FMS.

DOI: 10.1016/B978-0-443-06934-5.00018-8

INTRODUCTION

Fibromyalgia syndrome (FMS) is a common chronic muscular pain syndrome that is frequently treated by physiotherapists and occupational therapists. The classification criteria for FMS proposed by the American College of Rheumatology (Wolfe et al 1990) are

- at least a 3-month history of widespread pain, that is, pain in the left and right side of the body, pain above and below the waist and including the axial spine.
- Pain at a minimum of 11 of 18 specific musculoskeletal tender points on palpation of approximately $4 \, kg/cm^2$.

FMS is also often accompanied by a broad spectrum of other symptoms, e.g. fatigue, non-restorative sleep, anxiety and depression, and irritable bowel syndrome.

Although chronic musculoskeletal pain associated with tenderness, fatigue, sleeplessness and general malaise has been recognised for centuries (Smythe 1989), the authenticity of FMS generates (often vigorous) debate. It is argued that the FMS construct is flawed. The overlap between other conditions such as chronic fatigue syndrome and the absence of distinct pathological markers in FMS means the condition cannot be considered a discrete disorder. In the UK, researchers examined the relationship between tender points, pain and symptoms of distress such as depression, fatigue, and sleep quality. It was found that most participants with chronic widespread pain (CWP) had fewer than 11 tender points, and counts of 11 or more tender points were also found in participants with regional pain and no pain. Additionally there was a significant association between tender point count and scores for depression, fatigue, and sleep problems, independent of pain (Croft et al 1994). Consequently these authors concluded that high tender point count was a measure of general distress, and argued that the combination of CWP and high tender point count represented one end of a continuum of pain and tender points rather than a particular clinical condition.

In some respects the debate over the 'existence' of FMS is irrelevant. Patients with FMS or CWP may or may not have a high tender point count. Those that do generally are more distressed and have more somatic symptoms (McBeth et al 2001).

However, the strength of the ACR 1990 criteria is that they provide clinicians and researchers with a simple, uniform case definition for clinical investigation that has a high sensitivity (88.4%) and specificity (81.1%) for FMS (Wolfe et al 1990). For this reason the diagnostic label of FMS is useful.

PREVALENCE OF FMS AND CWP

The prevalence of FMS, using the ACR criteria is 2% overall but it is much more common in women (3.4%) than men (0.5%) and prevalence increases with age (Wolfe et al 1995). No population studies of the prevalence of FMS have been carried out in the UK, although the point prevalence of CWP has been reported to be 11–12%. When the more stringent 'Manchester definition' of CWP is used, the figure is 4.7% (Hunt et al 1999). The diagnosis of FMS appears to be increasing in the UK. However, this is perhaps due to a greater acceptance of the condition among GPs rather than a real increase. Additionally, wide geographical variations in diagnosis exist (Gallagher et al 2004, Hughes et al 2006).

The prognosis of FMS and CWP is poor (Papageorgiou et al 2002). It has been reported that when patients are followed up over a prolonged period, there was little change in pain, functional disability, fatigue, sleep disturbance, and psychological status from baseline. Once CWP is established it is likely to persist, to some extent, in most people.

DIFFERENTIAL DIAGNOSIS AND SPECIAL TESTS

Patients with FMS or CWP present with many symptoms and often have other musculoskeletal conditions. It is important such conditions are adequately screened to avoid unnecessary morbidity. Rheumatological conditions mimicking FMS include: mild systemic lupus erythematosus, polyarticular osteoarthritis, rheumatoid arthritis, polymyalgia rheumatica, hypermobility syndromes and perhaps osteomalacia. Non-rheumatological diseases mimicking FMS include neoplastic and neurological diseases such as: multiple sclerosis, thyroid dysfunction, chronic infections, and some psychiatric conditions. When considering a diagnosis of FMS all other possible diagnoses must be excluded. Standard blood tests include: full blood picture, erythrocyte sedimentation rate, nuclear

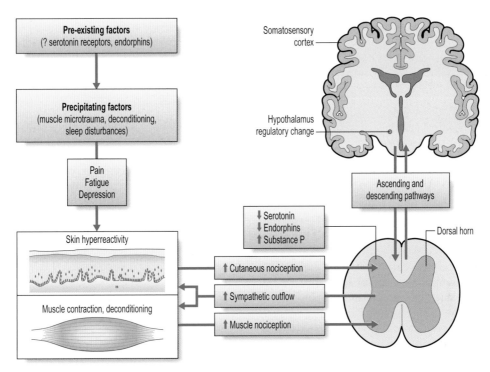

Figure 18.1 A possible pathophysiologic model of fibromyalgia. Adapted from Ch. 62, Figure 62.6 p 70, with permission from: Goldenburg DL 2003 Fibromyalgia and related syndromes. In: Hochberg MC et al (eds) Rheumatology (3rd edn), Elsevier, London.

antibody profile, creatine kinase, thyroid function tests and C2+.

PATHOLOGY OF FMS AND CWP

There is still no clear understanding of the pathogenesis of FMS or CWP. Early research examined muscle dysfunction and abnormalities, such as Type II muscle fibre atrophy and a 'moth-eaten' appearance of Type I fibres, were reported. But it is now accepted such changes are often seen in chronic neuromuscular conditions or could be attributed to deconditioning.

A summary for the possible pathophysiology of FMS and CWP is given in Figure 18.1 and the process considered below.

NEUROENDOCRINE DYSFUNCTION

FMS could be classified as a 'stress related syndrome'. The hypothalamic-pituitary-adrenal axis (HPA) plays a critical role in the body's response to threatening stimuli. Dysfunction of the normal stress

response can lead to the initiation and maintenance of FMS symptoms. In FMS a number of studies have investigated alterations of the HPA axis with some studies reporting elevated evening basal plasma cortisol levels and others reporting decreased 24-hour urinary free cortisol (Wingenfeld et al 2007). Alterations in the stress-response systems are thought to contribute to the development and maintenance of FMS and CWP (Crofford & Clauw 2002).

ABNORMAL PAIN PROCESSING

FMS may be related to altered central nervous system (CNS) processing of nociceptive stimuli. Noxious insult normally stimulates particular primary afferent nerve fibres. This information is then transmitted via the dorsal horn of the spinal cord to the thalamus and cerebral cortex where nociceptive information is consciously perceived, and interpreted in light of past experience. Injury and the activation of primary afferents, specifically A-delta and C fibres, results in the release of an 'inflammatory soup' which includes

---

BOX 18.1   Commonalities amongst people with FMS or CWP

- Tend to be women
- Will have widespread pain
- Will have allodynia and hyperalgesia
- May or may not have widespread tenderness points
- Will present with a multitude of symptoms (which may vary in their presentation)
- Often suffer from anxiety, distress or depression.

---

bradykinin, prostaglandins, histamine, potassium, adenosine, serotonin, substance P, and cytokines. The effect of this on nociceptors is hypersensitivity to noxious stimuli, associated with depolarisation and spontaneous discharge of nociceptors, commonly referred to as peripheral sensitisation (Bennett 2000). Increased neuronal barrage from peripheral pain generators to the CNS can result in increased excitability of spinal cord neurons, i.e. central sensitisation, and is responsible for increased spontaneous activity of the dorsal horn neurones, increased excitability to afferent inputs, prolonged after-discharge, and expansion of peripheral receptive field of the neurones of the dorsal horn.

The experience of allodynia (a painful response to a non-painful stimulus) and hyperalgesia (an increased response to a stimulus which is normally painful) in FMS are thought to be expressions of peripheral and central sensitisation in FMS. Vaerøy et al (1988) and Russell et al (1994) demonstrated a three-fold increase in the concentration of the neurotransmitter substance P in cerebrospinal fluid (CSF) of patients with FMS. Substance P modulates nociception and signalling intensity of noxious stimuli and so increased levels play a critical role in FMS symptoms, in conjunction with other neurotransmitters, e.g. serotonin. This neurotransmitter plays a key role in mood, cognition, deep sleep, and circadian and neuroendocrine rhythms, and also inhibits release of substance P in the spinal cord in response to peripheral stimuli. Reduced serotonin levels (or its precursor tryptophan) occur in FMS. Low serotonin and increased substance P could amplify painful sensory signals.

Chronic pain states may thus be the result of neuroendocrine dysfunction and aberrant nociceptive processing, resulting in muscular pain abnormality.

Commonalities amongst people with FMS or CWP are shown in Box 18.1. Other factors that have been linked to FMS include: being divorced, lower educational achievement, low household income, physical stress at work, being widowed, being disabled, and a family history of chronic pain.

ASSESSMENT OF THE PATIENT IN PAIN

Many with FMS complain their condition or symptoms are not taken seriously by health care providers. One way to address this, and gain the individual's confidence, is to conduct a comprehensive assessment including physical, psychological, social and environmental factors, which influence function and participation in normal activities.

The initial assessment helps build rapport, provides an opportunity to gain insight into the individual's perspective of their condition and its effect across all lifestyle areas. The physiotherapy and occupational therapy assessment will be slightly different although some aspects will be very similar. Both assessments are based on the biopsychosocial model; physiotherapists tend to focus their assessment on pain and the physical effects of this, while an occupational therapist will centre on the functional implications and consider physical, psychological, and environmental factors affecting occupational performance.

ASSESSMENT PROCEDURES FOR PHYSIOTHERAPISTS AND OCCUPATIONAL THERAPISTS

A full history, including past medical history and previous investigations, should be taken. It may be necessary to contact the referring physician to get a comprehensive picture of the patient's past medical history. The therapist should enquire about the history of the current episode. As it can sometimes be difficult to establish the 'current' episode with chronic pain conditions, note should be taken of when increasing problems started, precipitating factors and management to date. It may be necessary to conduct the assessment over several appointments because of activity tolerance and pain. As with all conditions it is important to ensure that 'red flags,' or indicators of serious pathology, are excluded, consequently the standard 'mandatory' questions should be asked (Box 18.2).

Pain

Identify with the person, on a body chart, areas of pain, paraesthesia or numbness, factors aggravating and easing pain, diurnal variation, and severity of pain.

BOX 18.2   Mandatory questions to identify 'red flags'

- General health: any rheumatoid arthritis, ischaemic heart disease, diabetes mellitus, history of cancer, recent surgery
- Unexplained weight loss >10 kg within 6 months
- Night pain or pain at rest
- Saddle anaesthesia or paraesthesia
- Bladder problems such as retention or incontinence
- Bowel symptoms - faecal incontinence
- Bilateral lower extremity weakness or numbness
- Progressive neurological deficit.

Table 18.1 Detailed recording of pain areas and pain sources

Local observations	Bony contours
	Colour changes
	Swelling
	Muscle atrophy
	Muscle spasm
Active and passive range of movements	Willingness to move
	Pain
	Range
	Joint end feel
Static muscle tests	Pain
	Muscle strength
	Muscle weakness
Special tests	Additional testing (e.g. ligaments) should be carried out as appropriate
Palpation	Painful areas should be gently palpated noting pain, temperature, and sympathetic changes such as sweating. Palpation should be conducted with regard to individual's increased sensitivity to pressure (allodynia and hyperalgaesia)
Other symptoms	Sleeplessness, fatigue, anxiety, and depression should be discussed and their impact recorded

Medications

People with CWP or FMS often take multiple medications, including narcotic based analgesics and antidepressants. Medications and sleeplessness can contribute to the experience of 'fibrofog' reported by many, i.e. difficulty with concentration, memory, and mental clarity.

PHYSIOTHERAPY ASSESSMENT

People with FMS and CWP can present with musculoskeletal problems in addition to their 'usual' pain. A comprehensive examination identifies these. The therapist should examine each area of pain and other structures that can cause referred pain to that area. This often means conducting full cervical and lumbar examinations including neurological, and multiple joint examinations. This can be time consuming. However, a comprehensive assessment will assist in identifying peripheral pain generators which contribute to widespread pain, allowing these to be correctly treated, to reduce overall pain levels.

A full description of joint examination techniques can be obtained from Petty (2006). However, the physiotherapist should ensure each area of pain and possible source of pain is assessed and details recorded (Table 18.1).

Manual tender point survey

Tender points (Fig. 18.2A-F) should be examined manually or with a pressure algometer (Fig. 18.3). Tender points are considered 'positive' if the patient complains of pain at approximately 4 kg/cm^2 of pressure, which is about the pressure required to blanch the nail bed of the thumb. Okifuji et al (1997) have described a standardized procedure for examining tender points, which is described in a booklet and CD developed by Sinclair et al (2003).

Cardiovascular fitness

Often people with FMS and CWP are sedentary and deconditioned. Their baseline fitness should be identified and used in future exercise prescription. The 6-minute walk test has been demonstrated to correlate significantly with aerobic fitness in patients with FMS (King et al 1999).

OCCUPATIONAL THERAPY ASSESSMENT

Occupational therapists assess the functional impact of FMS, and factors limiting performance including: physical, psychological, social and environmental influences. Extending the assessment over more than one session will encourage a therapeutic relationship, initially focusing on activities of daily living, and later progress to more sensitive issues such as psychological changes.

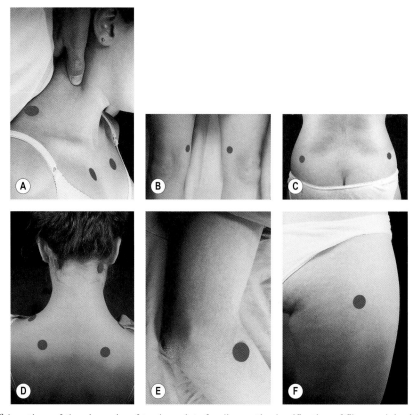

Figure 18.2 (A-F) Locations of the nine pairs of tender points for diagnostic classification of fibromyalgia. Adapted from Ch. 62 Figure 62.1 p702 with permission from: Goldenburg DL 2003 Fibromyalgia and related syndromes. In: Hochberg MC et al (eds.) Rheumatology (3rd edn), Elsevier, London.

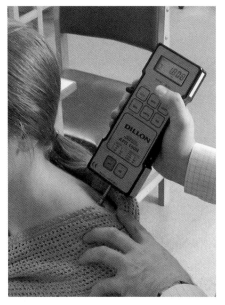

Figure 18.3 Pressure algometer for testing tender points.

Physical assessment

The following should be observed and recorded:

- Are they ambulant?
- Do they use walking aids?
- Do they have a normal gait?
- Do they appear slow/cautious?
- Do they appear in pain?

  Upper limb function can be observed through:

- How they remove a jacket
- What they do with their hands throughout the assessment
- Any evidence of wasting/muscle imbalance/contractures

Using a wheelchair:

- Is it manual or powered?

A more detailed examination may be necessary for some. The Gait Arms Legs and Spine (GALS) assessment is a relatively quick physical assessment

---

BOX 18.3   Psychological factors to observe and record

- Presentation and eye contact e.g. general neglect may indicate low mood or reduced volition
- Do they respond to questions, and elaborate on the effect of the condition?
- Flat speech with little/no intonation
- Do they speak quietly?
- Does their expression change, for example, do they smile?
- Are there any lapses in concentration?
- Do they become visibly upset/tearful?
- Do they show enthusiasm for any activity/hobby etc?

BOX 18.4   Social and environmental assessment

- Type of accommodation
- Surrounding area in relation to amenities
- Access to property
- Location of bedroom
- Location of bathroom
- Living area
- Do they live alone?
- Any support, if so from whom?
- Any young children?
- Are elderly parents living locally?
- Any statutory services or privately paid assistance involved?

---

to perform. Details of how to perform this and a training video are available at www.jointzone.org, in the musculoskeletal examination section.

Psychological assessment

Establishing rapport and developing a therapeutic relationship assists the therapist in evaluating psychological status, and careful observation and pertinent discussion can give an indication of psychological well-being (Box 18.3).

Direct questioning can also provide information. For example, asking about how they spend their day will indicate their activity level. If they do not get dressed they may be experiencing low mood. People with chronic conditions can feel anxious about their ability, and may avoid challenging activities, or only carry these out when environmental influences are likely to be less. For example, they may go shopping but only during off peak times, as shopping at peak times may heighten anxiety. In chronic conditions, people can become short tempered and frustrated by their inability to undertake 'normal' activities. Anger can be expressed towards family and carers, which can add to the complexity of the situation.

Social/environmental assessment

A social/environmental assessment will contextualise an individual's roles (Box 18.4). Given the potential complexity of social situations it may be appropriate to gain understanding as the intervention progresses rather than on initial assessment.

BOX 18.5   Leisure assessment

- Is the hobby physically demanding?
- Does is require cardiovascular exertion?
- Does it require lower/upper body strength, flexibility, and endurance?
- Are they still doing it?
- If not, when was the last time they did it?
- How long do they do it for?
- How many times per week did they do it?
- Has the frequency, duration or way they engaged with the hobby changed?
- Was their last experience positive or negative?

Leisure assessment

How people spent their leisure time pre-onset is very useful and informative. The combination of life roles and leisure interests can identify meaningful lifestyle areas or activities, which can be incorporated into a treatment intervention. Discussing hobbies may result in a change in affect if the individual recalls particularly enjoyable memories. Conversely, it may also reinforce their limitations. The therapist should try to establish how frequently they participated in these as this is a useful marker of meaningfulness. It is also valuable to identify when they last 'did' the hobby and whether adaptive of compensatory strategies were used, and if so what was their success (Box 18.5).

Treatment should be individual, focusing on their roles and leisure activities, as this is likely to increase motivation and engagement. Short and long term goals can be set, as this can increase the individual's sense of achievement and make intervention meaningful. For example, a person who enjoyed rambling previously is likely to find this exceeds their physical capabilities. A short term goal could be to identify short walks over flat terrain, such as canal walks, as the physical demands will be less. As activity tolerance improves the activity and location can be revised.

Work assessment

People with FMS and CWP may continue to work either in the same job, or in a modified capacity. Gaining information about their employment and current status is important. For example, are they working in the same capacity, modified capacity, off sick, or have they lost their job as a result of the condition. Balancing employment with other lifestyle areas is likely to be difficult and has been described as 'walking a tightrope' (Löfgren et al 2006). Box 18.6 identifies work questions which can be asked.

OUTCOME MEASURES

Therapists should measure the effectiveness of treatment using validated outcome measures. The most commonly used outcome measure in FMS is the Fibromyalgia Impact Questionnaire (FIQ).

BOX 18.6   Work questions

- What is the nature of the work?
- How many hours a week do they work usually?
- Do they work shifts or day time only?
- Did they do overtime prior to onset if so are they still doing this?
- Is it manual or administrative?
- If manual, what does the work involve?
- Does it involve lifting, bending, climbing?
- It is repetitious?
- Does it require fixed postures?
- Are they able to change posture e.g. from sitting to standing?
- How many breaks do they get during the day?
- How long is the lunch break?
- Have they received any specialist advice or equipment to optimise their performance?
- Do they/did they enjoy their job?
- Are their employers supportive?

This is a reliable and valid measure of health status (Burckhardt et al 1991). It is a short, self-administered 10-item questionnaire measuring physical function, job difficulty, depression, anxiety, sleep, pain, stiffness, fatigue and well-being. Scores range from 0–100, where a higher score indicates a greater impact of FMS on the individual. Bennett (2005) has reported FIQ scores for the 'average fibromyalgia patient' of around 50, with severely affected patients scoring 70+. A recent report from OMERACT (Outcome Measures in Rheumatology Clinical Trials; Mease et al 2005) recommended that key domains to be assessed in FMS are: pain, global wellbeing, fatigue, health related quality of life, function, sleep, depression and treatment side-effects.

MANAGEMENT OF FMS AND CWP

Management of people with FMS and CWP is complex and presents a major challenge for therapists. Guidelines for management have recently been developed by the European League against Rheumatism (EULAR; Carville et al 2008). They outline nine recommendations including: comprehensive assessment and multidisciplinary management (which may include aerobic exercise), strength training, cognitive behavioural therapy, relaxation, and psychological support.

INFORMATION FOR PEOPLE WITH FMS

People with FMS may have experienced pain, fatigue and sleep disturbance for a number of years. FMS is associated with high rates of health care resource use and visits to doctors for a broad range of symptoms for at least 10 years prior to diagnosis (Hughes et al 2006). Patients may have had extensive investigations and participated in treatment which has had little or no positive impact. It is therefore important to give a comprehensive explanation about FMS/CWP including pathologies and contributing factors, symptoms, possible treatments and likely outcome. Individuals respond differently to information, and therapists should be mindful of the range of responses the person may demonstrate. Initially a diagnosis of FMS may relieve anxiety and be viewed as a positive outcome. After the initial diagnosis the individual may want more detailed information which allows the therapist to introduce positive coping strategies and strategies to optimise functional performance.

ADHERENCE

In chronic conditions the success of any intervention is often dependent on an individual's treatment adherence. Although not often monitored in clinical trials, adherence is problematic and may contribute to the lack of long term improvement (Wigers et al 1996). Non-adherence is complex and not entirely understood. However, commonly reported barriers in FMS include: lack of time due to family or employment commitments, travel difficulties, increased pain, fatigue, or stress, and concomitant medical problems.

Physiotherapy and occupational therapy interventions require the individual to make lifestyle changes to improve functional performance. Self-efficacy (SE) is an important determinant of treatment success. Self-efficacy is an individual's belief in their own ability to succeed in accomplishing the desired outcome, and is associated with motivation and affect (Bandura 1997) (see Chs 5 & 6). People with low SE doubt their ability, and experience low motivation, they focus on personal deficiencies and the implications of failure. As a consequence performance is poor and failure is reinforced. Recovery from these experiences is difficult and stress and depression can result. In contrast people who have higher SE perceive difficult tasks as challenges to be mastered. Self efficacy can be enhanced through performance accomplishments, vicarious experience (modeling), persuasion, and changing physiological state (see Ch. 6).

Another important factor to consider is the person's readiness to change. People with FMS or CWP may find changing well established behaviour difficult. The process of behavioural change has been described by Prochaska & DiClemente (1983) and is known as the Transtheoretical Model of Behavioural Change. There are five stages to the model which are discrete and include: precontemplation, contemplation, preparation, action and maintenance. Each stage is completed (often a number of times) before the behaviour is fully adopted (see Ch. 6).

Identifying the person's stage of change provides a useful indicator regarding the likelihood of behavioural change. If they have no desire to change, or do not recognise change will positively affect their lifestyle, it is unlikely they will engage in the intervention. Readiness to change varies and additional factors such as family perception influence this. If the family are overly protective and 'do everything' for those with FMS/CWP, illness behaviour may be reinforced resulting in less desire to change. However, if they are perturbed by the amount of family assistance, and feel a 'burden' they may be more receptive to change and embrace therapy intervention wholeheartedly.

EXERCISE MANAGEMENT

A number of systematic reviews have evaluated the effectiveness of non-pharmacological interventions, in particular exercise interventions, in FMS and CWP (Busch et al 2007, Mannerkorpi & Henriksson, 2007, McVeigh et al 2008, Sim & Adams, 2002). A broad range of interventions have been examined including cycling or whole body exercise, walking, pool exercise, strength training and movement therapies. The evidence suggests that such physical therapy interventions can improve aerobic capacity, physical function, well-being, quality of life and tender point tenderness in patients with FMS. However, there is little consensus regarding which interventions work best. Indeed there is little standardization of the type of exercise, the duration, or frequency of interventions used in FMS. Reasons for the inconsistency include: the wide variety of exercise programmes used, large variation in baseline function, severity of symptoms and psychosocial wellbeing of participants, large drop out rates from studies, and differences in outcomes measured.

The American College of Sports Medicine (ACSM) recommend that in order to promote and maintain health, people aged 18 to 65 years should engage in aerobic exercise at moderate intensity for a minimum of 30 minutes 5 days per week, or alternatively should engage in vigorous aerobic exercise for at least 20 minutes, 3 days per week (Haskell et al 2007).

Accepting that these recommendations are for healthy people, this level of activity seems ambitious for people with FMS or CWP, and there is some evidence that patients do not tolerate high intensity exercise programmes well. High intensity exercise programmes can result in increased pain and fatigue post exercise, and can also exacerbate problems with programme adherence (van Santen et al 2002).

However, there is a growing consensus in the literature that lower intensity exercise interventions in FMS (40-50% maximum heart rate) are more likely to be tolerated by patients, and that the rate of exercise progression should be gradual (perhaps twice as long as that for healthy individuals; Jones et al 2006). In view of the time required for individuals with FMS/CWP to accommodate to exercise, programmes should be individualised and prolonged rather than short term, 'over months rather than weeks'. This has important implications for clinical practice in physiotherapy. Most physiotherapists treating people with FMS see them for between five to eight treatment sessions (McVeigh et al 2004). Delivering prolonged treatment interventions will have obvious financial and service delivery implications.

Maintenance of regular aerobic exercise is of key importance if benefits are to be achieved and maintained (Haskell et al 2007). Therefore, understanding what helps or hinders continued exercise participation in FMS is crucial. A number of factors have been identified that contribute to exercise adherence in FMS such as higher self-efficacy for exercise, previous exercise engagement, lower depression scores, and a wide social support network. These have been reported as accurately identifying almost 80% of those who demonstrated exercise adherence in a large group of people with FMS (Oliver & Cronan 2002). Factors that mitigate against exercise adherence are: increased pain during treatment, higher stress at baseline, and increased stress during treatment (Dobkin et al 2005).

If those with FMS are to benefit from interventions, barriers to engagement must be identified and overcome. Strategies have been proposed to ensure exercise adherence in FMS. For example, education on the benefits of exercise and how to initiate and continue exercise are important. Additionally, identifying individual barriers to exercise, and planning strategies to overcome them should be part of the initial therapeutic intervention. Keeping daily exercise logs, or improving support through regular telephone calls or e-mail can be used. Indeed these methods have been used with some success in other client groups, including chronic pain. However, unless an individual has the self-belief that they can complete a task, and that completing that task will produce desired outcomes, they have little incentive to act or persevere in the face of difficulties. This again emphasises the importance of improving self efficacy in FMS (Jones et al 2004).

EXERCISE PRESCRIPTION IN FMS/CWP

In prescribing exercises the therapist needs to reflect on what the most appropriate type of exercise is, including frequency, intensity, and duration.

Exercises should be individualised, i.e. consider:

- baseline function and current fitness level
- current pain and fatigue

- prior experiences and knowledge about exercise
- time availability, support network, financial costs
- exercise should be started at very low intensity and progressed slowly
- symptoms closely monitored
- progress should be viewed in the long term.

Exercise prescriptions should be written and include the dosage, duration and frequency of exercise. Exercise programmes should be reviewed regularly and progressed slowly. In order to enhance motivation and ensure long-term adherence the programme should be pleasant and enjoyable. Exercising in a group may enhance social support (Dawson & Tiidus 2005, Jones & Clark 2002).

In terms of the type of exercise used in FMS a variety of exercise interventions have been demonstrated to improve various aspects of FMS, such as physical function, pain and general wellbeing. Exercise interventions have included aerobic exercise (e.g. walking, dance training), strength training and various forms of hydrotherapy. The content of an individual exercise is not necessarily the most import aspect of the intervention rather that the exercise is tailored to the individual and delivered at a level that is acceptable.

LIFESTYLE MODIFICATION

The pain, fatigue and sleeplessness experienced by people with FMS means that simple activities become difficult or impossible; this can result in de-conditioning which further affects performance. Lifestyle modification incorporating activity analysis, compensatory techniques, including pacing techniques and energy conservation, and relaxation and stress/anxiety management are frequently used by occupational therapists. People with FMS/CWP need to pace activity to reduce fatigue. Löfgren et al (2006) found that working women tended to participate in leisure activities at the weekends only and allowed sufficient time for rest afterwards. For people who do not work opportunities for leisure activities may be less restricted, but will be dependent on the individual and the activity.

Strategies to enable people with FMS to continue working include:

- planning the working week
- reducing the length of the working day
- modification of work patterns or responsibilities, and ergonomic solutions

- working more during the warmer summer months
- taking short periods of sick leave (Löfgren et al 2006).

Occupational participation is engagement in meaningful activity and thus encompasses physically demanding and sedentary activities. It is possible therefore to have high levels of occupational participation and high levels of fatigue or symptom severity.

ACTIVITY ANALYSIS

People with FMS or CWP will experience difficulty completing daily living activities across many lifestyle areas. Pain, fatigue and sleep disturbance can affect their ability to carry out domestic activities, e.g. shopping, housework, laundry, meal preparation, and childcare. Symptoms may affect their ability at work depending on their role. Consequently, they may be unable to continue, or need to modify their role at work. It is necessary to break down activities into component parts and so identify specific individual difficulties.

The nature of these will vary but may include:

- performance requirements, e.g. motor, sensory, cognitive function
- sequence of the activity, i.e. fixed or flexible.
- structured or unstructured activity
- identifying the complexity of the activity
- positive or negative factors which affect performance
- defining the tools, materials and environment required
- identification of any risk factors or precautions necessary (Hagedorn 2000).

A detailed activity analysis will identify the components limiting performance, e.g. difficulty getting to the shops may be as a result of pain, limited muscle strength and tolerance of activity. Adaptation to improve performance is necessary and potential solutions could include: use of transport to reduce the amount of walking necessary, going to a shop closer to home, or for someone else to hold responsibility for this activity.

COMPENSATORY TECHNIQUES

Occupational therapists may advocate using compensatory techniques to allow optimum functional performance. This involves identifying the most appropriate compensatory technique and practicing this initially during intervention (see Ch. 10).

Energy conservation

People with FMS and CWP experience reduced activity tolerance which affects their ability to engage in everyday activities. Energy conservation techniques enable the individual to recognise their physical limitations and to work within these. The principle is to reduce the amount of energy expended during activities, and can be achieved by:

- re-organisation of the home environment, for example in the kitchen having all the equipment used regularly within easy reach.
- use of labour saving devices, e.g. dishwasher, washing machine and combined tumble drier reducing need to hang laundry and iron clothes.
- adapting the person's position when carrying out the activity, e.g. sitting reduces energy expended.

Activity pacing

The therapist should be conscious of the impact of activity on the person's independence. Information can be gained through observation, assessment and treatment and also by asking them how long they usually 'do things for'.

Activity diaries

An activity diary can be valuable for therapists as they can be used to gain a greater insight into individual's lifestyle. Patients can record:

- activities undertaken and time required
- physical and emotional symptoms on completion

A written record will assist people with FMS/CWP to recount the events of their week. It will also assist them to self monitor their progress and can serve as a positive re-enforcer as ability, rather than inability, is documented.

Too much activity can have adverse effects, i.e. if an individual engages in activities exceeding their physical capabilities they are likely to experience a reduction in function because of subsequent fatigue. Conversely too little activity can also affect performance and result in de-conditioning and a further reduction in tolerance and stamina in addition to a loss of muscle strength and joint range of motion. The principle underpinning pacing is to develop an individual's awareness of the amount of activity they can participate in and to work within these boundaries.

Goal setting

Goal setting is useful when encouraging pacing techniques. Goals should be:

- set jointly between the individual and therapist
- be relevant and meaningful
- achievable
- enhance self-efficacy.

The process should begin with specific simple goals but with improvement the number and demands of the goals may increase.

ACTIVITY TOLERANCE

An individual's tolerance will be dependent on the nature of the activity, for example, gardening is much more demanding physically than dusting. Therefore it is likely they will be able to do less gardening than dusting. Changing the nature of the activity is also important and alternating between more and less strenuous activities. The occupational therapist works with the client to establish their activity tolerance, factors affecting this, and encourages them to work slightly below this. Once they are using pacing techniques it is also important to encourage them to take frequent breaks from the activity or 'microbreaks', e.g. when using a computer take a couple of minutes break to stretch and change position. Some people may feel pacing is not acceptable as they may have always completed activities in a certain way, for example cleaning the entire house on Saturday. The therapist may be faced with resistance to change as it is habitual behaviour, developed over many years, which will be changed. People with chronic conditions can experience feelings of grief and loss for their former self, and their former body, life roles and responsibilities (Löfgren et al 2006). Therapists should consider the impact of these strategies carefully as they can influence the individual's psychological response to the condition.

ADAPTATION

Adapting the task or environment can improve functional performance. Adaptation can range from provision of small items of equipment such as dressing aids to installation of large specialist equipment. Very often, compensatory techniques involve a combination of: learning a new method, energy conservation and pacing techniques and the use of small items of equipment.

A person with FMS/CWP may experience difficulty preparing a meal and advice could include the following:

- cooking an easy meal rather than Sunday roast each week
- using prepared vegetables (fresh or frozen), or ready meals
- using a microwave to reheat meals
- carrying out parts of the activity throughout the day. Peeling vegetables in the morning sitting down, allows an opportunity to rest using small items of equipment such as cooking basket, vegetable steamer, perching stool (to sit whilst cooking), having a split level oven at waist height (to reduce the need to bend).

People can attribute very different values to simple everyday activities such as preparing a meal. If the activity is important to the individual strategies to maintain their participation should be incorporated and may include energy conservation, pacing and delegating demanding aspects, for example, lifting items from the oven or straining vegetables. People can also have very firm views on how an activity should be completed, e.g. using fresh rather than frozen vegetables. The occupational therapist should discuss the individual's values and identify the benefits of alternatives.

In some instances it may be necessary for the person to be assisted, especially for those demanding activities. For example, difficulty shopping because of reduced activity tolerance, muscle strength and pain may be reduced by:

- shopping for fresh items every couple of days (pacing)
- using door to door transport (energy conservation/adaptation)
- assistance whilst shopping to carry the basket/ push the trolley (energy conservation)
- using the internet to shop (adaptation)
- someone else does their shopping (compensation).

Provision of equipment can reinforce sick role behaviour. Fibromyalgia and chronic pain syndrome are complex in nature, and it is the interplay of physical and psychological factors which impacts on functional performance. Over provision of equipment can emphasise disability and have a negative effect on the individual's independence. Equipment may confirm limitations, which can result in less motivation to maintain current function, and further de-conditioning and reduced independence can result. Occupational therapists should be mindful of the positive and negative effect of equipment, if it may reinforce sick role behaviour and the question of appropriateness should be considered. Provision may be limited to key lifestyle areas.

RELAXATION AND STRESS/ANXIETY MANAGEMENT

People with FMS experience anxiety and depression, and often report significant stressors in the period preceding onset. An important aspect of intervention is relaxation and stress/anxiety management. Relaxation techniques help relieve stress, and provide coping mechanisms to allow thinking to become clearer. Cognitive behavioural therapy (CBT) aims to promote behavioural change through restructuring of conscious thoughts. The approach is designed to give a greater sense of control.

Guided imagery and passive neuromuscular relaxation

Guided imagery is a non-invasive technique effective in reducing stress and anxiety. The group facilitator describes a pleasant scene, providing details such as the time of year, weather, sounds and scents, which the group is guided through (Payne et al 2000). Passive neuromuscular relaxation (Everly & Rosenfield 1981) involves focusing on one muscle group at a time, and releasing any tension within these. No physical activity is involved. (This contrasts to progressive relaxation which involves tensing and releasing muscles which may influence levels of fatigue in some with FMS). These techniques are suited to an individual or group setting and the environment should be specifically designed to promote a sense of relaxation. However, these methods do not provide 'on the spot' strategies to deal with everyday stressful situations.

Quick fixes

'Quick fix' relaxation techniques are designed to reduce anxiety on the spot. Examples of these include Lichstein's breathing technique to relieve stress in a crisis situation, imagining the body is being swept by a large soft paintbrush to release body tension, and transformations using imagery from a substance which is harsh to a second, smooth substance, for example, burnt toast to baking bread (Fanning 1988, Lichstein 1988, Kermani 1990). Participants should be encouraged to practice the techniques as effectiveness improves with practice (Borkovec & Matthews 1983). A relaxation diary including when a technique was used and their feelings prior to and following, provides useful information regarding possible triggers which increase stress or anxiety and the effectiveness of the method. It also identifies if relaxation is not being used, which can facilitate further discussion regarding the reasons. Some may feel uncomfortable using such techniques as they may feel the condition is solely physical.

Consideration of the link between psychological and physical well-being is important. For some people, referral to a clinical psychologist is appropriate. People with FMS/CWP experience limited activity tolerance and some avoid physical activity for fear of increasing symptoms. The importance of exercise within their physical limitations should be stressed, and the physical and psychological benefits discussed.

MULTIDISCIPLINARY MANAGEMENT OF FMS AND CWP

Although individually physiotherapists and occupational therapists can effectively manage most people with FMS or CWP in a uni-disciplinary setting, best evidence suggests that this group should be offered multimodal treatment interventions, tailored to individual needs, delivered by a multidisciplinary team. Education programmes are designed to improve people's health status, self-efficacy and functional performance. In FMS and CWP the primary aims are: improving the ability of those affected to cope and manage symptoms, to change perceptions from despondency and helplessness to a more positive outlook, and improve quality of life (Burckhardt 2005). An important outcome is that the individual is able to self-manage their condition.

A number of systematic reviews have evaluated multimodal treatment programmes in FMS (Carville et al 2008, Goldenberg et al 2004, Hadhazy et al 2000, Sim & Adams 2002, van Koulil et al 2006). Treatment interventions reviewed included a combination of education programmes, cognitive behavioural treatment, relaxation, stress management, pain management, 'mind-body therapies' (i.e. those interventions that address the people's cognitions, beliefs, emotions and behaviours), and variety of exercise based interventions. The broad recommendations of these reviews were that exercise interventions, combined with interventions addressing behavioural and psychological aspects of chronic pain, were effective in reducing the impact of the condition on the individual, particularly in the short-term. Improvements have been noted in pain, function, quality of life, depression, and work capacity. However, there is little standardization in the interventions used or the mode of delivery. Nevertheless there is strong evidence that multidisciplinary treatment, using a cognitive-behavioural approach, is effective in treating FMS (Goldenberg et al 2004).

Hammond & Freeman (2006) evaluated a community based cognitive-behavioural education programme compared with relaxation. The programme included information on FMS, self-management, goal setting, stress management and relaxation, activity pacing, exercise (postural training, stretch, Tai Chi and strengthening exercises using light weights), sleep problems and medication. Participants were assessed at baseline, and four and eight months later. At 4 months there was a significant difference between groups score on the FIQ, the treatment group had better self-efficacy and less pain compared to the relaxation group. The authors recommended that people should be selected based on their perceived self-efficacy and readiness to change, as poorer self-efficacy was associated with fewer improvements.

Multidisciplinary interventions for those with FMS or CWP should be tailored to individual needs, however, in general the content of programmes may include:

- physical activity (e.g. pool-based exercise, walking, Tai Chi)
- patient education (diagnostic issues, prognosis, management strategies, medications)
- self-monitoring and goal setting

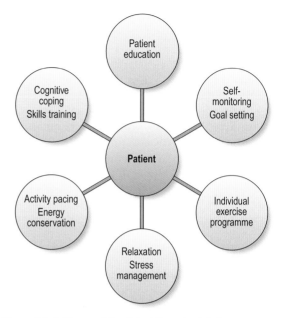

Figure 18.4 Fibromyalgia clinical flow chart. Patient management should be individual, based on a comprehensive assessment and the needs of the patient at that time. Treatment may comprise any combination of these interventions.

- activity pacing
- energy conservation
- cognitive coping skills training
- relaxation and stress management
- work and leisure
- interpersonal relationships (Fig. 18.4).

CONCLUSION

Fibromyalgia is a complicated and controversial pain syndrome, often associated with a complex myriad of associated symptoms; patients who present with widespread pain without the requisite number tender points, can simply be classified as having chronic widespread pain. Management of FMS and CWP is not easy, and is best treated using a multidisciplinary, multimodal treatment programme. Treatment needs to address the physical and psychological aspects of the condition, with due regard to the impact chronic pain has across all life areas including work, leisure, and family life.

STUDY ACTIVITIES

1. Outline the clinical picture of a person with FMS.
2. Describe the pathology that is thought to account for FMS and CWP.
3. Describe the factors that the therapist needs to consider when developing a management programme for a person with FMS.

CASE STUDY 18.1 FIBROMYALGIA

A 38-year-old women presents complaining of a 5 year history of various pains[1] but has only recently been diagnosed with fibromyalgia by her GP[2]. Sally's main problem at present is neck pain radiating to both arms and hands[3]. However, when her pain is severe she also experiences thoracic and low back pain radiating into both legs. She states that, when her pain is at its worst, even carrying her handbag or the weight of her bed clothes at night are excruciating[4]. Additional symptoms include overwhelming fatigue[5], headaches, cold intolerance and restless legs at night. Sally has two children aged 5 and 7 years, she is a home worker and has recently been divorced[6]. Current medications include Amitriptyline, Paracetamol and Ibuprofen[7]. She had a neck x-ray 2 years ago but no other investigations[8]. Sally is tearful during assessment[9] and says that she does not know what fibromyalgia is[10] although her friend told her it is a type of rheumatism.

Important points to note and management considerations:

1. In assessing this patient it is worth noting that patients with FMS often go undiagnosed for a number of years.
2. As this patient has only recently been diagnosed, she will still have many unanswered questions about the condition. The first stage of management is a complete and detailed explanation of what FMS is, the likely prognosis, and management options. Patient education is an important first step in the management of FMS and CWP.
3. It is important that other possible sources of pain have been excluded (see Table 18.1).
4. In order to allay anxieties about the cause of spontaneous pain, explanations about allodynia and hyperalgesia are important.
5. Again it is important to note that fatigue can be a symptom of many conditions. Other conditions must be excluded.
6. Individual social circumstances should be taken into account during assessment. Having a young family and recently divorced might indicate that this person

has a lot of stress in her life. Factors such as these can be used as indicators for treatment, e.g. a stress management programme. It is also worth noting individual factors when considering prescribing an exercise programme.
7. There is some evidence to support the role of amitriptyline in FMS and Paracetamol is often used as a rescue medication. However there is no evidence for the role of ibuprofen.
8. It is important that appropriate blood tests are carried out to exclude other conditions.
9. This gives an indication of the psychological aspects of FMS but may also be an indicate depression; discussion with the referring doctor might be advisable.
10. Again this highlights the importance of a comprehensive education programme.

Sally's management started with a comprehensive assessment from OT and PT. Although many people with FMS complain of a broad range of symptoms, there is little on objective examination other than widespread tenderness. Nevertheless, comprehensive examination reassured her that symptoms were being taken seriously and other pathologies excluded. Due to the pain referral pattern described, a thorough neurological examination was essential. Additionally, because she has not had investigations, other than x-ray 2 years ago, the appropriateness of further blood tests was discussed with her doctor.

The aims of treatment were to increase: her understanding of and ability to cope with her condition; and her physical activity and quality of life. Consequently, her pain is more likely to diminish. Education, cognitive-behavioural approaches and exercise are the mainstay of FMS treatment programmes. However, introducing exercise too early is likely to result in increased pain and possible treatment failure. The PT and OT worked collaboratively to assess Sally's receptiveness and willingness to engage actively in an

(Continued)

exercise programme. They determined treatment should initially focus on cognitive and behavioural aspects of the condition. She attended educational and stress management sessions with OT over the next 6 weeks. The condition and likely prognosis (emphasising positive outcomes) were explained and coping strategies taught, such as goal setting and pacing, increasing her self-efficacy. Relaxation and stress/anxiety management training were included. She was taught and practised relaxation skills over five sessions, and given a home relaxation programme, including quick fixes, such as breathing techniques for use in stressful situations. Practice frequency and effectiveness were reviewed as treatment progressed.

Energy conservation training helped her develop techniques to minimise energy expenditure during daily living activities to reduce fatigue. She was enabled to recognise her activity tolerance and pace accordingly, engaging in activity up to her threshold, but not exceeding this. Sally was having some difficulties with kitchen activities. The OT and PT together carefully considered whether recommending small items of equipment to help reduce energy expenditure was needed. Consideration should be given to not over- providing equipment as this may reinforce disability in the complex interplay of physical and psychological factors. As Sally was now ready to engage in an exercise programme, kitchen gadgets and a perch stool were recommended, with a view to

encouraging her to stop using the stool as endurance improved.

The OT and Sally discussed difficulties related to childcare and her work and jointly problem-solved solutions. The OT helped Sally set weekly action plans to make gradual changes. Additionally, she was encouraged to prioritise occupations in terms of meaningfulness. For example, she decided cleaning the house was less meaningful than going swimming with her children and prioritised her time accordingly. This helped her develop goals and strategies to increasingly engage in and achieve her meaningful occupations whilst having strategies to manage less meaningful ones.

By week 6 she was ready to engage in gentle progressive aerobic exercise and hydrotherapy was offered once a week. By week 8, exercise goals outside of the hydrotherapy sessions were additionally set collaboratively between the PT and Sally, starting with a walking programme (short distances initially), gradually increasing week by week, and by week 10 to go swimming at the local pool on one other occasion. The OT continued to see Sally every 2, then 3 weeks to help her with reviewing progress with her action plans/goals. By week 16, Sally was feeling much more in control of her condition, her mood was significantly improved, she was regularly walking and swimming and able to fulfil her work and care roles much better. On review, the PT and OT determined she was ready for discharge.

International MYOPAIN Society
http://www.myopain.org/
Fibromyalgia information foundation
http://wwwmyalgia.com/

The British Pain Society
http://www. britishpainsociety.org/
The Fibromyalgia Research Blog
http://www.fibroresearch.blogspot.com/

References and further reading

Bandura, A., 1997. The anatomy of stages of change. Am. J. Health. Promot. 12 (1), 8–10.

Bennett, G.J., 2000. Update on the neurophysiology of pain transmission and modulation: focus on the NMDA-receptor. J. Pain.

Symptom. Manage. 19 (Suppl), S2–S6.

Bennett, R., 2005. The Fibromyalgia Impact Questionnaire (FIQ): a review of its development, current version, operating characteristics and uses. Clin.

Exp. Rheumatol. 23 (Suppl. 9), S154–S162.

Borkovec, T.D., Matthews, A., 1983. Treatment of non-phobic anxiety disorders: a comparison of non-directive cognitive and coping densensitisation therapy.

J. Consult. Clin. Psychol. 56 (6), 877–884.

Burckhardt, C.S., 2005. Educating patients: self-management approaches. Disabil. Rehabil. 27, 703–709.

Burckhardt, C.S., Clark, S.R., Bennett, R.M., 1991. The fibromyalgia impact questionnaire: development and validation. J. Rheumatol. 18, 728–733.

Busch, A.J., Barber, K.A., Overend, T.J., et al., 2007. Exercise for treating fibromyalgia syndrome. Cochrane Database Systematic Reviews, Issue 4. Art. No.: CD003786. DOI: 10. 1002/14651858.CD003786. pub2.

Carville, S.F., Arendt-Nielsen, S., Bliddal, H., et al., 2008. EULAR evidence-based recommendations for the management of fibromyalgia syndrome. Ann. Rheum. Dis. 67 (4), 536–541.

Crofford, L.J., Clauw, D.J., 2002. Fibromyalgia: where are we a decade after the American College of Rheumatology classification criteria were developed? Arthritis Rheum. 46 (5), 1136–1138.

Croft, P., Schollum, J., Silman, A., 1994. Population study of tender point counts and pain as evidence of fibromyalgia. Br. Med. J. 309, 696–699.

Dawson, K.A., Tiidus, P.M., 2005. Physical activity in the treatment and management of fibromyalgia. Crit. Rev. Phys Rehabil Med. 17, 53–64.

Dobkin, P.L., 2005. A randomized clinical trial of an individualized home-based exercise programme for women with fibromyalgia. Rheumatology 44, 1422–1427.

Everly, G.S., Rosenfield, R., 1981. The Nature and Treatment of the Stress Response. Plenum Press, New York.

Fanning, P., 1988. Visualization for Change. New Harbinger, Oakland.

Gallagher, A.M., Thomas, J.M., Hamilton, W.T., White, P.D., 2004. Incidence of fatigue symptoms and diagnoses presenting in UK primary care from 1990 to 2001. J. R. Soc. Med. 97, 571–575.

Goldenberg, D.L., Burckhardt, C., Crofford, L., 2004. Management of fibromyalgia syndrome. JAMA 292, 2388–2395.

Hadhazy, V.A., Ezzo, J., Creamer, P., Berman, B.M., 2000. Mind-body therapies for the treatment of fibromyalgia. A systematic review. J. Rheumatol. 27, 2911–2918.

Hagedorn, R., 2000. Foundations for Practice in Occupational Therapy. Churchill Livingstone, Edinburgh.

Hammond, A., Freeman, K., 2006. Community patient education and exercise for people with fibromyalgia: a parallel group randomized controlled trial. Clin. Rehabil. 20 (10), 835–846.

Haskell, W.L., Lee, I.M., Pate, R.R., et al., 2007. Physical activity and public health: updated recommendation for adults from the American College of Sports Medicine and the American Heart Association. Med. Sci. Sports Exerc. 39 (8), 1423–1434.

Hughes, G., Martinez, C., Myon, E., et al., 2006. The impact of a diagnosis of fibromyalgia on health care resource use by primary care patients in the UK: an observational study based on clinical practice. Arthritis Rheum. 54, 177–183.

Hunt, I.M., Silman, A.J., Benjamin, S., et al., 1999. The prevalence and associated features of chronic widespread pain in the community using the 'Manchester' definition of chronic widespread pain. Rheumatology 38 (3), 275–279.

Jones, K.D., Clark, S.R., 2002. Individualizing the exercise prescription for persons with fibromyalgia. Rheum. Dis. Clin. North Am. 28, 419–436.

Jones, K.D., Burckhardt, C.S., Bennett, J. A., 2004. Motivational interviewing may encourage exercise in persons with fibromyalgia by enhancing self efficacy. Arthritis Rheum. 51, 864–867.

Jones, K.D., Adams, D., Winters-Stone, K., Burckhardt, C.S., 2006. A comprehensive review of 46 exercise treatment studies in fibromyalgia (1988-2005). Health Qual. Life Outcomes 4, 67.

Kermani, K.S., 1990. Autogenic Training. Souvenir Press, London.

King, S., Wessel, J., Bhambhani, Y., et al., 1999. Validity and reliability of the 6 minute walk in persons with fibromyalgia. J. Rheumatol. 26, 2233–2237.

Lichstein, K.L., 1988. Clinical Relaxation Strategies. John Wiley, New York.

Löfgren, M., Ekholm, J., Ohman, A., 2006. 'A constant struggle': successful strategies of women in work despite fibromyalgia. Disabil. Rehabil. 28 (7), 447–455.

McBeth, J., Macfarlane, G.J., Hunt, I.M., Silman, A.J., 2001. Risk factors for persistent chronic widespread pain: a community-based study. Rheumatology 40, 95–101.

McVeigh, J.G., Archer, S., Hurley, D., et al., 2004. Physiotherapy management of fibromyalgia syndrome: a survey of practice in Northern Ireland. Int. J. Ther. Rehabil. 11, 71–77.

McVeigh, J.G., McGaughey, H., Hall, M., Kane, P., 2008. The effectiveness of hydrotherapy in the management of fibromyalgia syndrome: a systematic review. Rheumatol. Int. 29 (2), 119–130.

Mannerkorpi, K., Henriksson, C., 2007. Non-pharmacological treatment of chronic widespread musculoskeletal pain. Best Pract. Res. Clin. Rheumatol. 21 (3), 513–534.

Mease, P.J., Clauw, D.J., Arnold, L.M., et al., 2005. Fibromyalgia syndrome. J. Rheumatol. 32, 2270–2277.

Okifuji, A., Turk, D.C., Sinclair, J.D., et al., 1997. A standardized manual tender point survey. I. Development and determination of a threshold point for the identification of positive tender points in fibromyalgia syndrome. J. Rheumatol. 24 (2), 377–383.

Oliver, K., Cronan, T., 2002. Predictors of exercise behaviors among fibromyalgia patients. Preventative Med. 35, 383–389.

Papageorgiou, A., Silman, A.J., Macfarlane, G.J., 2002. Chronic widespread pain in the population: a seven year follow-up study. Ann. Rheum. Dis. 61, 1071–1074.

Payne, R.A., 2000. Relaxation Techniques. A Practical Handbook for the Health Care Professional, second ed. Churchill Livingstone, London.

Petty, N.J., 2006. Neuromusculoskeletal Examination and Assessment: A Handbook for Therapists, third ed. Churchill Livingstone, London.

Prochaska, J., DiClemente, C., 1983. Stages and processes of self-change in smoking: toward an integrative model of change. J. Consult. Clin. Psychol. 5, 390–395.

Russell, I.J., Orr, M.D., Littman, B., et al., 1994. Elevated cerebrospinal fluid levels of substance P in patients with fibromyalgia syndrome. Arthritis Rheum. 37, 1593–1601.

Sim, J., Adams, N., 2002. Systematic review of randomised controlled trials of nonpharmacological interventions for fibromyalgia. Clin. J. Pain. 18, 324–336.

Sinclair, J.D., Starz, T.W., Turk, D.C., 2003. The Manual Tender Point Survey (Booklet and DVD/CD). National Fibromyalgia Research Association, Salem, Oregon.

Smythe, H., 1989. Fibrositis syndrome: a historical perspective. J. Rheumatol. 19 (Suppl), 2–6.

Vaerøy, H., Helle, R., Førre, O., et al., 1988. Elevated CSF levels of substance P and high incidence of Raynaud phenomenon in patients with fibromyalgia: new features for diagnosis. Pain 32, 21–26.

van Koulil, S., Effting, M., Kraaimaat, F.W., et al., 2007. Cognitive-behavioural therapies and exercise programmes for patients with fibromyalgia: state of the art and future directions. Ann. Rheum. Dis. 66 (5), 571–581.

van Santen, M., Bolwijn, P., Landewe, R., et al., 2002. High or low intensity aerobic fitness training in fibromyalgia: does it matter? J. Rheumatol. 29, 582–587.

Wigers, G.H., Stiles, T.C., Vogel, P.A., 1996. Effects of aerobic exercise versus stress management in fibromyalgia: a 4.5 year prospective study. Scand. J. Rheumatol. 25, 77–286.

Wingenfeld, K., Wagner, D., Schmidt, I., et al., 2007. The low-dose dexamethasone suppression test in fibromyalgia. J. Psychosom. Res. 62 (1), 85–91.

Wolfe, F., Smythe, H.A., Yunus, M.B., et al., 1990. The American College of Rheumatology 1990 criteria for the classification of fibromyalgia: Report of the multicenter criteria committee. Arthritis Rheum. 33, 160–172.

Wolfe, F., Ross, K., Anderson, J., et al., 1995. The prevalence and characteristics of fibromyalgia in the general population. Arthritis Rheum. 38, 19–28.

Chapter 19

Ankylosing spondylitis and the seronegative spondyloarthopathies

Mark L. Clemence MPhil Grad Dip Phys MCSP Physiotherapy Department, Torbay Hospital, Torquay, UK

CHAPTER CONTENTS

KEY POINTS

- There are a group of disorders collectively known as the spondyloarthropathies: ankylosing spondylitis, psoriatic arthritis, reactive arthritis and Reiter's disease, and enteropathic arthritis
- Clinical features of the spondyloarthropathies can overlap and can include low back pain and stiffness, restriction of chest expansion, inflammation of the sacroiliac joints, enthesitis, peripheral joint involvement and extraarticular manifestations (e.g. inflammation in the eye)
- Ankylosing spondylitis is considered the prototype of the spondyloarthropathies
- Treatment includes both pharmacological and nonpharmacological interventions
- Physical activity and exercise form key components of treatment and self management approaches.

INTRODUCTION

This chapter will describe the group of disorders collectively known as the spondyloarthropathies a group of interrelated but heterogenous conditions (Boonen et al 2004). The treatment of these conditions will be considered using ankylosing spondylitis (AS) as the exemplar. A number of different terms have been used to describe the same group of conditions including spondarthritides (Moll 1987), spondylarthropathies (Hakim & Clunie 2002), seronegative spondlyloarthritides (Olivieri et al 2002) and spondyloarthropathies (Wordsworth 2002). The last term has been adopted for use in this chapter. The chapter will cover ankylosing spondylitis, psoriatic arthritis, reactive arthritis and Reiter's disease, and enteropathic arthritis.

There is a degree of disagreement over the grouping and classification of the conditions within the group collectively known as the spondyloarthropathies (SpA) (Nash et al 2005). It was once thought that different entities of the SpA group represent variable expressions of the major characteristics of the same disease. Patients with SpA commonly test negative for rheumatoid factor hence the term 'seronegative'. In addition there is a common but

© 2010 Elsevier Ltd
DOI: 10.1016/B978-0-443-06934-5.00019-X

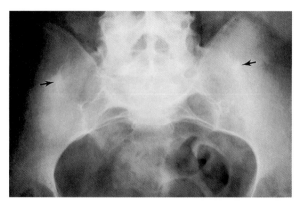

Figure 19.1 Anterior-posterior view of the sacroiliac joints in long-standing ankylosing spondylitis shows total ankylosis. Ossification of the ligaments connecting the posterior superior aspect of the sacroiliac joints is evident (arrows). From Hochberg MC et al (2008) Fig. 108.6, with permission.

variable association with the genetic factor HLA-B27, although some evidence suggests that there are also close associations with other HLA gene factors in this group (Said-Nahal et al 2002). There are racial variations in HLA B27 distribution with corresponding variations in the prevalence of SpA within the same racial grouping. Box 19.1 lists the common features associated with the SpA group of conditions.

ANKYLOSING SPONDYLITIS

Ankylosing spondylitis (AS) is an inflammatory disease that affects the axial skeleton causing characteristic inflammatory back pain, which can lead to structural and functional impairments and a decrease in quality of life (Braun & Sieper 2007). Fibrosis and ossification of ligament, tendon and capsule insertion (the entheses) mainly in the regions of the intervertebral discs and sacroiliac joints are hallmarks of the condition (Hakim & Clunie 2002). Inflammatory changes can also occur in the cartilagenous joints of the axial skeleton (symphysis pubis, discovertebral junction and manubrio sternal joint). The disease can sometimes affect the hip joints.

Initial changes usually begin in the sacroiliac joints, lumbosacral and thoracolumbar joints with later change progressing throughout the axial skeleton. The inflammatory process results in ligament ossification and the formation of vertical outgrowths of bone called syndesmophytes. Progressive syndesmophye growth results in bony union between adjacent vertebrae. In

moderate and severe cases there is progressive and irreversible stiffening of the vertebral column (Fig. 19.1). The disease has an insidious onset and typically continues over many years. Left untreated it will usually result in severe spinal deformity and functional limitation.

There is lack of universal agreement over the current classification system for AS (Braun et al 2002). A range of diagnostic criteria have been developed although in the early stages of the disease a person might be diagnosed as having AS without fulfilling all the criteria. The following is a description of the Modified New York criteria (Van der Linden et al 1984):

- Low back pain of at least 3 months duration with inflammatory characteristics
- Limitation of lumbar spine movement in saggital and frontal planes
- Reduced chest expansion (relative to normal for sex and age)
- Bilateral sacroiliitis grade 2 or higher on x-ray
- Unilateral sacroiliitis grade 3 or higher on x-ray.

Definite ankylosing spondylitis is said to be present when the 4th or 5th criteria is present with one of the clinical criteria (1–3), probable AS can be defined if three clinical criteria are present or the radiographic criterion is present in the absence of signs and symptoms.

PREVALENCE

Estimates of AS prevalence have been reported between 0.1–0.2% (McVeigh & Cairns 2006), 0.25–1% (Calin 2004) and 0.5% (Wordsworth 2002). This means

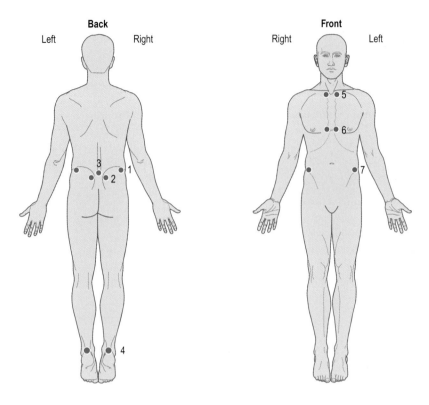

Maastricht Ankylosing Spondylitis Enthesitis Score (MASES)
(Heuft–Dorenbosch et al 2003)

1. Iliac crest right/left
2. Posterior superior iliac spine right/left
3. L5 spinous process
4. Achilles tendon insertion right/left
5. 1st costochondral junction right/left
6. 7th costochondral junction right/left
7. Anterio-superior iliac spine right/left

Tenderness on palpation of these points converts to a score ranging from 0 (no point tender) to 13 (maximal score, all points tender)

Figure 19.2 An example of an enthesitis index.

that whilst patients with AS are commonly seen within rheumatology units AS is relatively uncommon in the community as a whole. The ratio of males to females ranges from 3:1 (Symmons & Bankhead 1994), 2.5:1 (Calin 2004) and 5:1 (McVeigh & Cairns 2006).

MAIN FEATURES OF AS

The key characteristics of AS are listed below. They can be grouped under the headings: clinical, non-musculoskeletal and radiographic features.

Clinical features:

● Pain; low back pain, alternating buttock pain

● Night pain; woken in second half of night with pain and often needing to get up and move about before resuming sleep

● Improvement of pain on exercise

● Spinal stiffness, predominantly in the morning or after rest

● Postural changes - progressive postural change with an increasingly flexed posture, loss of lumbar lordosis, increase thoracic kyphosis and limitation of trunk lateral flexion and rotation

● Muscle spasm

● Enthesitis (see Fig. 19.2 for common sites).

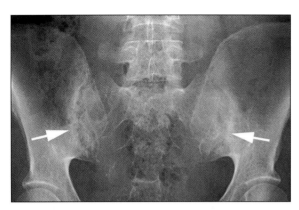

Figure 19.3 Anterior-posterior view of the sacroiliac joints in a patient with ankylosing spondylitis. There is bilateral, symmetrical involvement with succinct erosions (arrows). From Hochberg MC et al (2008) Fig. 108.5, with permission.

Non-musculoskeletal features:

- Fatigue
- Iritis
- Lung disease (less than 1%)
- Cardiac disease (less than 1%).

  Radiographic features (Fig. 19.3):

- Symmetrical and bilateral changes of sacroiliac joints (sacroiliitis) is usual in cases of established disease
- Vertebral squaring
- Syndesmophyte formation with or without vertebral fusion.
- Calcification of vertebral discs.

The first radiological signs of AS are usually evident as x-ray changes in the sacroiliac joints. However in early disease these changes are not always apparent on pelvic x-ray but can be detected on an MRI scan. In severe cases the progressive formation of syndesmophytes and ossification throughout the axial skeleton can lead to a so called 'bamboo spine'. In addition to affecting the lumbar spine AS commonly affects the thoracic and cervical spine and less commonly the hip joints.

PSORIATIC ARTHRITIS

Psoriatic arthritis (PsA) is a chronic heterogeneous disease whose pathogenesis is unknown, although genetic, environmental and immunological factors play major roles (Mease & Goffe 2005). It is a progressive condition and without appropriate treatment results in irreversible joint destruction with resultant disability and functional loss. Psoriasis is a skin disorder affecting 2% of the population characterised by plaques of hyperkeratonic skin commonly on extensor surfaces and in the scalp and occasionally more generalised (Veale & Fitzgerald 2002). The skin disease usually pre-dates the arthritis but in as many as 25% of subjects the arthritis might be synchronous or pre-date the skin disease (Wordsworth 2002). If there is a family history of psoriasis a patient can be diagnosed as having psoriatic arthritis without skin disease being present.

The prevalence of PsA is not well known (Boonen at al 2004). Estimates range from 0.04%–1.2% (Gladman 2006). Sixty percent of patients with PsA will be HLA-B27 positive (Wordsworth 2002). It affects men and women equally, usually between the ages of 20 and 40 years (Hakim & Clunie 2002). PsA may present in one of a number of clinical patterns, the following is based on the description by Gladman (2006):

- Oligoarticular pattern in which four or less large joints are involved in usually an asymmetric distribution.
- Polyarticular pattern (multiple joints) which can appear similar to rheumatoid arthritis (although it is not considered the same condition).
- Predominantly spinal pattern, with sacroiliitis and spondylitis.
- Arthritis mutilans-a form of the disease with severe joint destruction showing characteristic features on x-ray affecting distal interphalangeal joints of hands and feet.
- Distal joint pattern affecting distal interphalangeal joints of hands and feet.

Points 1 and 2 are the commonest presentations. There is some doubt about how strictly PsA exists within these clinical forms (Marsal et al 1999) although four of the five categories can assist in establishing a differential diagnosis (see Ch. 16 to contrast with the features of rheumatoid arthritis).

The clinical and radiographic features are listed below. Patients will not necessarily display all these features especially in early disease.
Clinical features of PsA

- Psoriasis
- Nail lesions (e.g. pitting)
- Asymmetrical distribution of arthritis
- Peripheral joint arthritis with or without axial skeletal involvement
- Distal interphalangeal joint arthritis
- Enthesitis
- Dactylitis.

The radiographic (x-ray) features of established psoriatic arthritis

- Erosions of distal interphalageal joints
- Unilateral or bilateral sacroiliac joint changes
- Spondylitis.

REACTIVE ARTHRITIS AND REITER'S DISEASE

Reactive arthritis (ReA) is a sterile inflammatory arthopathy, which may develop after bacterial or viral infection. A healthy but genetically predisposed individual develops it following an immune system response to an infection. In the gut this is commonly Shigella, Salmonella or Campylobacter infection, and in the genital tract Chlamydia trachomatis (Toivanen 2000). Typically 60–80% of patients with ReA are HLA-B27 positive (Yu & Fan 2001). Reactive arthritis differs from infectious (septic) arthritis in that the infectious organism cannot be cultured from the joint fluid or synovium.

Reiter's disease (or Reiter's syndrome) is currently the term applied to a reactive arthritis displaying specific signs. These are the classic triad of arthritis, urethritis (urethral inflammation) and conjunctivitis (Yu & Fan 2001). The common clinical features are listed below.

Common clinical features (Yu & Fan 2001)
- Asymmetrical synovitis of lower limb joints (especially ankle and knee although wrist and other joints can be involved)
- Dactylitis
- Sacroiliitis- 5–10% of patients in early disease and up to 70% if it becomes chronic
- Enthesitis
- Spondylitis.

ReA tends to be a self-limiting condition and 90% of patients recover in the first year (Yu & Fan 2001). It is very important to treat the underlying cause of infection as this settles the arthritis. Treatment is also directed at the joint manifestations of the disease. When reactive arthritis develops as the result of sexually acquired infection it can be called sexually acquired reactive arthritis (SARA). Treatment guidelines are provided for SARA by the British Association for Sexual Health and HIV (2001). It is always important to consider the implications of discussing the history of SARA with the patient when members of their family or friends are present.

ENTEROPATHIC ARTHRITIS

Enteropathic arthritis is an inflammatory arthritis of peripheral joints and axial skeleton associated with chronic inflammatory bowel disease. Peripheral arthritis is relatively common in inflammatory bowel disease and its incidence is 10% in ulcerative colitis and 15–20% in Crohn's disease (Jewell 1993, Shearman & Finlayson 1989, Wollheim 2001). Axial skeletal involvement has been reported as having an incidence of 10–15% in ulcerative colitis and 15–20% in Crohn's disease (Wollheim 2001). Peripheral arthritis tends to be asymmetrical and affect the larger joints (hips, knees, ankles and wrists). If there is a spondylitis (inflammation of spinal joints) or sacroiliitis the course of the disease is independent of the bowel condition. In addition to joint features some patients also experience enthesopathies and inflammatory eye conditions.

ASSESSMENT

This section will outline the principles of assessing the spondyloarthropathies and will relate this to intervention by the therapist. Ankylosing spondylitis (AS) is the prototype of the spondyloarthropathies (Braun et al 2002) so this section will focus on assessing AS. The principles of assessing peripheral joint arthritis in SpA and peripheral joint arthritis of other diagnostic types are almost identical so the reader should refer to Chapters 3 and 16 for further detail.

The four clinical features of AS, enthesitis, axial involvement, peripheral articular disease, and extra articular features should be assessed (Dougados & van der Heijde 2002). Some areas of potential extra articular problems (skin, eyes, gut) are outside the normal remit of therapists' roles and require other members of the team to assess and manage them. The assessment and treatment of foot and ankle problems arising from arthritis or enthesitis is sometimes undertaken by a podiatrist rather than a physiotherapist (see Ch. 13). Box 19.2 highlights the elements of a therapist's assessment.

It is important for the therapist to remember the context in which they are undertaking their assessment and to gather data relevant to the purpose of the assessment. Often, time will be a factor affecting the amount of data that can be collected but selective use of validated outcome measures can make the process more efficient and effective (see Ch. 4). The emphasis of assessment is likely to vary in different situations; a potential case of undiagnosed SpA is likely to need a different approach to a person newly diagnosed with AS or assessment undertaken as part of monitoring long term follow up. Therapists can facilitate the rapid referral of suspected SpA to rheumatologists as recommended by the Arthritis and Musculoskeletal Alliance (ARMA 2004). This is especially important in situations of patient self referral for therapy where the patient's GP has not been consulted. A systematic, analytical process is required to differentiate other forms of spinal pain from AS (Fruth 2006). A simple screening tool, such as the one used in a therapy service in South Devon, may be useful in identifying potentially undiagnosed individuals with early AS presenting directly to therapy services (Box 19.3). Such screening tools warrant further evaluation in clinical practice.

HISTORY TAKING IN AS

Thorough history taking is an important part of any assessment. General principles are covered in Chapter 3. In AS and other SpA, certain aspects of history taking such as a description of the problem, its duration and medication used are shared with other clinical conditions. There are certain responses which are suggestive of AS in new referrals lacking definitive diagnosis and they may also be useful in determining the severity of the condition in a known case of AS (Calin et al 1977, Rudwaleit et al 2005).

1. How old were you when it began?
2. Do any close relatives have an inflammatory arthritis?
3. Have you had inflammatory gut problems (Crohn's disease, ulcerative colitis), inflammatory eye problems (iritis) or psoriasis?
4. Do you have variable buttock pain in both sides? (This pain is associated with AS).

BOX 19.2   Issues to be addressed by a therapist assessment

- Disease activity
- Function
- Pain
- Mobility
- Fatigue
- Global assessment
- Work status
- Activities of daily living
- Patient beliefs and knowledge

BOX 19.3   Ankylosing spondylitis therapy screening tool

Screening questionnaire

1. In patients under 45 who have had pain for more than 4 months, does the patient have:

■ Early morning stiffness (back +/– neck) > 30 mins?	Yes	☐	No	☐
■ Back pain improves with exercise?	Yes	☐	No	☐
■ Awake second half of night with pain/stiffness?	Yes	☐	No	☐
■ Buttock pain (alternating)	Yes	☐	No	☐

In patients answering **yes** in at least two questions HLA-B27 screening is recommended and refer back to GP

Supplementary questions:

2. Has the patient ever had iritis (red painful eye)?	Yes	☐	No	☐
3. Has the patient ever had Achilles tendonitis?	Yes	☐	No	☐
4. Has the patient ever had plantar fasciitis?	Yes	☐	No	☐
5. Does the back pain improve with NSAIDs?	Yes	☐	No	☐
6. Is there a family history of AS?	Yes	☐	No	☐
7. Does the patient have psoriasis?	Yes	☐	No	☐
8. Does the patient have Crohns or ulcerative colitis?	Yes	☐	No	☐
9. Has the patient ever had a peripheral inflammatory arthritis?	Yes	☐	No	☐
10. Has the patient experienced central chest pain?	Yes	☐	No	☐

These questions are based on Calin et al (1977) and Rudwaleit et al (2005)

5. Do you wake in the second half of the night because of pain? (Common in AS).

6. Are your joints (especially your back) stiff in the morning? If yes how long? (Signs of stiffness longer than half hour are considered significant).

7. Have you had a warm and swollen joint?

8. Are you better after resting or moving around?

9. Is your back stiff after sitting down?

Box 19.4 provides a comparison of the common features of inflammatory and mechanical back pain.

SPINAL MEASUREMENT

Measurements less than the normal range for spinal and other joint movements can implicate AS but as far as possible these must be differentiated from non inflammatory causes. In the lumbar, thoracic and cervical spines this presents as limitation of flexion, extension, rotation and lateral flexion. If peripheral joint limitation is present it most commonly affects the hip and shoulder joints (Fig. 19.4). Measures commonly collected during general assessment of AS (e.g. Fig. 19.5) are published in a handbook provided by the National Ankylosing Spondylitis International Federation (Ankylosing Spondylitis: Assessment Scores, Classification and Diagnostic Criteria) (www.spondylitis-international.org). The measures selected are commonly affected by the disease and therefore data are collected to serve as a baseline by which to measure change and as a way of identifying problems which might need therapeutic intervention (Fig. 19.5). It might be desirable to undertake a more extensive assessment including peripheral joints and this can be done using standard musculoskeletal examination techniques.

OUTCOME MEASURES IN AS

The selection of an appropriate outcome measure can be a challenging task. Historically measures have been developed to capture the biomedical impairments of AS, e.g. the Stoke Ankylosing Spondylitis Spinal Score (SASSS) (Averns et al 1996). There is now a greater appreciation of other dimensions important to patients (see Ch. 4) and individualised measures (Haywood et al 2003).

THE BATH INDICES

A suite of measures developed in Bath has been adopted in many UK rheumatology departments.

BOX 19.4 Comparison of AS and mechanical back pain	
Ankylosing Spondylitis	**Mechanical Back Pain**
Early age of onset (under 45)	Older age (often over 45)
Insidious onset	Often sudden onset
Morning stiffness of more than 30 minutes	Morning stiffness less than 15 minutes, pain often worse than stiffness
Better on activity	No better/worse on
Worse on rest	activity
Stiff after sitting	Often worse pain on sitting, better on standing
Sacroiliac involvement causing alternating buttock pain	Pain tends not to alternate
Frequently - pain on movement in all directions, no clear positional/ movement preference	Some movements tend to be more painful than others, frequently some directions preferred over others
Bilateral movement limitation	Frequent unilateral limitation

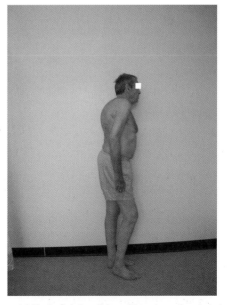

Figure 19.4 Typical deformities of long standing Ankylosing Spondylitis with loss of normal spinal posture and flexion deformity of the hip.

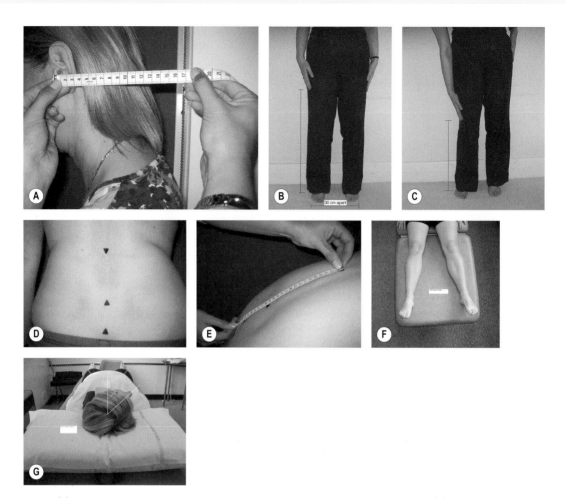

Figure 19.5 (A) Tragus to wall measure from the tragus cartilage above the earlobe to the wall. (B) Starting position for side flexion measurement and (C) finishing position of side flexion measurement, middle finger tip to floor distance. (D) Starting position for measurement of the Modified Schober measurement. Mark dimples of Venus (Posterior Superior Iliac Spines) and draw a dot where they intersect. Draw dots 10 cm and 5 cm below this dot. The actual measurement is the increase in length in this line during flexion, normally 5 cm or more (E). (F) Intermalleolar distance. (G) Cervical rotation.

The Bath indices are a range of outcome measures, which can be used to assess function, disease activity, movement and overall patient assessment of their condition (Fig. 19.5 A–G). The Bath Ankylosing Spondylitis Functional Index (BASFI) is a questionnaire with 10 questions scored on 10 cm visual analogue scales (VAS) (Calin et al 1994). The Bath Ankylosing Spondylitis Disease Activity Index (BASDAI) and the Bath Ankylosing Spondylitis Patient Global Score (BAS-G) are also self-completed questionnaires using visual analogue scales and with the BASFI have all been validated for use in AS (Garrett et al 1994, Jones et al 1996). They are useful not only in establishing baselines on initial presentation but can also be used in ongoing monitoring of disease and function. The Bath Ankylosing Spondylitis Metrology Index (BASMI) was developed to determine the most appropriate clinical measurements for the assessment of AS (Jenkinson et al 1994). The assessor is required to undertake a series of eight measurements in a standardised way. With all four of the Bath indices the individual measurements or responses convert into a score. These can be recorded on each visit and used as a measure of progress. Details of these indices are published by the National Ankylosing Spondyltis Society (NASS) with instructions about how to undertake the scoring (Irons & Jeffries 2004).

In addition to the Bath indices described above, there is the Bath Ankylosing Spondylitis Radiology

Table 19.1 Ankylosing spondylitis assessment

DATE

Tragus to wall Right *	CM
Tragus to wall Left *	CM
Chest Expansion	CM
Modified Schobers index flexion *	CM
Modified Schober index extension	CM
Lumbar side flexion Right *	CM
Lumbar side flexion Left *	CM
Cervical flexion	Degrees
Cervical extension	Degrees
Cervical side flexion right	Degrees
Cervical side flexion left	Degrees
Cervical rotation lying right *	Degrees
Cervical rotation lying left *	Degrees
Hip intermalleolar distance *	CM
Hip lateral rotation right	Degrees
Hip lateral rotation left	Degrees
Hip medial rotation right	Degrees
Hip medial rotation left	Degrees
Hip flexion right	Degrees
Hip flexion left	Degrees
Shoulder flexion right	Degrees
Shoulder flexion left	Degrees
SIGNED	

Name..................... Ref Number.....................Date of Birth...................

Items with asterisk [*] comprise measures used in the Bath Ankylosing Spondylitis Metrology Index (BASMI). BASMI consists of scores derived from: tragus to wall distance (left and right), lumbar side flexion in standing (left and right) modified Schober's index on flexion, cervical rotation in supine lying (left and right) and intermalleolar distance in supine lying. The positions for measuring BASMI measurement are illustrated in Figure 19.5. Refer to Irons & Jefferies (2004) to convert these measure to the scores used in BASMI. However they are also useful as stand alone measures.

Index (BASRI) and the Bath Ankylosing Spondylitis Radiology Hip Index (BASRI-h) which are validated measures for grading the radiographic changes observed in AS (MacKay et al 1998, 2000).

GENERAL ASSESSMENT OF FUNCTION AND MOVEMENT

The Bath indices are extremely valuable for monitoring patients and for research. However they are sometimes not sufficiently broad to cover all potential problems. For example, they will not detect movement limitation on lumbar extension or trunk rotation, both common problems in AS, and are amenable to treatment through exercises. For this reason when undertaking initial assessment it might be preferable to use a wider range of measures in addition to the Bath indices. An example of a more extensive range of motion measure is given in Table 19.1.

The 13 point enthesitis score (Maastricht Ankylosing Spondylitis Enthesitis Score or MASES) proposed by Heuft-Dorenbosch et al (2003) provides additional useful information (Fig. 19.2). An assessment format containing a range of measures (including modified versions of the Bath indices) is available on the Assessment in AS Working Group (ASAS) website listed at the end of the chapter under useful websites. The assessment of clinical outcome in AS patients present challenges attributable to both the disease process and the measures themselves (Ward 2006). Measures designed for research and classification purposes (e.g. Modified New York Criteria) might not be sufficiently sensitive to detect early or atypical presentations of AS. As with other types of inflammatory arthritis patients with AS and PsA can also have osteoarthritis The clinical presentation of osteoarthritis in the hands (Ch. 17) can sometimes appear similar to early PsA and it is important not to confuse the two conditions.

TREATMENT OF AS AND THE SPONDYLOARTHROPATHIES

Reactive arthritis and enteropathic arthritis tend to affect limited numbers of peripheral joints. The principles of therapy are similar for people affected by other types of arthritis. This current section will mainly concentrate on therapy for ankylosing spondylitis.

The medical management of AS is a continually developing area. Early diagnosis is difficult but important and patients with inflammatory back pain should be referred at an early stage to a rheumatologist (ARMA 2004, McVeigh & Cairns 2006). Conventional treatment consists of non-steroidal anti-inflammatory drugs (NSAIDs), intra-articular corticosteroid injections and limited use of surgery where there is significant spinal deformity (Dougados & van der Heijde 2002). Exercise (including hydrotherapy) is also an established part of conventional treatment. Therapy needs to be coordinated with medical treatment to benefit from the optimal effect of medication and to ensure an integrated team approach. More severe cases would need a timely referral to occupational therapy.

Assessment in AS Working Group (ASAS)/EULAR recommendations for the management of AS include:

- Individually tailored treatment programmes
- Use of appropriate methods of disease monitoring
- A combined approach based on pharmacological and non-pharmacological treatments
- Non-pharmacological treatments should include patient education, exercise, and patient self help strategies
- Pharmacological approaches should be based on the best evidence (Zochling et al 2006).

Current best evidence for pharmacological treatment includes limited evidence for conventional disease modifying therapy (e.g. Methotrexate, Sulfasalazine) in patients with axial disease alone. However there is evidence of benefit for Sulfasalazine (SAS), Methotrexate (MTX) and Leflunomide in treating peripheral joint disease in AS, psoriatic arthritis and enteropathic arthritis (see Ch. 15). There is also good evidence of benefit for the use of biologic therapies (e.g. Infliximab, Adalimubab, Etanercept) in AS, PsA and enteropathic arthritis (BSR 2004, Chen & Liu 2005, Chen et al 2006, Jones et al 2000, NICE 2006, 2007, Woolacott et al 2006). The reader should refer to Chapter 15 for a general review of pharmacological approaches in rheumatology.

Non-pharmacological interventions can be targeted to the following:

- Pain
- Spinal mobility
- Stiffness
- Function
- Fatigue
- Peripheral joint involvement
- Enthesitis
- Patient education
- Patient long term monitoring.

Health education and advice are central to therapists' interventions. Chapter 6 addresses the principles more fully.

EXERCISE THERAPY IN ANKYLOSING SPONDYLITIS

Compared to the medical treatment of AS and PsA evidence for physiotherapy and occupational therapy in these conditions is more limited (Fransen 2004). The majority of research focuses on exercise therapy and it forms a central component in managing the disease. There is limited evidence to support the efficacy of exercise therapy for AS patients, although there is the need for further research (Dagfinrud et al 2004). In addition to mobility exercises, patients with AS potentially benefit from cardiovascular exercise and exercises to improve their breathing (Ince et al 2006). Current opinion favours the use of exercise programmes combining trunk, neck and peripheral range of movement exercises. These should be performed on a daily basis with additional limited numbers of stretches when possible being performed after sustaining any fixed posture. The National Ankylosing Spondylitis Society (NASS) provides a guide to a basic exercise programme in their education booklet (NASS 2007) and on their website (www.nass.co.uk). It is important to emphasise stretches to improve the movement limitation specific to an individual patient as well as promoting the importance of routine exercise as a way of preventing long term deformity especially the kyphotic postural deformity which can occur. Exercise in water is a useful addition to a home exercise programme and there is evidence to support its use in AS (van Tubergen & Hidding 2002). Water-based exercise is useful for mobility, cardiovascular fitness and strength. There are many NASS groups around the UK, which use hospital facilities for water based and gym exercise classes. Exercise needs to become part of the daily lifestyle of a person with AS, not something they perform on rare occasions, and such groups can provide peer support.

Adequate pre-exercise assessment of patients should be undertaken to screen for risks associated with AS. These include

- Pseudoarthrosis
- Osteoporosis (including vertebral crush fractures)
- Heart abnormalities
- Joint replacements (total hip replacement is the commonest in AS)
- Severely restricted breathing
- Atlanto-occipital/atlanto-axial subluxation.

(Dziedzic 1999)

None of these is an absolute barrier to exercise but if present only appropriate exercises should be performed. In these situations (and in rare cases when AS is combined with another condition affecting movement e.g. Parkinson's disease) it is important to gain the opinion of a therapist specialising in such conditions for additional advice.

The Arthritis Research Campaign (arc) also publishes literature on AS, PsA and a wide range of other rheumatological conditions (www.arc.org.uk).

FUNCTIONING IN ANKYLOSING SPONDYLITIS

Closely associated with education about exercise is the promotion of good posture as a way of preventing pain, stiffness and long term deformity. Advice about sitting positions and other static postures should also be included. This is very relevant to patients who undertake large amounts of driving or whose work is office based. Sitting reinforces the flexed spinal deformity of AS as a result of the naturally slumped posture adopted when sat for long periods. Research demonstrates the major impact of AS on employment (e.g. Boonen et al 2001, Boonen et al 2002). Technical and ergonomic adaptation of the workplace can reduce the risk of withdrawal from the workforce due to AS (Chorus et al 2002). Therapists should be able to advise about the principles of workplace ergonomics especially in jobs involving prolonged static postures such as sitting or flexed standing. Office seating for employees with AS can affect the levels of comfort experienced when sat at work (Sweeney & Clarke 1990). Patients might need individual assessment of their seating as well as assessment of workstation design and layout. Night time posture should be addressed by attention to pillows and mattresses (Gall et al 2000).

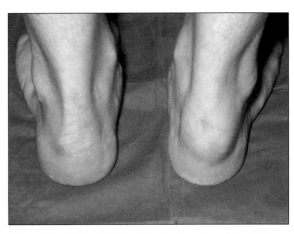

Figure 19.6 Enthesitis involving the insertion of the right tendo Achilles. From Hochberg MC et al (2008) Fig. 110.7, with permission.

OTHER CONSIDERATIONS IN PSORIATIC ARTHRITIS

Peripheral joint arthritis associated with AS and other conditions in the SpA group can be approached by therapists in a similar way to inflammatory arthritis of other types. When enthesitis is present (Fig. 19.6) it imposes a potentially modifying

---

BOX 19.5   Intervention plan for patients with spondyloarthropathies

Pain	Exercise, hydrotherapy, relaxation, external modalities (e.g. TENS), thermal treatment (hot/cold), correction of posture, use of appliances, ergonomic improvement
Spinal mobility & Stiffness	Exercise, correction of posture
Function	Activities of daily living assessment, ergonomic assessment and adaptation, use of appropriate appliances
Fatigue	Pacing, energy conservation, improved sleep posture
Peripheral joint involvement	As for spinal involvement
Enthesitis	Orthoses for foot/ankle enthesitis
Patient education	One-to-one advice, use of literature, patient education groups, patient self help groups (e.g. NASS)
Patient long-term monitoring	Use of validated measures (e.g. Bath indices), regular contact, clinics combined with other health professionals (e.g. rheumatologists, clinical nurse specialists).

CASE STUDY 19.1 PATIENT WITHOUT A PREVIOUS DIAGNOSIS OF SPONDYLOARTHROPATHY (SpA)

Mr Worth is a 31-year-old with low back, neck and scapular pain. The GP's surgery gives an option of self-referral to the practice-based physiotherapy service instead of making an appointment with one of the GPs. Mr Worth decided to see the physiotherapist with his problem as he was finding it hard to cope with the physical demands of working in a local hospital. On his initial assessment he described a 10 year history of intermittent back pain. The recent episode of neck and back pain began in the last 6 months without any specific trauma. Although he liked sport he had stopped playing squash during the last few months because of the pain it caused afterwards. Mornings were his worst time of the day for pain and stiffness, and he was getting up an hour earlier than usual to allow time to dress. It took at least an hour for the back stiffness to improve once he got up. He was trying to avoid sitting too long at work because it made his pain and stiffness worse when he got up, and he felt

better keeping moving. His general health was good but reported one episode of what he described as iritis 3 years earlier.

On examination the physiotherapist found reduced lumbar spine flexibility with a modified Schober's index on flexion of 5 cms, reduced lumbar side flexion and a small reduction in cervical rotation. There was normal range of motion in the hips but low back pain was elicited at end of range on hip rotation. Some muscle spasm was present on palpation of the lumbar region. Chest expansion was within normal range but caused some thoracic pain. The physiotherapist suspected that the problems might be arising from an inflammatory arthritis and after giving advice about posture, pain relief and gentle range of movement exercises, made an urgent appointment for Mr Worth with the GP. The GP referred him to the rheumatology department and the patient was diagnosed as having AS within 13 weeks of referring himself to the physiotherapist.

CASE STUDY 19.2 PATIENT WITH ESTABLISHED ANKYLOSING SPONDYLITIS (AS)

Mr Butters is a 35-year-old office manager who was referred by the rheumatologist to the specialist rheumatology physiotherapist in the rheumatology multidisciplinary team. Mr Butters had stopped attending yearly rheumatology clinic reviews for his AS about three years ago but had been referred back by his GP because he had been signed off sick from work due to the pain he was having and because of deteriorating function. Mr Butters had found it hard to fit regular rheumatology reviews in with work. He had also gradually reduced the amount of exercises he had been doing until he had stopped them altogether. His job involved prolonged sitting so during the day he was working in a fixed posture for hours at a time.

On assessment he displayed increased tragus to wall distance, reduced chest expansion and a flexed posture. Modified Schober's index on flexion was 2 cm. and there was reduced range of lumbar side flexion. Cervical movement was reduced in all directions. There was some restriction of hip range of movement with

intermalleolar distance reduced. The physiotherapist initiated an intensive course of hydrotherapy and exercises. His home exercise programme was reviewed and modified to allow him to do some at work. The patient was introduced to evening hydrotherapy sessions run by the local NASS branch to allow him to have regular hydrotherapy when he returned to work. He was also encouraged to access the NASS website to gain more information about AS. The occupational therapist gave advice about seating, pillows and how to pace his physical activity.

In addition to addressing the patient's pain and function the rheumatologist requested that the physiotherapists undertook an assessment of the patient using the Bath indices. These were used to determine the patient's eligibility to receive anti TNF therapy according to NICE guidelines. As the patient was eligible for treatment, regular reviews in the rheumatology clinic were required. The physiotherapist supported the rheumatologist in the review process.

factor on the advice, exercise and functional adaptation used in inflammatory arthritis. The pain of enthesitis can be helped through orthoses (eg heel pads) as left untreated it can cause gait disruption as a result of the pain (see Ch. 13). Appropriate exercises such as Achilles tendon stretches might be helpful. Deformities of PsA are often treated with

splints and supports (see Ch. 12). Some degree of splint modification might be required if psoriatic plaques are irritated by splint contact (Melvin 1989).

Box 19.5 summarises a nonpharmacological intervention plan for patients with Spondyloarthropathies. Further information on interventions can be found in the preceding chapters. General information on spondyloarthropathies, latest editions of guidelines and most recent evidence can be accessed via the websites listed at the end of this chapter. In addition a number of authoritative associations and organisations are given to facilitate searches for recent evidence. The internet contains large amounts of unreliable information about AS and psoriatic arthritis so it is important to become familiar with the information provided by organisations such as the National Ankylosing Spondylitis Society (NASS), Ankylosing Spondylitis International Federation (ASIF), the British Society for Rheumatology (BSR), Arthritis Research Campaign (arc), the European League Against Rheumatism (EULAR) and the American College of Rheumatology (ACR).

ACKNOWLEDGEMENTS

The author gratefully acknowledges the invaluable support given by Dr. Kirsten MacKay during the writing of this chapter. The author would also like to thank the models used for the illustrations.

STUDY ACTIVITIES

1. Describe the possible impact of ankylosing spondylitis in a female who
   - has sedentary occupation (eg taxi driver, call centre worker)
   - is self-employed shop owner
   How might regular hospital appointments for physiotherapy and occupational therapy affect a) and b)? Would adaptations in the workplace be helpful?
2. What advice would you give about exercise to a newly diagnosed patient with ankylosing spondylitis? Which website(s) or resources might you recommend to the patient?
3. Which website(s) and sources could you use to get the most up to date guidelines on the treatment of psoriatic arthritis?

USEFUL WEBSITES

The following websites are useful sources of information. All accessed March 2009.
General.
http:/www.library.nhs.uk/Default.aspx/ accessed March 2009.
http:/nice.org.uk/ accessed March 2009.
http://www.nlm.nih.gov/medlineplus/ accessed March 2009.
http:/www.eular.org/ accessed March 2009.
http:/www.rheumatology.org/ accessed March 2009.
http:/www.rheumatology.org.uk/ accessed March 2009.
http:/www.csp.org.uk/ accessed March 2009.
http:/www.cot.co.uk/ accessed March 2009.
http:/www.arma.uk.net/pdfs/ia06.pdf/ accessed March 2009.
Ankylosing spondylitis.
http:/www.arc.org.uk/ accessed March 2009.
http:/www.nass.co.uk/ accessed March 2009.
http:/www.spondylitis-international.org/ accessed March 2009.
http:/www.arc.org.uk/arthinfo/patpubs/6001/6001.asp.
http:/www.asresearch.co.uk.
http:/www.asas-group.org.
http:/www.astretch.co.uk.
http:/www.library.nhs.uk/musculoskeletal/ViewResource.aspx?resID=5112.

http:/www.nice.org.uk/page.aspx?o=98339.
http:/www.rheumatology.org/public/factsheets/as.asp,
http:/www.rheumatology.org/public/factsheets/as.asp.
http:/www.rheumatology.org/public/factsheets/diseases_and_conditions/spondyloarthritis.asp?aud=pat.
http:/www.rheumatology.org.uk/guidelines/guidelines_as.
http:/www.rheumatology.org.uk/search?SearchableText=ankylosing+spondylitis.
http:/www.uhce.ox.ac.uk/epidembase2/atlases/trends/England/Ankylosing%20spondylitis_England.pdf.
Psoriatic arthritis.
http:/www.arc.org.uk/arthinfo/patpubs/6029/6029.asp.
http:/www.nice.org.uk/enter/ search term "psoriatic arthritis".
http:/www.psoriasis-association.org.uk/arthritis.html/
http:/www.rheumatology.org/public/factsheets/diseases_and_conditions/psoriaticarthritis.asp?aud=pat/
http:/www.rheumatology.uk/search?SearchableText=psoriatic+arthritis.
Reactive arthritis/SARA.
http:/www.arc.org.uk/arthinfo/patpubs/6034/6034.asp.
http:/www.bashh.org/ enter search term "arthritis".
Crohns disease and colitis.
http:/www.nacc.org.uk/content/home.asp.
http://www.nlm.nih.gov/medlineplus/ enter search term "IBD arthritis"

References and further reading

ARMA, 2004. Standards of care for people with inflammatory arthritis. Arthritis and Musculoskeletal Alliance London. http://www.arma.uk.net/pdfs/ia06.pdf/ (accessed March 2009).

Averns, H.L., Oxtoby, J., Taylor, H.G., et al., 1996. Radiological outcome in ankylosing spondylitis: use of the Stoke Ankylosing Spondylitis Spine Score (SASSS). Br. J. Rheumatol. 35, 373–376.

Boonen, A., Chorus, A., Miedema, H., et al., 2001. Employment, work disability and work days lost in patients with ankylosing spondylitis: a cross sectional study of Dutch patients. Ann. Rheum. Dis. 60, 353–358.

Boonen, A., Chorus, A., Landewe, R., et al., 2002. Manual jobs increase risk of patients with ankylosing spondylitis withdrawing from the labour force also when adjusted for job related withdrawal in the general population. Ann. Rheum. Dis. 61, 658.

Boonen, A., van Tubergen, A., van der Linden, S., et al., 2004. Spondyloarthropathies. In: Tugwell, P., Shea, B., Boers, M., Brooks, P., Simon, L.S., Strand, V., Wells, G. (Eds.), Evidence Based Rheumatology. BMJ Publishing Group, London.

Braun, J., Sieper, J., 2007. Ankylosing spondylitis. Lancet 369, 1379–1390.

Braun, J., Sieper, J., 2002. Building consensus on nomenclature and disease classification for ankylosing spondylitis: results and discussion of a questionnaire prepared for the International Workshop on New Treatment Strategies in Ankylosing Spondylitis, Berlin, Germany. Ann. Rheum. Dis. 61 (suppl III), ii61–iii67.

Braun, J., van der Heijde, D., Douados, M., et al., 2002. Staging patients with ankylosing spondylitis: a preliminary proposal. Ann. Rheum. Dis. 61 (Suppl. III), iii19–iii23.

British Association for Sexual Health and HIV, 2001. National Guideline on the Management of Sexually Acquired Reactive Arthritis. http://www.bashh.org/guidelines/

BSR, 2004. Guidelines for prescribing TNF α blockers in adults with ankylosing spondylitis. British Society for Rheumatology, London.

Calin, A., Porta, J., Fries, J.F., et al., 1977. Clinical history as a screening test for ankylosing spondylitis. J. Am. Med. Assoc. 237 (24), 2613–2614.

Calin, A., Garrett, S., Whitelock, H., et al., 1994. A new approach to defining functional ability in ankylosing spondylitis: the development of the Bath Ankylosing Spondylitis Functional Index. J. Rheumatol. 21 (12), 2281–2285.

Calin, A., et al., 2004. Ankylosing spondylitis. In: Isenburg, D.A., Maddison, P.J., Woo, P. (Eds.), Oxford Textbook of Rheumatology. Oxford University Press, Oxford.

Chen, J., Liu, C., 2005. Sulfasalazine for ankylosing spondylitis. Coch. Database Syst. Rev. (2) Art No. CD004800.

Chen, J., Liu, C., Lin, J., 2006. Methotrexate for ankylosing spondylitis. Coch. Database Syst. Rev. (4) Art No. CD004525.

Chorus, A.M.J., Boonen, A., Miedema, H.S., et al., 2002. Employment perspectives of patients with ankylosing spondylitis. Ann. Rheum. Dis. 61, 693–699.

Dagfinrud, H., Hagen, K.B., Kvien, T.K., 2004. Physiotherapy interventions for ankylosing spondylitis. Coch. Database Syst. Rev. (4) Art No. CD002822.

Dougados, M., van der Heijde, D., 2002. Ankylosing spondylitis: how should the disease be assessed? Best Pract. Res. Clin. Rheumatol. 16 (4), 605–618.

Dziedzic, K., 1999. Ankylosing spondylitis. In: David, C.,

Lloyd, J. (Eds.), Rheumatolgical Physiotherapy. Mosby, London.

Fransen, M., 2004. When is physiotherapy appropriate? Best Pract. Res. Clin. Rheumatol. 18 (4), 477–489.

Fruth, S.J., 2006. Differential diagnosis and treatment in a patient with posterior upper thoracic pain. Phys. Ther. 86 (2), 254–268.

Gall, V., Arnett, F.C., Slonaker, D., 2000. Ankylosing spondylitis. In: Mevin, J.L., Ferrell, K.M. (Eds.), Adult Rheumatic Diseases Rheumatologic Rehabilitation Series, vol. 2. American Occupational Therapy Association, Bethesda.

Garrett, S., Jenkinson, T., Kennedy, L.G., et al., 1994. A new approach to defining disease status in ankylosing spondylitis; the Bath Ankylosing Spondylitis Disease Activity Index. J. Rheumatol. 21 (12), 2286–2291.

Gladman, D.D., 2006. Clinical, radiological and functional assessment in psoriatic arthritis: is it different from other inflammatory joint diseases? Ann. Rheum. Dis. 65 (Suppl III), iii22–iii24.

Hakim, A., Clunie, G., 2002. Oxford Handbook of Rheumatology. Oxford University Press, Oxford.

Heuft-Dorenbosch, L., Spoorenberg, A., van Tubergen, A., et al., 2003. Assessment of enthesitis in ankylosing spondylitis. Ann. Rheum. Dis. 62, 127–132.

Ince, G., Sarpel, T., Durgun, B., et al., 2006. Effect of a multimodal exercise programme for people with ankylosing spondylitis. Phys. Ther. 86 (7), 924–935.

Irons, K., Jefferies, C., 2004. The Bath Indices-Outcome Measures for use with Ankylosing Spondylitis. NASS, East Sussex.

Jenkinson T.R., Mallorie P.A., Whitelock H.C., et al. 1994. Defining spinal mobility in ankylosing spondylitis

(AS). The Bath AS Metrology Index. J. Rheumatol. 21 (9), 1694–1698.

Jewell, D.P., 1993. Ulcerative Colitis. In: Sleisenger, M.H., Fordtran, J. S. (Eds.), Gastrointestinal Disease, fifth ed, vol. 2. WB Saunders Company, Philadelphia.

Jones, G., Crotty, M., Brooks, P., 2000. Interventions for treating psoriatic arthritis. Coch. Database Syst. Rev. (1) Issue 3 Art No. CD 000212.

Jones, S.D., Steiner, A., Garrett, S.L., et al., 1996. The Bath Ankylosing Spondylitis Patient Global Score (BAS-G). Br. J. Rheumatol. 35 (1), 66–71.

MacKay, K., Mack, C., Brophy, S., et al., 1998. The Bath Ankylosing Spondylitis Radiology Index (BASRI); a new, validated approach to disease assessment. Arthrit. Rheum. 41 (12), 2263–2270.

MacKay, K., Brophy, S., Mack, C., et al., 2000. The development and validation of a radiographic grading system for the hip in ankylosing spondylitis; the Bath Ankylosing Spondylitis Radiology Hip Index. J. Rheumatol. 27 (12), 2866–2872.

Marsal, S., Armadans-Gil, L., Martinez, M., et al., 1999. Clinical, radiographic and HLA associations as markers for different patters of psoriatic arthritis. Rheumatology 38, 332–337.

Mease, P., Goffe, B.S., 2005. Diagnosis and treatment of psoriatic arthritis. J. Am. Acad. Dermatol. 52 (1), 1–19.

Melvin, J.L., 1989. Rheumatic Disease in the Adult and Child; Occupational Therapy and Rehabilitation, third ed. FA Davis Company, Philadelphia.

McVeigh, C.M., Cairns, P., 2006. Diagnosis and management of ankylosing spondylitis. Br. Med. J. 333, 581–585.

Moll, J.H.M., 1987. Rheumatology in Clinical Practice. Blackwell Scientific Publications, Oxford.

Nash, P., Mease, P.J., Braun, J., et al., 2005. Seronegative spondyloarthropathies: to lump or split? Ann. Rheum. Dis. 64 (Suppl II), ii9–ii13.

National Ankylosing Spondylitis Society, 2007. Guidebook for Patients. A Positive Response to Ankylosing Spondylitis. NASS, Richmond, UK.

NICE, 2006. Ankylosing spondylitis, adalimumab, etancecept and infliximab: appraisal consultation document. TA104. Available: National Institute of Clinical Excellence http:// guidance.nice.org.uk.

NICE, 2007. Psoriatic arthritis (moderate to severe) – adalimumab: guidance. TA125 Available: National Institute of Clinical Excellence http://guidance.nice. org.uk.

Olivieri, I., Van Tubergen, A., Salvarani, C., et al., 2002. Seronegative Spondyloarthritides. Best Pract. Res. Clin. Rheumatol. 16 (5), 723–739.

Rudwaleit, M., Khan-Muhammad, A., Sieper, J., 2005. The challenge of diagnosis and classification in early ankylosing spondylitis: do we need new criteria? Arthrit. Rheum. 52 (4), 1000–1008.

Said-Nahal, R., Miceli-Richard, C., Gautreau, C., et al., 2002. The role of HLA genes in familial spondyloarthropathy: a comprehensive study of 70 multipex families. Ann. Rheum. Dis. 61, 201–206.

Shearman, D.J.C., Finlayson, N.D.C., 1989. Diseases of the Gastrointestinal Tract and Liver, second ed. Churchill Livingstone, Edinburgh.

Sweeney, G.M., Clarke, A.K., 1990. Office seating for people with rheumatoid arthritis, ankylosing spondylitis and low back pain. Physiotherapy 76 (4), 203–206.

Symmons, D., Bankhead, C., 1994. Health care needs assessment for musculoskeletal diseases. ARC Epidemiology Unit, University of Manchester, Manchester.

Toivanen, A., 2000. Managing reactive arthritis. Rheumatology 39, 117–121.

Van der Linden, S., Valkenburg, H. A., Cats, A., 1984. Evaluation of diagnostic criteria for ankylosing spondylitis: a proposal for modification of the New York criteria. Arthrit. Rheum. 27, 361–368.

van Tubergen, A., Hidding, A., 2002. Spa and exercise treatment in ankylosing spondylitis: fact or fancy? Best Pract. Res. Clin. Rheumatol. 16 (4), 653–666.

Veale, D., Fitzgerald, O., 2002. Psoriatic arthritis. Best Pract. Res. Clin. Rheumatol. 16, 523–525.

Ward, M.M., 2006. Outcomes in ankylosing spondylitis : what makes the assessment of treatment effects in ankylosing spondylitis different? Ann. Rheum. Dis. 65 (suppl III), iii25–iii28.

Woolacott, N., Bravo Vergel, Y., Kainth, A., et al., 2006. Etanercept and inflximab for the treatment of psoriatic arthritis; a systematic review and economic evaluation. Health Technol. Assess. 10 (31), 1–258.

Wollheim, F. A., 2001. Enteropathic arthritis. In: Ruddy, S., Harris, E.D., Sledge, C.B. (Eds.). Kelleys Textbook of Rheumatology, second ed. WB Saunders, Philadelphia.

Wordsworth, P., et al., 2002. Spondyloarthropathies. In: Bulstrode, C., Carr, A., Marsh, L. (Eds.), Oxford Textbook of Orthopaedics and Trauma, vol. 2. Oxford University Press, Oxford.

Yu, D.T.Y., Fan, P.T., 2001. Reiter's syndrome and undifferentiated spondyloarthropathy. In: Ruddy, S., Harris, E.D., Sledge, C.B. (Eds.) Kelly's Textbook of Rheumatology, sixth ed, vol. 2. WB Saunders, Philadelphia.

Zochling, J., van der Heijde, D., Burgos-Vargas, R., et al., 2006. ASAS/EULAR recommendations for the management of ankylosing spondylitis. Ann. Rheum. Dis. 65, 442–452.

Chapter 20

Osteoporosis

Caitlyn Dowson MBChB FRCP Haywood Hospital, Stoke on Trent NHS Primary Care Trust, High Lane, Stoke-on-Trent, UK

Rachel Lewis MCSP SRP HT Physiotherapy Department, Southmead Hospital, Bristol, UK

CHAPTER CONTENTS

KEY POINTS

- Osteoporosis increases the risk of fractures, particularly the wrist, spine and hip.
- Osteoporosis affects one in five women and one in 12 men over the age of 50.
- Over the age of 80, one in three women and one in five men will suffer a hip fracture.
- Only 25% of people suffering a hip fracture regain their previous level of independence and up to 20% die within 6 months.
- Low bone density measurements strongly predict high fracture risk.
- Secondary causes of osteoporosis must be considered.
- Management of osteoporosis and Paget's disease requires a multidisciplinary approach.

© 2010 Elsevier Ltd
DOI: 10.1016/B978-0-443-06934-5.00020-6

INTRODUCTION

Osteoporosis is a condition in which gradually decreasing bone mass and deteriorating bone structure leads to increased bone fragility and increased risk for fractures, particularly of the wrist, hip and spine (WHO 1994). This process progresses without symptoms until fractures occur or kyphosis becomes apparent. Thus osteoporosis is often described as a silent menace.

Once fractures and deformities have occurred, pain may become a prominent problem and a challenge for people with osteoporosis and everyone involved with their care. Such established osteoporosis is a major cause of morbidity, mortality and reduced quality of life (Lips et al 2005).

INCIDENCE

Osteoporosis affects one in three women and one in twelve men over the age of 50 years (Barlow 1994). The incidence of osteoporotic fractures rises with increasing age. In particular, the incidence of hip fractures rises sharply beyond the age of 65 years in both men and women (Cooper & Melton 1992). Of people surviving to 80 years of age, one in three women and one in five men will suffer a hip fracture. Each year in the UK there are about 60,000 hip fractures, 50,000 wrist fractures and 40,000 clinically diagnosed vertebral fractures (Compston et al 1995, Donaldson et al 1990). The annual NHS cost for managing these is estimated to be in excess of £2.1 billion pounds per year (Cooper 1993). As only 25% of people suffering a hip fracture regain their previous level of independence and up to 20% die within six months, the cost to society is much greater (Jensen & Tondevold 1979).

Interventions to reduce fracture risk have been shown to be clinically and cost effective and should be implemented for those at greatest risk. Women are as likely to suffer an osteoporotic fracture in their lifetime as they are coronary heart disease and the cost effectiveness for interventions are similar for both diseases (Johnell et al 2005).

AETIOLOGY

Bone undergoes a repetitive cycle of remodelling. Osteoclasts break down the bone (resorption) and osteoblasts rebuild it (formation) (Fig. 20.1).

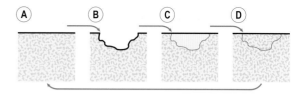

A. Quiescence – the bone is in a resting state
B. Resorption – osteoclasts create a cavity by resorption of bone mineral and matrix
C. Formation – osteoblasts refill the cavity with new matrix
D. Mineralisation – the new matrix is mineralised

Figure 20.1 Diagram of bone metabolism.

Throughout childhood bone formation exceeds resorption and bone mass increases. Peak bone mass is achieved by the age of 20 to 30 years and plateaus for approximately 10 years before declining gradually by about 1% per year. During the menopause the rate of bone loss is greater as bone resorption exceeds formation.

Adult bone mass may be lower than average due to impaired acquisition during childhood or a greater than average rate of bone loss later in life. Impaired peak bone mass acquisition accounts for approximately two thirds of the variance in bone mass seen at any age. Genetic factors have the greatest influence on this (Nguyen et al 2003). Suppressed oestrogen, testosterone or growth hormone production and environmental factors such as poor dietary calcium intake and lack of exercise also delay or diminish bone mass acquisition during childhood and adolescence.

Beyond the age of 40 years, hormonal and environmental factors, rather than genetic factors, have the greatest impact on the rate of bone loss (Seeman 2002). A combination of oestrogen deprivation, calcium and vitamin D deficiency and secondary hyperparathyroidism account for the rapid loss seen in postmenopausal women (Cummings et al 1995). Many other epidemiological factors have been identified (Box 20.1). However, the impact of each factor, or combinations of factors, on an individual requires further clarification.

DIAGNOSIS

As osteoporosis causes no symptoms until fractures or kyphosis occur, it may remain undiagnosed for many years. Whilst the strongest predictive factors for sustaining osteoporotic fractures are a previous

---

BOX 20.1   Risk factors for osteoporotic fractures

* Indicates the risk factors referred to within NICE guidance (2008)

- Low trauma fracture*
- Corticosteroid therapy
- Hypogonadism
  - delayed menarche or puberty
  - prolonged amenorrhoea
  - untreated premature menopause*
  - testosterone deficiency
- Low body mass index less than 22 kg/m^2*
- Parental hip fracture*

- Medical conditions
  - Rheumatoid arthritis, ankylosing spondylitis, Crohn's disease*
  - Others indicated in Box 21.2
- Low dietary calcium intake
- Lack of vitamin D
- Prolonged immobility*
- Cigarette smoking
- Excess alcohol consumption, >4 units per day*
- Excess caffeine consumption

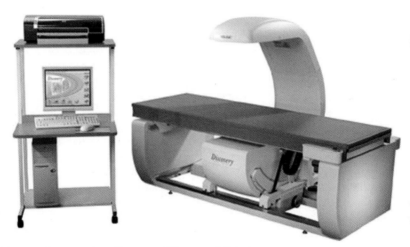

Figure 20.2 DEXA Scanner. Image on loan Courtesy of Vertec and Hologic.

fracture and a low bone mass measurement (Bouxesin 2003, Cummings et al 1995), diagnosis may predate fractures if individuals and health care professionals routinely consider the risks for osteoporosis, fractures and falls. A variety of tools, such as paper or electronic questionnaires, are available to facilitate the identification of patients at risk (Kanis et al 2002, Kanis & Gluer 2000).

The gold standard method for diagnosis is to measure bone mass, or bone mineral density (BMD), using dual energy x-ray absorptiometry (DEXA). DEXA scans are quick, comfortable and relatively cheap to perform and involve minimal radiation exposure (equivalent to about a days background radiation) (Fig. 20.2). DEXA results correlate strongly with fracture risk (Kanis & Gluer

2000) but other bone qualities such as elasticity and architecture, not measurable with DEXA, also contribute.

Bone density readings of the hip and spine are given as the number of standard deviations below the mean peak bone mass of a 20 to 30 year old woman (T-score), the standard deviations below the age matched mean (Z-score) (Fig. 20.3A,B) and as a reading of g/cm^2. A woman has normal bone density if her T-score is no lower than 1 standard deviation below the young adult mean (T-score higher than −1). Osteopaenia (mild thinning of the bones) is present if density lies between 1 to 2.5 standard deviations below the young adult mean. Readings representing osteoporosis are more than 2.5 standard deviations below the young adult mean (T-score

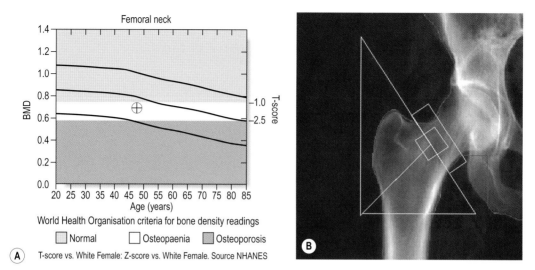

Figure 20.3 DEXA report showing normal hip bone density of a 42-year-old female. The light green shaded area represents normal bone density (T-score above −1), the white osteopaenia (T-score between −1 and −2.5) and the darker green osteoporosis (T-score below −2.5). Image on loan courtesy of Vertec and Hologic.

below –2.5) and established osteoporosis is present if at least one fragility fracture has occurred at this low level (WHO 1994). If the Z-score is low, bone density is lower than expected for the patient's age and other risk factors or underlying disease must be considered. The same criteria are used for men but further work is required to determine the relationship between these scores and fracture risk.

Bone biochemistry (consisting of corrected calcium, alkaline phosphatase and inorganic phosphate) is normal in osteoporosis. Serum and urinary bone marker measurements are used to determine osteoblast and osteoclast activity, but may only be available in research departments. Other diagnostic tools used for diagnosis, screening, or research purposes include heel ultrasonography, quantitative computed tomography (QCT) and bone biopsy. Bone biopsy provides a definitive diagnosis of osteoporosis but is rarely required. Axial DEXA is recommended to confirm a diagnosis of osteoporosis following a positive finding on peripheral imaging e.g. heel ultrasonography.

DIFFERENTIAL DIAGNOSIS

Low bone density can be assumed to be due to osteoporosis only if other causes have been excluded (Box 20.2). For this reason screening blood tests for

metabolic, endocrine and malignant disease are often performed in patients with low bone density. Typically, these tests include full blood count, erythrocyte sedimentation rate (ESR), urea and electrolytes, liver function, bone biochemistry, thyroid function, testosterone and gonadotrophins (in men) and perhaps parathyroid hormone and vitamin D levels (depending on the history and other findings). Serum immunoglobulins and electrophoresis and urinary Bence-Jones proteins should be measured if myeloma is suspected.

Calcium and vitamin D deficiency can occur in specific populations e.g. those from the Indian sub continent including teenage girls, and is common amongst older people, particularly those in long-term nursing or residential care. This is often due to poor dietary intake, lack of adequate sunlight exposure, reduced intestinal absorption or renal impairment and leads to impaired mineralisation of bone, known as osteomalacia. The bones become soft, prone to fracture and appear less dense on DEXA. Blood tests may show low/normal calcium, high/normal alkaline phosphatase, low phosphate, and a high parathyroid hormone level (secondary hyperparathyroidism) (Fig. 20.4).

An elevated serum corrected calcium level should raise suspicion of underlying malignancy (primary or metastatic), myeloma or primary hyperparathyroidism due to a parathyroid adenoma.

Box 20.2   Secondary causes of osteoporosis

Drugs
- Corticosteroids
- Anticonvulsants
- Heparin
- Aromatase inhibitors (breast cancer)
- Testosterone suppression (prostate cancer)

Endocrine disorders
- Hyperparathyroidism
- Thyrotoxicosis
- Cushing's syndrome
- Hyperprolactinaemia

Malignancy
- Myeloma
- Lymphoma
- Leukaemia

Associated chronic disease
- Malabsorption, e.g. coeliac disease
- Chronic renal disease/transplant
- Chronic liver disease
- Rheumatoid arthritis
- Immobility
- Alcohol abuse

Connective tissue disease
- Osteogenesis imperfecta
- Marfan's syndrome
- Ehler's-Danlos syndrome
- Homocysteinuria

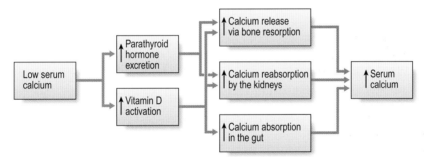

Figure 20.4 Simplified diagram of the metabolic response to low serum calcium levels.

CLINICAL PRESENTATION

Patients may express concern that they have osteoporosis because they have heard or read about it, entered the menopause early (before 42 years), taken steroid therapy or have a family history of osteoporosis or fractures. The incidental finding of radiological osteopaenia, meaning a fainter appearance of the bones on a plain x-ray, also raises suspicion, but does not confirm the presence of osteoporosis. However patients mostly present with a low trauma fracture (e.g. fall from own body height), sudden severe back pain from a vertebral fracture, or the development of kyphosis and loss of height due to asymptomatic vertebral fractures. Only about a third of vertebral fractures come to medical attention (Gallacher et al 2000, Gehlbach et al 2000).

The vast majority of patients who present with their first or subsequent low trauma fractures are not assessed for osteoporosis (RCP 2007). Years later, women who have sustained wrist fractures go on to suffer hip fractures which are associated with high morbidity and mortality rates. Patients with severe osteoporosis may also suffer vertebral, pelvic or rib fractures spontaneously or from minimal trauma such as coughing or rolling over in bed.

CLINICAL EVALUATION

HISTORY

A detailed medical history is essential to assess a patient's risks for osteoporosis (Box 20.1), falls and fractures and to consider the possibility of underlying metabolic bone disease or malignancy (Box 20.2). Patients at greatest risk for suffering an osteoporotic fracture are those who have already fractured and those with known low bone mass. For instance, the relative risk for sustaining a new vertebral fracture is more than doubled for a patient with a previous vertebral fracture and quadrupled if the patient also has low bone density. A woman who has just sustained a vertebral fracture has a one in five chance of sustaining another within one year (Lindsay et al 2001).

Fracture liaison services have been shown to improve identification of high-risk patients (McClellan et al 2003). Without these services in place, less than 10% of high-risk patients attending fracture clinics are identified, diagnosed or treated for osteoporosis (RCP 2007). As many fractures occur following falls, patients' risks for falls must also be assessed in detail and referrals made to physiotherapists or specialist falls clinics as appropriate. Reduction of the risk for falls among the older age group requires a comprehensive multidisciplinary falls risk evaluation and multifactorial intervention (NICE 2004).

EXAMINATION

Whilst some fractures may be painfully obvious others may be detected only after careful examination and investigation. Thoracic kyphosis (Fig. 20.5A,B) may develop gradually as one vertebra after another fractures (or is compressed) or more suddenly if one or more severe wedge fractures occur. The development of the Dowager's hump is a well recognised but late sign of osteoporosis. As this becomes more pronounced, the lower ribs impinge on the iliac crests and the abdomen protrudes. An exaggerated cervical lordosis is apparent when the patient attempts to look straight ahead. Evidence of a previous wrist fracture may also be seen such as the classical dinner fork deformity of a Colle's fracture. A shortened externally rotated leg is highly suggestive of a fractured neck of femur.

Examination of the locomotor system includes inspection followed by palpation and then assessment of movement and function. Palpation of the spine for instance may reveal marked tenderness at the site of a fractured vertebra or associated powerful spasm of the paravertebral muscles. Movement of the spine is likely to be globally reduced following an acutely painful vertebral fracture. Pain increases with flexion or with increased intrathoracic pressure such as coughing, patients' balance, gait and ability to perform simple activities of daily living, including dressing may be significantly impaired.

In addition to examination of the locomotor system it is imperative that patients suspected of suffering with osteoporosis also undergo a full medical examination to elicit signs of any underlying cause for their low bone density (Box 20.2).

RADIOGRAPHY

PLAIN RADIOGRAPHY

The incidental x-ray finding of radiological osteopaenia or vertebral fractures, warrants further assessment for osteoporosis. These incidental vertebral

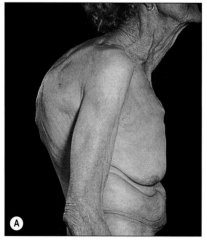 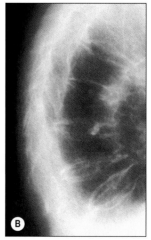

Figure 20.5 (A), (B) Thoracic kyphosis. (Dowager's hump) (A) Marked thoracic kyphosis due to multiple osteoporotic fractures in an elderly woman with (B) corresponding radiograph. With permission Hochberg MC (2008). Elsevier.

fractures may have been spontaneous and painless or due to trauma many years ago. Previous x-rays may reveal the age of the fracture and progression of the condition. Confusion sometimes arises when reporting which vertebra has fractured. The same fracture may be reported as a T4 vertebral fracture on one x-ray and a T3 compression fracture on another occasion. However, vertebral deformities do not resolve. On a lateral view, they are described as a compression or crush fracture when the vertebra is reduced in height, a wedge fracture when the anterior portion is compressed, or a biconcave fracture if the height of the central portion of the vertebra is reduced superiorly and inferiorly.

BONE DENSITOMETRY

As bone density changes only gradually over years, and DEXAs have a margin of error of a couple of percent, there is nothing to be gained by monitoring patients more frequently than every three to five years. Exceptions include patients with severe established osteoporosis in whom response to treatment is in doubt because of ongoing medical problems, numerous ongoing risk factors, difficulties tolerating medication, further fractures and in whom a deteriorating scan result is likely to influence their management.

SPINAL MORPHOMETRY

Spinal morphometry using bone densitometry can also be used and although less information is provided by these images compared with plain x-ray, the radiation dose is much lower (Fig. 20.6).

TECHNETIUM ISOTOPE SCANS

Isotope bone scans may highlight a recent fracture, such as a pelvic insufficiency fracture, not evident on plain x-ray.

MAGNETIC RESONANCE IMAGING

Magnetic resonance imaging (MRI) scans of the spine or pelvis are indicated when there is clinical suspicion of underlying malignancy or significant neurological compromise. The difficulties of performing an MRI scan on patients with severe back pain and kyphosis must be considered carefully. Extra analgesia and sedation may be required.

QUANTITATIVE COMPUTED TOMOGRAPHY

Quantitative computed tomography (QCT) of the spine have been used mainly in research settings and are reported to give additional information regarding bone quality that is not detected on bone densitometry (Engelke et al 2008).

PROGRESSION AND PROGNOSIS

Osteoporosis cannot be cured but the rate of bone loss may be slowed and the risk for further fractures reduced (but not eliminated). Gradual bone loss is a normal feature of ageing, thus interventions may be deemed to be successful if bone density remains stable. Although most treatments offer only a small increase in bone density of up to about five percent during the first year or two, fracture risk reduction may be up to seventy percent (Black et al 1996, 2007).

Difficulties arise when patients sustain further fractures despite treatment. This may reflect lack of efficacy, or conversely, even more fractures may have occurred had treatment not been given. Poor adherence is common and reasons include the development of side-effects, difficulties following the administration instructions and inappropriate expectations and then disappointment when, for example, the medication fails to relieve back pain.

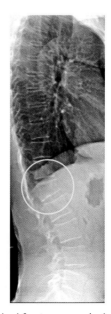

Figure 20.6 Vertebral fractures on spinal morphometry. Images on loan courtesy of Vertec and Hologic.

As osteoporosis does not affect morbidity or mortality until fractures occur, there is a danger of diagnosing people too early and creating a large population of worried well. However, if patients remain undiagnosed and subsequently fracture, the outcome can be devastating. Patients visit their GP approximately 14 times in the first year following a vertebral fracture and quality of life reduces significantly with each subsequent vertebral fracture (Dolan & Jorgensen 1998). Worst still, only 25% of people suffering a hip fracture regain their previous level of independence and up to 20% die within 6 months.

AIMS AND PRINCIPLES OF MANAGEMENT

General population screening for osteoporosis is neither clinically appropriate nor cost effective. Selective screening of patients at high risk for osteoporotic fractures, however, is worthwhile (NICE 2008a, 2008b, NOGG 2008, SIGN 2003). Tools that predict a patient's absolute risk for fracture over 10 years are particularly useful for directing treatment appropriately (Kanis 2008).

Treatment may be indicated for patients with osteoporosis to reduce their risks for sustaining their first fracture (primary prevention) or subsequent fractures if they have already suffered one (secondary prevention). Treatment is also recommended to prevent the development of osteoporosis (prophylaxis) such as that occurring with longterm corticosteroid use.

NICE Technology Appraisal Guidelines for primary prevention and secondary prevention of osteoporotic fractures in postmenopausal women, recommend treatment only for women of certain age groups, with specific numbers of given risk factors and bone density T-scores (NICE 2008a, 2008b). NICE Clinical Guidance for the management of osteoporosis affecting younger women, men and people on corticosteroids is awaited. Guidance for the prevention and treatment of corticosteroid-induced osteoporosis is available from The Royal College of Physicians (RCP 2000). The National Osteoporosis Guideline Group (NOGG) give guidance on the management of osteoporosis in men and women based on the use of FRAX, an on-line 10-year probability of fracture risk assessment tool that incorporates the main risk factors identified by the World Health Organisation (NOGG 2008).

Whilst recommendations regarding who should receive medication differ, all agree that lifestyle risk factors for osteoporosis, fractures and falls should be addressed and deficiency in calcium and vitamin D avoided.

PATIENT EDUCATION

At risk patients should be educated about osteoporosis prior to diagnosis if prophylaxis or lifestyle changes are required. Once a diagnosis of osteoporosis has been established, the patient requires an explanation of the condition, what they can do to help themselves and how long term treatment slows progression but cannot offer a cure. Clear instructions regarding how to take the medication are essential, including dosage and duration.

Patients should be informed of resources available to them for advice, psychological and social support and further information. A wide variety of information is available from The National Osteoporosis Society (NOS 2003) and Arthritis Research Campaign (http://www.arc.org.uk/). Additional information may also be available at GP surgeries, hospital outpatient clinics or osteoporosis department help lines. Local National Osteoporosis Groups are established in many parts of the UK.

SELF-MANAGEMENT

Lifestyle risk factors for osteoporosis, fractures and falls vary in significance and some are more amenable to modification than others (Box 20.1). Currently patients are advised that they should not smoke at all and should not drink more than 1 or 2 units of alcohol a day. A healthy balanced diet including adequate amounts of calcium is important and excessive caffeine consumption should be reduced.

Approximately ten minutes of sunlight exposure to the face and forearms reduces the risk for vitamin D deficiency. Weight-bearing exercise delivered in a variety of ways, slows or prevents further bone loss, in postmenopausal women (Martyn-St James & Carroll 2008) and physiotherapy improves pain and functional performance (Malmros et al 1998).

THERAPY MANAGEMENT OF OSTEOPOROSIS

Physiotherapists and occupational therapists often have a high profile within the osteoporosis team. Therapists can undertake specialist roles for education and treatment and may adopt a modern matron approach to ensuring all eligible patients are given appropriate treatment, advice and preventative strategies.

AIMS OF TREATMENT

The aims of treatment are outlined below:

- Prevention of fracture
- Maintain/optimise bone quality/micro-architecture
- Reduce the rate of bone loss
- Fall prevention
- Maintain/improve balance
- Pain relief
- Postural stability
- Ergonomic advice
- Maintain independence/activities of daily living
- Education.

GUIDELINES

The Physiotherapy Management of Osteoporosis Physiotherapy guidelines (CSP 1999, and recently updated in 2007) were accompanied by an audit tool (CSP 2002).

ASSESSMENT

Assessment should include metrology, function, pain, general mobility, aerobic testing, and quality of life. The principles of assessment are covered in Chapters 3 and 4. In this section specific reference is made to assessments that have been adopted for people with osteoporosis.

METROLOGY

Height is an easy way to assess patients over time, particularly as patients will lose height with each vertebral fracture. Height does vary with other factors, such as diurnal rhythms - patients will often regain height after rehabilitation - therefore some of the height loss may be postural. Tragus or occiput to wall measurement or a flexi curve can be used to assess posture and evaluate the effects of treatment interventions (Laurent et al 1991).

A measurement of posture is important as a kyphotic posture leads to loss of balance, which is exacerbated by muscle weakness, so rehabilitation can be targeted to such problems (Mika et al 2005, Sinaki et al 2005). Trunk lateral flexion can be assessed with a tape measure to evaluate spinal mobility (Moll et al 1972) and highlight balance restrictions or pain limitation. Care should be taken as patients may become unsteady when tested. Upper and lower limb mobility and range of movement should be tested. Due to increasing kyphosis shoulder range of movement and function can be limited (Pearlmutter et al 1995).

FUNCTION

Functional tests are numerous and there are many validated tools (Ch. 4). One of the simplest tests is the timed up and go test (TUG) (Podsiadlo & Richardson 1991). The TUG times a patient standing from a chair with no arms, walking 5 metres and returning to sit down. The average time to complete this test is 15 seconds (Podsiadlo & Richardson 1991). Patients may vary from 12 seconds up to 85 seconds. The TUG can demonstrate clinical improvement following an intervention. Other tests to be considered include functional reach, and timed stairs climb and dressing activities (Helmes et al 1995, Lyles et al 1993).

PAIN

Pain should be monitored. A visual analogue score is quick (Melzack 1983, Scott & Huskisson 1976) where a pain diary can be time consuming. Physiotherapists may use a manual therapy assessment protocol to evaluate symptoms. However, accessory mobilisations of the spine should be excluded due to the potential risk of further fracture and increase in pain levels.

GENERAL MOBILITY

Many patients with osteoporosis are at risk of falls. This could be due to altered proprioceptive and kinaesthetic awareness resulting from kyphosis and altered posture. A record should be maintained of the number of falls, including reason for fall and injuries sustained (NICE 2004).

AEROBIC TESTING

Aerobic testing is not performed routinely by therapists. However, it can form part of a special test in some individuals who would benefit from an intervention improving aerobic capacity.

QUALITY OF LIFE

Quality of life can be assessed using generic measures (Ch. 4) or specific measures, e.g. the European Foundation for Osteoporosis Quality of Life Measure (Qualetto) (Lips et al 1996).

INTERVENTIONS

Osteoporosis is a multi-factorial condition as is the risk of fracture and undertaking an early intervention with the multi-disciplinary team is essential. The high risk areas for fracture are areas of high trabecular bone content, e.g. hip and spine. Treatment and exercises must be targeted to these vulnerable areas. Trunk flexion should be avoided as this can provide a high risk of vertebral fracture due to the biomechanics of the trabecular tissue (Myers & Wilson 1997).

PAIN RELIEF

Following assessment the therapist aims to control pain levels, gain the patient's trust and confidence and willingness to continue with further treatment. Modalities for pain relief are varied and include management of both acute post-fracture pain and management of chronic pain from altered posture and kyphosis. Treatments should be simple to enable patients to continue at home and self-management should be a priority.

The following interventions may be appropriate for people with osteoporosis pain:

- TENS
- Acupuncture and non-invasive acupuncture
- Heat (with all the adequate safety instructions)
- Exercise
- Hydrotherapy
- Postural correction.

Many patients try alternative treatments such as aromatherapy and reflexology. Further information on pain relief is available within the National Osteoporosis Society booklet (NOS 2003).

POSTURAL CORRECTION

Kyphosis can be due to a combination of muscle weakness and muscle imbalance. Patients with vertebral fracture have a further biomechanical alteration with a reduction in anterior vertebral height in comparison to the posterior height, increasing with multiple fractures (Genant et al 1993, Myers & Wilson 1997). Fractures can exacerbate muscle imbalance and a vicious cycle of muscle pain and weakness can perpetuate increasing kyphosis and further fracture (Huang et al 2006).

By addressing posture correction and giving ergonomic advice, a more muscle-efficient posture can be adopted, pain can be reduced and overall biomechanics improved. This is often demonstrated by an increase in patient activities of daily living and improvement in metrology. Advice should be given regarding sleeping positions with particular attention to the cervical spine and hips, which are common sites of discomfort. The use of lumbar rolls for the spine should be advised for sitting and travelling to improve posture and relieve discomfort. Ergonomic advice regarding sitting positions should be given as basic information, and advice on office seating and armchair design should be highlighted. Patients should be made aware of their local resource centres, e.g. the Disabled Living Foundation.

Osteoporosis does not only affect retired postmenopausal women, therefore occupational therapists may need to perform fit-for-work assessment. Further self-management advice on postural correction is applicable in some cases, e.g. the Alexander technique, Pilates etc.

TAPING

Taping can be used for pain relief and proprioceptive feedback. It is important to assess skin viability as taping may be contraindicated in those with hypersensitivity or susceptibility to skin tears. Glucocorticoid induced osteoporosis needs careful assessment due to possible drag of the tape. The proprioceptive input should be accompanied by suitable home exercise programme for the thoracic spine and shoulder to maximise the benefits of taping.

ORTHOTIC BRACING

The debate for and against bracing continues due to lack of evidence. Orthoses have been shown to reduce deformity and bracing of the trunk may reduce postural sway, pain and possibly reduce risk of falls as well as improving quality of life (Pfiefer et al 2004).

BREATHING EXERCISES

Breathing exercises are important for many patients. Some people experience more pain from vertebral fractures on deep inhalation and coughing. Consequently, they reduce the depth of inhalation and are at further risk of chest infection.

RELAXATION

Relaxation can be very beneficial for patients with osteoporosis and the occupational therapist may lead this aspect of management (Chs 9 & 11). The Laura Mitchell method can be very useful (Bell & Saltikov 2000).

PACING

Pacing may be used as part of a pain management strategy. A gradual increase in exercise repetitions as well as exercise intensity and amount of resistance used can be beneficial. Patients frequently require reassurance that they are increasing their exercise intensity correctly (Harding & Watson 2000).

EXERCISE

There is good evidence for the benefit of exercise as a treatment for osteoporosis and as a prevention strategy (Berard et al 1997, Chow et al 1989, Joakimsen et al 1997, Kemper et al 2000, Wolff et al 1999). Studies in men are also becoming more common (Kelley et al 2000, Maddslozzo & Snow 2000).

Patients worry that if they do too much exercise they will sustain fractures but they need to load trabecular bone areas with gravity and weight to stimulate osteoblast activity. Physiotherapists must therefore reassure patients that movements in the correct patterns, e.g. avoiding flexion, are beneficial not detrimental. Many patients are surprised at how strenuously they can exercise without causing or exacerbating pain. People with osteoporosis can lift surprising amounts of weight (Kerr et al 1996) and weights and spinal loading are recommended for both prevention and treatment (Sinaki et al 2005).

Exercise should be viewed as a lifestyle change and should be undertaken for the rest of their lives and not only for the duration of the intervention. Studies have demonstrated that exercise can improve quality of life following vertebral fracture (Gardner et al 2000, Steinberg et al 2000). It is important to advise the whole family on exercise to prevent osteoporosis.

HYDROTHERAPY

In the hydrotherapy pool the risk of falling and fracturing is much reduced, as long as patients are safely managed in the surrounding pool area. The physiological effects of immersion need to be considered (Hall et al 1990) for example in patients with renal problems.

Immersed patients experience pain relief and buoyancy of the water assists range of movement. Patients progress to resisted movement for muscle strengthening (Levine 1984). The action of a muscle/tendon 'pull' on a bone will also stimulate osteoblast activity (Nordin & Frankel 1989). Exercises without resistance including trunk rotation can be very beneficial for pain relief in osteoporosis (Hall et al 1990). Such exercises are easy to perform when standing, improve the patient's confidence in the water, allow the trunk to be supported by hydrostatic pressure and facilitate spinal column lengthening.

Patients can perform exercises to correct postural alignment, stretch pectoral muscle groups, perform trunk extension with or without equipment and increase the buoyancy, resistance and stamina. Cardiovascular fitness and respiratory exertion can be facilitated more easily in water due to the physiological demands of the immersion (Levine et al 1984). Hydrotherapy alone does not increase bone density and consequently patients also need a land-based exercise programme.

GENERAL MOBILITY AND BALANCE RE-EDUCATION

Balance and mobility need to be addressed to prevent further falls and fracture. Balance exercise is important in preventing fracture (Gardner et al 2000, Steinberg et al 2000) and patients should be advised how to continue their exercise programmes once discharged. Tai Chi is an effective technique for fall prevention. Tai Chi classes, Alexander technique, Pilates and Yoga, may be available locally. Further details can be obtained from the NICE Falls Guideline (NICE 2004).

COMMON PHARMACOLOGICAL APPROACHES

BISPHOSPHONATES

Bisphosphonates reduce the rate of bone resorption and significantly reduce the risk for fracture. Generic alendronate is the first line agent for osteoporosis. Large randomised placebo controlled clinical trials have shown that treatment with alendronate significantly increases bone mineral density and reduces risk for hip fracture by 53% and clinical vertebral fracture by 45% (Black et al 2000). When used for ten years, alendronate remained effective and did not lead to significant deterioration in bone quality, despite the prolonged inhibition of bone resorption (Bone et al 2004). As bisphosphonates bind to bone and continue to exert an antiresorptive effect for years after discontinuation, further studies are required to determine longer-term safety. Some specialists suggest that a break from therapy, after 5 years, may be appropriate for patients at lower risk for fractures (Black et al 2006).

In order to reduce the risk for developing oesophagitis, alendronate should be taken (usually once weekly) with a large glass of water first thing in the morning before having anything to eat or drink. The patient must then keep their oesophagus upright for at least 30 minutes, but preferably 60 minutes, before lying down or having anything else to eat or drink. Some patients misinterpret the instructions and spend the whole hour standing up when sitting upright would suffice.

Other bisphosphonates are available but are not yet generic and therefore much more expensive, e.g. Risedronate (McClung et al 2001), Ibandronate (Delmas et al 2006) and Zoledronate (Black et al 2007). A rare, but potentially severe, side effect of bisphosphonate therapy is osteonecrosis of the jaw in which the bone of the mandible or maxilla becomes exposed and necrotic. Patients are encouraged to maintain good dental hygiene and to inform their dentist that they are taking bisphosphonates. For patients with poor oral hygiene, a dental examination is advisable before commencing therapy. Extractions are not contraindicated but root filling is preferred (Arrain & Masud 2008).

CALCIUM AND VITAMIN D

Calcium and vitamin D supplements are often required in addition to the bisphosphonates to treat, or prevent the development of, osteomalacia. This is particularly important for older people with limited sunlight exposure. Numerous supplements are available, some being more palatable than others. Correction of vitamin D deficiency has also been shown to improve muscle strength and may reduce frequency of falls (Venning 2005).

OTHER THERAPEUTIC AGENTS FOR OSTEOPOROSIS

For some patients, who are unable to take bisphosphonates or fail to respond to them, alternative agents are available, although guidelines may restrict their use. Raloxifene, a selective oestrogen receptor modulator (or SERM) is recommended by NICE as an alternative to bisphosphonate therapy for the secondary prevention of osteoporotic fractures (Ettinger et al 1999).

Strontium ranelate is reported to have both antiresorptive and anabolic (bone building) effects (Meunier et al 2004, Reginster et al 2005). NICE recommend strontium ranelate as a third line agent (after alendronate and risedronate) for primary and secondary prevention but again only if certain clinical and bone density criteria are met (NICE 2008a, 2008b). Teriparatide leads to significant increases in bone mineral density, improved bone architecture and a reduction in risk for vertebral and non-vertebral fractures (Neer et al 2001). The significant cost and potential adverse effects however restrict its use (NICE 2008a, 2008b).

Long-term calcitonin therapy has been shown to increase bone mineral density and reduce the risk for vertebral fractures in postmenopausal women. Calcitonin also has analgesic properties and is given, for up to 2 weeks, to patients with painful vertebral fractures and to facilitate rehabilitation in the acute phase (Knopp et al 2005). Although effective, hormone replacement therapy (HRT) is no longer recommended for the treatment of osteoporosis due to associated increased cardiovascular, cerebrovascular and cancer risks (WHI 2002). However HRT is still indicated for women suffering a premature menopause or severe postmenopausal symptoms.

ANALGESIA

Although osteoporosis itself is a painless condition, many patients who have sustained fractures suffer acute or chronic pain. Increasing potency of analgesics may be required alongside the physical therapies described above.

MANAGEMENT OF FRACTURES

General principles for the management of fractures apply, but are more challenging to implement due to poor bone quality and other comorbidity. Hip fractures require surgical fixation or replacement to enable early mobilisation. A multidisciplinary care package is essential for rehabilitation and to reduce the associated high morbidity and mortality in older people (Morrison et al 1998, Roche et al 2005).

Symptomatic vertebral fractures are usually managed medically, with analgesia and perhaps calcitonin. For patients who fail to respond to conservative measures, the injection of cement into the fractured vertebral body, directly (vertebroplasty) or using a balloon (kyphoplasty), may provide some pain relief and structural support in the short term (Diamond 2006 et al, Grafe et al 2005). Long-term benefits are unclear and these procedures should be performed only in units supported by a spinal surgeon (NICE 2003, 2006).

PREVENTION OF FALLS AND FRACTURES

National guidelines emphasise the need for an integrated approach to the management of osteoporosis and falls in order to reduce the rate of fracture amongst older people (DOH 2001, NICE 2004). Thus, fracture liaison services and falls services must work together to provide education and support for health professionals, patients and their carers.

PAGET'S DISEASE

Paget's disease is the second most common metabolic bone disease after osteoporosis (ARMA 2007). It affects about 2% of the UK population above the age of 55 years and increases with advancing age (ARMA 2007, Paget 1887). However, only 5% of people with Paget's disease are symptomatic (ARMA 2007). Despite its prevalence, it is often neglected as some health care practitioners consider it to be a benign condition of older adults for which there is no treatment (ARMA 2007, Cooper et al 1999, Whyte 2006).

In Paget's disease there is a marked increase in bone turnover in parts of the skeleton, resulting in the development of structurally weak abnormal bone, with an increased risk of pain, fracture, deformity, osteoarthritis of the large joints and deafness (ARMA 2007) (Fig. 20.7). Over the last few years a number of highly effective bisphosphonate treatments have been developed which can effectively suppress the symptoms and may prevent the development of complications (ARMA 2007).

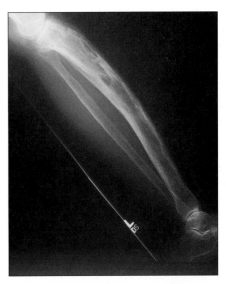

Figure 20.7 Lateral radiograph of the lower extremity. Classic changes of Paget's disease are present in the bowing deformity of the tibia, with marked cortical thickening and mixed lytic and sclerotic lesions. The fibula is spared. With permission Hochberg MC (2008). Rheumatology edition Elsevier.

CONCLUSION

Osteoporosis is a common condition and causes significant morbidity and mortality. It is often called the silent epidemic. It increases the risk of fractures and only a quarter of people suffering a hip fracture regain their previous level of independence and up to 20% die within six months. Low bone density measurements strongly predict high fracture risk.

Paget's disease is the second most common metabolic bone disease after osteoporosis.

Management of osteoporosis and Paget's disease requires a combination of pharmacological and non-pharmacological approaches and, as members of the multidisciplinary team, therapists have a key role in the management of these conditions.

ACKNOWLEDGEMENT

We would like to acknowledge Hilary Jones from the Arthritis Research Campaign National Primary Care Centre for her secretarial support with the therapy manuscript.

CASE STUDIES

Write a treatment plan using the recommended guidance for each of the following cases:
- A post menopausal woman with risk factors for osteoporosis (NICE guidance on primary prevention, Physiotherapy guidelines for osteoporosis)
- A twenty-two year old woman with Systemic Lupus Erythematosus on 7.5 mg prednisolone and

a family history of osteoporosis (NICE guidance on secondary prevention, Physiotherapy guidelines for osteoporosis)
- A man with severe established osteoporosis and recurrent falls (falls guidance, physiotherapy guidelines for osteoporosis).

STUDY ACTIVITIES

1. Look up the latest physiotherapy guidelines for osteoporosis and the latest NICE guidance for falls and osteoporosis. Suggest appropriate amendments to the physiotherapy guidelines to incorporate the latest NICE guidance on falls and osteoporosis.
2. Should NICE include more guidance on physiotherapy and occupational therapy in their documents regarding falls and osteoporosis? If so, what would you suggest they recommend and what evidence is available to support this inclusion?
3. Perform a search of qualitative studies to identify the impact of osteoporosis on the individual. Give a summary of their findings and suggest areas that warrant further study.

USEFUL WEBSITES

www.sign.ac.uk/guidelines/fulltext/71/index.html/ (accessed March 2009).

www.shef.ac.uk/NOGG/downloads.html/ (accessed March 2009).

www.nice.org.uk/TA160/ (accessed March 2009).

www.nice.org.uk/TA161/ (accessed March 2009).

www.arma.uk.net/pdfs/mbdweb.pdf/ (accessed March 2009).

www.arc.org.uk/ search for: "osteoporosis" (accessed March 2009).

www.csp.org.uk/uploads/documents/OSTEOgl.pdf (accessed March 2009).

http://www.csp.org.uk/uploads/documents/OsteoAudit.pdf accessed March 2009.

References and further reading

ARMA, 2007. Standards of Care for people with metabolic bone diseases. www.arma.uk.net/pdfs/mbdweb.pdf/ date (accessed March 2009).

Arrain, Y., Masud, T., 2008. Recent recommendations on bisphosphonate-associated osteonecrosis of the jaw. Dent. Update 35 (4), 238–240.

Barlow, D.H., 1994. Report of the Advisory Group on Osteoporosis. Department of Health, London.

Bell, J.A., Saltikov, J.B., 2000. Mitchell's relaxation technique: is it effective? Physiotherapy 86 (9), 473–478.

Berard, A., Bravo, G., Gauthier, P., 1997. Meta-analysis of the effectiveness of physical activity for the prevention of bone loss in post-menopausal women. Osteoporos. Int. 7, 331–337.

Black, D.M., Cummings, S.R., Karpf, D.B., et al., 1996. Randomised trial of effect of alendronate on risk of fracture in women with existing vertebral fractures. Fracture intervention trial research group. Lancet 348, 1535–1541.

Black, D.M., Delmas, P.D., Eastell, R., et al., 2007. Once yearly zoledronic acid for the treatment of postmenopausal osteoporosis. N. Engl. J. Med. 356 (18), 1809–1822.

Black, D.M., Schwarz, A.V., Ensrud, K.E., et al., 2006. Effects of continuing or stopping alendronate after 5 years of treatment. The fracture intervention trial long-term extension (FLEX): A randomized

trial. J. Am. Med. Assoc. 296 (24), 2927–2938.

Black, D.M., Thompson, D.E., Bauer, D.C., et al., 2000. Fracture risk reduction with alendronate in women with osteoporosis: The fracture intervention trial. J. Clin. Endocrinol. Metab. 85 (11), 4119–4124.

Bone, H.G., Hosking, D., Devogelaer, J.P., et al., 2004. Ten years' experience with alendronate for osteoporosis in post-menopausal women. N. Engl. J. Med. 18; 350 (12), 1189–1199.

Bouxesin, M.L., 2003. Bone quality: where do we go from here?. Osteoporos. Int. 14 (Suppl. 5), 118–127.

Chow, R., Harrison, J., Dornan, J., 1989. Prevention and rehabilitation of osteoporosis program. Exercise and osteoporosis. Int. J. Rehabil. Res. 1, 49–56.

Compston, J.E., Cooper, C., Kanis, J.A., 1995. Bone densitometry in Clinical Practice. Br. Med. J. 310, 1507–1510.

Cooper, C., 1993. Epidemiology and public health impact of osteoporosis. Baillière's Clin. Rheumatol. 7, 459–477.

Cooper, C., Melton, L.J., 1992. Epidemiology of osteoporosis. (3rd edn).Trends Endocrinol. Metab. 3, 224–229.

Cooper, C., Schafheutle, K., Dennison, E., et al., 1999. The epidemiology of Paget's disease in Britain: Is the prevalence decreasing. J. Bone Miner. Res. 14, 192–197.

CSP, 1999. Physiotherapy Guidelines for the Management of Osteoporosis. Chartered Society of Physiotherapists, London Available at http://www.csp.org/uk/ uploads/documents/OSTEOgl.pdf. (accessed March 2009).

CSP, 2002. Physiotherapy Guidelines for the Management of Osteoporosis. Osteoporosis Audit Pack. Chartered Society of Physiotherapists, London Available at http://www.csp.org.uk/ uploads/documents/OsteoAudit. pdf (accessed March 2009)..

Cummings, S.R., Nevitt, M.C., Browner, W.S., et al., 1995. Risk factors for hip fracture in white women. Study of osteoporotic fractures research group. N. Engl. J. Med. 332, 767–773.

Delmas, P.D., Adami, S., Strugala, C., et al., 2006. Intravenous ibandronate injections in postmenopausal women with osteoporosis: one-year results from the dosing intravenous administration study. Arthritis Rheum. 54 (6), 1838–1846.

Diamond, T.H., Bryant, C., Browne, L., et al., 2006. Clinical outcomes after acute osteoporotic vertebral fractures: a 2-year non-randomised trial comparing percutaneous vertebroplasty with conservative therapy. Med. J. Aust. 184 (3), 113–117.

DOH, , 2001. National Service Framework for Older People. Department of Health, London Accessed on 31/01/09 at http://www.dh.gov.uk/en/ publicationsandstatistics/ publications/ publicationspolicyandguidance/ DH_4003066. (accessed March 2009).

Dolan, P., Jorgensen, D.J., 1998. The cost of treating osteoporotic fractures in the United Kingdom female population. Osteoporos. Int. 8, 611–616.

Donaldson, L.J., Cook, A., Thompson, R.G., 1990. Incidence of fractures in a geographically defined population. J. Epidemiol. Commun. Health 44, 241–245.

Engelke, K., Adams, J.E., Armbrecht, G., et al., 2008. Clinical use of quantitative computed tomography and peripheral quantitative computed tomography in the management of osteoporosis in adults: the 2007 ISCD Official Positions. J. Clin. Densitomet. 11 (1), 123–162.

Ettinger, B., Black, D.M., Mitlak, B.H., 1999. Reduction of vertebral fracture risk in postemenopausal women with osteoporosis treated with raloxifene: results from a 3 year randomised clinical trial. Multiple Outcomes of Raloxifene Evaluation (MORE) Investigators. J. Am. Med. Assoc. 18; 282 (7), 637–645.

Gallacher, S.J., Gallagher, A.P., McQuillan, C., et al., 2000. The prevalence of vertebral fracture amongst patients presenting with non-vertebral fractures. Osteoporos. Int. 18, 185–192.

Gardner, M.M., Robertson, M.G., Campbell, A.J., 2000. Exercise in preventing falls and fall related injuries in older people: a review of randomised controlled trials. Br. J. Sports Med. 34 (1), 7–17.

Gehlbach, S.H., Bigelow, C., Heimisdottir, M., et al., 2000. Recognition of vertebral fracture in a clinical setting. Osteoporos. Int. 11, 577–582.

Genant, H.K., Wu, C.Y., van Kuijk, C., et al., 1993. Vertebral fracture assessment using a semi-quantitative technique. J. Bone Miner. Res. 8, 1137–1148.

Grafe, I.A., Da Fonseca, K., Hillmeier, J., et al., 2005. Reduction of pain and fracture incidence after kyphoplasty: 1-year outcomes of a prospective controlled trial of patients with primary osteoporosis. Osteoporos. Int. 16 (12), 2005–2012.

Hall, J., Bisson, D., O'Hare, P., 1990. The physiology of immersion. Physiotherapy 76, 517–521.

Harding, V., Watson, P., 2000. Increasing activity and improving function in chronic pain management. Physiotherapy 86 (12), 619–630.

Helmes, E., Hodsman, A., Lazowski, D., et al., 1995. A questionnaire to evaluate disability in osteoporotic patients with vertebral compression fractures. J. Gerontol. Series A Biolog. Med. Sci. 50 (2), M91–M98.

Huang, M.H., Barrett-Connor, E., Grendale, G.A., et al., 2006. Hyperkyphotic posture and risk of future osteoporotic fracture-Rancho Bernado Study. J. Bone Miner. Res. 21 (3), 419–423.

Jensen, J.S., Tondevold, E., 1979. Mortality after hip fractures. Acta Orthop. Scand. 50 (2), 161–167.

Joakimsen, R.M., Magnus, J.H., Fonnebo, V., 1997. Physical activity and predisposition for hip fractures: a review. Osteoporos. Int. 7, 503–513.

Johnell, O., Kanis, J.A., Jonsson, B., et al., 2005. The burden of hospitalised fractures in Sweden. Osteoporos. Int. 16, 222–228.

Kanis, J.A., 2008. on behalf of the National Osteoporosis Guideline Group. Case finding for the management of osteoporosis with FRAX – assessment and intervention thresholds for the UK. Osteoporos. Int. 19, 1395–1408.

Kanis, J.A., Gluer, C.C., 2000. For the committee of scientific advisors, International Osteoporosis Foundation. An update of the diagnosis and assessment of osteoporosis with densitometry. Osteoporos. Int. 11, 192–202.

Kanis, J.A., Johnell, O., Oden, A., et al., 2002. Ten-year risk of osteoporotic fracture and the effect of risk factors on screening strategies. Bone 30, 251–258.

Kelley, G.A., Kelley, K.S., Tran, Z.V., 2000. Exercise and bone mineral density in men: a meta-analysis. J. Appl. Physiol. 88 (5), 1730–1736.

Kemper, H.G.C., Bakker, I., van Tulder, M.W., et al., 2000. Exercise for Preventing Low Bone Mass in Young Males and Females (Protocol). The Cochrane Library, issue 4, Oxford 2000.

Kerr, D., Morton, A., Dick, I., et al., 1996. Exercise effects on bone mass in postmenopausal women are site specific and load dependent. J. Bone Miner. Res. 11, 218–225.

Knopp, J.A., Diner, B.M., Blitz, M., et al., 2005. Calcitonin for treating acute pain of osteoporotic vertebral compression fractures: a systematic review of randomised controlled trials. Osteoporos. Int. 16 (10), 1281–1290.

Laurent, M.R., Buchanon, W.W., Bellamy, N., 1991. Methods of assessment used in ankylosing spondylitis clinical trials: a review. Br. J. Rheumatol. 30, 326–329.

Levine, B., 1984. Use of hydrotherapy in reduction of anxiety. Psychol. Rep. 55, 526.

Lindsay, R., Silverman, S.L., Cooper, C., et al., 2001. Risk of new vertebral fracture in the year following a fracture. J. Am. Med. Assoc. 285, 320–323.

Lips, P., Agnusdei, D., Caulin, F., et al., 1996. The development of a European questionnaire for quality of life in patients with vertebral osteoporosis. Scand. J. Rheumatol. 103 (Suppl.), 84–85.

Lips, P., Van Schoor, N.M., 2005. Quality of life in patients with osteoporosis. Osteoporos. Int. 16 (5), 447–455.

Lyles, K.W., Gold, D.T., Shipp, K. M., et al., 1993. Association of osteoporotic vertebral compression fractures with impaired functional status. Am. J. Med. 94, 595–601.

Maddslozzo, G.F., Snow, C.M., 2000. High intensity resistance training: effects on bone in older men and women. Calcif. Tissue Int. 66 (6), 399–404.

Malmros, B., Mortensen, L., Jensen, M.B., et al., 1998. Positive effects of physiotherapy on chronic pain and performance in osteoporosis. Osteoporos. Int. 8 (3), 215–221.

Martyn-St James, M., Carroll, S., November 3, 2008. A meta-analysis of impact exercise on postmenopausal bone loss: the case for mixed loading exercise programmes. Br. J. Sports Med. [Epub ahead of print].

McClellan, A.R., Gallacher, S.J., Fraser, M., et al., 2003. The fracture liaison service: success of a program for the evaluation and management of patients with osteoporotic fracture. Osteoporos. Int. 14, 1028–1034.

McClung, M.R., Geusens, P., Miller, P.D., et al., 2001. Effect of risedronate on the risk of hip fracture in elderly women. Hip Intervention Program Study Group. N. Engl. J. Med. 344 (5), 333–340.

Melzack, R. 1983. The McGill pain questionnaire in: Pain measurement and assessment. Raven Press, New York, pp. 41–46.

Meunier, P.J., Roux, C., Seeman, E., et al., 2004. The effects of strontium ranelate on the risk of vertebral fracture in women with osteoporosis. N. Engl. J. Med. 350 (5), 459–468.

Mika, A., Unnithan, M.P., 2005. Differences in thoracic kyphosis and back muscle strength in women with bone loss due to osteoporosis. Spine 30 (2), 241–246.

Moll, J.M.H., Liyanage, S.P., Wright, V., 1972. An objective clinical method to measure spinal extension. Rheumatol. Phys. Med. 67, 668–673.

Morrison, R.S., Chassin, M.R., Siu, A.L., et al., 1998. The medical consultant's role in caring for patients with hip fracture. Ann. Intern. Med. 128 (12), 1010–1020.

Myers, E.R., Wilson, S.E., 1997. Biomechanics of osteoporosis and vertebral fracture. Spine 22 (245), 25S–31S.

National Osteoporosis Society, , 2003. Living with Osteoporosis. Coping after Broken Bones. National Osteoporosis Society Bath. www.nos.org.ukaccessedMarch 2009o://ww.

Neer, R.M., Arnaud, C.D., Zanchetta, J.R., et al., 2001. Effect of parathyroid hormone (1-34) on fractures and bone mineral density in postmenopausal women with osteoporosis. N. Engl. J. Med. 10; 344 (19), 1434–1441.

Nguyen, T.V., Livshits, G., Centre, J.R., et al., 2003. Genetic Determination of Bone Mineral Density: Evidence for a Major Gene. J. Clin. Endocrinol.Metab. 88 (8), 3614–3620.

NICE, 2003. Percutaneous Vertebroplasty. Interventional Procedure Guidance 12. National Institute for Clinical Excellence, London www.nice.org.uk/guidance/IPG12 (accessed March 2009).

NICE, 2004. NICE Clinical Guidance 21 Falls: The Assessment and Prevention of Falls in Older People. National Institute for Clinical Excellence, London http://www.nice.org.uk/CG021NICEguideline. (accessed 29.01.09).

NICE, 2006. Balloon Kyphoplasty for Vertebral Compression Fractures. Interventional Procedure Guidance 166. National Institute for Health and Clinical Excellence, London Available at www.nice.org.uk/download-aspx?0=1PG166publicinfo (accessed March 2009).

NICE, 2008a. Alendronate, etidronate, risedronate, raloxifene and strontium ranelate for the primary prevention of osteoporotic fragility fractures in postmenopausal women. NICE technology appraisal guidance 160. Available at www.nice.org.uk/TA160/ (accessed March 2009).

NICE, 2008b. Alendronate, etidronate, risedronate, raloxifene, strontium ranelate and teriparatide for the secondary prevention of osteoporotic fragility fractures in postmenopausal women. NICE technology appraisal guidance 161. Available at www.nice. org.uk/TA161 (accessed March 2009).

NOGG, 2008. National Osteoporosis Guideline Group on behalf of the Bone Research Society, British Geriatrics Society, British Orthopaedic Association, British Society of Rheumatology, National Osteoporosis Society, Osteoporosis 2000, Osteoporosis Dorset, Primary Care Rheumatology Society, and Society for Endocrinology. London Available at www.shef. ac.uk/NOGG/downloads.html/ (accessed March 2009).

Nordin, M., Frankel, V.H., 1989. Basic Biomechanics of the Musculoskeletal System, second ed. Lea & Febiger, Philadelphia Ch 1, 3–31.

Paget, J., 1887. On a form of chronic inflammation of bones (osteitis deformans). Med.-Chir. Trans. 16, 37–63.

Pearlmutter, L., Bode, B., Wilkinson, W., et al., 1995. Shoulder range of motion in patients with osteoporosis. Arthritis Care Res. 8 (3), 194–199.

Pfiefer, M., Begerow, B., Minne, H.W., 2004. Effects of a newly developed spinal orthosis on posture, trunk muscle strength and quality of life in women with postmenopausal osteoporosis: a randomized controlled trial. Am. J. Phys. Med. Rehabil. 83 (3), 177–186.

Podsiadlo, D., Richardson, S., 1991. The timed up and go: a test of functional mobility for frail elderly persons. J. Am. Geriat. Soc. 39, 142–148.

RCP, 2000. Osteoporosis – clinical guidelines for prevention and treatment. Update on pharmacological interventions and an algorithm for management. Royal College of Physicians & Bone and Tooth Society of Great Britain, London.

RCP, 2007. The Clinical Effectiveness and Evaluation Unit, Royal College of Physicians. The National Clinical Audit of Falls and Bone Health in Older People Report. London. Available at http:// www.rcplondon.ac.uk/clinical-standards/ceeu/Documents/ fbhop-execsummary.pdf. (accessed March 2009).

Reginster, J.Y., Seeman, E., De Vernejoul, M.C., et al., 2005. Strontium ranelate reduces the risk of nonvertebral fractures in postmenopausal women with osteoporosis: Treatment of Peripheral Osteoporosis (TROPOS) study. J. Clin. Endocrinol. Metab. 90 (50), 2816–2822.

Roche, J.J.W., Wenn, R.T., Sahota, O., et al., 2005. Effects of comorbidities and postoperative complications on mortality after hip fracture in elderly people: prospective observational cohort study. Br. Med. J. 331 (7529), 1374–1376.

Scott, J., Huskisson, E.C., 1976. Graphic representation of pain. Pain 2, 175–184.

Seeman, E., 2002. Pathogenesis of bone fragility in women and men. Lancet 359, 1841–1850.

SIGN, 2003. Management of Osteoporosis. Guideline 71. Scottish Intercollegiate Guidelines Network, Edinburgh Available from http:// www.sign.ac.uk/guidelines/ fulltext/71/index.html (accessed 24.01.09).

Sinaki, M., Brey, R.H., Hughes, C.A., et al., 2005. Balance Disorders and Muscle Strength. Osteoporos. Int. 16 (8), 1004–1010.

Steinberg, M., Cartwright, C., Peel, N., et al., 2000. A sustainable programme to prevent falls and near falls in community dwelling older people: results of a randomised controlled trial. J. Epidemiol. Commun. Health 54 (3), 227–232.

Venning, G., 2005. Recent developments in Vitamin D deficiency and muscle weakness in elderly people. Br. Med. J. 330, 524–526.

WHO, 1994. Assessment of Fracture Risk and its Application to Screening for Postmenopausal Osteoporosis Report of a WHO Study Group. World Health Organisation, Geneva.

Whyte, M.P., 2006. Pagets Disease of Bone. N. Engl. J. Med. 355, 593–600.

Wolff, I., van Croonenborg, J.J., Kemper, H.C., et al., 1999. The effect of exercise training programs on bone mass: a meta analysis of published controlled trials in pre and post menopausal women. Osteoporos. Int. 9 (1), 1–12.

Chapter 21

Connective tissue disorders

Janet L. Poole PhD OTR/L FAOTA Occupational Therapy Graduate Program, University of New Mexico, Albuquerque, NM, USA

Jane S. Brandenstein PT Freedom, Pennsylvania, USA

CHAPTER CONTENTS

© 2010 Elsevier Ltd
DOI: 10.1016/B978-0-443-06934-5.00021-8

KEY POINTS

- Connective tissue disorders are uncommon conditions compared to other rheumatic diseases such as rheumatoid arthritis, osteoarthritis and fibromyalgia but just as debilitating.
- Fatigue is a universal symptom of all of the disorders and thus patients could benefit from instruction in energy conservation.
- Range of motion and strengthening exercises are appropriate for all patients; however, extreme care should be taken during periods of flare as in myositis and dermatomyositis. During a flare, rest and active-assisted to active exercises are indicated. As symptoms subside, gentle strengthening may be incorporated into the programme.
- Patient education regarding the disease process and the medical and therapeutic management is key to the management of persons with connective tissue disorders.

INTRODUCTION

This chapter will provide an overview of the connective tissue disorders including scleroderma, systemic lupus erythematosus, dermatomyositis, polymyositis, and mixed connective tissue disease. These diseases are characterized by the presence of spontaneous overactivity of the immune system which results in the production of extra antibodies into the circulation. Each of these diseases has a 'classic' presentation with typical findings and can evolve slowly or rapidly from very subtle abnormalities before demonstrating the classic features which help in the diagnosis.

SCLERODERMA

Systemic sclerosis (SSc) or scleroderma is a connective tissue disease characterized by thickening of the skin, fibrosis, and vascular and internal organ involvement. Scleroderma literally means 'thick skin'.

PREVALENCE AND INCIDENCE

The prevalence of scleroderma is estimated to be 300,000 in the USA; 4000 to 5000 new cases are diagnosed each year. The disease is four times more common in women than men and the average age of onset is between the third and fifth decade of life (Silman 1997). Scleroderma affects all racial groups but the onset of scleroderma is more likely to occur at a younger age in African American women who are more likely to develop diffuse disease, and have a poorer age-adjusted survival rate (Greidinger et al 1998, Laing et al 1997). In the UK, the prevalence has been reported to range from 3.08 per 100,000 (West Midlands area) (Silman et al 1988) to 8.8/100,000 in Northeast England (Allock et al 2004) to 14.6 per 100,000 in south and west London (Silman et al 1990).

AETIOLOGY, PATHOLOGY, IMMUNOLOGY

The cause of scleroderma is not known. Some precipitating event causes cells to start making collagen as if some injury has occurred. However, once the production has begun, the cells do not turn off. The excess collagen interferes with functioning of the skin, lungs, heart, muscles and gastrointestinal tract as well as other organs. Factors that are related to higher rates of scleroderma include ethnicity, geography, gender, and age.

DIAGNOSIS, DIFFERENTIAL DIAGNOSIS, SPECIAL TESTS

Many of the symptoms of scleroderma are similar to other diseases and there are no definitive blood tests that confirm a diagnosis of scleroderma. However, serum anti-topoisomerase (SCL-70) is present in 30% of people with diffuse scleroderma and anticentromere antibody (ACA) is present in 70–80% of people with limited cutaneous scleroderma (Medsger 2004). Other special tests that may be indicated for those with scleroderma are pulmonary function tests, echocardiograms and visualization of nailfold capillaries by microscope.

CLINICAL PRESENTATION, CLINICAL FEATURES, CLINICAL SUBSETS

The two main forms of scleroderma are localized scleroderma and systemic scleroderma (Box 21.1). In localized scleroderma, the skins changes are confined to a specific area of the skin and the internal organ systems are not involved (Medsger 2004). In systemic scleroderma, the internal organ systems are involved and the skin involvement is less localized. There are two subsets of systemic scleroderma: diffuse scleroderma and limited cutaneous scleroderma.

BOX 21.1 Clinical subsets of scleroderma

Localized scleroderma

- Morphea (patches of thickened skin)
- Linear (thickened skin in a linear pattern attached to underlying muscle and bone)
- Scleroderma en coup de saber (meaning "cut of the saber", linear scleroderma involving the head)

Systemic scleroderma

- Diffuse scleroderma
  - Extensive thickening of the skin proximal to the elbows and knees
  - Early internal organ involvement
- Limited cutaneous scleroderma
  - Skin thickening limited to the fingers, hands and distal forearms.
  - Later involvement of internal organs
  - Other early symptoms include Raynaud's phenomenon, puffiness in the fingers and heartburn (Medsger 2004).
  - The CREST syndrome falls into the limited cutaneous subset
    - Calcinosis
    - Raynaud's phenomenon
    - Esophageal dysfunction
    - Sclerodactyly
    - Telengiectasias

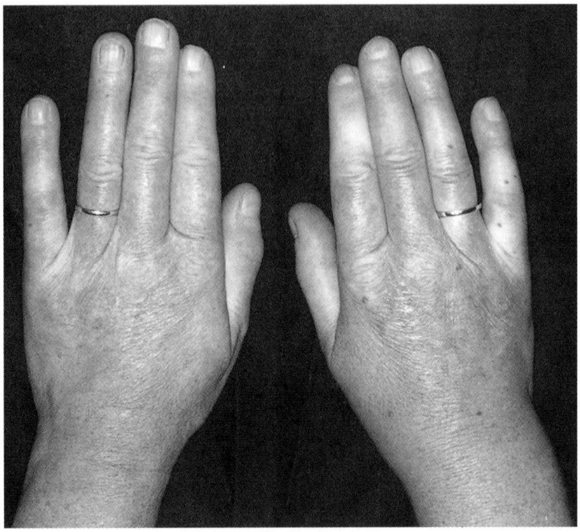

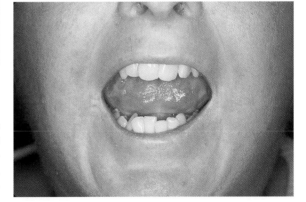

Figure 21.1 Raynaud's phenomenon in a patient with scleroderma (Note: white discoloration and telangectasia). With permission from Al-Alluf AW, Belch JF 2003 Ch. 136 Raynaud's Phenomenon. In: Hochberg MC et al (eds) Rheumatology (3rd edn), Elsevier, London, Fig. 136.1 p1509.

Figure 21.2 Microstomia in sclerdoderma (Note the taut smooth skin and reduced oral aperture). With permission from: Wigley FM, Hummers LK 2003 Ch. 133 Clinical features of systemic sclerosis. In: Hochberg MC et al (eds.) Rheumatology (3rd edn), Elsevier, London, Fig. 133.12 p1469.

SYMPTOMS AND SIGNS

Common symptoms of scleroderma include Raynaud's phenomenon (Fig. 21.1), skin thickening, and involvement of the musculoskeletal, pulmonary, gastrointestinal, cardiac and renal systems. Musculoskeletal involvement, such as non inflammatory arthralgias and myalgias, can be an early symptom in people with scleroderma (Blocka 2004). Skin tightening and fibrosis can lead to contractures in the hand (Entin & Wilkinson 1973). The most common contractures are a loss of flexion of the metacarpal phalangeal joints, loss of extension of the proximal interphalangeal joints and a loss of thumb abduction. Mandibular resorption is also a common symptom as well as thickening of the periodontal membrane. These oral changes may lead to microstomia (Fig. 21.2) and dental problems.

Symptoms of lung involvement in scleroderma are shortness of breath and coughing. Some persons develop pulmonary fibrosis of the lungs, that in the later stages, may cause death (White 2004). Initial gastrointestinal symptoms include gastroesophegeal reflux disease (GERD) which consists of difficulty swallowing, nausea, vomiting and bloating after meals (Weinstein & Kadell 2004). Symptoms progress from the upper to the lower GI tract with symptoms of diarrhoea and/or constipation. Cardiac problems are more subtle and symptoms may not occur until later in the disease (Follansbee & Marroquin 2004). Later cardiac involvement may consist of arrythmias, heart failure and pericarditis. Many people with scleroderma also have kidney involvement. However, the most important clinical manifestation is an accelerated hypertension with resultant decrease or lack of urine output precipitating a scleroderma renal crisis (Steen 2004, Wollheim 2004).

DISEASE ACTIVITY, PROGRESSION, PROGNOSIS

The course of scleroderma is variable and prognosis dependent on the subtype of scleroderma and timing, site and degree of internal organ involvement (Medsger 2004). With early diagnosis and the introduction of new medications such as ACE inhibitors, some of the complications from scleroderma, such as renal crisis, have been decreased.

CLINICAL EVALUATION/ASSESSMENT/ EXAMINATION – SUBJECTIVE AND OBJECTIVE

A clinical evaluation must consist of range of motion, hand function, pain, fatigue, and ability to perform daily activities (ADL), including basic ADL, work and leisure activities. In addition, the patient's hand should be inspected for digital ulcers, calcium deposits, extent of skin thickness, and Raynaud's phenomenon. Table 21.1 describes assessments that have been shown to be reliable and valid with persons with scleroderma.

AIMS AND PRINCIPLES OF MANAGEMENT

Exercise and splinting

Range of motion exercises should be started before there is any observed loss of motion. The exercises should be performed frequently and aggressively and patients are encouraged to maintain a position of stretch. Specific exercises for the hand and face can be found in Poole (2004). In general the exercises should emphasize flexion of the metacarpophalangeal joint, extension of the proximal interphalangeal joints, and flexion and abduction of the thumb. Stretching exercises for the hand were shown to increase motion and subsequent function in daily tasks (Mugii et al 2006) and several studies have found stretching exercises for the mouth increase oral aperture and ease of oral hygiene (Naylor & Douglass 1984, Poole, Cante & Brewer, et al in press). Hand splints to increase joint motion must be used very carefully as dynamic splints were shown to exacerbate Raynaud's (Seeger & Furst 1987). Static splints may be useful if clients have inflammation but should only be worn at night until the inflammation decreases.

Those patients with weakness can benefit from strengthening and conditioning programmes monitoring blood pressure and other vital signs. Warm water swimming programmes can be especially helpful. The only concern has been that chlorine in the water may act as a drying agent for skin. To minimize this, it is recommended to shower after being in the water, rinse off, and rub the skin with moisturizing skin creams. There is scant information regarding the effectiveness of conditioning exercises in people with scleroderma but because of limitations

Table 21.1 Assessments specific to scleroderma		
ASSESSMENT	**WHAT IS MEASURED?**	**TYPE OF ASSESSMENT**
Health Assessment Questionnaire (Fries et al 1980, Poole & Steen 1991)	Ability to perform daily tasks	Self-report
United Kingdom Scleroderma Questionnaire (Poole & Brower 2004, Silman et al 1998)	Ability to perform daily tasks	Self-report
The Hand Mobility in Scleroderma Test (Sandqvist & Eklund 2000a, 2000b)	Functional joint motion test for the fingers and wrists and forearm	Performance test
The Arthritis Hand Function Test (Backman & Mackie 1997, Poole et al 2000)	Assesses hand strength (grip and pinch), dexterity, applied dexterity and applied strength. Normative data provided. Some training and equipment are required	Performance test

in physical capacity and decreased lung functioning, general conditioning exercise programs are recommended in moderation with periodic rests.

Energy conservation

People with scleroderma should be instructed in energy conservation due to the fatigue associated with pulmonary and cardiac involvement. The general principles of pacing, planning, prioritizing and positioning are appropriate for persons with scleroderma (see Ch. 10).

Modalities

Heat modalities, such as paraffin, in conjunction with exercise programmes, have been shown to be effective in increasing or maintaining joint motion and hand function (Mancuso & Poole 2009, Pils et al 1991, Sandqvist et al 2004) (see Ch. 8).

Assistive/adapted devices

Persons with scleroderma have been shown to have difficulty performing daily tasks and may benefit from devices to compensate for decreased manipulation (built up handles, button hooks, electric can openers), reach (long handled equipment, reachers), and weakness (raised toilet seats, grab bars) (Poole 2004). Patients and families/caregivers also need education about devices, preventative techniques for Raynaud's, fatigue and wound care. Splints may help protect digital ulcers.

Some people diagnosed with scleroderma have psychosocial impairments due to uncertainties regarding disease progression and ability to work, disfigurement, and impact on their families. Malcarne (2004) provides some suggestions ranging from support groups, patient self-management programmes, individual/family therapy and/or pharmacotherapy. Although there are few studies examining the effectiveness of self-management programmes for people with scleroderma, two studies found that these provided practical information to manage activities, stress, fatigue and improved sense of control (Brown et al 2004, Samuelson & Ahlmen 2000).

SYSTEMIC LUPUS ERYTHEMATOSUS

Systemic lupus erythematosus (SLE) is a multisystem, highly inflammatory autoimmune disease. The disease can be mild or life threatening. The course is unpredictable in that different systems can be affected at different times.

PREVALENCE AND INCIDENCE

The incidence of SLE varies between and within countries. In the United States is estimated to be 9.4 per 100,000) in women and 1.54 per 100,000 in men. In the UK, incidence is 7.89 per 100,000 in women and 1.53 per 100,000 in men. SLE is more common in women with a ratio of 9:1 in the US and 5.2:1 in the UK (Petri, 2006, Somers et al 2007). Disease onset usually occurs between the ages of 20–30 years of age but may occur at any other point across the lifespan as well. In the USA, SLE is more common in African Americans and Hispanics than in Caucasians.

AETIOLOGY, PATHOLOGY, IMMUNOLOGY

The cause of SLE is not known. However, genetic factors and environmental factors such as ultraviolet light, medications, smoking, infections and toxin exposure, have been implicated (Petri 2006).

DIAGNOSIS, DIFFERENTIAL DIAGNOSIS, SPECIAL TESTS

Although the majority of persons with SLE have a positive antinuclear antibody (ANA) test, a positive test is not sufficient for diagnosis (Petri 2006) as this is seen in other diseases and can be caused by medications. Therefore, other criteria such as organ involvement and other immunological tests help establish a diagnosis of SLE. To be classified as having SLE, four or more of the 11 symptoms in Box 21.2 must be present (Tan et al 1982). These are intended as guidelines not diagnostic criteria.

CLINICAL PRESENTATION, CLINICAL FEATURES, SIGNS AND SYMPTOMS

The clinical presentation and features of SLE are listed above under Classification and in Box 21.2. The major symptoms are the facial rash over the cheeks and bridge of the nose (i.e. the malar or 'butterfly rash'; Fig. 21.3), photosensitivity and ulcers in the nose and mouth. The major organ system manifestations are musculoskeletal, renal, neuropsychiatric, serous, gastrointestinal, pulmonary and cardiac (Buyon 2008). Musculoskeletal manifestions may consist of arthralgias, arthritis and muscle weakness. Some patients

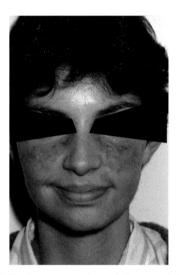

Figure 21.3 Erythematous malar rash in systemic lupus erythematosus. With permission from: Gladman DD, Urowitz MB 2003 Ch. 122 Clinical features: Systemic Lupus Erythematosus. In: Hochberg MC et al (eds.) Rheumatology (3rd edn), Elsevier, London, Fig. 122.2 p1361.

develop ulnar deviation and swan neck deformities of the fingers, called 'Jaccoud's arthopathy' (Fig. 21.4) (Petri 2006). Clinical features of renal involvement may not be noticed until there is advanced kidney disease. A common neuropsychiatric manifestation is headache. Less common are seizures, strokes, cranial and peripheral neuropathy, organic brain syndrome

and psychosis. Studies of neurocognitive function report that more than 80% have active or inactive neuropsychological involvement (Denburg et al 1993). Serositis in SLE may present as pleurisy, pericarditis or peritonitis. Gastrointestinal manifestations are common and include abdominal pain, anorexia, and nausea. Pulmonary manifestions include pneumonitis, pulmonary haemorrhage, pulmonary embolism, and pulmonary hypertension. Cardiac manifestations include pericarditis, myocarditis, endocarditis or coronary artery disease.

DISEASE ACTIVITY, PROGRESSION, PROGNOSIS

The progression of SLE is highly variable and depends on the organs involved. Early detection and aggressive intervention before major organ damage occurs increases life expectancy (Hahn 2001).

CLINICAL EVALUATION, ASSESSMENT AND EXAMINATION – SUBJECTIVE AND OBJECTIVE

A clinical evaluation must consist of range of motion, pain, fatigue, stress, cognitive function, and ability to perform daily activities, including basic ADL, work and leisure activities. There are some specific assessments for people with SLE but the majority of these are measures of organ damage (Ramsey-Goldman & Isenberg 2003). The Fatigue Severity Scale (Krupp et al 1989) was developed especially to measure fatigue in persons with SLE and the Health Assessment Questionnaire (Fries et al 1980, Milligan et al 1993) has been widely used to measure disability in persons with SLE.

AIMS AND PRINCIPLES OF MANAGEMENT

The management of SLE is challenging due to the involvement of multiple systems and unpredictable nature of the disease. Patient education is crucial as well as empowering the person with SLE to ensure open communication between the patient, family and health professionals.

Exercise

Before starting an exercise programme, people with SLE should have their physician's approval.

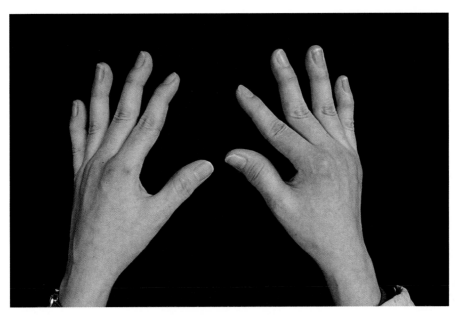

Figure 21.4 Jaccoud's arthropathy. Swan-neck deformities in systemic lupus erythematosus. With permission from: Gladman DD, Urowitz MB 2003 Ch. 122 Clinical features: Systemic Lupus Erythematosus. In: Hochberg MC et al (eds.) Rheumatology (3rd edn), Elsevier, London, Fig. 122.10 p1363.

In clinically stable patients with mild to moderate disease activity, conditioning exercises of high to moderate intensity have been shown to be effective in increasing aerobic capacity without exacerbating symptoms (Carvalho et al 2005, Clarke-Jenssen et al 2005, Daltroy et al 1995, Ramsey-Goldman et al 2000, Robb-Nicholson et al 1989, Strombeck & Jacobsson 2007, Tench et al 2003). Heart rate and blood pressure should be monitored. Petri (2006) provided the following considerations for rehabilitation. For patients with positive antiphospholipid antibody or cardiac history, patients should be monitored for deep vein thrombosis. For patients with avascular necrosis, loading weight bearing joints should be avoided; aquatic exercises would be indicated. In persons with muscle involvement, use eccentric exercise with caution (Petri 2006).

Energy conservation

Fatigue is a common debilitating complaint in persons with SLE. A healthy diet, exercise, rest and managing stress may lessen the fatigue. In addition, incorporating energy conservation techniques into daily life can also help manage fatigue. Patients can identify activities that cause fatigue and create

a plan to complete activities and pace more fatiguing ones throughout a day or week. Energy conservation is also important when patients have cognitive impairments. When cognitive impairment is present, patients should plan their days so that they perform more cognitively challenging tasks earlier in the day when they are more fresh and alert. Using memory devices such as schedule books or palm pilots can also help to compensate for memory impairments. Several studies have shown that aerobic conditioning exercise programs reduce fatigue (Robb-Nicholson et al 1989, Tench et al 2003). Self-management programmes that teach coping and techniques to manage fatigue have resulted in decrease fatigue (Sohng 2003).

Modalities

For patients who have arthralgias, heat modalities such as hot packs and paraffin wax treatments may be helpful. Those with ulnar deviation and swan neck deformities of the fingers ('Jaccoud's arthopathy') should be taught joint protection. Entrapment of the median nerve (carpel tunnel) occurs in some patients. In this case, wrist splints may help alleviate symptoms.

Assistive/adapted devices

Assistive devices to compensate for reach (long handled equipment, reachers), and weakness (raised toilet seats, grab bars) may be indicated. Electrical appliances such as dishwashers, food choppers and processors, microwaves and crockpots (slow cookers) may help save energy.

DERMATOMYOSITIS

Dermatomyositis is classified as an idiopathic inflammatory myopathy. It is clearly related to polymyositis (see later). It is characterized by chronic muscle inflammation and muscle weakness. The accompanying rash looks patchy. There are bluish-purple or red discolorations, classically on the eyelids) and over muscles which extend joints.

PREVALENCE AND INCIDENCE

Because it is rare and does not have a universally accepted diagnostic criteria, it is difficult to estimate its prevalence. A rough estimate would be between 5.5 cases per million individuals. The incidence seems to be increasing, but this may be reflective of increased awareness of its presence (Callen 2009).

AETIOLOGY, PATHOLOGY, IMMUNOLOGY

The pathology is similar to polymyositis. It shows a perivascular infiltration of inflammatory cells composed of higher percentages of B lymphocytes and CD4+ T-helper lymphocytes. Biopsies reveal perifascicular atrophy. This may in fact be a diagnostic criteria. About 10% of all cases have no evidence of muscle disease. Fatigue may be a dominant complaint and testing by magnetic resonance spectroscopy shows abnormal muscle energy metabolism and altered exercise capacities when energy containing compounds (ATP) are examined. There may be an increased prevalence of neoplasia associated with this presentation of the disease.

DIAGNOSIS, DIFFERENTIAL DIAGNOSIS, SPECIAL TESTS

Three of four of the following criteria plus the rash must be present to be definitely diagnosed as dermatomyositis.

1. Symmetrical weakness (proximal to trunk muscles and anterior neck flexors progressing to dysphagia or respiratory muscle involvement).
2. Muscle biopsy evidence - evidence of necrosis of Type I and II fibres and phagocytosis.
3. Elevation of muscle enzymes – increased serum of skeletal muscle enzymes (creatine phosphokinase and others).
4. Electromyographic (EMG) evidence – the EMG triad of short, small, polyphasic motor units, fibrillations, positive sharp waves, and insertional irritability.

CLINICAL PRESENTATION, CLINICAL FEATURES, CLINICAL SUBSETS

In adult dermatomyositis, rashes may precede the muscle weakness by a year or so. Skin involvement varies widely from person to person. This tends to be symmetrical and classically includes the heliotrope (lilac) discoloration on the eyelids (Fig. 21.5) with oedema and macular erythema of the back of the shoulders and neck (shawl sign). Other dermatologic features include: scaly skin patches over the knees, elbows, and medial malleoli; face, neck and upper torso erythematosus; and dermatitis over the dorsum of the hands, especially the MCP and PIP joints (Fig. 21.6). Symptoms may include telangectasias periungually and nail-fold capillary changes similar

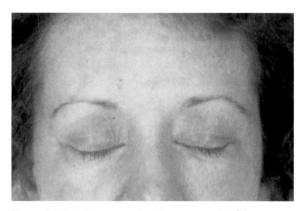

Figure 21.5 Heliotrope rash of dermatomyositis (Note: the rash over the eyelids is a characteristic feature). With permission from: Oddis CV, Medsger TA (2003) Ch.139 Inflammatory muscle disease: clinical features. In: Hochberg MC et al (eds.) Rheumatology (3rd edn), Elsevier, London. Fig. 139.3 p1540.

to those in scleroderma or systemic lupus erythematosus. Raynaud's phenomenon may also be seen. Hand deformities may also occur (Fig. 21.7A,B).

Many adults also experience low-grade fevers, have inflamed lungs, and may be sensitive to light (National Institute of Neurological Disorders and Stroke 2009). Juvenile cases generally show muscle inflammatory processes first. These include vasculitis, ectopic calcification, lipodystrophy, and muscle weakness. There is great variety from patient to patient.

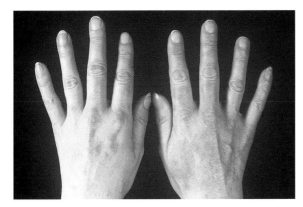

Figure 21.6 Scaling rash over the knuckles and dorsum of the hand in dermatomyositis. With permission from: Oddis CV, Medsger TA (2003) Ch.139 Inflammatory muscle disease: clinical features. In: Hochberg MC et al (eds.) Rheumatology (3rd edn), Elsevier, London, Fig. 139.1 p1540.

SYMPTOMS AND SIGNS

As stated above, the rash and muscle weakness are generally indicative that a problem exists. Calcinosis often occurs 1–3 years after the beginning of the disease. The deposits are more often seen in children than adults. They appear as hard bumps under the skin or in the muscle.

DISEASE ACTIVITY, PROGRESSION, PROGNOSIS

Disease activity is varied in both adults and juveniles. In some cases remission is complete with little or no therapy. Most cases do respond to therapies. When accompanied with vasculitis the disease may be devastating despite therapies. It is also generally more severe and therapy resistant for individuals with cardiac or respiratory problems.

CLINICAL EVALUATION, ASSESSMENT AND EXAMINATION – SUBJECTIVE AND OBJECTIVE

Physical evaluation must include range of motion, strength as well as assessment of functional activities. Patient complaints and information are important to guide development of therapeutic goals. Knowledge of muscle enzyme activity is imperative to drive any therapeutic intervention. During periods

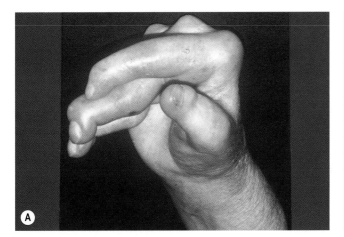
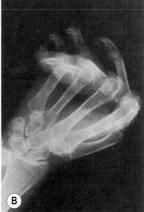

Figure 21.7 (A), (B) Deforming arthropathy of polymyositis. (Note: the rheumatoid-like deformities. The radiograph shows numerous subluxations but minimal erosive changes). With permission from Oddis CV, Medsger TA (2003) Ch.139 Inflammatory muscle disease: clinical features. In: Hochberg MC et al (eds.) Rheumatology (3rd edn), Elsevier, London, Fig. 139.7 p1542.

of severe inflammation bed rest may be required with passive range of motion to preserve joint integrity.

AIMS AND PRINCIPLES OF MANAGEMENT

Exercise

This must be targeted at information gained during evaluation and to the patient's disease activity. When appropriate, patients can progress to active and gentle resisted exercises targeted at maintaining or improving function. Assistive devices for gait may be helpful and require proper fitting and instruction. Patient and family education must include instructions for all levels of the disease process. They need to understand how to modify activity levels appropriately accounting for disease activity at the time. For instance, resisted activities should not be included during periods of active muscle inflammation.

Energy conservation

Instruction is imperative for these patients. It is important to decrease activity in times of flare. Use of assistive devices for ADL will allow best use of muscle strength and energy.

Modalities

Gentle use of mild heat is helpful for painful muscles with consideration to the skin in affected areas.

Medical management

Corticosteroids are the standard first-line medication. Initially prednisolone is generally given daily, but may be switched to IV methylprednisolone if needed. Improvements may be noted in the early weeks and gradually over 3 to 6 months. As many as 90% of patients improve at least partially and 50–75% achieve complete remission of symptoms. If the patient does not respond, immunosuppressant drugs such as methotrexate or azathioprine may be added by the physician if symptoms do not subside. Topical ointments may be helpful for the skin symptoms.

Sunscreen and protective clothing

This may be helpful to decrease damage due to sun exposure.

Surgery

This may be necessary to remove calcium deposits that may cause nerve pain or recurrent infections.

POLYMYOSITIS

Polymyositis is another inflammatory muscle disease and is characterized by symmetrical proximal muscle weakness. It can be accompanied by systemic symptoms like fatigue, morning stiffness, and anorexia.

PREVALENCE AND INCIDENCE

Polymyositis is uncommon, being seen in approximately eight individuals per 100,000.

AETIOLOGY, PATHOLOGY, IMMUNOLOGY

At this time, there is no known cause of polymyositis, but consideration is given to environmental factors triggering the disease in genetically susceptible individuals. The autoimmunity factor is supported by its association with other autoimmune diseases, including Hashimoto's thyroiditis, Grave's disease, myasthenia gravis, type I diabetes mellitus and connective tissue diseases. Also the high prevalence of circulating autoantibodies associated with polymyositis and dermatomyositis include the myositis-specific autoantibodies (MSAs) found commonly in myositis. These are nonspecific and are also found in overlap syndromes.

Genetic factors are evident in mouse models. Individuals with HLS-DR3 are at increased risk for developing inflammatory muscle diseases. Also suspicious are those carrying anti-Jo-1 antibodies, as well as HLS-138, HLA-DR3 and DR6, HLA-DR1, DR6, AND DQ1. Pathologic changes in muscle provide the strongest evidence these diseases are immune-mediated. Research findings suggest the pathology of polymyositis involves recognition of an antigen on the surface of muscle fibres by antigen-specific T cells.

DIAGNOSIS, DIFFERENTIAL DIAGNOSIS, SPECIAL TESTS

Diagnosis is initiated by the patient complaining of muscle weakness and fatigue. Laboratory investigation reveals elevated serum enzymes derived from skeletal muscle, especially creatine kinase (CK), CPK, aldolase, SGOT, SGPT, and LDH. Electromyography (EMG) demonstrates myopathic changes consistent with inflammation which is also shown in muscle histology. Muscle biopsy is used to confirm muscle inflammation. Muscles commonly used for biopsy include quadriceps, biceps, and deltoid. A pathologist examines the tissue under a microscope. No single feature is specific or diagnostic, and a variety of patterns can occur.

CLINICAL PRESENTATION, CLINICAL FEATURES AND CLINICAL SUBSETS

Weakness of proximal muscles is most commonly seen in this disease. Patients report difficulty with sit-to-stand, navigating stairs, and lifting above shoulder height. It could also include difficulty swallowing or lifting the head from the pillow. Heart and lung involvement can lead to irregular heart rhythm, heart failure and shortness of breath. It may sometimes be associated with cancers, including lymphoma, breast, lung, ovarian and colon cancer. Patients must be monitored for possible cancer occurrence.

SYMPTOMS AND SIGNS

Muscle weakness is the most common symptom, generally in muscles close to the trunk. About 25% of patients complain of fatigue, a general feeling of discomfort and weight loss and low grade fever.

DISEASE ACTIVITY, PROGRESSION AND PROGNOSIS

Onset can be gradual or rapid, with varying degrees of loss, muscle power and atrophy.

MEDICAL MANAGEMENT

Patients are treated with high doses of corticosteroids either by mouth or intravenously, in order to decrease the inflammatory process in muscles. Patients must be monitored for the many potential side effects of steroids. If management is not effective on corticosteroids alone, immunosuppressive medications may be added. These could include methotrexate, azathioprine, cyclophosphamide, chlorambucil or cyclosporine. These also have side effects that require monitoring.

CLINICAL EVALUATION, ASSESSMENT AND EXAMINATION – SUBJECTIVE AND OBJECTIVE

Evaluations by therapists include examination of medical information and physical examination including range of motion, muscle strength and physical function. Subjective information from the patient is helpful to guide treatment and appropriate goal setting. Exercise management will need to be lifelong, and patient education is paramount to successful management. Patients need to understand appropriate lifestyle adjustment depending on symptoms present at any given time.

AIMS AND PRINCIPLES OF MANAGEMENT

Exercise

Therapeutic exercises are dependent on patient's symptoms and muscle enzymes at the time. When in flare, rest and active-assisted to active exercises are indicated. As symptoms subside, gentle strengthening may be incorporated into the programme.

Energy conservation

Patients need instruction in pacing and energy conservation to decrease unnecessary muscle use, especially when in flare. Training may need to be repeated at periodic intervals as patients improve.

Modalities

Moist heat may be used with careful supervision during times of flare and muscle achiness. Warm shower or baths are especially helpful if morning stiffness is present. Careful monitoring of the skin is imperative for any heat modalities.

MIXED CONNECTIVE TISSUE DISEASE

Mixed Connective Tissue Disease (MCTD) was first described in 1972 and is considered to be an 'overlap' or 'mix' of three specific connective tissue diseases. These are systemic lupus erythematosis (SLE), scleroderma and polymyositis. Patients with MCTD display features of the three conditions. Some patients even demonstrate features of rheumatoid arthritis.

PRESENTATION OF MCTD SYMPTOMS

Symptoms include high quantities of antinuclear antibodies (ANAs), and antibodies to ribonucleoprotein (anti-RNP) detectible by blood testing. In most cases the symptoms become dominated by features of one of the above three diseases, most commonly scleroderma.

MEDICAL MANAGEMENT

Management is similar to that for the most common diseases which are presenting. MCTD is often considered as a subset of SLE. Children with MCTD tend to have an increased incidence of Raynaud's phenomenon and hypergammaglobulinemia, but a lower incidence of hypocomplementemia. They are less likely to develop severe nephritis or require immunosuppressive therapies. A significant number of children with MCTD develop scleroderma. As above, treatment of children with MCTD is identical to that for SLE.

THERAPEUTIC EVALUATION AND MANAGEMENT

The therapist's evaluation of clients with MCTD must include evaluation of medical information, patient's subjective information, and objective measurements of range of motion, strength, endurance and physical function. Treatment is designed to improve the deficits noted and includes patient education about the disease process and careful monitoring of symptoms to determine the appropriate activity level. Management will follow the advice given earlier for management of SLE, scleroderma and polymyositis.

CONCLUSION

This chapter has provided an overview of the connective tissue disorders including scleroderma, systemic lupus erythematosus, dermatomyositis, polymyositis, and mixed connective tissue disease. Although these disorders are very different, persons with these disorders could benefit from occupational and physical therapy to improve the performance of daily tasks, manage fatigue and maintain or improve joint motion and muscle strength.

STUDY ACTIVITIES

1. Compare and contrast the symptoms of scleroderma, systemic lupus erythematosus, dermatomyositis, polymyositis, and mixed connective tissue disease.
2. How would physical and occupational therapy intervention be similar or different for these disorders?
3. Why is management of fatigue so important for these disorders?

CASE STUDY 21.1 SCLERODERMA

Alyson is a 38-year-old white female referred to physical therapy and occupational therapy. She was diagnosed with systemic sclerosis (scleroderma). She was an insurance underwriter, married and lived out of town. Three months later, she stopped working, went on disability and returned to Pittsburgh with her husband to be closer to her family and medical care. At that time, she was disheartened about her disease and needed assistance with many activities of daily living (ADLs).

Alyson's disease was progressing rapidly from diagnosis to evaluation in physical therapy. She also had involvement in kidneys, hypertension and problems with swallowing in addition to the tight skin over hands, face and upper extremities to the shoulder. She complained of joint stiffness which limited her functional activities mostly in the upper extremities, but also in her right hip. She has problems with sit to stand and with gait due to her hip. Her complaint as she stated was "I cannot do anything, dressing or any household chores and the itching is driving me crazy". Management of her disease to this time has been medical. She has stopped all physical activities and has help with all ADLs.

Therapy intervention - Range of motion measurements were taken of all joints while instructing her in a programme of range of motion/stretching exercises. She had limitations of 45 degrees in all shoulder planes, elbows were −40 degrees of extension and −30 degrees of full flexion bilaterally. Both wrists flexed 70 degrees and lacked hyperextension. Supination and pronation were about half of her range and she was 1" from touching fingers to palm. She had similar degrees of lower extremity limitations, but was not as aware of these until the evaluation. She had hip flexion contractures of 30 degrees and knee contractures of 20 degrees, therefore walking forward flexed. Her posture was poor with rounded shoulders and forward head. Her general strength fell in the 3+ to 4− range in her available ranges. Her endurance was not tested, but was reported to be poor. Alyson reported her pain in the 7–9/10 range most of the time. She was emotionally frustrated and hopeless. Her family was supportive, perhaps too much so. Alyson was seen for five therapy sessions focusing on patient education to teach her a programme of heat (electric heating pad) to larger joints and paraffin wax for the hands prior to exercise to decrease pain, stiffness and skin tightness. She was then instructed in range of motion with hold at maximum end range to all joints. We suggested 15–20 second hold beginning with two to three repetitions increasing to 10. We also instructed her in a walking programme, beginning with 5 minutes two to three times daily.

Alyson was also observed performing her ADLs and it was recommended that she use a long handled sponge for bathing and to put a bathroom caddy over her showerhead to hold shampoo, conditioner, and soap. Alyson had difficulty with dressing and was encouraged to wear pull over tops and pants. She was issued a button hook to help with buttoning some of her favorite shirts. Alyson was also provided with education in energy conservation to pace herself throughout the day, delegate tasks to family members and consider using smaller appliances such as the microwave and table top (or toaster) oven in the kitchen. Although Alyson was not working, her computer set up at home was evaluated and recommendations made to lower her keyboard and to try a smaller size keyboard.

Alyson returned for a 'tune-up' a year later. At that time, she was still stiff, but more positive emotionally, she had increased her physical activity and reported decreased itching and improved kidney function. Her shoulder, elbow and hip mobility had increased at that time. She was also independent in dressing and bathing and doing most of her home management tasks. She was also enjoying using the computer and thinking of trying to work part time. Stretches to hip, hamstring, cervical and chest areas and fingers were increased at that time.

Emma presented to physical therapy and occupational therapy with a prescription from her Rheumatologist for 'strengthening exercises and ADL training' Dx. Dermatomyositis.

Emma is 58 years old and has had complaints of fatigue, generalised muscle aches and weakness off and on for several years. Recently, she had developed a red/purple rash on her eyelids and muscles. Three months ago, her GP suggested she see a rheumatologist to better diagnose her problems.

After a series of tests, including blood tests, finally a magnetic resonance spectroscopy showed abnormal muscle metabolism and Emma was diagnosed with Dermatomyositis. Her past medical history is significant for weight gain, mild hypertension and the above rash and fatigue.

On evaluation, Emma's proximal muscles of both upper and lower extremities scored 3/5 in shoulders and hips, but the distal muscles were in the 4/5 range. She needed to use hand assist to rise from a chair and used the rails to go up and down stairs at home. She required assistance with chores for overhead activities and had

difficulty putting her dishes in the cabinets. She felt she needed a rest by mid-day and was exhausted following shopping trips. Emma demonstrated difficulty trying to stand on one leg and she was nervous walking.

Following a call to Emma's rheumatologist to check she could perform strengthening exercises, she was instructed in range of motion exercises to all joints and isometric exercises for gluteal and quadriceps muscles. Her programme was to be done daily beginning with five repetitions and increasing slowly to ten. She was shown use of a cane for longer distances, but had already learned to use a shopping trolley (or buggy) on shopping trips. It was also recommended that Emma get a raised toilet seat and grab bars for her bathroom and a long sponge for bathing. To conserve energy and compensate for her shoulder weakness, it was recommended that her kitchen be arranged so that the more frequently used items were put on lower shelves that could be reached easily. Emma was also issued and shown how to use a dressing stick to get clothes over her shoulders, and to get her trousers over her feet and a long handed shoe horn to put on her shoes.

(Continued)

CASE STUDY 21.2 (CONTINUED)

Emma was seen once a week for 3 weeks and once a month for two more sessions to gently increase her programme. Gradually, she was able to add resistance bands three times per week and begin a walking programme. She was cautioned many times to go slow, pace herself, use energy saving appliances, and pay attention to her fatigue level. Emma was quite pleased to transfer sit to stand without use of hands.

USEFUL WEBSITES

Information about these conditions, clinical guidelines and patient education materials can be found at (use the search facility for condition specific information):

http://www.rheumatology.org
http://www.arthritis.org/disease-center.php
http://www.medicinenet.com
http://www.nlm.nih.gov/medlineplus
http://www.healthline.com
http://www.mayoclinic.com/health
http://www.ninds.nih.gov

Condition-specific websites include:

http://www.myositis.org
http://www.scleroderma.org
http://www.sclerodermasociety.co.uk
http://www.raynauds.org.uk/
(Raynauds and Scleroderma Society)
http://www.sclero.org
http://www.lupus.org
http://www.lupusresearchinstitute.org
http://www.lupusuk.com

References and further reading

Allock, R.J., Forrest, I., Corris, P.A., et al., 2004. A study of the prevalence of systemic sclerosis in northeast England. Rheumatology 43 (5), 596–602.

Backman, C., Mackie, H., 1997. Arthritis hand function test: test manual. University of British Columbia, Vancouver, BC.

Blocka, K.L.N., 2004. Musculoskeletal involvement in systemic sclerosis. In: Clements, P.J., Furst, D.E. (Eds.) Systemic sclerosis. Lippincott Williams & Wilkins, Philadelphia, pp. 249–260.

Brown, S.J., Somerset, M.E., McCabe, C.S., et al., 2004. The impact of group education on participants' management of their disease in lupus and scleroderma. Musculoskelal Care 2 (4), 207–217.

Buyon, J.P., 2008. Systemic lupus erythematosus: clinical and laboratory features. In: Klippel, J. H. (Ed.), Primer on the Rheumatic Diseases. Springer, New York, pp. 303–318.

Callen, J.P., 2009. Dermatomysositis. http://emedicine.medscape.com/article/332783-overview/ (accessed 9.2.09).

Carvalho, M.R., Sato, E.I., Tebexreni, A. S., et al., 2005. Effects of supervised cardiovascular training program on exercise tolerance, aerobic capacity, and quality of life in patients with systemic lupus erythematosus. Arthritis Rheum. 53, 838–844.

Clarke-Jenssen, A., Fredriksen, P. M., Lilleby, V., et al., 2005. Effects of supervised aerobic exercise in patients with systemic lupus erythematosus: a pilot study. Arthritis Care Res. 53 (2), 308–312.

Daltroy, L.H., Robb-Nicholson, C., Iversen, M.D., et al., 1995. Effectiveness of minimally supervised home aerobic training in patients with systemic rheumatic disease. Br. J. Rheumatol. 34, 1064–1069.

Denburg, S.D., Denburg, J.A., Carbotte, R.M., et al., 1993. Cognitive deficits in systemic lupus erythematosus. Rheum. Dis. Clin. North Am. 19, 815–831.

Entin, M.A., Wilkinson, R.D., 1973. Scleroderma hand: a reappraisal. Orthop. Clin. North Am. 4, 1031–1038.

Follansbee, W.P., Marroquin, O. C., 2004. Cardiac involvement in systemic sclerosis. In: Clements, P.J., Furst, D.E. (Eds.) Systemic sclerosis. Lippincott Williams & Wilkins, Philadelphia, pp. 195–220.

Fries, J.F., Spitz, P.V., Kraines, R.G., et al., 1980. Measurement of patient outcome in arthritis. Arthritis Rheum. 23, 137–145.

Greidinger, E.L., Flaherty, K.T., White, B., et al., 1998. African-American race and antibodies to topoisomerase I are associated with increased severity of scleroderma lung disease. Chest 114 (3), 801–807.

Hahn, B.H., 2001. Management of systemic lupus erythematosus. In: Ruddy, S., Harris, E.D., Sledge, C.B. (Eds.) Kelly's textbook of rheumatology. WB Saunders, Philadelphia, 6th ed. pp. 1125–1143.

Krupp, L.B., LaRocca, N.G., Muir-Nash, J., et al., 1989. The fatigue severity scale: application to patients with multiple sclerosis and systemic lupus erythematosus. Arch. Neurol. 46, 1121–1123.

Laing, T.J., Gillespie, B.W., Toth, M.B., et al., 1997. Racial differences in scleroderma among women in Michigan. Arthritis Rheum. 40, 734–742.

Malcarne, V.L., 2004. Psychosocial adjustment in systemic sclerosis. In: Clements, P.J., Furst, D.E. (Eds.) Systemic sclerosis. Lippincott Williams & Wilkins, Philadelphia, pp. 331–350.

Mancuso, T., Poole, J.L., 2009. The effect of paraffin and hand exercises on hand function in persons with scleroderma. J. Hand Ther. 22 (1), 71–78.

Medsger Jr., T.A., 2004. Classification, prognosis. In: Clements, P.J., Furst, D.E. (Eds.) Systemic sclerosis. Lippincott Williams & Wilkins, Philadelphia, pp. 17–28.

Milligan, E.D., Horn, D.L., Ballou, S.P., et al., 1993. An assessment of the Health Assessment Questionnaire functional Ability Index among women with systemic lupus erythematosus. J. Rheumatol. 20, 972–976.

Mugii, N., Hasegawa, M., Matsushita, T., et al., 2006. The efficacy of self-administered stretching for finger joint motion in Japanese patients with systemic sclerosis. J. Rheumatol. 33 (8), 1586–1592.

Naylor, W.P., Douglass, S.W., 1984. The non-surgical treatment of microstomia in scleroderma: a pilot study. Oral Surg. Oral Med.Oral Pathol. 57 (5), 508–511.

National Institute of Neurological Disorders and Stroke, 2009. Dermatomyositis information page. http://www.ninds.nih.gov/disorders/dermatomyositis/dermatomyositis.htm/ (accessed 9.2.09).

Petri, M.A., 2006. Systemic lupus erythematosus. In: Bartlett, S.

J. (Ed.), Clinical Care in the Rheumatic Diseases. ACR, Atlanta, GA, pp. 187–191.

Pils, K., Graninger, W., Sadil, F., 1991. Paraffin hand bath for scleroderma. Phys. Med. Rehabil. 1, 19–21.

Poole, J.L., 2004. Occupational and physical therapy in systemic sclerosis: an experiential approach. In: Clements, P.J., Furst, D.E. (Eds.) Systemic sclerosis. Lippincott Williams & Wilkins, Philadelphia, pp. 261–268.

Poole, J.L., Steen, V.D., 1991. The use of the Health Assessment Questionnaire (HAQ) to determine physical disability in systemic sclerosis. Arthritis Care Res. 4, 27–31.

Poole, J.L., Brower, L.M., 2004. Validity of the scleroderma functional assessment questionnaire. J. Rheumatol. 31 (2), 402–403.

Poole, J.L., Gallegos, M., O'Linc, S., 2000. Reliability and validity of the Arthritis Hand Function Test in adults with systemic sclerosis (scleroderma). Arthritis Care Res. 13, 69–73.

Poole, J.L., Conte, C., Brewer, C., et al., In press. Oral hygiene in scleroderma: The effectiveness of a multi-disciplinary intervention program. Disabil. Rehabil.

Ramsey-Goldman, R., Isenberg, D.A., 2003. Systemic lupus erythematosus measures. Arthritis Care Res. 49, S225–S233.

Ramsey-Goldman, R., Schilling, E.M., Dunlop, D., et al., 2000. A pilot study on the effects of exercise in patients with systemic lupus erythematosus. Arthritis Care Res. 13, 262–269.

Robb-Nicholson, C., Daltroy, L., Eaton, H., et al., 1989. Effects of aerobic conditioning in lupus fatigue: a pilot study. Br. J. Rheumatol. 28, 500–505.

Samuelson, U.K., Ahlmen, M.E., 2000. Development and evaluation of a patient education programme for persons with systemic sclerosis. Arthritis Care Res. 13 (3), 141–148.

Sandqvist, G., Akesson, A., Eklund, M., 2004. Evaluation of paraffin bath treatment in patients with systemic sclerosis. Disabil. Rehabil. 26, 981–987.

Sandqvist, G., Eklund, M., 2000a. Hand mobility in scleroderma (HAMIS) test: the reliability of a novel hand function test. Arthritis Care Res. 13, 382–387.

Sandqvist, G., Eklund, M., 2000b. Validity of HAMIS: a test of hand mobility in scleroderma. Arthritis Care Res. 13, 382–387.

Seeger, M.W., Furst, D.E., 1987. Effects of splinting in the treatment of hand contractures in progressive systemic sclerosis. Am. J. Occup. Ther. 41, 118–121.

Silman, A.J., 1997. Scleroderma-demographics and survival. J. Rheumatol. 48, 58–61.

Silman, A.J., Howard, Y., Hicklin, A.J., et al., 1990. Geographical clustering of scleroderma in south and west London. Br. J. Rheumatol. 29 (2), 93–96.

Silman, A., Akesson, A., Newman, J., et al., 1998. Assessment of functional ability in patients with scleroderma: a proposed new disability instrument. J. Rheumatol. 25, 79–83.

Silman, A., Jannini, S., Symmons, D., et al., 1988. An epidemiological study of scleroderma in the West Midlands. Br. J. Rheumatol. 27 (4), 286–290.

Sohng, K.Y., 2003. Effects of a self-management course for patients with systemic lupus erythematosus. J. Adv. Nurs. 42 (5), 479–486.

Somers, E.C., Thomas, S.L., Smeeth, L., et al., 2007. Incidence of systemic lupus erythematosus in the United Kingdom 1990–1999. Arthritis Rheum. 57 (4), 612–618.

Strombeck, B., Jacobsson, L.T.H., 2007. The role of exercise in the rehabilitation of patients with systemic lupus erythematosus and patients with primary sjogren's syndrome. Curr. Opin. Rheumatol. 19, 197–203.

Tan, E.M., Cohen, A.S., Fries, J.F., et al., 1982. The 1982 revised criteria for the classification of systemic lupus erythematosis. Arthritis Rheum. 25, 1271–1277.

Tench, C.M., McCarthy, J., McCurdie, I., et al., 2003. Fatigue in systemic lupus erythematosus: A randomized controlled trial of exercise. Rheumatology 42, 1050–1054.

Weinstein, W.M., Kadell, B.M., 2004. The gastrointestinal tract in systemic sclerosis. In: Clements, P.J., Furst, D.E. (Eds.) Systemic sclerosis. Lippincott Williams & Wilkins, Philadelphia, pp. 293–308.

White, B., 2004. Pulmonary fibrosis in systemic sclerosis. In: Clements, P.J., Furst, D.E. (Eds.) Systemic sclerosis. Lippincott Williams & Wilkins, Philadelphia, pp. 163–183.

Wollheim, F.A., 2004. Scleroderma renal crisis. J. Clin. Rheumatol. 10 (5), 234–235.

Chapter 22

Physiotherapy and occupational therapy for children and young people with juvenile idiopathic arthritis

Janine Hackett MSc BA(Hons) Dip.COT Department of Occupational Therapy, University of Derby, Derby, UK

Bernadette Johnson MCSP Children's Physiotherapy Service, South Staffordshire PCT, Samuel Johnson Hospital, Lichfield, Staffordshire, UK

CHAPTER CONTENTS

KEY POINTS

Key principles of therapy management with children

- Training in paediatrics is essential to have an understanding of how development impacts upon disease. Patients with JIA are not 'little adults'.
- Talk directly to the child/young person to determine treatment aims and goals and ensure treatments are realistic
- Ensure that the child is an active participant in the design and implementation of any treatment plans. Offer choices and 'decriminalise' non-adherence
- Provide developmentally appropriate disease education in a variety of mediums. Ensure interventions are ongoing and reflect the child/young person's changing stage of cognitive development.
- Signpost patients and families to organisations which can offer support and education.

© 2010 Elsevier Ltd
DOI: 10.1016/B978-0-443-06934-5.00022-X

INTRODUCTION

Although musculoskeletal pains are common in childhood, Juvenile Idiopathic Arthritis (JIA), or Juvenile Chronic Arthritis (JCA) as it was formerly known, is a fairly uncommon condition with a prevalence of one in a 1000. This is similar to that of childhood diabetes but more common than cystic fibrosis. American literature will refer to Juvenile Rheumatoid Arthritis (JRA). JIA is a chronic auto-immune disease characterized by persistent joint inflammation in children and young people with onset before their 16th birthday.

AETIOLOGY

The aetiology of JIA is still unclear although a genetic pre-disposition has been suggested (Thomas et al 2000).

SIGNS AND SYMPTOMS OF JIA

These are:

- Joint swelling persisting longer than 6 weeks
- Joint pain
- Joint stiffness
- Functional difficulties e.g. walking, writing, dressing
- Fatigue, particularly in those with systemic disease
- Fever in systemic onset JIA
- Rash – in systemic onset and psoriatic JIA.

CLASSIFICATION AND FEATURES OF JIA

There are several different sub-groups of JIA and, although primarily designed for research purposes, the International League against Rheumatism Classification (Petty et al 2004) is now in general usage globally, with the exception of North America (see Table 22.1).

DIFFERENTIAL DIAGNOSIS

JIA's relative rarity can make it difficult to diagnose. Some children and young people may have seen many doctors and therapists before receiving their diagnosis as there are many conditions which present with joint pain and/or swelling (Allen 1993). The diagnosis is often one of clinical presentation and exclusion. There are no specific blood tests which will confirm the diagnosis although some may be helpful in establishing the presence of inflammation.

MULTI-DISCIPLINARY TEAM APPROACH

Although there is no cure for JIA many of the disease's consequences are preventable with good medical management. Referral to a paediatric rheumatologist is therefore essential. Since JIA is an unpredictable chronic disease a team of professionals attending to the global needs of patients can help mediate many of the disease's effects. A multi-disciplinary team (MDT) approach is therefore viewed as the most beneficial for the child/young person and their family (Lady Hoare Trust 1997, Southwood & Malleson 1993).

THE CHANGING ROLE OF PHYSIOTHERAPY AND OCCUPATIONAL THERAPY

Traditionally, splinting and exercise played a dominant role in physiotherapy and occupational therapy management of JIA (Ansell & Swann 1983, Hackett et al 1996, Jarvis & Lawton 1985). However, the role of these two professions has changed dramatically over the years with the advent and earlier use of second line disease modifying drugs, such as methotrexate and the subsequent reduction in morbidity. The introduction of biologics, such as etanercept and infliximab, has also offered hope to those who have not responded to methotrexate. This has been an exciting time for therapists who have been forced to evaluate their practice and develop new roles for themselves, as well as design treatment interventions which meet the emerging needs of patients. The focus is now firmly on equipping the child/young person with the skills to manage their own condition and to lead to a healthy and meaningful life.

ASSESSMENT

Delays in diagnosis of JIA often result in anxiety and frustration for the family and may lead to mistrust of health care professionals. Therapists are therefore encouraged to spend time at the start of their initial assessment listening to the patient's and family's 'journey to diagnosis', acknowledging any distress or unhelpful delays in diagnosis, as a way of building trust and positive relationships

Table 22.1 The subgroups and features of JIA

SUB GROUP	SEX DIFFERENCES	FEATURES (ILAR CLASSIFICATION)
Systemic arthritis	Usually occurs in younger children M = F	Arthritis with once to twice daily spikes of fever and one or more of the following: rash, lymph node enlargement, hepatomegaly, splenomegaly, serositis
Oligoarthritis: Persistent	Most common in 1-3 year old white girls Girls:boys 4:1	Affects one to four joints during first 6 months Most common type of JIA Knee most commonly affected joint Associated with chronic anterior uveitis particularly those who are ANA positive
Extended		If > four joints after first 6 months then defined as extended oligoarthritis
Polyarthritis (rheumatoid factor negative)	Girls:boys 3:1	Affects five or more joints in first 6 months Usually symmetrical Often involves small joints
Polyarthritis (rheumatoid factor positive)	Most common in adolescent girls	Affects five or more joints in first 6 months Rheumatoid factor positive Usually symmetrical Often involves small joints of hands
Psoriatic arthritis	Girls slightly more affected than boys Onset between 7 and 10 years of age	Arthritis and psoriasis or arthritis plus two of: dactylitis, nail abnormalities, family history of psoriasis in 1st degree relative
Enthesitis related arthritis	More common in boys over the age of 8	Arthritis and/or enthesitis and at least two from: Sacro-iliac joint tenderness, HLA-B27 positive, 1st degree relative with HLA-B27 disease, anterior uveitis or onset of arthritis in a boy >8 years
Other arthritis Unclassified		Arthritis persisting > 6 weeks that does not meet criteria for other categories or fulfils criteria for more than one of other categories

Key: ILAR – International League Against Rheumatism (Petty et al 2004)

(Britton & Moore 2002a) which are likely to be long term due to the chronic nature of the disease.

In paediatrics it is often tempting to talk solely to the parent who, we might assume, will be able to give a quick and accurate account of the symptoms of JIA and the impact this has on their child's life. However, children and young people spend a considerable amount of time away from their parents from an early age and experience their JIA on a daily basis. Parents may also not be the most reliable reporters and indeed may be unaware of some of the issues affecting their child.

OUTLINE OF ASSESSMENT

Introduction

After eliciting information on a range of topics including: history of the condition, the child/young person's past medical/developmental history, as well as drug history, it is important to gain insight into the family/social history. This will allow therapists to identify potential support systems as well as any social/housing issues. The British Society of Paediatric and Adolescent Rheumatology (BSPAR) Allied Health Professional Guidelines for

Assessment of Children and Young People can be obtained from the Society's website (BSPAR 2002).

SUBJECTIVE ASSESSMENT

The Childhood Health Assessment Questionnaire (CHAQ) (Nugent et al 2001, Singh et al 1994) is a standardised assessment which quantifies levels of functional ability in a number of domains including dressing, walking and reach, and is commonly used in rheumatology clinics in the UK. Although this may be a useful tool for screening for functional deficits, it should not replace a comprehensive therapy assessment. It is however a valuable tool for audit/research and is one of the core outcome variables used by medics to determine drug efficacy.

Early morning stiffness (EMS)

This characteristic feature of JIA provides an indication of disease activity. Establish which joints are affected, the severity, duration and impact on function.

Pain

There are many paediatric pain scales available. However, a 100mm visual analogue scale (VAS) with zero (no pain) to 100 (severe pain), is the favoured method in UK rheumatology centres and is another core outcome variable. It is also important to establish the type of pain, and the areas affected, including what exacerbates or relieves it.

Daily occupations and lifestyle

A detailed assessment of the child/young person's occupations will reveal activity levels and integration and participation in their communities. This is important, even in the absence of active disease, as children and young people with no active signs of JIA also report functional difficulties (Miller et al 1999), suggesting psychosocial factors or poor fitness may play a role. The four main areas of daily occupation should be included:

(i) Self care
Establish the level of independence with self-care activities (including washing, dressing, transfers, and mobility). Elicit how much assistance, if any, is required. Consider the variability of their abilities throughout the day and in differing contexts, such as at home and school.

(ii) Productivity
If developmentally appropriate, domestic activities of daily living (ADL) should also be considered, including household chores, making hot drinks and snacks. Promoting household chores as a normal occupation for young people is important as it has been shown to be a strong prognostic indicator for resilience in later life (Werner 1989).

Discussion about school is essential as it occupies a considerable amount of the child/young person's time and involves a wide range of activities. Explore the specific demands of each activity, rather than ask, "How are you getting on at school?" as this often elicits the answer of "fine". Ask about, for example; attendance; mode of transport to school; mobility around school; hand writing; fatigue; science lessons; Physical education (P.E.); break times.

(iii) Play/leisure
Since play and leisure are principal occupations of childhood, evaluating the impact of JIA is essential. Children and young people with JIA have been found to experience a number of barriers to play and leisure, both as a direct and an indirect consequence of their JIA (Hackett 2003). These include the obvious symptoms of the disease, such as pain, stiffness and fatigue. However fear, overprotection and inaccurate beliefs about JIA have also been shown to limit participation. By asking about play and leisure activities therapists can gain important insight into lifestyle, patterns of activity and inactivity, as well as social relations and peer support.

(iv) Rest
Sleep is often a neglected area of assessment. Problems are seldom recognised or documented, yet it is an important daily occupation which can greatly impact on quality of life. Ask about any difficulties with getting off to sleep, as well as sleeping throughout the night and whether they wake refreshed. This may reveal difficulties with night pain, anxiety or poor sleep hygiene.

Disease knowledge and education

Gaining an understanding of the child's and family's level of knowledge of their disease and its management helps support concordance with therapy. Care should be taken not to 'test' patients and families. Instead patients/carers could be asked if they have told others about their child's condition. This can then be followed up with the supplementary question, "what have you told them?" This helps elicit their understanding. Therapists should also review what educational resources the family have already received and provide education and other suitable resources as appropriate.

Mood

To avoid upsetting parents, some children/young people choose not to disclose their true feelings about their arthritis. Patients therefore need an opportunity to express themselves in a safe and supported environment. This is important for screening for any mental health issues. Possible questions could include; "some young people tell us they feel very frustrated/angry/sad/tearful. Do you ever feel like this?"

Developmental status

Full developmental assessments are not normally indicated as global delay is unusual. However, any concerns regarding the patient's cognitive, physical and emotional developmental status should be identified. Deficits affecting communication and understanding will impact on how treatment programmes are provided as well as affecting the patients communication and learning styles.

Future aspirations

Of course, young people will eventually become adults, assuming adult roles and responsibilities. Consideration therefore should be given to assessing their potential future occupations and what they hope to achieve in life. For example, ask what their career plans are and whether they are planning on living away from home. Vocational planning is particularly important as this has been highlighted as a need by young people with JIA (McDonagh et al 2007).

OBJECTIVE ASSESSMENT

Baseline measurements include height and weight. This establishes whether JIA is having an adverse effect on growth and development.

Joint/soft tissue examination

Compare the left and right sides to identify if any true abnormalities exist. Observation of the joints and soft tissue should include: skin colour, swelling, deformity and muscle wasting.

Palpation of the joint/soft tissue

This may elicit some or all of the following: temperature change, swelling, joint margin tenderness, instability of the joint, subluxation, crepitus and enthesitis related pain.

Range of movement

It is important to record both active and passive range of movement, painful movements, fluidity, end feel and the type and severity of any deformity. Record if there is any joint hypermobility as this can also give rise to pain and intermittent swelling.

Muscle strength

Muscle wasting is common during a flare of arthritis or when there has been ongoing or poorly controlled disease. Wasting should be noted and manual muscle testing will determine any weakness.

Posture and gait

Leg length discrepancy resulting from arthritis in the lower limb is common, particularly in asymmetric disease. It may cause a limp, back pain and/or a postural scoliosis. Remember to identify whether there is any hip or knee flexion deformity which might account for apparent leg length discrepancy. A gait assessment, including speed, fluency and heel-toe pattern, should also be performed.

Assessment of daily occupations

Wherever possible these should be done in context, i.e. the home, school. This provides information about the interaction between the person and their environment and highlights any specific environmental, physical and psychosocial challenges of tasks.

SPLINTS, ORTHOSES, WHEELCHAIRS AND ASSISTIVE DEVICES

Some children/young people may already have a range of equipment including: mobility aids, splints, orthoses or assistive devices purchased from local shops, inherited from others or provided from other agencies. It is important to assess whether they are best meeting the needs of the child or young person or whether another treatment approach may be better utilised.

MANAGEMENT

PRINCIPLES OF TREATMENT

There is little research-based evidence available at present to support best practice; rather it is largely shaped by clinical expertise and experience. Patients should always be active participants in the design of their programmes.

DRUG THERAPY

A summary of the drugs used in JIA is shown in Figure 22.1 and further details are provided in Chapter 15.

Pain management

Although pain may be a predominant feature of JIA it can be under-recognised by health professionals and disease activity may not be the only predictor of pain (Anthony & Shanberg 2003). Therapists should therefore develop their understanding of pain theory and management and be aware of factors increasing perceptions of pain. Therapists need to equip children and young people with the skills to manage their pain at home and school (see Chs 5, 10 & 11). Please note however it is important to seek further guidance as there may be some specific precautions to consider in children. For example, the use of ultrasound over growth plates (Chartered Society of Physiotherapy 2006).

Exercise

Disease specific exercise programmes have historically played a major role in the management of

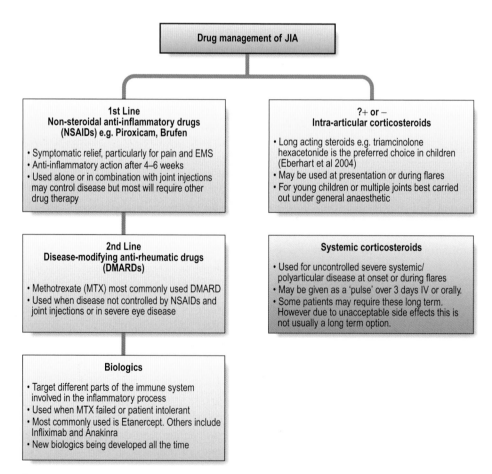

Figure 22.1 Drug management of juvenile idiopathic arthritis.

JIA. Today exercise is still very important, but with advances in drug therapies and improved morbidity for many patients these tend to be less regimented. Short term programmes may be required in times of specific need and are a more realistic and manageable option. For example, when muscle weakness affects function or disease is poorly controlled and there is a danger of contractures.

As yet, there is no good evidence to determine how often exercises need to be performed to be most effective and, clinically, opinions differ. When designing an exercise programme, the therapist must work with the patient and their family on goal setting and designing realistic programmes that fit in with daily life, rather than dominating it, as exercise routines can greatly reduce leisure time for children with JIA and affect family activities (Britton & Moore 2002b). Any programme should be regularly reviewed and modified as necessary.

Active, rather than passive, exercise is preferred by most young people as it gives them a sense of control. Gentle passive exercise is generally only used with very small children (or older children/young people carrying out stretching regimes). However, even with this age group therapists can be inventive to encourage more active exercise for example, making up games and using music and action songs. Resisted exercise may be included for muscle strengthening. However, it may be contraindicated during a severe flare as it may increase pain levels. If pain is poorly controlled therapists should discuss options with the doctor or try simple remedies, such as hot-packs, prior to exercise.

Young people with JIA may also be less physically active than their healthy peers (Henderson et al 1995, Takken et al 2003) resulting in deconditioning, decreased aerobic capacity and muscle weakness, which may further reinforce an inactive lifestyle. Greater emphasis is therefore placed on encouraging children/young people with JIA to lead a normal active lifestyle for general health reasons e.g. cardiovascular fitness, bone density, co-ordination, and fun. It has also been reported that lack of fitness is not related to disease activity (Klepper et al 1992) thus other factors, such as family anxiety about the risks of exercise, must be considered. Most young people with JIA can participate in low-impact fitness programmes without any adverse effects (Klepper 1999, Takken et al 2001), with the possible exception of those with severe hip disease (Singh-Grewal et al 2006). If a child or young person has severe neck disease it may be inappropriate to participate in activities placing their necks at risk, for example rugby, trampolining and some gymnastic activities. A child with severe polyarticular JIA might find it difficult to join in some games classes, so therapists need to be inventive and help find suitable activities to avoid sedentary lifestyles. Liaison with schools, particularly PE staff, to solve such issues is important.

Aquatic therapy

Aquatic therapy has been a commonly used modality in the management of JIA. Improved medical management and financial constraints mean it is used less today. Although there is little evidence to show that the physical benefits of aquatic therapy are any greater than land based interventions (Epps et al 2005), it is preferred by patients, parents and therapists as it is an enjoyable form of therapy (Scott 2000, Epps et al 2005). It should therefore be considered as a treatment option, particularly where disease is unremitting.

Splints

There is little evidence to support splinting in JIA. With effective medical management splints are often unnecessary, however anecdotally they may be beneficial when: joints are very painful, significant EMS interferes with function, or when deformity e.g. wrist subluxation (see Fig. 22.2) or deviation is present. Soft collars may also be useful to give symptomatic relief to the neck during an acute flare in the neck (see Ch. 12).

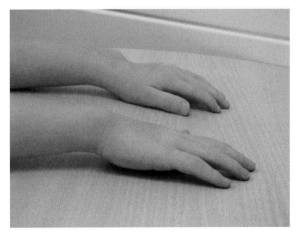

Figure 22.2 A subluxed wrist.

Serial splinting and casting

This is used occasionally when contractures have not responded to other interventions, such as exercise, resting splints and/or joint injections. Clinical experience suggests that casting is more effective than serial splinting, possibly because an optimum position can be maintained, since the child/young person is unable to remove it Prior to serial casting therapists should remind themselves of the specific associated contra-indications and take care when stretching (Fig. 22.3).

Foot orthoses

Children/young people with foot and ankle arthritis may benefit from foot orthoses and should be referred to an experienced orthotist or podiatrist. Therapists can offer advice however, on sensible, supportive and shock absorbing footwear. Trainers are ideal. In order not to set them apart from their peers, it is important to 'give permission' for the child/young person to wear 'party shoes' for special occasions.

Assistive devices and adaptations

When a deficit in occupational performance has been identified the first course of action is to analyse the activity to identify the specific cause. This may be due to a physical limitation. However, it could be due to other factors such as poor technique, lack of confidence or simple overprotection. Firstly, ensure the patient is on their optimum drug treatment.

Secondly, take steps to remediate the problem rather than provide assistive devices to compensate for the deficit. Interventions may include specific range of movement or strengthening exercises, education and confidence building. Devices should not be considered unless absolutely necessary and should never be the first course of action as they can reinforce feelings of disability, and limit independence to one particular context. This prevents children/young people from maximising their full potential. Assistive devices may be indicated in some instances, for example when damage has occurred to the joints resulting in permanent limitation in range of movement.

PATIENT EDUCATION

Education should be an integral part of all consultations and ongoing throughout the course of the disease since needs will change over time as the child/young person develops. Education about the disease, its management, as well as generic health information, such as exercise, smoking, alcohol and diet, should be provided in a variety of formats (written and verbal) and therapists should ensure the environment is conducive to learning (Table 22.2, Fig. 22.4).

PSYCHOSOCIAL INTERVENTIONS

Social aspects of the young person's life should be considered alongside their physical and psychological needs (Shaw et al 2004) as children/young people with JIA have been found to have limited social participation and report an overwhelming need to

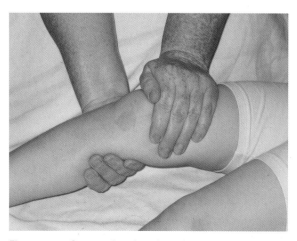

Figure 22.3 Care needs to be taken when applying a passive stretch to the knee prior to serial casting.

Table 22.2 Effective strategies and barriers to learning	
BARRIERS TO LEARNING	**FACILITATING LEARNING**
Fear/anxiety	Trusting/friendly relationships
Distractions	Calming environments
Hurried consultations	Adequate time for discussions
Uni-directional communication	Interactive learning
Language/cultural barriers	Use of interpreters and a culturally sensitive approach
Learning difficulties	Developmentally appropriate
Developmentally inappropriate information	Regular educational updates using multiple methods, e.g. verbal, written, internet

meet similar others with JIA (Shaw 1998). Health professionals should pay attention to issues such as bullying, social isolation and the loss of valued social activities. In a healthcare setting discussion of such topics can help develop rapport and build trusting relationships. Developing interventions to address these issues is also important. Group work can be a useful method, for introducing patients to similar others, as well as addressing specific issues such as transition to secondary school, back care, independence, hydrotherapy or be purely social.

Therapists can also be instrumental in enabling children and young people to disclose their JIA to others. Many may not possess the skills and confidence to do this and thus not receive appropriate support and understanding from those around them. This is an important skill to acquire however, and is particularly important when entering the workforce or embarking on a long-term relationship. Increasing knowledge of the disease, their rights under the Disability Discrimination Act (1995), confidence building, assertiveness training and facilitating communication skills are extremely useful.

ADHERENCE AND CONCORDANCE

Insufficient or non-adherence with treatment can contribute to increased morbidity. However, it is not uncommon for disease management to prove particularly demanding during the period of adolescence (McDonagh et al 2000). The challenge for healthcare professionals is to ensure treatment

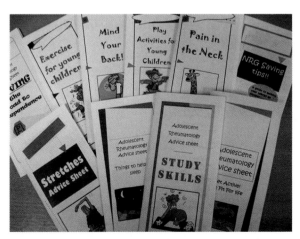

Figure 22.4 Patient information can help children and young people gain useful self management skills.

programmes are realistic and involve young people as active participants in their disease management and in informed decision making regarding their treatment.

PROGNOSIS

Prognosis tends to vary for the different sub-groups of JIA and outcomes are ever changing with the introduction of new drugs. Generally, it is expected that at least one third of children with JIA will continue to have active disease into adult life. Those who do not have active disease but have permanent joint damage or localized growth abnormalities, may still have some functional limitations as adults. Overall, up to 60% of children with JIA will have some functional limitation as adults (Andersson-Gare & Fasth 1995, Minden et al 2002, Packham & Hall 2002a). As well as functional limitations, it is important for therapists to consider that general health status, quality of life and employment might also be affected (Foster et al 2003, Packham & Hall 2002b). Generally, the sub-group with the best outcome is persistent oligoarticular arthritis.

CONCLUSION

Early identification and referral to a paediatric rheumatology service is essential as untreated or poorly controlled JIA can have a potentially devastating long-term effect on the child and young person. Physical, social and psychological impairments can also limit engagement in meaningful occupations, therefore a holistic and collaborative biopsychosocial approach which equips children/young people and their families with the skills to manage their condition is advocated to promote inclusion/participation and optimise quality of life.

ACKNOWLEDGEMENTS

We would like to thank our colleagues at Birmingham Childrens' Hospital for all their support. Special thanks go to Jan Scott MA, BSc, MCSP, Rosanne Wilshire MCSP, and Dr Janet McDonagh for their valuable input and insightful comments. We would also like to express our thanks to our patient and family for allowing us to use their photograph.

STUDY ACTIVITIES

1. Write a comprehensive list of differential diagnoses for JIA (see Allen 1993).
2. Obtain a copy of the Paediatric Gait Arms Legs Spine DVD (pGALS 2006). This can be ordered or down loaded from The Arthritis Research Campaign at www.arc.org.uk/arthinfo/medpubs/6965/6965.asp. Review the assessment and write notes about the key movements being assessed. Practice the assessment with one of your peers.
3. Review the BSPAR guidelines on the use of aquatic therapy and identify the benefits for patients with JIA. www.bspar.org.uk/downloads/other/hydrotherapy_standard_bspar_june_2007_final.pdf
4. Download resources on disclosure from the following websites and consider the advantages and disadvantages of disclosing a chronic illness.
www.skill.org.uk
www.dreamteam-uk.org

CASE STUDY 22.1

Charlotte: Polyarticular JIA

Charlotte's parents took her to the GP at 12 months of age after noticing difficulty weight bearing and crawling. She appeared stiff in the mornings and her parents believed she was in pain. For the next 3½ years she saw a variety of doctors and underwent several investigations including MRI under general anaesthetic, EMG, nerve conduction studies and muscle biopsy. Initially, a diagnosis of Cerebral Palsy was made and Charlotte received Botulinum toxin injections followed by casting on two occasions. She received no benefit from these and continued to deteriorate. Eventually, she required an electric wheelchair and adaptations to the house. Finally, at the age of 4½, Charlotte was referred to a paediatric rheumatologist who diagnosed JIA. Unfortunately, by this time, Charlotte was confined to a wheelchair, had bilateral subluxed wrists, fixed flexion deformities (FFDs) of both knees of 80°, elbow flexion deformities (FD's) and FD's of all her finger joints. Medical treatment was immediately instigated consisting of joint injections and methotrexate.

What interventions were considered?

Initially, much time was spent with the family offering support and reassurance. The disease education process was also initiated consisting of face to face meetings, and the provision of written resources and web addresses. As she was initially fearful of health professionals, time was spent playing with Charlotte and more active therapy was commenced once rapport was established. Wrist splints were provided to support the wrists in a functional position, provide pain relief and encourage participation in activities. She was also encouraged to remain as active as possible to prevent gelling. Advice on pain relief was offered to her parents including warm baths and hot packs. Following joint injections there was an immediate decrease in pain and more active exercise, including hydrotherapy, was commenced. This did not result in any improvement in her knee FFD's so many months of serial casting followed. The subsequent provision of night resting splints and advice regarding seating ensured gains made during casting were not lost during leisure/sleep time. As Charlotte made gains in her knee extension through casting she was able to stand and appropriate walking aids were also used to build confidence and encourage mobility. Charlotte was visited at school on numerous occasions to assess her environment and her participation in activities. Modifications, particularly in the bathroom, were implemented. Teachers were educated about JIA and how they might increase her participation levels. An appropriate Special Educational Needs (SEN) programme was initiated into which the physiotherapist and occupational therapist had input. Eventually, Charlotte was able to take her first proper steps which served to motivate her further and she improved to the point where she no longer needed her electric wheelchair. Although Charlotte has been left with significant deformities and damage to her wrists and hands her progress to date has been excellent. She still struggles with some fine motor skills (e.g. jean buttons, toothpaste tubes) due to poor hand strength which is to be addressed by further OT input. Charlotte also continues to be monitored by physiotherapy and further interventions will be offered as necessary.

CASE STUDY 22.2

Molly. Oligoarticular JIA

Molly is a 2-year-old girl recently diagnosed with oligoarticular onset JIA, affecting her wrist and knee. Mother and father are terribly upset and feel guilty as they failed to notice that she had any swelling or pain. However, they had noticed difficulties crawling initially and had visited the GP. Molly has a nursery placement three mornings a week but her mother is finding it difficult to get her there due to Molly's significant early morning stiffness. Molly is mobile but walks with a limp and trips frequently. She has been reluctant to engage in some play activities and appears unwilling to scribble or pick up a crayon. Older siblings are reluctant to play with her for fear of hurting her.

1. What is the first course of action?

The first course of action is to support and reassure the parents and to try to reduce some of their guilt and anxiety which may impact upon their willingness to play and handle Molly for fear of further pain or damage. Advice and information about the condition should be provided, as well as strategies to alleviate some of Molly's pain and discomfort. A thorough assessment should be carried out in a child friendly environment which will allow you to assess her mobility and function at play. This will enable you to build rapport and facilitate later handling to formally assess range of movement etc.

2. What steps can be taken to manage Molly's early morning stiffness?

Several things can be considered including night resting splints if she is unable to walk or use her hand first thing in the morning. You might also advise the parent to give Molly a warm bath first thing in the morning and then warm her clothes on the radiator, or to take analgesia, such as paracetamol, followed by a short rest. You should also liaise with the nursery to provide information about the condition and suggest an afternoon placement rather than morning to optimize her participation and enjoyment.

3. What factors are considered when assessing walking?

Firstly, Molly should be observed walking. A history from the parents is important at it may be reveal that the limp wears off throughout the morning and is due to early morning stiffness. If a persistent limp is evident it may be wise to assess her for any knee flexion contractures, or leg length discrepancy which is highly likely if there has been uncontrolled disease activity in one knee joint. A shoe raise may be indicated if a leg length difference is found.

4. How is the issue of play addressed with peers and parents?

Play is a very important issue to discuss with parents. It is important to reassure parents it is safe for them to play with their child and to encourage him/her to be as independent as possible. Suggestions which therapists might make to parents could include the following:

- Outline the importance of play. Not only is it great fun and can help children develop important skills and stay active, it can also distract them from pain and improve their mood.
- Encourage the child to be active.
- Involve brothers and sisters.
- Consider tumble tots/nursery, or council-run schemes.
- When playing protect the joints that have arthritis, e.g. do not weight bear through small fingers and the hand.
- Try to incorporate large movements into games which move the joint through its full range of movement.

If Molly enjoys scribbling but her wrist is painful you may want to try a work splint to provide some support.

5. How can you encourage a child of 2 or 3 years old to do exercises?

When young children have joint problems it is often very difficult, if not impossible, to persuade them to carry out formal exercise programmes. Battles over exercises can lead to anxiety and unhappiness for both child and parents. However there are lots of fun activities which can benefit them in much the same way. Offering rewards such as star charts might work for some young children.

References and further reading

Allen, R., 1993. Differential diagnosis of arthritis in childhood. In: Southwood, T.R., Malleson, P. (Eds.) Clinical Paediatrics 1:3: Arthritis in Children and Adolescents. Bailliere Tindall, London, pp. 665–694.

Andersson-Gare, B., Fasth, A., 1995. The natural history of juvenile chronic arthritis: a population based cohort study II. Outcome. J. Rheumatol. 22, 308–319.

Anthony, K.A., Shanberg, L.E., 2003. Pain in children with arthritis: a review of the current literature. Arthritis Rheum. 49 (2), 272–279.

Ansell, B., Swann, M., 1983. The management of chronic arthritis of children. J. Bone Joint Surg. (British volume) 65 (5), 536–543.

British Society for Paediatric and Adolescent Rheumatology (BSPAR) 2002 Standard assessment for juvenile idiopathic arthritis. http://www.bspar.org.uk/downloads/other/Standard_Assessment_Juvenile_Ideopathic_Arthritis.pdf. (accessed 8.12.08).

Britton, C., Moore, A., 2002a. Views from the inside, Part 1: routes to diagnosis – families experience of living with a child with arthritis. Br. J. Occup. Ther. 65 (8), 374–379.

Britton, C., Moore, A., 2002b. Views from the inside, Part 3: How and why families undertake prescribed exercise and splinting programmes and a new model of the families experience at living with Juvenile Arthritis. Br. J. Occup. Ther. 65 (10), 453–460.

Chartered Society of Physiotherapy, 2006. Guidance for the Clinical use of Electrophysical Agents. Chartered Society of Physiotherapists, London.

Disability Discrimination Act, 1995, HMSO, London.

Eberhardt, B., Sison, M.C., Gottlieb, B.S., Ilowite, N.T., 2004. Comparison of the intraarticular effectiveness of triamcinolone hexacetonide and triamcinolone acetonide in treatment of juvenile rheumatoid arthritis. J. Rheumatol. 12 (31), 2507–2512.

Epps, H., Ginnelly, L., Utley, M., et al., 2005. Is hydrotherapy cost-effective? A randomised controlled trial of combined hydrotherapy programmes compared with physiotherapy land techniques in children with juvenile idiopathic arthritis. Health Technol. Assess. 9 (39), 1–59.

Foster, H., Marshall, N., Myers, A., et al., 2003. Outcome in adults with juvenile idiopathic arthritis. A quality of life study. Arthritis Rheum. 48 (3), 767–775.

Hackett, J., Johnson, B., Parkin, A., et al., 1996. Physiotherapy and occupational therapy for juvenile chronic arthritis: custom and practice in five centres in the UK USA and Canada. British J. Rheumatol. 35 (7), 695–699.

Hackett, J., 2003. Perceptions of play and leisure in junior school aged children with JIA: what are the implications for occupational therapists. Br. J. Occup. Ther. 66 (7), 303–310.

Henderson, C., Lovell, D., Specker, B., et al., 1995. Physical activity in children with juvenile rheumatoid arthritis, quantification and evaluation. Arthritis Care Res. 8 (2), 114–125.

Jarvis, R.E., Lawton, D.S., 1985. The Management of JCA. Association of Paediatric Chartered Physiotherapists, London.

Klepper, S.E., Darbee, J., Effgen, S.K., et al., 1992. Physical fitness levels in children with polyarticular juvenile rheumatoid arthritis. Arthritis Care Res. 5 (2), 93–100.

Klepper, S.E., 1999. Effects of eight week physical conditioning on disease signs and symptoms in children with chronic arthritis. Arthritis Care Res. 12 (1), 52–60.

Lady Hoare Trust, , 1997. Key Findings and Actions in Living with JCA. Lady Hoare Trust, London.

McDonagh, J., Southwood, T., Ryder, C., 2000. Bridging the gap in rheumatology. Ann. Rheum. Dis. 59, 575–584.

McDonagh, J.E., Southwood, T.R., Shaw, K.L., 2007. The impact of a coordinated transitional care programme on adolescents with juvenile idiopathic arthritis. Rheumatology 46 (1), 161–168.

Miller, M., Kress, A., Berry, C., 1999. Decreased physical function in JRA. Arthritis Care Res. 12 (5), 309–313.

Minden, K., Niewerth, M., Listing, J., et al., 2002. Long-term outcome in patients with juvenile idiopathic arthritis. Arthritis Rheum. 46 (9), 2392–2401.

Nugent, J., Ruperto, N., Grainger, J., et al., 2001. for the Paediatric Rheumatology International Trials Organisation (PRINTO). The British version of the Childhood Health Assessment Questionnaire (CHAQ) and the Childhood Health Questionnaire (CHQ). Clin. Exp. Rheumatol. 19 (Suppl. 23), s163–s167.

Packham, J., Hall, A., 2002a. Long-term follow-up of 246 adults with juvenile idiopathic arthritis: functional outcome. Rheumatology 41 (12), 1428–1435.

Packham, J., Hall, A., 2002b. Long-term follow up of 246 adults with JIA: education and employment. Rheumatology 41 (12), 1436–1439.

Petty, R.E, Southwood, T.R., Manners, P., et al., 2004. International League of Associations for Rheumatology classification of juvenile idiopathic arthritis: second revision,

Edmonton 2001. J. Rheumatol. 31 (2), 390–392.

Scott, J.M., 2000. Hydrotherapy or land-based exercises: a patient satisfaction survey. Ann. Rheum. Dis. 59, 9. abstract.

Shaw, K., 1998. The experience of children with juvenile chronic arthritis. J. Natl. Assoc. Rheumatol. Occup. Ther. 12 (1), 20–23.

Shaw, K., Southwood, T., McDonagh, J., 2004. It's not about arthritis is it? It's about living with it. Users' perspective of transitional care for adolescents with juvenile idiopathic arthritis. Rheumatology 43, 770–778.

Singh, G., Arthreya, B.H., Fries, J.F., Goldsmith, D.P., 1994. Measurement of health status in children with rheumatoid Arthrits. Arthritis Rheum. 37, 1761–1769.

Singh-Grewal, D., Wright, V., Bar-Or, O., Feldman, B.M., 2006. Pilot study of fitness training in polyarticular childhood arthritis. Arthritis Rheum. 55 (3), 364–372.

Southwood, T.R., Malleson, P., 1993. The team approach. In: Southwood, T.R., Malleson, P. (Eds.), Clinical Paediatrics 1:3: Arthritis in Children and Adolescents. Bailliere Tindall, London, p. 729–743.

Takken, T., van der Nett, J.J., Helders, P.J., 2001. Do juvenile idiopathic arthritis patients benefit from an exercise program? A pilot study. Arthritis Care Res. 45, 81–85.

Takken, T., Van der Net, J., Kuis, W., Helders, P.J., 2003. Physical activity and health related physical fitness in children with juvenile idiopathic arthritis. Ann. Rheum. Dis. 62 (9), 885–889.

Thomas, E., Barrett, J.H., Donn, R.P., et al., 2000. Subtyping of juvenile idiopathic arthritis using latent class analysis. British Paediatric Rheumatology Group. Arthrit. Rheum. 43, 1496–1503.

Werner, E., 1989. High risk children in young adulthood: a longitudinal study from birth to thirty-two. Am. J. Orthopsych. 59, 72–81.

Chapter 23

Miscellaneous conditions

Edward Roddy DM MRCP(UK) Arthritis Research Campaign National Primary Care Centre, Primary Care Sciences, Keele University, Keele, UK

David G.I. Scott MD FRCP Department of Rheumatology, Norfolk & Norwich University Hospital, Norwich, UK

CHAPTER CONTENTS

KEY POINTS

- Septic arthritis is a medical emergency requiring urgent referral for joint aspiration and appropriate intravenous antibiotic therapy
- Non-pharmacological management of acute gout and pseudogout includes application of ice-packs to the affected joint and initial rest followed by rapid mobilisation
- Lifestyle modification advice regarding weight loss, restriction of alcohol and purine-rich foods is a key component of the management of gout
- Neuropathic arthropathy is an uncommon complication of diabetes mellitus; a high index of suspicion is necessary to avoid delay in treatment and permanent disability
- An assessment of physical functioning and activities of daily living is needed in patients with vasculitis to determine appropriate rehabilitation.

© 2010 Elsevier Ltd
DOI: 10.1016/B978-0-443-06934-5.00023-1

INTRODUCTION

This chapter outlines the clinical presentation of some of the miscellaneous rheumatological conditions: Part 1 covers septic arthritis, gout, pyrophosphate arthropathy, sarcoidosis, diabetes mellitus and in Part 2 the vasculitidies are described.

Part 1: Septic arthritis, gout, pyrophosphate arthropathy, sarcoidosis and diabetes mellitus

Edward Roddy

Septic arthritis is an uncommon but important medical emergency. Although less common than other causes of the acute, hot, swollen joint (Box 23.1); it remains the most important diagnosis to make and treat appropriately. Despite appropriate treatment, septic arthritis is associated with joint destruction and long-term morbidity and functional loss. The incidence of septic arthritis is approximately two to six cases per 100,000 population per year and is highest at extremes of age (Cooper & Cawley 1986, Kaandorp et al 1997a).

AETIOLOGY AND PATHOLOGY

Organisms may enter a joint from several routes. The most frequent modes are haematogenous spread, spread from an infected local focus, e.g. osteomyelitis or cellulitis, and direct penetrating injury (Nade 2003).

BOX 23.1 Differential diagnosis of the acute, hot, swollen joint

- Septic arthritis
- Acute gout
- Acute pseudogout
- Reactive arthritis (Reiter's syndrome)
- Haemarthrosis
- Monoarticular presentation of inflammatory arthritis.

The most common causative organisms are staphylococcal and streptococcal species with *Staphylococcus aureus* being the most common (Gupta et al 2001, Kaandorp et al 1997a, Weston et al 1999). *Methicillin-resistant staphylococcus aureus* (MRSA) septic arthritis is becoming increasingly prevalent (Nixon et al 2007). Gram-negative organisms are less frequently implicated: *Haemophilus influenzae* is most frequently seen in children. Less frequently encountered organisms include enterobacteria, *Pseudomonas aeruginosa* and *Mycobacterium tuberculosis*.

Risk factors for septic arthritis include underlying joint disease (especially rheumatoid arthritis), prosthetic joints, low socioeconomic class, intravenous drug abuse, alcoholism, diabetes mellitus, previous intra-articular injection and cutaneous ulceration (Mathews et al 2007).

CLINICAL PRESENTATION AND CLINICAL FEATURES

The classical presentation of septic arthritis is with a short history of a painful, hot, swollen, tender single joint with reduced range of movement (Mathews et al 2007). The most frequently affected joint is the knee. However, involvement is polyarticular in 22% of cases. Fever may be present but is absent in approximately 50% of cases.

DIAGNOSIS AND DIFFERENTIAL DIAGNOSIS

The diagnosis of septic arthritis relies upon prompt aspiration of the affected joint prior to commencing antibiotic therapy (Coakley et al 2006). Gram stain, culture and crystal examination of synovial fluid should be performed. A possible infected prosthetic joint requires referral to an orthopaedic surgeon for aspiration in theatre. Blood cultures should always be taken and may identify a causative organism in 33% of cases (Weston et al 1999). Inflammatory markers such as white cell count, erythrocyte sedimentation rate and C-reactive protein should be measured but may not be raised in a significant number of cases (Gupta et al 2001, Weston et al 1999). The important differential diagnoses of septic arthritis include crystal arthropathies, e.g. gout and pseudogout, haemarthrosis, reactive arthritis and a monoarticular presentation of an inflammatory arthritis (Box 23.1).

MANAGEMENT

As soon as the joint has been aspirated, intravenous antibiotics should be commenced. The choice of antibiotics will usually be guided by local microbiologists and should be modified in light of the results of Gram stain and culture. Conventionally, the duration of intravenous antibiotic therapy is 2 weeks followed by 4 weeks of oral therapy (Coakley et al 2006). Regular aspiration to dryness should be performed and arthroscopic aspiration may be required.

PROGNOSIS

Septic arthritis is associated with considerable mortality and morbidity (Gupta et al 2001, Kaandorp et al 1997b, Weston et al 1999). The mortality of septic arthritis is approximately 11%. Adverse functional outcome is seen in 21–24% of cases. Factors predicting poor outcome include older age, pre-existing joint disease and the presence of synthetic material within the joint (Mathews et al 2007).

GOUT

Gout is a crystal deposition disease caused by the formation of monosodium urate (MSU) crystals in and around joints. It is one of the most common inflammatory arthropathies having a prevalence of 0.52–1.39% and incidence of approximately 13 cases per 10,000 patient-years (Harris et al 1995, Lawrence et al 1998, Mikuls et al 2005, Wallace et al 2004). The prevalence and incidence of gout are thought to be rising (Arromdee et al 2002, Wallace et al 2004). Gout is traditionally subdivided into primary and secondary gout according to clinical features and risk factors (Table 23.1).

AETIOLOGY AND PATHOLOGY

The primary risk factor for the development of gout is an elevated serum urate (uric acid) level (SUA) or hyperuricaemia. Uric acid is the end-product of purine metabolism in humans. Hyperuricaemia arises from overproduction or renal under-excretion of uric acid, or a combination of both. As hyperuricaemia develops, and body tissues become supersaturated with urate, the formation of MSU crystals leads to clinical gout.

Several independent risk factors for the development of gout are recognised (Table 23.1). Primary gout occurs almost exclusively in men and displays a familial tendency: several genetic factors have been identified (Cheng et al 2004, Huang et al 2006, Taniguchi et al 2005, Wang et al 2004). Further independent risk factors include hypertension, obesity and lifestyle factors (excess alcohol consumption, especially beer, and a diet rich in animal purines, for example red meat and seafood) (Choi et al 2004a, 2004b, 2005, Mikuls et al 2005). Gout associates with other features of the metabolic syndrome including hyperlipidaemia, insulin resistance and cardiovascular disease (Abbott et al 1988, Mikuls et al 2005). Diuretic therapy and renal failure are risk factors for secondary gout (Choi et al 2005, Mikuls et al 2005). Osteoarthritis (OA) predisposes to local MSU crystal deposition (Roddy et al 2007).

CLINICAL PRESENTATION AND CLINICAL FEATURES

Clinical gout is sub-divided into acute gouty arthritis, interval (intercritical) gout and chronic tophaceous gout. Acute gouty arthritis typically manifests as acute mono-arthritis characterised by severe pain with associated redness, warmth, swelling and tenderness. The first metatarsophalangeal (MTP) joint is affected most frequently followed by the mid-foot, ankle, knee, finger interphalangeal joints, wrist and elbow. Attacks occur rapidly,

Table 23.1 Comparison of the clinical features and risk factors of primary and secondary gout

	PRIMARY GOUT	SECONDARY GOUT
Age	Middle-aged	Elderly
Gender	Males	Equal gender distribution
Acute attacks	Common	Less common May present with tophi alone
Distribution	Predominantly lower limb	Equal upper and lower limb
Risk factors	Family history of gout Metabolic syndrome Hypertension Obesity Hyperlipidaemia Insulin resistance Excess alcohol consumption Purine-rich diet	Diuretics Renal failure

often overnight, peaking within 24 hours, before resolving completely over a 2–3 week period. A variable period elapses before the next attack occurs (interval gout). With time, attacks become more frequent, more severe and are more often pauci- or polyarticular leading to chronic tophaceous gout characterised by chronic arthropathy and chalky-white subcutaneous deposits of MSU crystals (tophi). Typical sites for tophi include the toes (Fig. 23.1A), Achilles' tendons, fingers, elbows (Fig. 23.1B) and, less commonly, the helix of the ear.

DIAGNOSIS AND DIFFERENTIAL DIAGNOSIS

Definitive diagnosis of gout requires compensated polarised light microscopy of aspirated synovial fluid or tophaceous material to demonstrate MSU crystals which appear needle-shaped with strong negative birefringence. The differential diagnosis includes septic arthritis, pseudogout, reactive arthritis and palindromic rheumatism (Box 23.1). Crystal arthropathies and septic arthritis can be readily differentiated by crystal examination, Gram stain and culture of synovial fluid.

Measurement of serum urate level (SUA) is an important investigation both to confirm hyperuricaemia and monitor response to treatment. However, the SUA level must be interpreted with caution. Many hyperuricaemic individuals do not develop gout (Campion et al 1987) and SUA is frequently lowered during an attack of acute gout (Schlesinger et al 1997).

MANAGEMENT

Acute gout

Treatment of the acute attack of gout aims to relieve pain by reducing inflammation and intra-articular hypertension. Local application of ice packs four times per day has been shown to reduce pain associated with acute gouty arthritis (Schlesinger et al 2002). Rest and elevation of the affected joint during an acute attack and the use of a bed-cage have been recommended (Jordan et al 2007). Joint aspiration reduces intra-articular hypertension and often provides rapid pain relief. Effective pharmacological therapies for acute gout include non-steroidal anti-inflammatory drugs (NSAIDs), both non-selective and COX-2 selective agents, low-dose colchicine and systemic and intra-articular corticosteroids (Alloway et al 1993, Fernandez et al 1999, Morris et al 2003, Rubin et al 2004, Schumacher et al 2002).

LONG–TERM MANAGEMENT

Gout is potentially curable. The aim of long-term management is lowering of SUA to facilitate crystal dissolution (Zhang et al 2006).

Modification of provoking factors including lifestyle

Risk factor modification is a key component of the management of gout. Advice regarding weight loss, restriction of alcohol (especially beer) and purine-rich foods should be offered to all patients with

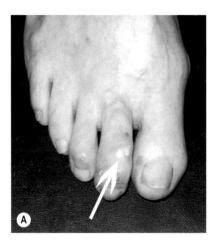
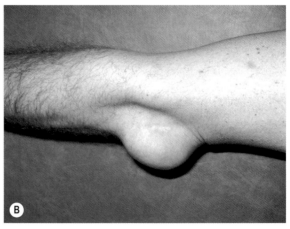

Figure 23.1 Tophaceous deposits of subcutaneous monosodium urate crystals on (A) the right 2nd toe (white arrow) and (B) elbow.

primary gout (Jordan et al 2007, Zhang et al 2006). In diuretic-induced gout the diuretic should be stopped or the dose reduced wherever possible.

Urate–lowering therapy

The aim of urate-lowering therapy is to reduce SUA below the saturation threshold of urate (Li-Yu et al 2001). The most commonly used drug in the UK is allopurinol. Other options include uricosuric agents such as sulphinpyrazone, probenecid and benzbromarone. New drugs in development include febuxostat and recombinant uricase.

PYROPHOSPHATE ARTHROPATHY

Calcium pyrophosphate dihydrate (CPPD) crystal deposition is a common age-related phenomenon that has three main clinical manifestations: (1) acute synovitis (pseudogout), (2) chronic pyrophosphate arthropathy and (3) the incidental finding of cartilage calcification (chondrocalcinosis) on plain radiographs. Over 40 years of age, the UK community prevalence of pyrophosphate arthropathy is 2.4% and chondrocalcinosis is 4.5% (Neame et al 2003, Zhang et al 2004).

AETIOLOGY

CPPD deposition is most commonly idiopathic being more common in females and with increasing age. In the context of chronic pyrophosphate arthropathy, it associates with OA (Dieppe et al 1982, Zhang et al 2004). CPPD deposition may also occur as a consequence of metabolic disease; most importantly, haemochromatosis, hyperparathyroidism, hypomagnesaemia and hypophosphatasia (Jones et al 1992). Familial CPPD deposition is uncommon although genetic mutations associating with chondrocalcinosis have been identified (Pendleton et al 2002, Williams et al 2003).

CLINICAL PRESENTATION AND CLINICAL FEATURES

Pseudogout is a common cause of acute monoarthritis in the elderly. As occurs with gout, the joint appears swollen, tender, red and warm. Onset is rapid, peaking within 24 hours, with resolution occurring within 2–3 weeks. The most commonly affected site is the knee followed by the wrist, ankle and shoulder. Systemic upset is common.

Chronic pyrophosphate arthopathy presents with features of OA (chronic pain and stiffness, crepitus, bony swelling and restricted movement) with or without superimposed attacks of acute synovitis. The knee is again the most frequently affected site. Chondrocalcinosis is a common asymptomatic incidental radiographic finding in the elderly.

CPPD crystals can be identified by compensated polarised light microscopy of aspirated synovial fluid as rhomboid or rod-shaped crystals with weak positive birefringence. Plain radiographs may show chondrocalcinosis or the structural changes of OA. Chondrocalcinosis mainly affects fibrocartilage and is most commonly seen at the knee (Fig. 23.2), wrist and symphysis pubis. Screening for haemochromatosis, hyperparathyroidism, hypomagnesaemia and hypophosphatasia is indicated under the age of 55 years and when radiographic chondrocalcinosis is particularly striking and widespread (Wright & Doherty 1997).

The most important differential diagnoses of pseudogout include septic arthritis and gout (Box 23.1). Chronic pyrophosphate arthropathy may be confused for rheumatoid arthritis (RA) or polymyalgia rheumatica depending on the sites involved.

MANAGEMENT

The evidence for non-pharmacological management of pseudogout is sparse but treatment options are similar to those for gout: application of ice-packs

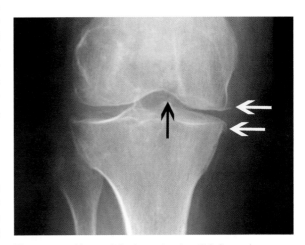

Figure 23.2 X-ray of the knee showing tibiofemoral chondrocalcinosis (black arrow), medial compartment loss of joint space and medial osteophytes (white arrows) - pyrophosphate arthropathy.

and initial rest of the affected joint with rapid mobilisation once improving. Pharmacological options include NSAIDs (with caution in the elderly), low-dose colchicine and systemic and intra-articular corticosteroids.

There is no specific therapy for chronic pyrophosphate arthropathy. Treatment principles are as for OA and may include education, exercise, weight loss, walking aids, analgesics and surgery with superimposed attacks of acute synovitis treated as above.

SARCOIDOSIS

Sarcoidosis is a multisystem disorder of unknown aetiology characterised by non-caseating granulomatous inflammation of affected organs. A recent UK study found the incidence of sarcoidosis to be 5.0 per 100,000 person-years between 1991 and 2003 (Gribbin et al 2006). The incidence is higher in females and Afro-Caribbean individuals and peaks between the ages of 20 and 49 years (Rybicki et al 1997).

CLINICAL PRESENTATION AND CLINICAL FEATURES

Almost any body system can be involved although the lungs, skin, lymph nodes and eyes are most frequently affected (Baughman et al 2001). Musculoskeletal involvement, including arthritis, tenosynovitis, myopathy and bony lesions, occurs in 10–25% of cases (Gumpel et al 1967, Perruquet et al 1984, Rybicki et al 1997). Sarcoid arthritis has acute and chronic forms. Acute sarcoid arthritis presents with acute swelling, warmth, erythema and tenderness characteristically affecting the ankles or knees (Gumpel et al 1967, Visser et al 2002). It is often accompanied by fever, bilateral hilar lymphadenopathy and erythema nodosum (Löfgren's syndrome) (Mana et al 1999, Visser et al 2002). Chronic sarcoid arthropathy is more common in Afro-Caribbean subjects and targets the same joints as acute sarcoid arthritis manifesting as an oligo- or polyarthritis (Gumpel et al 1967). Affected patients tend to have evidence of chronic disease in other body systems, for example, the skin or interstitial lung disease.

DIAGNOSIS AND DIFFERENTIAL DIAGNOSIS

The diagnosis of acute sarcoidosis may be made on clinical grounds when the presentation is typical, for example, Löfgren's syndrome (Mana et al 1994, Mana et al 1999). Erythrocyte sedimentation rate and C-reactive protein are often elevated (Visser et al 2002). Hypercalcaemia or hypercalciuria may also be present. Radiography and computed tomography (CT) of the chest may reveal bilateral hilar lymphadenopathy or evidence of interstitial lung disease. In many cases, a biopsy specimen of an affected organ is required to make a tissue diagnosis, for example, transbronchial lung biopsy or lymph node biopsy. Angiotensin-converting enzyme (ACE), which is produced by macrophages within granulomata, is elevated in 40–90% but may be normal in acute sarcoid arthritis.

Given the protean manifestations of sarcoidosis, the differential diagnosis is wide and depends upon which organs are affected. Important diagnoses to consider include tuberculosis, lymphoma and malignancy. The differential diagnosis of acute sarcoid arthritis includes reactive arthritis and gout. Chronic sarcoid arthropathy may mimic RA.

MANAGEMENT

The treatment of acute sarcoid arthritis is largely symptomatic. Symptoms are often responsive to NSAIDs (Visser et al 2002) although corticosteroids may be necessary in a small number of patients. Corticosteroids are the mainstay of treatment for patients with significant symptomatic severe pulmonary and extra-pulmonary disease (Paramothayan et al 2005, Pettersson et al 2000). Steroid-sparing agents such as methotrexate, antimalarials or ciclosporin are often tried although the evidence-base for their use is limited (Paramothayan et al 2006). Response of sarcoidosis to infliximab is reported (Doty et al 2005, Saleh et al 2006, Sweiss et al 2005) although these findings were not replicated in a recent phase II randomised trial (Baughman et al 2006).

PROGNOSIS

Acute sarcoidosis is usually a benign condition (Demirkok et al 2007, Glennas et al 1995, Perruquet et al 1984, Visser et al 2002) with 90% of cases achieving remission within 2 years (Mana et al 1999). A small number of cases progress to develop chronic disease (Gran & Bohmer 1996, Neville 1983). Mortality is infrequent but is usually due to pulmonary involvement (Reich 2002).

DIABETES MELLITUS

Diabetes mellitus is associated with several musculoskeletal conditions including septic arthritis, adhesive capsulitis, Dupuytren's contracture, palmar flexor tenosynovitis, carpal tunnel syndrome, neuropathic (Charcot) arthropathy and cheiroarthropathy (Cagliero et al 2002, Geoghegan et al 2004, Mathews et al 2007). The latter two are discussed below.

DIABETIC NEUROPATHIC (CHARCOT) ARTHROPATHY

Diabetic neuropathic arthopathy is a destructive arthropathy which occurs almost exclusively in the presence of a dense lower limb sensorimotor peripheral neuropathy. It affects 0.1–0.4% of diabetics (Rajbhandari et al 2002). Peak onset is in the 6th decade with an equal gender distribution. Diabetes has usually been long-standing. An acute neuropathic joint typically presents with local swelling, warmth and erythema that may not be referrable clinically to a particular joint. Although pain may be present, it is usually painless. Diabetic neuropathic arthropathy most commonly affects the foot. Foot pulses are usually present and are often hyperdynamic. There may be accompanying ulceration.

A high index of suspicion is necessary to avoid delay in treatment and permanent disability. The diagnosis of neuropathic arthopathy is made largely on clinical grounds although plain radiographs, isotope bone scans and MRI may help to differentiate the main differential diagnoses which include osteomyelitis, cellulitis and acute gout. Causes other than diabetes mellitus include leprosy and tabes dorsalis (syphilis). Management of the acute neuropathic joint aims to reduce weight-bearing of the affected limb and may require plaster casts or orthoses (Armstrong et al 1997). Bisphosphonates may also be of benefit (Jude et al 2001). Management of the chronic neuropathic joint relies upon adaptation of footwear. Surgical correction of deformity may also play a role.

DIABETIC CHEIROARTHROPATHY

Diabetic cheiroarthropathy is characterised by an inability to fully extend the metacarpophalangeal joints and scleroderma-like skin thickening (Crispin & Cocer-Varela 2003). It is seen more frequently in insulin-dependent disease and associates with disease duration and vascular complications (Frost & Beischer 2001). The characteristic clinical sign is a positive "prayer" sign which describes the inability to flatten the hands together as in prayer (Crispin & Cocer-Varela 2003). Treatment can be challenging and consists of physiotherapy, wax therapy, corticosteroid injection or, in severe cases, surgery.

Part 2: Vasculitis

David G. I. Scott

DEFINITION

Vasculitis literally means inflammation of blood vessels and indicates that the vessel wall itself is the site and target of inflammation. This results in damage (necrosis) of the vessel wall, hence the term sometimes used-necrotizing vasculitis.

The consequence of vasculitis depends on the size, site and number of blood vessels involved and a number of different clinical patterns are recognised (Scott & Watts 1994) (Table 23.2). Symptoms range from benign skin rashes to life threatening diseases involving vital internal organs. The most serious types of vasculitis are those that involve small/medium arteries. It is also important to recognise that vasculitis can occur as a primary event (arising de novo/primary vasculitis) or in association with a number of infections and connective tissue diseases, including rheumatoid arthritis, Sjögren's syndrome and systemic lupus erythematosus.

EPIDEMIOLOGY/AETIOLOGY

The primary systemic vasculitides are rare. Giant cell arteritis is probably the most common, but the primary ANCA-associated vasculitides (Wegener's granulomatosis, Churg-Strauss syndrome and microscopic polyangiitis) have an incidence of approximately 20 million/year. If all the vasculitides are lumped together, the incidence is approximately 150 million/year but this may still be an under-estimate as many cases of giant cell arteritis are seen in the community, and mild small vessel skin vasculitis (e.g. drug reaction) may go unrecognised or unreported.

The cause of vasculitis is in most circumstances unknown. Important infections linked to vasculitis

Table 23.2 Classification of systemic vasculitis

DOMINANT VESSELS INVOLVED	PRIMARY	SECONDARY
Large arteries	Giant cell arteritis	
	Takayasu arteritis	Aortitis associated with RA
	Isolated CNS angiitis	Infection (e.g. syphilis)
Medium arteries	Classical PAN	Infection (e.g. Hepatitis B)
	Kawasaki disease	Hairy cell leukaemia
Small vessels and medium arteries	Wegener's granulomatosis[a]	Vasculitis 2° to RA, SLE, SS
	Churg-Strauss syndrome[a]	Drugs, malignancy
	Microscopic polyangiitis[a]	Infection (e.g. HIV)
		Drugs[b]
Small vessels (leukocytoclastic)	Henoch-Schönlein purpura	Infection (e.g.hepatitis B, C)
	Essential mixed cryoglobulinaemia	
	Cutaneous leukocytoclastic angiitis	

[a]Diseases most commonly associated with ANCA (anti-myeloperoxidase and anti-proteinase 3 antibodies), a significant risk of renal involvement, and which are most responsive to immunosuppression with cyclophosphamide.
[b]e.g. sulphonamides, penicillins, thiazide diuretics, and many others.
CNS, central nervous system; HIV, human immunodeficiency virus; PAN, polyarteritis nodosa; RA, rheumatoid arthritis; SLE, systemic lupus erythematosus; SS, Sjögren's syndrome.
Reproduced from Scott & Watts (1994) with permission

include hepatitis B (classic polyarteritis nodosa) and hepatitis C (cryoglobulinaemic vasculitis). A number of drugs may trigger vasculitis, usually small vessel vasculitis. The ANCA-associated vasculitides have only recently come into the group of conditions thought to be autoimmune because of the presence of ANCA – an antibody directed against neutrophil cytoplasmic antigens, where the specificity for proteinase 3 is strongly linked to Wegener's granulomatosis and myeloperoxidase to microscopic polyangiitis. These antibodies form part of the immunological investigations carried out in cases where vasculitis is suspected.

LARGE VESSEL VASCULITIS

Giant cell arteritis is commonly linked to polymyalgia rheumatica. It is a disease affecting particularly an older population over the age of 50, and usually over the age of 60, presenting commonly with severe temporal headaches, temporal artery tenderness and a high ESR. It is important that this diagnosis is recognised as it is very sensitive to steroid treatment, but untreated can lead to blindness because of involvement of blood vessels affecting the optic nerve (ciliary artery and branches). Takayasu's arteritis by contrast affects a much younger population, is very rare in the UK and presents with non-specific systemic symptoms which later lead to loss of pulses and claudication, especially of the upper limbs.

MEDIUM VESSEL VASCULITIS

Polyarteritis nodosa is a term that has been around for over 140 years and was loosely applied to many cases of systemic vasculitis. Recent reviews and the introduction of testing for the ANCA antibodies has led to a reclassification of this as a disease restricted to medium sized vessels which is now quite rare. It is characterised by the formation of aneurysms in medium sized arteries. Patients can present with systemic symptoms, rash (particularly livido reticularis), nerve damage (mononeuritis multiplex), hypertension and internal organ infarction. The disease when triggered by hepatitis B is best treated with anti-viral treatment plus plasma exchange.

Kawasaki disease (mucocutaneous lymph node syndrome) is an acute inflammatory disease affecting children, usually under the age of 5 years, presenting with fever, rash, swollen lymph glands and palmoplantar erythema. In about a quarter of untreated children the coronary arteries can be involved, leading to a small but significant mortality (approx 2%) and sometimes later in life myocardial ischaemia and infarction.

MEDIUM AND SMALL VESSEL VASCULITIDES

This group is also sometimes known as the primary systemic vasculitides. They are separated from pure small vessel vasculitis because they can involve larger vessels and be associated with aneurysms, they are also particularly associated with ANCA and are not infrequently associated with significant renal impairment due to an inflammatory glomerulonephritis. Although they occur at any age, the peak incidence is 60–70 years.

Wegener's granulomatosis is the most common of the three diseases in the UK and northern Europe (microscopic polyangiitis is commoner in southern Europe and Japan). It is characterised by granuloma formation involving the upper and lower airways and glomerulonephritis. The lungs are involved in about 45% with nodules which can cavitate, leading to haemoptysis. Upper airway involvement, particularly in the naso-pharynx, leads to destruction of the sinuses and presents often with epistaxis, crusting and also complications such as deafness. The prognosis of Wegener's granulomatosis in terms of mortality relates to kidney involvement, but the upper airway involvement can lead to very significant morbidity and be difficult to treat.

Microscopic polyangiitis (MPA) is characterised by vasculitis that usually presents with kidney involvement, but sometimes presents with lung haemorrhage due to small vessel bleeding from vasculitis. The kidney changes are identical to Wegener's-glomerulonephritis with few immune deposits ('pauci immune' glomerulo-nephritis). Churg-Strauss syndrome is characterised by allergy, particularly late onset asthma followed by systemic vasculitis with flitting pulmonary shadowing (presenting like pneumonia) with increased numbers of eosinophils in the circulation and in tissues involved with vasculitis. Asthma can pre-date the vasculitis by many years. Kidney involvement is rarer than (but identical to that seen) in Wegener's and MPA, but particular features more common in Churg-Strauss syndrome are heart problems (peri/myocarditis) and neuropathy.

SMALL VESSEL VASCULITIS

This type of vasculitis is usually confined to the skin. It is important to recognise that if a patient presents with vasculitic skin rash this can be part of the other diseases outlined above. There are a number of very specific patterns of small vessel vasculitis known as Henoch-Schönlein purpura (HSP), cutaneous leukocytoclastic vasculitis and cryoglobulinaemia. Henoch-Schönlein purpura is mainly seen in children who present with a purpuric rash, arthritis (usually involving large joints), abdominal pain, and haematuria. The kidney disease is usually mild in comparison with the ANCA-associated vasculitides. Immunoglobulin A is detected in involved tissue, particularly the kidney. When HSP involves adults the kidney involvement can be more severe, and it may be difficult sometimes to differentiate from microscopic polyangiitis.

Cryoglobulins are proteins which precipitate in the cold. Cryoglobulinaemic vasculitis usually presents with a skin rash, but also digital ischaemia and ulcers, arthralgia and mild neuropathy. It is strongly linked to hepatitis C infection.

INVESTIGATIONS OF VASCULITIS

These can be split into different sections as follows:

- Tests to assess the degree of inflammation include blood count and the acute phase response (ESR, CRP).
- Investigations to assess specific involvement include urinalysis for kidney involvement, formal renal function (such as creatinine clearance, 24 hour urine protein excretion and biopsy), chest X-ray, liver function tests, nerve conduction studies, ECG, echo and occasionally angiography.
- Immunological tests are undertaken with aetiology in mind. ANCA, as outlined above, is particularly useful for Wegener's and microscopic polyangiitis. The presence of other antibodies such as rheumatoid factor, ANA and anticardiolipin antibodies is useful to exclude secondary vasculitis (see below). Complement levels are usually low in SLE, cryoglobulinaemic vasculitis and infection but are raised or normal in all the other vasculitides.

DIFFERENTIAL DIAGNOSIS

The important diagnoses to exclude in a patient with suspected vasculitis include infection, particularly bacterial endocarditis (urgent echocardiography is therefore essential in all cases), and cholesterol embolism in the elderly can mimic vasculitis with skin infarction, as can antiphospholipid syndrome (clotting in blood vessels due to antiphospholipid antibodies). A very rare condition is atrial myxoma which is also detected by echocardiography.

The presence of protein or blood on urine dipstix is probably the most important investigation because kidney involvement can be sub-clinical and kidney damage can occur without any very specific symptoms. This in the presence of a systemic illness needs to be treated as an emergency. The white cell count can be useful when eosinophils are present, suggesting allergies such as Churg-Strauss syndrome. A low white count is usually suggestive of infection or a disease such as SLE. Very abnormal liver function tests raise the possibility of hepatitis (B or C).

Although ANCA is useful in aiding diagnosis (PR3 ANCA is highly specific (greater than 90%) for Wegener's granulomatosis), tissue biopsy is still important to confirm the diagnosis to target the organs clinically involved. Renal biopsy is perhaps the most useful because of the link between kidney involvement and prognosis (see below). In patients that are difficult to diagnose, then angiography can be useful to show aneurysms. Finally, in addition to echocardiography for investigating the differential diagnosis of vasculitis, blood cultures and viral serology are essential because of the important differential diagnosis of infection.

PROGNOSIS

The natural history of primary systemic vasculitis untreated is of a progressive, usually fatal disease. Survival improved with the introduction of steroids for some conditions, but the most dramatic improvement followed the introduction of cyclophosphamide in the late 1960s and early 1970s. For example, the median survival of Wegener's granulomatosis with no treatment was 5 months for those with renal involvement, 12.5 months with steroids alone but now the survival rate at 5 years is in excess of 80% in most series.

Small vessel vasculitis is usually associated with a good prognosis, as is large vessel vasculitis, except for specific problems such as blindness as outlined above.

TREATMENT

Treatment is dependent on the type of vasculitis. Small vessel vasculitis can often be treated with low dose corticosteroids and the large vessel vasculitides usually respond well to higher doses (oral prednisolone 40–60 mg per day). The duration of treatment is usually in excess of one year. Once symptoms settle the steroid dose can be rapidly reduced, titrated to clinical features and inflammatory markers such as the ESR/CRP.

Cyclophosphamide is almost always used to treat the primary systemic/ANCA-associated vasculitides combined with steroids. Cyclophosphamide can be given as continuous low dose oral therapy or intermittent pulse intravenous therapy. Both treatments are equally effective but pulse therapy is associated with a lower total cyclophosphamide dose and less toxicity. Particularly concerning problems with long-term oral cyclophosphamide are the risk of haemorrhagic cystitis and bladder tumours, but also infertility and infections. With intravenous cyclophosphamide bladder protection is enhanced by the addition of mesna and patients are often given trimethoprim-sulfamethoxazole to prevent infections with pneumocystis. Fertile males should be offered sperm storage before being given cyclophosphamide and ovarian function is often lost in females given cyclophosphamide, especially if over the age of 30–35. Corticosteroids are usually given at a dose of 1 mg/kg with rapid reduction after remission has been obtained within 2–3 months.

After remission has been induced, usually with cyclophosphamide and steroids, patients are switched to either azathioprine or methotrexate. Long-term treatment is usually advised because of a significant risk of relapse, higher in Wegener's granulomatosis than in microscopic polyangiitis. Plasmapheresis is sometimes given to patients with severe renal disease or pulmonary haemorrhage, intravenous immunoglobulin is effective treatment for Kawasaki disease and the role of the new biologic agents is currently being evaluated, but the results of treatment with rituximab in particular appear to be encouraging.

REHABILITATION

Even with effective medical treatment, e.g. low dose corticosteroids, patients with vasculitis may have difficulty with walking, impaired muscle strength, limitation of joint movement, reduced proprioception and limitation in activities of daily living (Seo 2006). Monitoring of joint stiffness and pain can determine when referral back to the Rheumatologist is required. In polymyalgia rheumatica, this is more common in the shoulder and pelvic girdle, and neck. Stiffness can be worse on wakening and on exertion. Muscle strength can be difficult to determine in patients with polymyalgia rheumatica because of muscle tenderness and pain (Paget & Spiera 2006). Tenderness can lead to muscle atrophy although in the absence of pain, muscle strength should be normal (Paget & Spiera 2006). Dynamic exercises need to be tailored to the individual to maintain physical functioning and core stability and are often targeted to the shoulder girdle and hips. In severe cases and in the elderly referral to occupational therapy is warranted.

STUDY ACTIVITY

- Familiarise yourself with on-line patient resources suggested below:

Patient UK
Septic arthritis-accessed February 2009
http://www.patient.co.uk/showdoc/27000235/

Arthritis Research Campaign (UK) patient information booklet
Gout- accessed February 2009
http://www.arc.org.uk/arthinfo/patpubs/6015/6015.asp

American College of Rheumatology patient information sheet
Gout- accessed February 2009
http://www.rheumatology.org/public/factsheets/diseases_and_conditions/gout.asp?aud=pat

National Institute of Arthritis and Musculoskeletal and Skin Diseases (USA) Health Topics
Questions and answers about gout-accessed February 2009
http://www.niams.nih.gov/hi/topics/gout/Gout.pdf

Arthritis Research Campaign (UK) patient information booklet
Pseudogout and calcium crystal diseases-accessed February 2009
http://www.arc.org.uk/arthinfo/patpubs/6051/6051.asp

The Sarcoidosis Charity (UK)
About sarcoidosis-accessed February 2009
http://www.sila.org.uk/

National Heart Lung and Blood Institute (USA)
What is sarcoidosis? - accessed February 2009
http://www.nhlbi.nih.gov/health/dci/Diseases/sarc/sar_whatis.html

Diabetes UK – the charity for people with diabetes
Long-term complications - Musculoskeletal conditions-accessed February 2009
http://www.diabetes.org.uk/Guide-to-diabetes/Complications/Long_term_complications/Musculoskeletal_Conditions/

CASE STUDY 23.1

Mr Addisson is a 51-year-old bricklayer. One day after being admitted to hospital with a myocardial infarction, he wakes with an acutely painful, swollen, red left knee. He reports several episodes of acute gout affecting his big toes in the past, which his GP has treated with non-steroid anti-inflammatory drugs. He has also recently been commenced on allopurinol 100 mg daily. He is overweight and drinks four pints of beer every day.

Investigation

An aspiration of the left knee is performed. Examination of synovial fluid using compensated polarised light microscopy identifies monosodium urate crystals confirming the diagnosis of gout. No organisms are identified on Gram stain and culture. Serum urate is 480 micromol/L (normal range 200–400).

Management

Ice-packs are applied locally to the joint. An intra-articular injection of corticosteroid into the left knee is performed providing rapid relief of his pain and swelling. The joint is rested initially and he is then mobilised as his cardiovascular status allows. He is advised to lose weight and to restrict his alcohol intake. Once he is discharged, follow-up is arranged to increase the dose of allopurinol with the aim of lowering the serum urate into the lower half of the normal range.

ACKNOWLEDGEMENT

Thanks to Dr Tasso Gazis (Consultant in Diabetes and Endocrinology, Nottingham University Hospitals) for his review and comments regarding diabetic neuropathic arthropathy.

References and further reading

Abbott, R.D., Brand, F.N., Kannel, W.B., et al., 1988. Gout and coronary heart disease: the Framingham Study. J. Clin. Epidemiol. 41, 237–242.

Alloway, J.A., Moriarty, M.J., Hoogland, Y.T., et al., 1993. Comparison of triamcinolone acetonide with indomethacin in the treatment of acute gouty arthritis. J. Rheumatol. 20, 111–113.

Armstrong, D.G., Todd, W.F., Lavery, L.A., et al., 1997. The natural history of acute Charcot's arthropathy in a diabetic foot specialty clinic. Diabet. Med. 14, 357–363.

Arromdee, E., Michet, C.J., Crowson, C.S., et al., 2002. Epidemiology of gout: is the incidence rising? J. Rheumatol. 29, 2403–2406.

Baughman, R.P., Drent, M., Kavuru, M., et al., 2006. Infliximab therapy in patients with chronic sarcoidosis and pulmonary involvement. Am. J. Respir. Crit. Care Med. 174, 795–802.

Baughman, R.P., Teirstein, A.S., Judson, M.A., et al., 2001. Clinical characteristics of patients in a case control study of sarcoidosis. Am. J. Respir. Crit. Care Med. 164, 1885–1889.

Cagliero, E., Apruzzese, W., Perlmutter, G.S., et al., 2002. Musculoskeletal disorders of the hand and shoulder in patients with diabetes mellitus. Am. J. Med. 112, 487–490.

Campion, E.W., Glynn, R.J., DeLabry, L.O., 1987. Asymptomatic hyperuricemia, risks and consequences in the normative aging study. Am. J. Med. 82, 421–426.

Cheng, L.S., Chiang, S.L., Tu, H.P., et al., 2004. Genomewide scan for gout in Taiwanese Aborigines reveals linkage to chromosome 4q25. Am. J. Human Genet. 75, 498–503.

Choi, H.K., Atkinson, K., Karlson, E.W., et al., 2005. Obesity, weight change, hypertension, diuretic use, and risk of gout in men: the health professionals follow-up study. Arch. Intern. Med. 165, 742–748.

Choi, H.K., Atkinson, K., Karlson, E.W., et al., 2004a. Alcohol intake and risk of incident gout in men: a prospective study. Lancet 363, 1277–1281.

Choi, H.K., Atkinson, K., Karlson, E.W., et al., 2004b. Purine-rich foods, dairy and protein intake, and the risk of gout in men. N. Engl. J. Med. 350, 1093–1103.

Coakley, G., Mathews, C., Field, M., et al., 2006. BSR & BHPR, BOA, RCGP and BSAC guidelines for management of the hot swollen joint in adults. Rheumatology 45, 1039–1041.

Cooper, C., Cawley, M.I., 1986. Bacterial arthritis in an English health district: a 10 year review. Ann. Rheum. Dis. 45, 458–463.

Crispin, J.C., Cocer-Varela, J., 2003. Rheumatologic manifestations of diabetes mellitus. Am. J. Med. 114, 753–757.

Demirkok, S.S., Basaranoglu, M., Akinci, E.D., et al., 2007. Analysis of 275 patients with sarcoidosis over a 38 year period; a single-institution experience. Respir. Med. 101, 1147–1154.

Dieppe, P.A., Alexander, G.J., Jones, H.E., et al., 1982. Pyrophosphate arthropathy: a clinical and radiological study of 105 cases. Ann. Rheum. Dis. 41, 371–376.

Doty, J.D., Mazur, J.E., Judson, M.A., 2005. Treatment of sarcoidosis with infliximab. Chest 127, 1064–1071.

Fernandez, C., Noguera, R., Gonzalez, J.A., et al., 1999. Treatment of acute attacks of gout with a small dose of intraarticular triamcinolone acetonide. J. Rheumatol. 26, 2285–2286.

Frost, D., Beischer, W., 2001. Limited joint mobility in type 1 diabetic patients: associations with microangiopathy and subclinical macroangiopathy are different in men and women. Diab. Care 24, 95–99.

Geoghegan, J.M., Clark, D.I., Bainbridge, L.C., et al., 2004. Risk factors in carpal tunnel syndrome. J. Hand Surg. (British) 29, 315–320.

Glennas, A., Kvien, T.K., Melby, K., et al., 1995. Acute sarcoid arthritis: occurrence, seasonal onset, clinical features and outcome. Br. J. Rheumatol. 34, 45–50.

Gran, J.T., Bohmer, E., 1996. Acute sarcoid arthritis: a favourable outcome? A retrospective survey of 49 patients with review of the literature. Scand. J. Rheumatol. 25, 70–73.

Gribbin, J., Hubbard, R.B., Le, J.I., et al., 2006. Incidence and mortality of idiopathic pulmonary fibrosis and sarcoidosis in the UK. Thorax 61, 980–985.

Gumpel, J.M., Johns, C.J., Shulman, L.E., 1967. The joint disease of sarcoidosis. Ann. Rheum. Dis. 26, 194–205.

Gupta, M.N., Sturrock, R.D., Field, M., 2001. A prospective 2-year study of 75 patients with adult-onset septic arthritis. Rheumatology 40, 24–30.

Harris, C.M., Lloyd, D.C., Lewis, J., 1995. The prevalence and prophylaxis of gout in England. J. Clin. Epidemiol. 48, 1153–1158.

Huang, C.M., Lo, S.F., Lin, H.C., et al., 2006. Correlation of oestrogen receptor gene polymorphism with gouty arthritis. Ann. Rheum. Dis. 65, 1673–1674.

Jones, A.C., Chuck, A.J., Arie, E.A., et al., 1992. Diseases associated with calcium pyrophosphate deposition disease. Semin. Arthrit. Rheum. 22, 188–202.

Jordan, K.M., Cameron, J.S., Snaith, M., et al., 2007. British Society for Rheumatology and British Health Professionals in Rheumatology guideline for the management of Gout. Rheumatology 46, 1372–1374.

Jude, E.B., Selby, P.L., Burgess, J., et al., 2001. Bisphosphonates in the treatment of Charcot neuroarthropathy: a double-blind randomised controlled trial. Diabetologia 44, 2032–2037.

Kaandorp, C.J., Dinant, H.J., van de Laar, M.A., et al., 1997a. Incidence and sources of native and prosthetic joint infection: a community based prospective survey. Ann. Rheum. Dis. 56, 470–475.

Kaandorp, C.J., Krijnen, P., Moens, H.J., et al., 1997b. The outcome of bacterial arthritis: a prospective community-based study. Arthrit. Rheum. 40, 884–892.

Lawrence, R.C., Helmick, C.G., Arnett, F.C., et al., 1998. Estimates of the prevalence of arthritis and selected musculoskeletal disorders in the United States. Arthrit. Rheum. 41, 778–799.

Li-Yu, J., Clayburne, G., Sieck, M., et al., 2001. Treatment of chronic gout. Can we determine when urate stores are depleted enough to prevent attacks of gout? J. Rheumatol. 28, 577–580.

Mana, J., Gomez-Vaquero, C., Montero, A., et al., 1999. Löfgren's syndrome revisited: a study of 186 patients. Am. J. Med. 107, 240–245.

Mana, J., Salazar, A., Manresa, F., 1994. Clinical factors predicting persistence of activity in sarcoidosis: a multivariate analysis of 193 cases. Respiration 61, 219–225.

Mathews, C.J., Kingsley, G., Field, M., et al., 2007. Management of septic arthritis: a systematic review. Ann. Rheum. Dis. 66, 440–445.

Mikuls, T.R., Farrar, J.T., Bilker, W.B., et al., 2005. Gout epidemiology: results from the UK General Practice Research Database, 1990–1999. Ann. Rheum. Dis. 64, 267–272.

Morris, I., Varughese, G., Mattingly, P., 2003. Colchicine in acute gout. Br. Med. J. 327, 1275–1276.

Mukhtyar, C., Guillevin, L., Cid, M.C., et al., 2008. EULAR recommendations for the management of large vessel vasculitis. Ann. Rheum. Dis. published online 15 Apr.

Mukhtyar, C., Guillevin, L., Cid, M.C., et al., 2008. EULAR recommendations for the management of primary small and medium vessel vasculitis. Ann. Rheum. Dis. Published online 15 Apr.

Nade, S., 2003. Septic arthritis. Bailliéres Best Prac. Res. Clin. Rheumatol. 17, 183–200.

Neame, R.L., Carr, A.J., Muir, K., et al., 2003. UK community prevalence of knee chondrocalcinosis: evidence that correlation with osteoarthritis is through a shared association with osteophyte. Ann. Rheum. Dis. 62, 513–518.

Neville, E., Walker, A.N., James, D.G., 1983. Prognostic factors predicting the outcome of sarcoidosis: an analysis of 818 patients. Quart. J. Med. 52, 525–533.

Nixon, J.C., Mortimer, K., Holden, S., et al., 2007. Clinical features of septic arthritis in patients admitted to hospital in Nottingham 1997–2001. Rheumatol. 46 (Suppl 1), i145.

Paget, S.A., Spiera, R.F.P., 2006. Polymyalgia Rheumatica. In: Clinical Care in the Rheumatic Diseases, third ed. Association of Rheumatology Health Professionals, pp. 153–156., third ed.

Paramothayan, N.S., Lasserson, T.J., Jones, P.W., 2005. Corticosteroids for pulmonary sarcoidosis. Coch. Database. Syst. Rev. CD001114-.

Paramothayan, S., Lasserson, T.J., Walters, E.H., 2006. Immunosuppressive and cytotoxic therapy for pulmonary sarcoidosis. Coch. Database. Syst. Rev. 3 CD003536-.

Pendleton, A., Johnson, M.D., Hughes, A., et al., 2002. Mutations in ANKH cause chondrocalcinosis. Am. J. Human Genet. 71, 933–940.

Perruquet, J.L., Harrington, T.M., Davis, D.E., et al., 1984. Sarcoid arthritis in a North American Caucasian population. J. Rheumatol. 11, 521–525.

Pettersson, T., 2000. Sarcoid and erythema nodosum arthropathies. Bailliéres Best Pract. Res. Clin. Rheumatol. 14, 461–476.

Rajbhandari, S.M., Jenkins, R.C., Davies, C., et al., 2002. Charcot neuroarthropathy in diabetes mellitus. Diabetologia 45, 1085–1096.

Reich, J.M., 2002. Mortality of intrathoracic sarcoidosis in referral vs population-based settings: influence of stage, ethnicity, and corticosteroid therapy. Chest 121, 32–39.

Roddy, E., Zhang, W., Doherty, M., 2007. Are joints affected by gout also affected by osteoarthritis? Ann. Rheum. Dis. Published Online First: 6 February 2007. doi:10.1136/ard.2006.063768.

Rubin, B.R., Burton, R., Navarra, S., et al., 2004. Efficacy and safety profile of treatment with etoricoxib 120 mg once daily compared with indomethacin 50 mg three times daily in acute gout: a randomized controlled trial. Arthrit. Rheum. 50, 598–606.

Rybicki, B.A., Major, M., Popovich, J., et al., 1997. Racial differences in sarcoidosis incidence: a 5-year study in a health maintenance organization. Am. J. Epidemiol. 145, 234–241.

Saleh, S., Ghodsian, S., Yakimova, V., et al., 2006. Effectiveness of infliximab in treating selected patients with sarcoidosis. Resp. Med. 100, 2053–2059.

Schlesinger Jr., N., Baker, D.G., Schumacher, H.R., 1997. Serum urate during bouts of acute gouty arthritis. J. Rheumatol. 24, 2265–2266.

Schlesinger, N., Detry, M.A., Holland, B.K., et al., 2002. Local ice therapy during bouts of acute gouty arthritis. J. Rheumatol. 29, 331–334.

Schumacher Jr., H.R., Boice, J.A., Daikh, D.I., et al., 2002. Randomised double blind trial of etoricoxib and indometacin in treatment of acute gouty arthritis. Br. Med. J. 324, 1488–1492.

Scott, D.G.I., Watts, R.A., 1994. Classification and epidemiology of systemic vasculitis. Br. J. Rheumatol. 33, 897–899.

Seo, P., 2006. Vasculitis. In: Clinical Care in the Rheumatic Diseases, third ed. Association of Rheumatology Health Professionals (third ed), pp. 199–202.

Sweiss, N.J., Welsch, M.J., Curran, J.J., et al., 2005. Tumor necrosis factor inhibition as a novel treatment for refractory sarcoidosis. Arthrit. Rheum. 53, 788–791.

Taniguchi, A., Urano, W., Yamanaka, M., et al., 2005. A common mutation in an organic anion transporter gene, SLC22A12, is a suppressing factor for the development of gout. Arthrit. Rheum. 52, 2576–2577.

Visser, H., Vos, K., Zanelli, E., et al., 2002. Sarcoid arthritis: clinical characteristics, diagnostic aspects, and risk factors. Ann. Rheum. Dis. 61, 499–504.

Wallace, K.L., Riedel, A.A., Joseph-Ridge, N., et al., 2004. Increasing prevalence of gout and hyperuricemia over 10 years among older adults in a managed care population. J. Rheumatol. 31, 1582–1587.

Wang, W.H., Chang, S.J., Wang, T.N., et al., 2004. Complex segregation and linkage analysis of familial gout in Taiwanese aborigines. Arthrit. Rheum. 50, 242–246.

Watts, R.A., Scott, D.G., Pusey, C.D., et al., 2000. Vasculitis – aims of therapy. A review. Rheumatology 39, 229–232.

Weston, V.C., Jones, A.C., Bradbury, N., et al., 1999. Clinical features and outcome of septic arthritis in a single UK Health District 1982–1991. Ann. Rheum. Dis. 58, 214–219.

Williams, C.J., Pendleton, A., Bonavita, G., et al., 2003. Mutations in the amino terminus of ANKH in two US families with calcium pyrophosphate dihydrate crystal deposition disease. Arthrit. Rheum. 48, 2627–2631.

Wise, C.M., 2007. Crystal-associated arthritis in the elderly. Rheum. Dis. Clin. N. Am. 33, 33–55.

Wright, G.D., Doherty, M., 1997. Calcium pyrophosphate crystal deposition is not always 'wear and tear' or aging. Ann. Rheum. Dis. 56, 586–588.

Zhang, W., Doherty, X., Bardin, T., et al., 2006. EULAR evidence based recommendations for gout. Ann. Rheum. Dis. 65, 1301–1311 Part I: Diagnosis. Report of a task force of the EULAR Standing Committee for International Clinical Studies Including Therapeutics (ESCISIT).

Zhang, W., Doherty, M., Bardin, T., et al., 2006. EULAR evidence based recommendations for gout. Part II: Management. Ann. Rheum. Dis. 65, 1312–1324 Part II: Management. Report of a task force of the EULAR Standing Committee for International Clinical Studies Including Therapeutics (ESCISIT).

Zhang, W., Neame, R., Doherty, S., et al., 2004. Relative risk of knee chondrocalcinosis in siblings of index cases with pyrophosphate arthropathy. Ann. Rheum. Dis. 63, 969–973.

Further reading

Nade, S., 2003. Septic arthritis. Bailliéres best practice in research. Clin. Rheumatol. 17, 183–200.

Jordan, K.M., Cameron, J.S. & Snaith, M., et al., 2007. BSR and BHPR guideline for the management of gout. Rheumatology 46, 1372–1374.

Zhang, W., Doherty, M. & Bardin, T., et al., 2006. EULAR evidence based recommendations for gout. Part I: Diagnosis. Ann. Rheum. Dis. 65, 1301–1311 Report of a task force of the EULAR Standing Committee for International Clinical Studies Including Therapeutics (ESCISIT).

Zhang, W., Doherty, M. & Bardin, T., et al., 2006. EULAR evidence based recommendations for gout. Part II: Management. Ann. Rheum. Dis. 65, 1312–1324 Report of a task force of the EULAR Standing Committee for International Clinical Studies Including Therapeutics (ESCISIT).

Wise, C.M., 2007. Crystal-associated arthritis in the elderly. Rheum. Dis. Clin. N. Am. 33, 33–55.

Pettersson, T., 2000. Sarcoid and erythema nodosum arthropathies. Bailliéres best practice in research. Clin. Rheumatol. 14, 461–476.

Crispin, J.C. & Cocer-Varela, J., 2003. Rheumatologic Manifestations of diabetes mellitus. Am. J. Med. 114, 753–757.

Mukhtyar, C., Guillevin, L. & Cid, M.C., et al., 2008. EULAR recommendations for the management of primary small and medium vessel vasculitis. Ann. Rheum. Dis. published online 15 Apr.

Mukhtyar, C., Guillevin, L. & Cid, M.C., et al., 2008. EULAR recommendations for the management of large vessel vasculitis. Ann. Rheum. Dis. published online 15 Apr.

Index